Fit & Well

FIFTH EDITION

Core Concepts and Labs in Physical Fitness and Wellness

ALTERNATE

Thomas D. Fahey
California State University, Chico

Paul M. Insel
Stanford University

Walton T. Roth
Stanford University

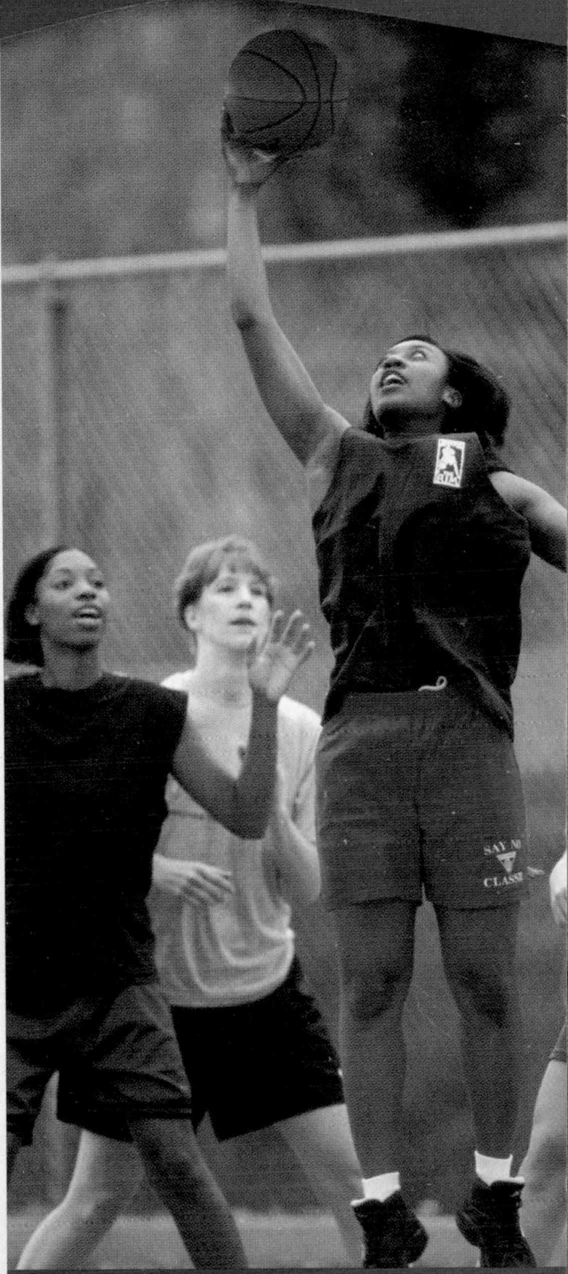

McGraw Hill

Boston Burr Ridge, IL Dubuque, IA Madison, WI New York
San Francisco St. Louis Bangkok Bogotá Caracas Kuala Lumpur
Lisbon London Madrid Mexico City Milan Montreal New Delhi
Santiago Seoul Singapore Sydney Taipei Toronto

McGraw-Hill Higher Education

A Division of The **McGraw-Hill** *Companies*

2 3 4 5 6 7 8 9 0 QPD/QPD 0 9 8 7 6 5 4 3 2

Library of Congress Cataloging-in-Publication Data

Fahey, Thomas D. (Thomas Davin), 1947–
Fit & well : core concepts and labs in physical fitness and wellness / Thomas D. Fahey, Paul M. Insel, Walton T. Roth—5th ed., Alternate ed.
p. cm.
Includes bibliographical references and index.
ISBN 0-7674-2948-6
1. Physical fitness. 2. Health. I. Title: Fit and well. II. Insel, Paul M. III. Roth, Walton T. IV. Title.
GV481.F26 2002b
613.7′043—dc21 2002016502

Vice president and editor-in-chief, Thalia Dorwick; Publisher, Jane E. Karpacz; Executive editor, Vicki Malinee; Senior developmental editor, Kirstan Price; Managing editor, Melissa Williams; Senior marketing manager, Pamela S. Cooper; Production editors, Jennifer Mills and Brett Coker; Manuscript editor, Sheryl Rose; Art director, Jeanne M. Schreiber; Design manager, Violeta Díaz; Text designer, Linda M. Robertson; Cover designer, Laurie Anderson; Art editor, Robin Mouat; Illustrators, Joan Carol, Emma Ghiselli, Robin Mouat, Kristin Mount, Susan Seed, John and Judy Waller; Manager, photo research, Brian J. Pecko; Proofreader, Julianna Scott Fein; Senior production supervisor, Pam Augspurger. Cover photograph © David Epperson/Getty Images/The Image Bank. The text was set in 10.5/12 Berkeley Book by The GTS Companies and printed on acid-free 45# Lighthouse Matte by Quebecor World, Dubuque.

The Internet addresses listed in the text were accurate at the time of publication. The inclusion of a Web site does not indicate an endorsement by the authors or McGraw-Hill Higher Education, and McGraw-Hill does not guarantee the accuracy of the information presented at these sites.

www.mhhe.com

Photo Credits

Title page © David Madison

Chapter 1 p. 1, © Myrleen Ferguson Cate/PhotoEdit; p. 16 © Eric Fowke/PhotoEdit

Chapter 2 p. 25, © Gary Conner/PhotoEdit; p. 31, © Robert Brenner/PhotoEdit; p. 33, © Spencer Grant/PhotoEdit

Chapter 3 p. 47, © Syracuse Newspapers/The Image Works; p. 53, © Alán Gallegos/AG Photograph; p. 58, 74, Courtesy Shirlee Stevens

Chapter 4 p. 79, © Bill Bachman/PhotoEdit; p. 84, © Dana White/PhotoEdit; p. 85, 91, Courtesy Neil A. Tanner; p. 98T, Courtesy Shirlee Stevens; p. 98B, Courtesy Joseph Quever; p. 99, Courtesy Neil A. Tanner; p. 100T, Courtesy Joseph Quever; p. 100M, 100B, Courtesy Shirlee Stevens; p. 101T, Courtesy Neil A. Tanner; p. 101M, Courtesy Joseph Quever; p. 101B, Courtesy Neil A. Tanner; p. 102T, Courtesy Neil A. Tanner; p. 102B, 103T, Courtesy Joseph Quever; p. 103B, 104T, Courtesy Neil A. Tanner; p. 104B, 105, Courtesy Joseph Quever; p. 106T, Courtesy Shirlee Stevens; p. 106B, Courtesy Joseph Quever; p. 107T, Courtesy Neil A. Tanner; p. 107B, Courtesy Joseph Quever; p. 108T, Courtesy Shirlee Stevens; p. 108B, Courtesy Neil A. Tanner; p. 113, 114, Photos furnished by Universal Gym Equipment, Inc. Cedar Rapids, Iowa; p. 115, 117, 118, Courtesy Neil A. Tanner; p. 120, Courtesy Joseph Quever

Chapter 5 p. 123, © Alán Gallegos/AG Photograph; p. 127, 129, 130, 131, 132, Courtesy Shirlee Stevens; p. 133, Courtesy Neil A. Tanner; p. 137, Courtesy Joseph Quever; p. 138, Courtesy Shirlee Stevens; p. 139T, Courtesy Shirlee Stevens; p. 139B, Courtesy Joseph Quever; p. 140T, Courtesy Neil A. Tanner; p. 140M, 140B, Courtesy Shirlee Stevens; p. 145, Courtesy Shirlee Stevens; p. 146, Courtesy Neil A. Tanner; p. 153, Courtesy Joseph Quever

Chapter 6 p. 155, © Sean Clayton/The Image Works; p. 163, © Nathan Benn/Stock Boston; p. 168, Courtesy Shirlee Stevens

Chapter 7 p. 175, © Jonathan Nourok/PhotoEdit; p. 176, © Rachel Epstein/PhotoEdit; p. 186, © Jose Carillo/PhotoEdit

Chapter 8 p. 203, © Joel Gordon; p. 211, © Bob Daemmrich/Stock Boston; p. 225, © Esbin-Anderson/The Image Works

Chapter 9 p. 253, © Richard Pasley/Stock Boston; p. 257, © Alán Gallegos/AG Photograph; p. 266, © Jeff Greenberg/PhotoEdit; p. 271, © Bob Daemmrich/The Image Works

Chapter 10 p. 283, © David Young-Wolff/PhotoEdit; p. 287, © Richard Lord/The Image Works; p. 293, © Joel Gordon

Chapter 11 p. 307, © Spencer Grant/PhotoEdit; p. 311, © Gary Conner/PhotoEdit; p. 320, © Lawrence Migdale/Stock Boston

Preface

For today's fitness-conscious student, *Fit and Well: Alternate Edition* combines the best of two worlds. In the area of physical fitness, *Fit and Well* offers expert knowledge based on the latest findings in exercise physiology and sports medicine, along with tools for self-assessment and guidelines for becoming fit. In the area of wellness, it offers accurate, current information on today's most important health-related topics and issues, again with self-tests and guidelines for achieving wellness. To create this book, we have drawn on our combined expertise and experience in exercise physiology, athletic training, personal health, scientific research, and teaching. This special Alternate Edition contains the first 11 of the 15 chapters that appear in the full version of *Fit and Well*.

OUR AIMS

Our aims in writing this book can be stated simply:

- To show students that becoming fit and well greatly improves the quality of their lives
- To show students how they can become fit and well
- To motivate students to make healthy choices and to provide them with tools for change

The first of these aims means helping students see how their lives can be enhanced by a fit and well lifestyle. This book offers convincing evidence of a simple truth: To look and feel our best, to protect ourselves from degenerative diseases, and to enjoy the highest quality of life, we need to place fitness and wellness among our top priorities. *Fit and Well* makes clear both the imprudence of our modern, sedentary lifestyle and the benefits of a wellness lifestyle.

Our second aim is to give students the tools and information they need to become fit and well. This book provides students with everything they need to create their own personal fitness programs, including instructions for fitness tests, explanations of the components of fitness and guidelines for developing them, descriptions and illustrations of exercises, sample programs, and more. In addition, *Fit and Well* provides accurate, up-to-date, scientifically based information about other key topics in wellness, including nutrition, weight management, stress, and cardiovascular health.

In providing this material, we have pooled our efforts. Thomas Fahey has contributed his knowledge as an exercise physiologist, teacher, and author of numerous exercise science textbooks. Paul M. Insel and Walton T. Roth have contributed their knowledge of current topics in health as the authors of the leading personal health textbook, *Core Concepts in Health*.

Because we know this expert knowledge can be overwhelming, we have balanced the coverage of complex topics with student-friendly features designed to make the book accessible. Written in a straightforward, easy-to-read style and presented in a colorful, open format, *Fit and Well* invites the student to read, learn, and remember. Boxes, labs, tables, figures, artwork, photographs, and other features add interest to the text and highlight areas of special importance.

Our third aim is to involve students in taking responsibility for their health. *Fit and Well* makes use of interactive features to get students thinking about their own levels of physical fitness and wellness. We offer students assessment tools and laboratory activities to evaluate themselves in terms of each component of physical fitness and each major wellness area, ranging from cardiorespiratory endurance and muscular strength to stress and heart disease.

We also show students how they can make difficult lifestyle changes by using the principles of behavior change. Chapter 1 contains a step-by-step description of this simple but powerful tool for change. The chapter not only explains the five-step process but also offers a wealth of tips for ensuring success. Behavior management aids, including personal contracts, behavior checklists, and self-tests, appear throughout the book. *Fit and Well*'s combined emphasis on self-assessment, self-development in each area of wellness, and behavior change ensures that students not only are inspired to become fit and well but also have the tools to do so.

When students use these tools to make significant lifestyle changes, they begin to realize that they are in charge of their health—and their lives. From this realization comes a sense of competence and personal power.

Perhaps our overriding aim in writing *Fit and Well* is to convey the fact that virtually everyone has the ability to understand, monitor, and make changes in his or her own level of fitness and wellness. By making healthy choices from an early age, individuals can minimize the amount of professional medical care they will ever require. Our hope is that *Fit and Well* will help people make this exciting discovery: that they have the power to shape their own futures.

CONTENT AND ORGANIZATION OF THE FIFTH EDITION

The basic content of *Fit and Well* remains unchanged in the fifth edition. Chapter 1 provides an introduction to fitness and wellness and explains the principles of behavior change. Chapters 2–7 focus on the various areas of fitness. Chapter 2 provides an overview, discussing the components of fitness, the principles of physical training, and the factors involved in designing a well-rounded, personalized exercise program. Chapter 3 provides basic information on how the cardiorespiratory system functions, how the body produces energy for exercise, and how individuals can create successful cardiorespiratory fitness programs. Chapters 4, 5, and 6 look at muscular strength and endurance, flexibility and low-back health, and body composition, respectively. Chapter 7 "puts it all together," describing the nature of a complete program that develops all the components of fitness. This chapter also includes complete sample exercise programs.

Chapters 8, 9, and 10 treat three important areas of wellness promotion: nutrition, weight management, and stress management, respectively. It is in these areas that individuals have some of the greatest opportunities for positive change. Chapter 11 focuses on one of the most important reasons for making lifestyle changes: cardiovascular disease, the leading cause of death among Americans. Students learn the basic risk factors for cardiovascular disease and how they can make lifestyle changes to reduce their risk.

For the fifth edition, each chapter was carefully reviewed, revised, and updated. The latest information from scientific and wellness-related research is incorporated in the text, and newly emerging topics are discussed. The following list gives a sample of some of the new and updated material included in the fifth edition of *Fit and Well:*

- *Healthy People 2010* objectives
- Performance aids and dietary supplement safety and labeling issues
- Links between lifestyle and quality of life
- Dietary Guidelines for Americans, 2000 edition, and Dietary Reference Intakes
- Fitness and fatness
- Body image and eating disorders
- Preventing and managing low-back pain
- Nutrition for athletes
- Diabetes
- Sleep
- Diet pills and diet aids
- Anger management
- College stressors and counterproductive coping methods
- Cholesterol testing and treatment recommendations
- Spiritual wellness

Research in the areas of health and wellness is ongoing, with new discoveries, advances, trends, and theories reported nearly every week. For this reason, no wellness book can claim to have the final word on every topic. Yet, within these limits, *Fit and Well* does present the latest available information and scientific thinking on important wellness topics. Taken together, the chapters of the book provide students with a complete, up-to-date guide to maximizing their well-being, now and through their entire lives.

Ww To help students obtain the most current wellness information, each chapter in the fifth edition is also closely tied to the Web site developed as a companion to the text. Boxes, illustrations, tables, labs, terms, and sections of text marked with the special new World Wide Web icon have corresponding links and activities on the Fit and Well Online Learning Center (www.mhhe.com/fahey5e).

FEATURES OF THE FIFTH EDITION

This edition of *Fit and Well* builds on the features that attracted and held our readers' interest in previous editions. These features are designed to help students increase their understanding of the key concepts of wellness and to make better use of the book.

Laboratory Activities

To help students apply the principles of fitness and wellness to their own lives, *Fit and Well* includes **laboratory activities** for classroom use. These hands-on activities give students the opportunity to assess their current level of fitness and wellness, to create plans for changing their lifestyle to reach wellness, and to monitor their progress. They can assess their daily physical activity, for example, or their level of cardiorespiratory endurance; they can design a program to improve muscular strength or meet weight-loss goals; and they can explore their risk of developing cardiovascular disease. Labs are found at the end of each chapter; they are perforated for easy use. New to the fifth edition, assessment labs end with a section labeled "Using Your Results," which guides students in evaluating their scores, setting goals for change, and moving forward.

Also new to the fifth edition, the laboratory activities are found in an interactive format on the Fit and Well Online Learning Center. For a complete list of laboratory activities, see pp. xv–xvi in the table of contents.

Illustrated Exercise Sections

To ensure that students understand how to perform important exercises and stretches, *Fit and Well* includes three **illustrated exercise sections,** one in Chapter 4 and two in Chapter 5. The section in Chapter 4 covers exercises for developing muscular strength and endurance, as performed both with free weights and on weight machines. One section in Chapter 5 presents stretches for flexibility, and the other presents exercises to stretch and strengthen the lower back. Each exercise is illustrated with one or more full-color photographs showing proper technique.

Sample Programs

To help students get started, Chapter 7 offers seven complete **sample programs** designed to develop overall fitness. The programs are built around four popular cardiorespiratory endurance activities: walking/jogging/running, bicycling, swimming, and in-line skating. They also include weight training and stretching exercises. Each one includes detailed information and guidelines on equipment and technique; target intensity, duration, and frequency; calorie cost of the activity; record keeping; and adjustments to make as fitness improves. The chapter also includes general guidelines for putting together a personal fitness program: setting goals; selecting activities; setting targets for intensity, duration, and frequency, maintaining a commitment; and recording and assessing progress.

Boxes

Boxes are used in *Fit and Well* to explore a wide range of current topics in greater detail than is possible in the text itself. Boxes fall into five different categories, each marked with a special icon and label.

Take Charge boxes distill from the text the practical advice students need to apply information to their own lives. By referring to these boxes, students can easily find information about such topics as becoming more active, rehabilitating athletic injuries, exercising in hot weather, adding whole-grain foods to the diet, judging serving sizes, helping a friend who has an eating disorder, breathing techniques for stress reduction, managing anger, boosting motivation for behavior change, and many others.

Critical Consumer boxes are designed to help students develop and apply critical thinking skills, thereby enabling them to make sound choices related to health and well-being. Critical Consumer boxes provide specific guidelines for choosing a fitness center and exercise footwear and equipment; for evaluating health information, diet pills and aids, and supplements; and for using food labels and dietary supplement labels to make informed dietary choices.

Dimensions of Diversity boxes focus on the important theme of diversity. Most wellness issues are universal; we all need to exercise and eat well, for example. However, certain differences among people—based on gender, educational attainment, socioeconomic status, ethnicity, age, and other factors—do have important implications for wellness. Dimensions of Diversity boxes give students the opportunity to identify special wellness concerns that affect them because of who they are, as individuals or as members of a group. Topics of Dimensions of Diversity boxes include fitness for people with disabilities, gender differences in muscular strength, and ethnic foods.

Wellness Connection boxes highlight important links among the different dimensions of wellness—physical, emotional, social/interpersonal, intellectual, spiritual, and environmental—and emphasize that all the dimensions must be developed in order for an individual to achieve optimal health and well-being. Topics include the effects of exercise on mental functioning, how social support affects overall health, paths to spiritual wellness, and expressive writing.

In Focus boxes highlight current topics and issues of particular interest to students. These boxes focus on such topics as the importance of lifestyle for young adults, exercise safety, exercise machines versus free weights, diabetes, fitness and fatness, and many others.

Vital Statistics

Vital Statistics tables and figures highlight important facts and figures in an accessible format. From tables and figures marked with the Vital Statistics label, students learn about such matters as the leading causes of death for Americans and the factors that play a part in each one; the relationship between lifestyle and quality of life; current levels of physical activity in the United States; and a wealth of other information. For students who learn best when material is displayed graphically or numerically, Vital Statistics tables and figures offer a way to grasp information quickly and directly.

Common Questions Answered

Sections called **Common Questions Answered** appear at the ends of Chapters 2–11. In these student-friendly sections, the answers to frequently asked questions are presented in easy-to-understand terms. Included are such questions as, Are there any stretching exercises I shouldn't do? Do I need more protein in my diet when

I train with weights? Are kickboxing and Tae Bo effective forms of exercise? Can working out with an exercise ball be useful in preventing and managing low-back pain? and, How can I tell if I'm allergic to a food?

Quick-Reference Appendixes

Included at the end of the book are four appendixes containing vital information in an easy-to-use format. **Appendix A, Injury Prevention and Personal Safety,** is a reference guide to preventing common injuries, whether at home, at work, at play, or on the road. It also provides information on giving emergency care when someone else's life is in danger.

Appendix B, Nutritional Content of Common Foods, allows students to assess their daily diet in terms of 11 nutrient categories, including protein, fat, saturated fat, fiber, added sugar, cholesterol, and sodium. **Appendix C, Nutritional Content of Popular Items from Fast-Food Restaurants,** provides a breakdown of the nutritional content of the most commonly ordered menu items at popular fast-food restaurants.

Appendix D, Monitoring Your Progress, is a log that enables students to record and summarize the results of the assessment tests they complete as part of the laboratory activities. With space for preprogram and postprogram assessment results, the log provides an easy way to track the progress of a behavior change program.

Built-in Behavior Change Workbook

The built-in Behavior Change Workbook contains 15 separate activities that complement the lifestyle management model presented in Chapter 1. The workbook guides students in developing a successful program by walking them through each of the steps of behavior change—from choosing a target behavior to completing and signing a contract. It also includes activities to help students overcome common obstacles to behavior change. The workbook is also found on the Online Learning Center.

OTHER FEATURES AND LEARNING AIDS

At the beginning of each chapter, under the heading **Looking Ahead,** five or six statements preview the main points of the chapter for the student and serve as learning objectives. New to the fifth edition, each chapter also opens with **Test Your Knowledge**—a series of three multiple choice and true-false questions, with answers. These self-quizzes facilitate learning by emphasizing key points, highlighting common misconceptions, and sparking debate. Within each chapter, important terms appear in boldface type and are defined on the same or facing page of text in a **running glossary,** helping students handle new vocabulary.

Other features and learning aids are found at the end of each chapter. **Tips for Today,** new to the fifth edition, provide a very brief distillation of the major message of the chapter, followed by suggestions for a few simple things that students can try right away. Tips for Today are designed to encourage students and to build their confidence by giving them easy steps they can take immediately to improve wellness. **For Further Exploration** sections, also new to the fifth edition, offer suggestions for using the free student supplements that accompany the text—the Online Learning Center, the Daily Fitness and Nutrition Journal, and the Health*Quest* CD-ROM—to build fitness and wellness. These sections also list recommended books, newsletters, organizations, hotlines, and Web sites. Finally, **chapter summaries** offer students a concise review and a way to make sure they have grasped the most important concepts in the chapter.

For more on the features of the book, refer to the illustrated **User's Guide to *Fit and Well,*** found on pp. xvii–xx.

TEACHING TOOLS

Available with the fifth edition of *Fit and Well* is a comprehensive package of supplementary materials designed to enhance teaching and learning.

Instructor's Resource Binder (ISBN 0-07-253058-8)

The Instructor's Resource Binder contains a variety of helpful teaching materials in an easy-to-use form:

- The **Course Integrator Guide** (ISBN 0-7674-2949-4) includes learning objectives, extended chapter outlines, lists of additional resources, and many other teaching tools. It also describes all the print and electronic supplements available with the text and shows how to integrate them into lectures and assignments for each chapter.
- More than 90 **Additional Laboratory Activities** supplement the labs that are included in the text.
- The printed **Test Bank** (0-07-253054-5) includes more than 1000 true/false, multiple choice, and essay questions.

Computerized Test Bank CD-ROM (ISBN 0-07-253050-2)

The Computerized Test Bank CD-ROM from Brownstone provides a powerful, easy-to-use test maker to create a print version, a computer lab version, or an Internet version of each test. The CD-ROM includes the Diploma program for Windows users and Exam VI for Macintosh users. The Diploma program also includes a built-in gradebook.

Visual Resources: PowerPoint Slides, Acetates, and Videos

A variety of visual resources is available for use with the fifth edition of *Fit and Well:*

- The **Image Presentation CD-ROM** (ISBN 0-07-253056-1) is an electronic library of visual resources. It includes images from the text displayed in PowerPoint as well as complete, ready-to-use PowerPoint presentations for each chapter.
- Expanded for the fifth edition, a set of 100 color **Transparency Acetates** (ISBN 0-07-253051-0) is available as a lecture resource.
- The new **McGraw-Hill Custom Video for Health** (ISBN 0-7674-2567-7) includes brief video segments with additional information on wellness topics such as nutrition, exercise, and heart disease.
- **Students on Health Custom Video** (ISBN 0-7674-0022-4) features students from college campuses across the country discussing how their daily lives are affected by their choices in such wellness areas as exercise, nutrition, and stress.
- The **Healthy Living Video Clips CD-ROM** (ISBN 0-07-238808-0) contains a collection of brief, digitized video clips that can be used to introduce a lecture or to spark classroom discussion. The segments are 2–4 minutes long, and links provide brief descriptions of each clip.

Videos from Films for Humanities and from the award-winning series *Healthy Living: Road to Wellness* are also available.

Digital Solutions

The ***Fit and Well*** **Online Learning Center (www.mhhe.com/fahey5e)** provides many additional resources for both instructors and students. Instructor tools include downloadable versions of the Course Integrator Guide and all the PowerPoint slides, links to professional resources, and a guide to using the Internet. For students, there are learning objectives, self-quizzes and glossary flashcards for review, interactive Internet exercises, and extensive links. The Online Learning Center also includes many tools for wellness behavior change, including interactive versions of the Behavior Change Workbook as well as lab activities from the text.

The **Health and Human Performance Web Site (www.mhhe.com/hhp)** provides monthly articles about current issues, downloadable supplements for instructors, a "how-to" technology guide, self-assessments, study tips, exam-preparation materials, and a wealth of other tools and resources for instructors and students. It also includes information about professional organizations, scholarship opportunities, conventions, and careers.

PageOut (www.pageout.net) is a free, easy-to-use program that enables instructors to quickly develop Web sites for their courses. PageOut can be used to create a course home page, an instructor home page, an interactive syllabus that can be linked to elements in the Online Learning Center, Web links, online discussion areas, an online grade book, and much more. The Online Learning Center can also be customized to work with products like WebCT and Blackboard.

PowerWeb (www.dushkin.com/online) is a student Internet resource of course-specific articles and current events. Students can visit PowerWeb and take self-scoring quizzes, complete interactive exercises, or check the daily news. Students using PowerWeb are also granted full access to Dushkin/McGraw-Hill's Student Site, where they can read study tips, conduct Web research, learn about different career paths, and follow Web links.

For more information about McGraw-Hill's digital resources, including how to obtain passwords for PageOut and PowerWeb, contact your local representative and visit McGraw-Hill on the World Wide Web (www.mhhe.com/solutions).

Student Resources Available with *Fit and Well*

In addition to the materials on the Online Learning Center, there are many resources available with *Fit and Well* designed to help students learn and apply key concepts.

- The **Daily Fitness and Nutrition Journal** (ISBN 0-07-253055-3) is a handy booklet that guides students in planning and tracking their fitness programs. It also helps students assess their current diet and make appropriate changes. It is packaged free with each copy of the text.
- **Health*Quest* 4.0** (ISBN 0-07-253052-9) is an interactive CD-ROM that helps students explore their wellness behavior. It includes tutorials, assessments, and behavior change guidance in such key areas as stress, fitness, nutrition, communicable diseases, cardiovascular disease, cancer, tobacco, alcohol, and other drugs. It is packaged free with each copy of the text.
- The **FoodWise CD-ROM** (ISBN 0-07-243775-8) is a dietary analysis program that includes food composition information based on USDA data. It offers a variety of functions, including the ability to add new foods to the database. FoodWise is available for both Windows and Macintosh and can also be networked.
- The **Quick View Guide to the Internet for Students of Health, Physical Education, and Exercise Science, Version 2.0** (ISBN 0-7674-2062-4) provides step-by-step instructions on how to access the Internet; how to find, evaluate, and use online information about fitness and wellness; and many other topics.
- **TestWell** (ISBN 0-69-721131-2) is a printed, self-scoring wellness assessment developed by the

National Wellness Institute in Stevens Point, Wisconsin. It can be used as a pre- and postcourse assessment tool.

Additional supplements and many packaging options are available; check with your local sales representative.

A NOTE OF THANKS

Fit and Well has benefited from the thoughtful commentary, expert knowledge, and helpful suggestions of many people. We are deeply grateful for their participation in the project.

Academic reviewers of the fifth edition:

Chris A. Ayres, East Tennessee State University
Tom Ball, DePauw University
Joan Barch, Lansing Community College
Joe D. Bell, Abilene Christian University
Evonne Bird, Truman State University
Laura L. Borsdorf, Ursinus College
Randy Deere, Western Kentucky University
J. Frederick Garman, Kutztown University of Pennsylvania
Beth Gebstadt, Central Oregon Community College
Steve Glass, Grand Valley University
Ron Holloway, Kennesaw State University
Robert Kostelnik, Indiana University of Pennsylvania
Alan M. Kramer, Abraham Baldwin College
Wayne Major, Eastern Kentucky University
Michelle Miller, Indiana University
Laurie A. Milliken, University of Massachusetts, Boston
Rich Schroeder, DeAnza College
Kenneth Sparks, Cleveland State University
Thaxton Springfield, St. Petersburg College
Lisa L. Watson, Gainesville College

Special fitness consultants for the fifth edition:

Glenn A. Gaesser, University of Virginia
Carol Ewing Garber, Northeastern University

Special thanks are due to Rich Schroeder, DeAnza College, for hosting the photo shoot for the fifth edition and to Gabriel Darden, Dennis Lin, and Graciela Blaum for their participation in the photo shoot. We are also grateful to the *Fit and Well* book team, without whose efforts the book could not have been published. Special thanks to Vicki Malinee, executive editor; Kirstan Price, developmental editor; Megan Scully, editorial assistant; Pam Cooper, marketing manager; Jason Dewey, field publisher; Jen Mills and Brett Coker, project managers; Melissa Williams, managing editor; Pam Augspurger, production supervisor; Violeta Díaz, design manager; Robin Mouat, art manager; Emma Ghiselli, art editor; Brian Pecko, photo researcher; and Marty Granahan, permissions editor.

Thomas D. Fahey
Paul M. Insel
Walton T. Roth

Brief Contents

Contents

CRITICAL CONSUMER

WELLNESS CONNECTION

DIMENSIONS OF DIVERSITY

IN FOCUS

W BEHAVIOR CHANGE WORKBOOK ACTIVITIES

PART 1 DEVELOPING A PLAN FOR BEHAVIOR CHANGE AND COMPLETING A CONTRACT

PART 2 OVERCOMING OBSTACLES TO BEHAVIOR CHANGE

W LABORATORY ACTIVITIES

Www The Behavior Change Workbook and the laboratory activities are also found in an interactive format on the *Fit and Well* Online Learning Center (www.mhhe.com/fahey5e).

A User's Guide to *Fit and Well*

Are you looking for ways to improve your lifestyle and become fit and well? Do you need help finding reliable wellness resources online? Would you like to boost your grade? *Fit and Well* can help you do all this and much more!

LABORATORY ACTIVITIES

These hands-on self-assessments help you determine your current level of wellness and create plans for making positive changes in your lifestyle. The Using Your Results sections guide you in setting goals and moving forward based on the results of the assessments. Lab activities are included at the end of every chapter on easy-to-use perforated pages.

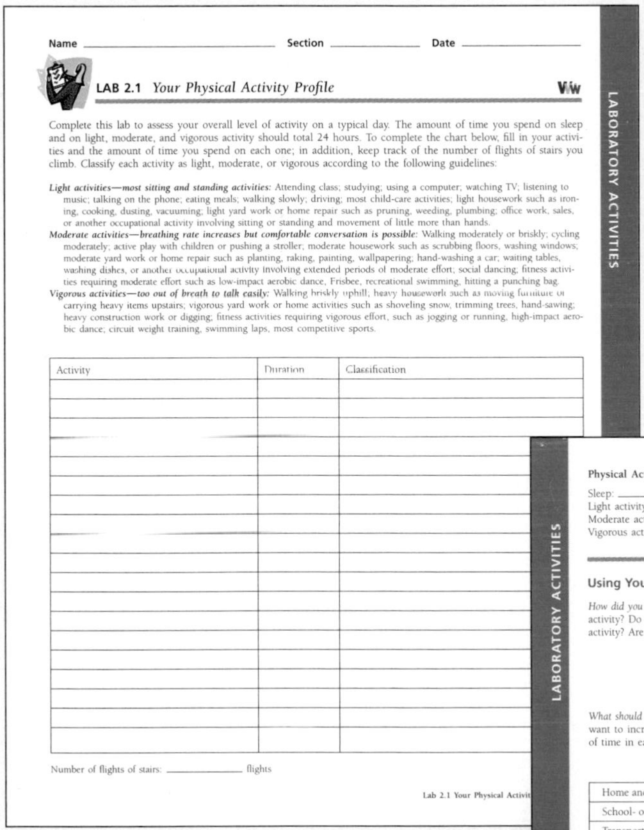

Name ________________ Section ________ Date ________

LAB 2.1 *Your Physical Activity Profile*

Complete this lab to assess your overall level of activity on a typical day. The amount of time you spend on sleep and on light, moderate, and vigorous activity should total 24 hours. To complete the chart below, fill in your activities and the amount of time you spend on each one; in addition, keep track of the number of flights of stairs you climb. Classify each activity as light, moderate, or vigorous according to the following guidelines:

Light activities—most sitting and standing activities: Attending class; studying; using a computer; watching TV; listening to music; talking on the phone; eating meals; walking slowly; driving; most child-care activities; light housework such as ironing, cooking, dusting, vacuuming; light yard work or home repair such as pruning, weeding, plumbing; office work, sales, or another occupational activity involving sitting or standing and movement of little more than hands.

Moderate activities—breathing rate increases but comfortable conversation is possible: Walking moderately or briskly; cycling moderately; active play with children or pushing a stroller; moderate housework such as scrubbing floors, washing windows; moderate yard work or home repair such as planting, raking, painting, wallpapering; hand-washing a car; waiting tables, washing dishes, or another occupational activity involving extended periods of moderate effort; social dancing; fitness activities requiring moderate effort such as low-impact aerobic dance, Frisbee, recreational swimming, hitting a punching bag.

Vigorous activities—too out of breath to talk easily: Walking briskly uphill; heavy housework such as moving furniture or carrying heavy items upstairs; vigorous yard work or home activities such as shoveling snow, trimming trees, hand-sawing; heavy construction work or digging; fitness activities requiring vigorous effort, such as jogging or running, high-impact aerobic dance; circuit weight training, swimming laps, most competitive sports.

Activity	Duration	Classification

Number of flights of stairs: ________ flights

Lab 2.1 Your Physical Activit

LABORATORY ACTIVITIES

Fit and Well ONLINE LEARNING CENTER (www.mhhe.com/fahey5e)

Look for the special World Wide Web icon throughout the text. Elements marked with the icon have corresponding activities and links on the *Fit and Well* Online Learning Center. The lab activities can be found online in an interactive format.

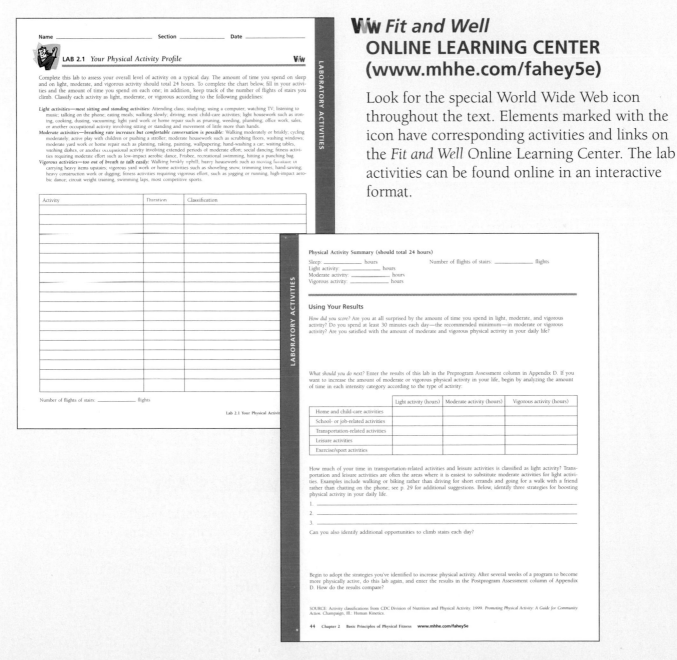

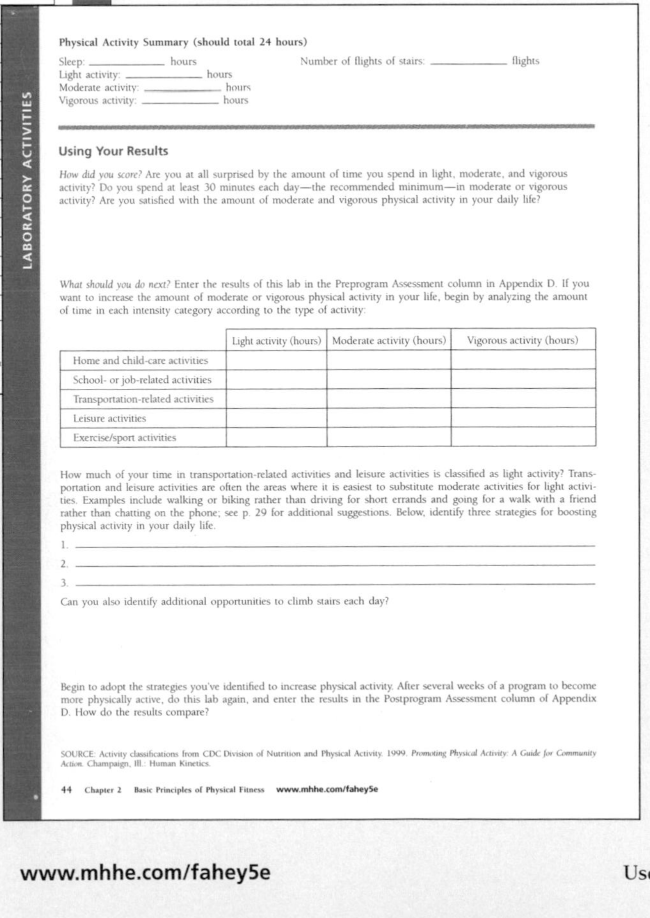

LABORATORY ACTIVITIES

Physical Activity Summary (should total 24 hours)

Sleep: ________ hours
Light activity: ________ hours
Moderate activity: ________ hours
Vigorous activity: ________ hours

Number of flights of stairs: ________ flights

Using Your Results

How did you score? Are you at all surprised by the amount of time you spend in light, moderate, and vigorous activity? Do you spend at least 30 minutes each day—the recommended minimum—in moderate or vigorous activity? Are you satisfied with the amount of moderate and vigorous physical activity in your daily life?

What should you do next? Enter the results of this lab in the Preprogram Assessment column in Appendix D. If you want to increase the amount of moderate or vigorous physical activity in your life, begin by analyzing the amount of time in each intensity category according to the type of activity:

	Light activity (hours)	Moderate activity (hours)	Vigorous activity (hours)
Home and child-care activities			
School- or job-related activities			
Transportation-related activities			
Leisure activities			
Exercise/sport activities			

How much of your time in transportation-related activities and leisure activities is classified as light activity? Transportation and leisure activities are often the areas where it is easiest to substitute moderate activities for light activities. Examples include walking or biking rather than driving for short errands and going for a walk with a friend rather than chatting on the phone; see p. 29 for additional suggestions. Below, identify three strategies for boosting physical activity in your daily life.

1. ________
2. ________
3. ________

Can you also identify additional opportunities to climb stairs each day?

Begin to adopt the strategies you've identified to increase physical activity. After several weeks of a program to become more physically active, do this lab again, and enter the results in the Postprogram Assessment column of Appendix D. How do the results compare?

SOURCE: Activity classifications from CDC Division of Nutrition and Physical Activity. 1999. *Promoting Physical Activity: A Guide for Community Action.* Champaign, Ill.: Human Kinetics.

44 Chapter 2 Basic Principles of Physical Fitness www.mhhe.com/fahey5e

TIPS FOR TODAY

Tips for Today sections, found at the end of each chapter, provide a brief summary of the major message of the chapter, followed by suggestions for a few easy steps you can try right away to improve your level of wellness.

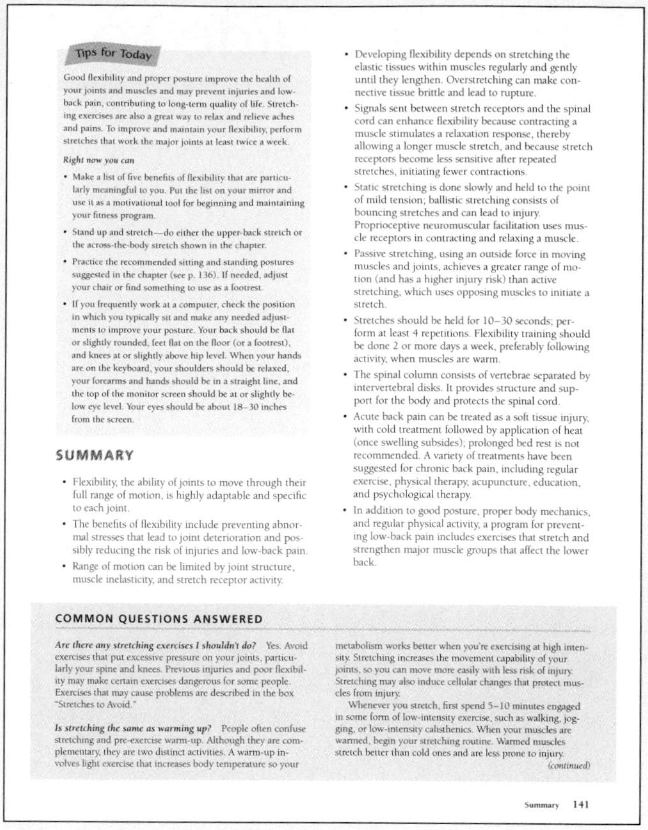

Tips for Today

Good flexibility and proper posture improve the health of your joints and muscles and may prevent injuries and low-back pain, contributing to long-term quality of life. Stretching exercises are also a great way to relax and relieve aches and pains. To improve and maintain your flexibility, perform stretches that work the major joints at least twice a week.

Right now you can

- Make a list of five benefits of flexibility that are particularly meaningful to you. Put the list on your mirror and use it as a motivational tool for beginning and maintaining your fitness program.
- Stand up and stretch—do either the upper-back stretch or the across-the-body stretch shown in the chapter.
- Practice the recommended sitting and standing postures suggested in the chapter (see p. 136). If needed, adjust your chair or find something to use as a footrest.
- If you frequently work at a computer, check the position in which you typically sit and make any needed adjustments to improve your posture. Your back should be flat or slightly rounded, feet flat on the floor (or a footrest), and knees at or slightly above hip level. When your hands are on the keyboard, your shoulders should be relaxed, your forearms and hands should be in a straight line, and the top of the monitor screen should be at or slightly below eye level. Your eyes should be about 18–30 inches from the screen.

SUMMARY

- Flexibility, the ability of joints to move through their full range of motion, is highly adaptable and specific to each joint.
- The benefits of flexibility include preventing abnormal stresses that lead to joint deterioration and possibly reducing the risk of injuries and low-back pain.
- Range of motion can be limited by joint structure, muscle inelasticity, and stretch receptor activity.
- Developing flexibility depends on stretching the elastic tissues within muscles regularly and gently until they lengthen. Overstretching can make connective tissue brittle and lead to rupture.
- Signals sent between stretch receptors and the spinal cord can enhance flexibility because contracting a muscle stimulates a relaxation response, thereby allowing a longer muscle stretch, and because stretch receptors become less sensitive after repeated stretches, initiating fewer contractions.
- Static stretching is done slowly and held to the point of mild tension; ballistic stretching consists of bouncing stretches and can lead to injury. Proprioceptive neuromuscular facilitation uses muscle receptors in contracting and relaxing a muscle.
- Passive stretching, using an outside force in moving muscles and joints, achieves a greater range of motion (and has a higher injury risk) than active stretching, which uses opposing muscles to initiate a stretch.
- Stretches should be held for 10–30 seconds; perform at least 4 repetitions. Flexibility training should be done 2 or more days a week, preferably following activity, when muscles are warm.
- The spinal column consists of vertebrae separated by intervertebral disks. It provides structure and support for the body and protects the spinal cord.
- Acute back pain can be treated as a soft tissue injury, with cold treatment followed by application of heat (once swelling subsides); prolonged bed rest is not recommended. A variety of treatments have been suggested for chronic back pain, including regular exercise, physical therapy, acupuncture, education, and psychological therapy.
- In addition to good posture, proper body mechanics, and regular physical activity, a program for preventing low-back pain includes exercises that stretch and strengthen major muscle groups that affect the lower back.

COMMON QUESTIONS ANSWERED

Are there any stretching exercises I shouldn't do? Yes. Avoid exercises that put excessive pressure on your joints, particularly your spine and knees. Previous injuries and poor flexibility may make certain exercises dangerous for some people. Exercises that may cause problems are described in the box "Stretches to Avoid."

Is stretching the same as warming up? People often confuse stretching and pre-exercise warm-up. Although they are complementary, they are two distinct activities. A warm-up involves light exercise that increases body temperature so your metabolism works better when you're exercising at high intensity. Stretching increases the movement capability of your joints, so you can move more easily with less risk of injury. Stretching may also induce cellular changes that protect muscles from injury.

Whenever you stretch, first spend 5–10 minutes engaged in some form of low-intensity exercise, such as walking, jogging, or low-intensity calisthenics. When your muscles are warmed, begin your stretching routine. Warmed muscles stretch better than cold ones and are less prone to injury.

(continued)

Summary 141

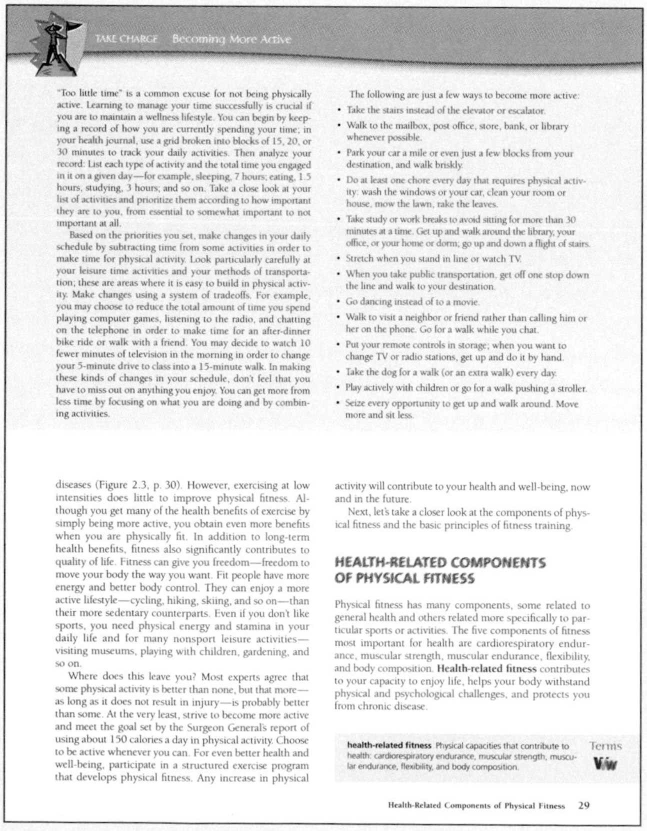

TAKE CHARGE Becoming More Active

"Too little time" is a common excuse for not being physically active. Learning to manage your time successfully is crucial if you are to maintain a wellness lifestyle. You can begin by keeping a record of how you are currently spending your time; in your health journal, use a grid broken into blocks of 15, 20, or 30 minutes to track your daily activities. Then analyze your record: List each type of activity and the total time you engaged in it on a given day—for example, sleeping, 7 hours; eating, 1.5 hours, studying, 3 hours; and so on. Take a close look at your list of activities and prioritize them according to how important they are to you, from essential to somewhat important to not important at all.

Based on the priorities you set, make changes in your daily schedule by subtracting time from some activities in order to make time for physical activity. Look particularly carefully at your leisure time activities and your methods of transportation; these are areas where it is easy to build in physical activity. Make changes using a system of tradeoffs. For example, you may choose to reduce the total amount of time you spend playing computer games, listening to the radio, and chatting on the telephone in order to make time for an after-dinner bike ride or walk with a friend. You may decide to watch 10 fewer minutes of television in the morning in order to change your 5-minute drive to class into a 15-minute walk. In making these kinds of changes in your schedule, don't feel that you have to miss out on anything you enjoy. You can get more from less time by focusing on what you are doing and by combining activities.

The following are just a few ways to become more active:

- Take the stairs instead of the elevator or escalator.
- Walk to the mailbox, post office, store, bank, or library whenever possible.
- Park your car a mile or even just a few blocks from your destination, and walk briskly.
- Do at least one chore every day that requires physical activity: wash the windows or your car, clean your room or house, mow the lawn, rake the leaves.
- Take study or work breaks to avoid sitting for more than 30 minutes at a time. Get up and walk around the library, your office, or your home or dorm; go up and down a flight of stairs.
- Stretch when you stand in line or watch TV.
- When you take public transportation, get off one stop down the line and walk to your destination.
- Go dancing instead of to a movie.
- Walk to visit a neighbor or friend rather than calling him or her on the phone. Go for a walk while you chat.
- Put your remote controls in storage; when you want to change TV or radio stations, get up and do it by hand.
- Take the dog for a walk (or an extra walk) every day.
- Play actively with children or go for a walk pushing a stroller.
- Seize every opportunity to get up and walk around. Move more and sit less.

diseases (Figure 2.3, p. 30). However, exercising at low intensities does little to improve physical fitness. Although you get many of the health benefits of exercise by simply being more active, you obtain even more benefits when you are physically fit. In addition to long-term health benefits, fitness also significantly contributes to quality of life. Fitness can give you freedom—freedom to move your body the way you want. Fit people have more energy and better body control. They can enjoy a more active lifestyle—cycling, hiking, skiing, and so on—than their more sedentary counterparts. Even if you don't like sports, you need physical energy and stamina in your daily life and for many nonsport leisure activities—visiting museums, playing with children, gardening, and so on.

Where does this leave you? Most experts agree that some physical activity is better than none, but that more—as long as it does not result in injury—is probably better than some. At the very least, strive to become more active and meet the goal set by the Surgeon General's report of using about 150 calories a day in physical activity. Choose to be active whenever you can. For even better health and well-being, participate in a structured exercise program that develops physical fitness. Any increase in physical activity will contribute to your health and well-being, now and in the future.

Next, let's take a closer look at the components of physical fitness and the basic principles of fitness training.

HEALTH-RELATED COMPONENTS OF PHYSICAL FITNESS

Physical fitness has many components, some related to general health and others related more specifically to particular sports or activities. The five components of fitness most important for health are cardiorespiratory endurance, muscular strength, muscular endurance, flexibility, and body composition. **Health-related fitness** contributes to your capacity to enjoy life, helps your body withstand physical and psychological challenges, and protects you from chronic disease.

health-related fitness Physical capacities that contribute to health: cardiorespiratory endurance, muscular strength, muscular endurance, flexibility, and body composition. Terms

Health-Related Components of Physical Fitness 29

TAKE CHARGE BOXES

Take Charge boxes, found throughout the text, provide practical advice that you can apply to your everyday life.

RUNNING GLOSSARY

Important terms appear in boldface type in the text and are defined in a running glossary on the same or facing page. A pronunciation guide to the glossary terms is found on the Online Learning Center.

CRITICAL CONSUMER BOXES

Critical Consumer boxes help you develop and apply critical thinking skills so you can make sound choices related to wellness. Additional resources for each Critical Consumer topic are found on the *Fit and Well* Online Learning Center.

CRITICAL CONSUMER Dietary Supplements: A Consumer Dilemma

"Builds lean muscle fast!" "Burns fat and gives you super energy!" "The most effective muscle-building product ever!" It's only human nature to want to feel, perform, and look as good as possible. But wading through advertising hype can be tricky when you are considering taking a dietary supplement. While drugs and food products undergo stringent government testing, dietary supplements can be freely marketed without testing for safety or effectiveness. There is no guarantee that advertising claims about dietary supplements are accurate or true.

What's the difference between a drug—which must be approved by the Food and Drug Administration (FDA)—and a dietary supplement? In some cases, the only real difference is in how the product is marketed. Some dietary supplements are as potentially dangerous as potent prescription drugs. For example, the male hormone testosterone, a powerful drug with many adverse affects, is closely regulated by the FDA. Androstenedione, a hormone converted in the body to testosterone (and estrogen), is readily available without a prescription as a dietary supplement. Androstenedione ("andro") is legal and can be purchased in thousands of stores and Internet sites. Andro disrupts the hormonal balance of its users and can increase the risk of heart disease. Teens who take andro are at risk for early closure of bone growth centers, which could limit their adult height. Other potential adverse effects of andro include acne, psychological disturbances, male breast development, baldness, and kidney and liver dysfunction. Advertisements for andro claim that it will increase muscle size, strength, and performance, but there are actually very few good studies of andro's effects on humans; the two best studies showed no significant difference in muscle growth and strength in andro users compared with nonusers. Most medical experts believe that andro is neither safe nor effective—yet it is used by thousands of athletes, most of whom are unaware of the risks.

Androstenedione is only one of the many popular dietary supplements that are of questionable benefit and safety. Ephedra is another common ingredient in dietary supplements, often touted as an "energy booster" and a "fat burner." Consumers might assume that ephedra is free of serious side effects since it is a natural herbal product and is available without a prescription. But ephedra has caused severe high blood pressure, heart attacks, strokes, and seizures, and has been implicated in numerous deaths. Adverse effects are much more likely when ephedra, which is a stimulant, is combined with other stimulants such as caffeine. Despite the risk, many ephedra-containing dietary supplements do contain caffeine or other stimulants—a fact that may not be clear from their labels. Many sports organizations, including the National Football League, have banned the use of ephedra because of safety concerns. However, it's estimated that more than 12 million Americans use ephedra-containing products. (Chapter 9 has more information about ephedra and other dietary supplements marketed for weight loss.)

Glowing reports about the supposed effects of dietary supplements may sound very enticing, but how can you determine if a particular supplement might be helpful? Ask yourself the following questions:

- *Do you really need a supplement at all?* Nutritional authorities agree that most athletes and young adults can obtain all the necessary ingredients for health and top athletic performance by eating a well-balanced diet and training appropriately. There is no dietary supplement that outperforms wholesome real food and a good training regimen. Remember, too, that athletic performance and appearance are not life and death issues. It's one thing to take a cancer chemotherapy drug with many known adverse effects if there is a reasonable chance that it will save your life. It's another to take a potentially dangerous dietary supplement that may not even work for you when your goal is to increase your sports performance.
- *Is the product safe and effective?* The fact that a dietary supplement is available in your local store is no guarantee of safety. As described above, the FDA doesn't regulate supplements in the same way as drugs. The only way to determine if a supplement really works is to perform carefully controlled research on human subjects. Testimonials from individuals who claim to have benefited from the product don't count. Few dietary supplements have undergone careful human testing, so it is difficult to tell which of them may actually work. Reliable resources for information on dietary supplements include the FDA Center for Food Safety and Applied Nutrition (http://www.cfsan.fda.gov/~dms/supplmnt.html) and the Nutritional Supplements for Athletes Web site from Kansas State University (http://www.oznet.ksu.edu/nutrition/supplements.htm).
- *Can you be sure that the specific product is of high quality?* There is no official agency that ensures the quality of dietary supplements. There is no guarantee that a supplement contains the desired ingredient, that dosages are appropriate, that potency is standardized, or that the product is free from contaminants (see Chapter 8 for more information on dietary supplement labeling).

A recent study of twelve over-the-counter brands of supplements containing androstenedione and related steroids found that one brand contained more and eleven brands contained less than the amount stated on the label; in addition, one brand contained a significant amount of a controlled steriod. The International Olympic Committee recently issued a warning to athletes based on a test of 634 different nutritional supplements; researchers found that 15% of the supplements tested contained unlabled substances that would cause an athlete to fail a drug test.

Many dietary supplements are ineffective and/or unsafe, but it is extremely difficult for consumers to get the information they need to make an informed decision. Once you have gathered the best information you can find, consider whether the potential benefits of the supplement appear to outweigh the risks and the cost. When in doubt, it's best not to buy or take the product. Remember that no supplement eliminates the need for proper training, and no supplement has been shown to be safe and effective in long-term weight loss. A product that is marginally effective, not proven safe, and expensive to boot is probably not worth the money or the risk.

94 Chapter 4 Muscular Strength and Endurance www.mhhe.com/fahey5e

Behavior Change Workbook

This workbook is designed to take you step by step through the process of behavior change. The first eight activities in the workbook will help you develop a successful plan—beginning with choosing a target behavior and moving through the program planning steps described in Chapter 1, including the completion and signing of a behavior change contract. The final seven activities will help you work through common obstacles to behavior change and maximize your program's chances of success.

Part 1 Developing a Plan for Behavior Change and Completing a Contract

1. Choosing a Target Behavior
2. Gathering Information About Your Target Behavior
3. Monitoring Your Current Patterns of Behavior
4. Setting Goals
5. Examining Your Attitudes About Your Target Behavior
6. Choosing Rewards
7. Breaking Behavior Chains
8. Completing a Contract for Behavior Change

Part 2 Overcoming Obstacles to Behavior Change

9. Building Motivation and Commitment
10. Managing Your Time Successfully
11. Developing Realistic Self-Talk
12. Involving the People Around You
13. Dealing with Feelings
14. Overcoming Peer Pressure: Communicating Assertively
15. Maintaining Your Program over Time

ACTIVITY 1 CHOOSING A TARGET BEHAVIOR

Use your knowledge of yourself and the results of Lab 1-2 (Lifestyle Evaluation) to identify five behaviors that you could change to improve your level of wellness. Examples of target behaviors include smoking cigarettes, not exercising regularly, eating candy bars every night, not getting enough sleep, getting drunk frequently on weekends, and not wearing a safety belt when driving or riding in a car. List your five behaviors below.

1. ____________________
2. ____________________
3. ____________________
4. ____________________
5. ____________________

For successful behavior change, it's best to focus on one behavior at a time. Review your list of behaviors and select one to start with. Choose a behavior that is important to you and that you are strongly motivated to change. If this will be your first attempt at behavior change, start with a simple change, such as wearing your bicycle helmet regularly, before tackling a more difficult change, such as quitting smoking. Circle the behavior on your list that you've chosen to start with; this will be your target behavior throughout this workbook.

www.mhhe.com/fahey5e W-1

BEHAVIOR CHANGE WORKBOOK

The Behavior Change Workbook takes you step by step through the process of behavior change. It helps you target a specific behavior, set goals, create a plan, and overcome common obstacles to change. The Workbook is available in an interactive format on the Online Learning Center, and a printed copy is included in the full and Alternate editions of the text.

SAMPLE EXERCISE PROGRAMS

Illustrated exercise programs in Chapters 4 and 5 show proper technique for exercises and stretches that develop muscular strength and endurance, flexibility, and low-back health. The complete sample fitness programs in Chapter 7 are built around popular endurance activities such as walking, jogging, cycling, and swimming.

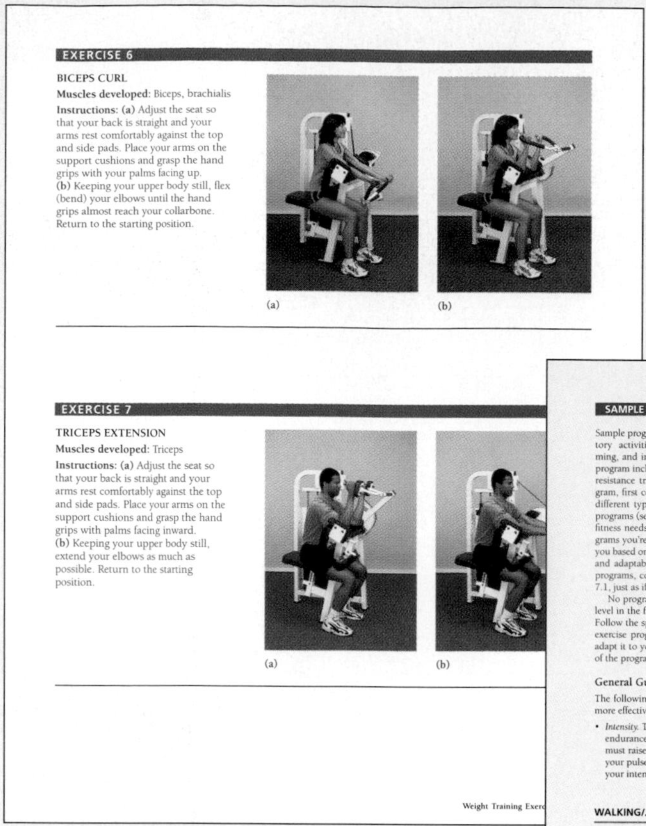

EXERCISE 6

BICEPS CURL

Muscles developed: Biceps, brachialis

Instructions: (a) Adjust the seat so that your back is straight and your arms rest comfortably against the top and side pads. Place your arms on the support cushions and grasp the hand grips with your palms facing up.
(b) Keeping your upper body still, flex (bend) your elbows until the hand grips almost reach your collarbone. Return to the starting position.

(a) (b)

EXERCISE 7

TRICEPS EXTENSION

Muscles developed: Triceps

Instructions: (a) Adjust the seat so that your back is straight and your arms rest comfortably against the top and side pads. Place your arms on the support cushions and grasp the hand grips with palms facing inward.
(b) Keeping your upper body still, extend your elbows as much as possible. Return to the starting position.

(a) (b)

Weight Training Exerc

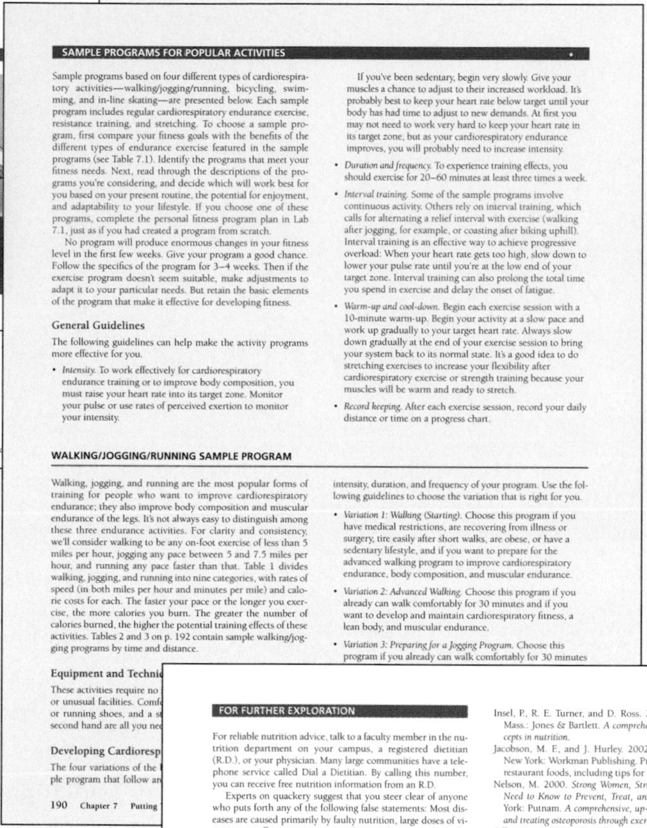

SAMPLE PROGRAMS FOR POPULAR ACTIVITIES

Sample programs based on four different types of cardiorespiratory activities—walking/jogging/running, bicycling, swimming, and in-line skating—are presented below. Each sample program includes regular cardiorespiratory endurance exercise, resistance training, and stretching. To choose a sample program, first compare your fitness goals with the benefits of the different types of endurance exercise featured in the sample programs (see Table 7.1). Identify the programs that meet your fitness needs. Next, read through the descriptions of the programs you're considering, and decide which will work best for you based on your present routine, the potential for enjoyment, and adaptability to your lifestyle. If you choose one of these programs, complete the personal fitness program plan in Lab 7.1, just as if you had created a program from scratch.

No program will produce enormous changes in your fitness level in the first few weeks. Give your program a good chance. Follow the specifics of the program for 3–4 weeks. Then if the exercise program doesn't seem suitable, make adjustments to adapt it to your particular needs. But retain the basic elements of the program that make it effective for developing fitness.

General Guidelines

The following guidelines can help make the activity programs more effective for you.

- *Intensity.* To work effectively for cardiorespiratory endurance training or to improve body composition, you must raise your heart rate into its target zone. Monitor your pulse or use rates of perceived exertion to monitor your intensity.

If you've been sedentary, begin very slowly. Give your muscles a chance to adjust to their increased workload. It's probably best to keep your heart rate below target until your body has had time to adjust to new demands. At first you may not need to work very hard to keep your heart rate in its target zone, but as your cardiorespiratory endurance improves, you will probably need to increase intensity.

- *Duration and frequency.* To experience training effects, you should exercise for 20–60 minutes at least three times a week.
- *Interval training.* Some of the sample programs involve continuous activity. Others rely on interval training, which calls for alternating a relief interval with exercise (walking after jogging, for example, or coasting after biking uphill). Interval training is an effective way to achieve progressive overload: When your heart rate gets too high, slow down to lower your pulse rate until you're at the low end of your target zone. Interval training can also prolong the total time you spend in exercise and delay the onset of fatigue.
- *Warm-up and cool-down.* Begin each exercise session with a 10-minute warm-up. Begin your activity at a slow pace and work up gradually to your target heart rate. Always slow down gradually at the end of your exercise session to bring your system back to its normal state. It's a good idea to do stretching exercises to increase your flexibility after cardiorespiratory exercise or strength training because your muscles will be warm and ready to stretch.
- *Record keeping.* After each exercise session, record your daily distance or time on a progress chart.

WALKING/JOGGING/RUNNING SAMPLE PROGRAM

Walking, jogging, and running are the most popular forms of training for people who want to improve cardiorespiratory endurance; they also improve body composition and muscular endurance of the legs. It's not always easy to distinguish among these three endurance activities. For clarity and consistency, we'll consider walking to be any on-foot exercise of less than 5 miles per hour, jogging any pace between 5 and 7.5 miles per hour, and running any pace faster than that. Table 1 divides walking, jogging, and running into nine categories, with rates of speed (in both miles per hour and minutes per mile) and calorie costs for each. The faster your pace or the longer you exercise, the more calories you burn. The greater the number of calories burned, the higher the potential training effects of these activities. Tables 2 and 3 on p. 192 contain sample walking/jogging programs by time and distance.

Equipment and Techni

These activities require no
or unusual facilities. Comf
or running shoes, and a s
second hand are all you ne

Developing Cardioresp

The four variations of the
ple program that follow ar

intensity, duration, and frequency of your program. Use the following guidelines to choose the variation that is right for you.

- *Variation 1: Walking (Starting).* Choose this program if you have medical restrictions, are recovering from illness or surgery, tire easily after short walks, are obese, or have a sedentary lifestyle, and if you want to prepare for the advanced walking program to improve cardiorespiratory endurance, body composition, and muscular endurance.
- *Variation 2: Advanced Walking.* Choose this program if you already can walk comfortably for 30 minutes and if you want to develop and maintain cardiorespiratory fitness, a lean body, and muscular endurance.
- *Variation 3: Preparing for a Jogging Program.* Choose this program if you already can walk comfortably for 30 minutes

190 Chapter 7 Putting

FOR FURTHER EXPLORATION

For Further Exploration sections at the end of each chapter describe books, newsletters, organizations, hotlines, and Web sites that you can turn to for additional advice and information. These sections also suggest ways to use the free tools available with *Fit and Well:*

- The Daily Fitness and Nutrition Journal gives you an easy way to plan and track a fitness program and a program for dietary improvement.
- The Health*Quest* CD-ROM includes interactive tutorials, self-assessments, review questions, and many other resources.
- The *Fit and Well* Online Learning Center (www.mhhe.com/fahey5e) provides interactive study guide questions, learning objectives, chapter outlines, glossary flashcards, Internet activities, links, and other useful study aids.

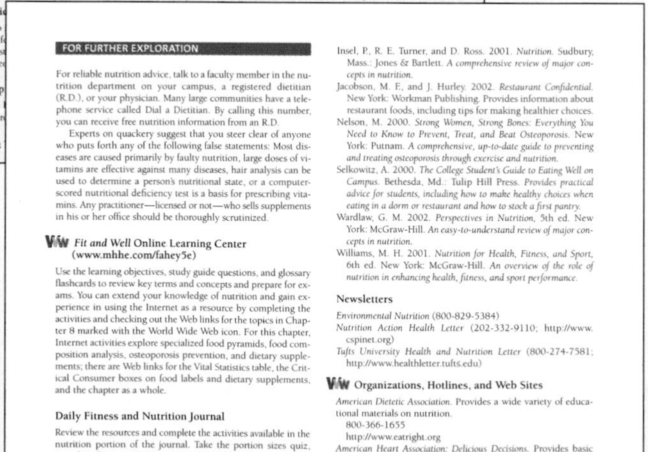

FOR FURTHER EXPLORATION

For reliable nutrition advice, talk to a faculty member in the nutrition department on your campus, a registered dietitian (R.D.), or your physician. Many large communities have a telephone service called Dial a Dietitian. By calling this number, you can receive free nutrition information from an R.D.

Experts on quackery suggest that you steer clear of anyone who puts forth any of the following false statements: Most diseases are caused primarily by faulty nutrition, large doses of vitamins are effective against many diseases, hair analysis can be used to determine a person's nutritional state, or a computer-scored nutritional deficiency test is a basis for prescribing vitamins. Any practitioner—licensed or not—who sells supplements in his or her office should be thoroughly scrutinized.

Fit and Well Online Learning Center (www.mhhe.com/fahey5e)

Use the learning objectives, study guide questions, and glossary flashcards to review key terms and concepts and prepare for exams. You can extend your knowledge of nutrition and gain experience in using the Internet as a resource by completing the activities and checking out the Web links for the topics in Chapter 8 marked with the World Wide Web icon. For this chapter, Internet activities explore specialized food pyramids, food composition analysis, osteoporosis prevention, and dietary supplements; there are Web links for the Vital Statistics table, the Critical Consumer boxes on food labels and dietary supplements, and the chapter as a whole.

Daily Fitness and Nutrition Journal

Review the resources and complete the activities available in the nutrition portion of the journal. Take the portion sizes quiz, complete the preprogram nutrition log, and analyze the results. Based on what you find, set healthy goals for change and complete the contract. Once you put your plan into action, complete the postprogram nutrition log to determine how successful you've been at improving your diet and moving toward the goals you've set.

Health*Quest*

Learn more about your current diet by completing the dietary assessment in the Nutrition and Weight Control module of the Health*Quest* CD-ROM (select How's Your Diet? from the Wellness Activities menu). Your scores will help you pinpoint dietary patterns that you could change to improve wellness. To determine if you are ready to make changes in your diet, complete the Stages of Change quiz (select Stages of Change from the Wellness Activities menu). You'll receive an assessment of your stage plus advice on moving forward toward the action and maintenance stages.

Books

American Dietetic Association. 1999. The *Essential Guide to Nutrition and the Foods We Eat: Everything You Need to Know About the Foods You Eat.* New York: HarperCollins. *An excellent review of current nutrition information and issues.*

Insel, P., R. E. Turner, and D. Ross. 2001. *Nutrition.* Sudbury, Mass.: Jones & Bartlett. *A comprehensive review of major concepts in nutrition.*

Jacobson, M. F., and J. Hurley. 2002. *Restaurant Confidential.* New York: Workman Publishing. Provides information about restaurant foods, including tips for making healthier choices.

Nelson, M. 2000. *Strong Women, Strong Bones: Everything You Need to Know to Prevent, Treat, and Beat Osteoporosis.* New York: Putnam. *A comprehensive, up-to-date guide to preventing and treating osteoporosis through exercise and nutrition.*

Selkowitz, A. 2000. *The College Student's Guide to Eating Well on Campus.* Bethesda, Md.: Tulip Hill Press. *Provides practical advice for students, including how to make healthy choices when eating in a dorm or restaurant and how to stock a first pantry.*

Wardlaw, G. M. 2002. *Perspectives in Nutrition,* 5th ed. New York: McGraw-Hill. *An easy-to-understand review of major concepts in nutrition.*

Williams, M. H. 2001. *Nutrition for Health, Fitness, and Sport,* 6th ed. New York: McGraw-Hill. *An overview of the role of nutrition in enhancing health, fitness, and sport performance.*

Newsletters

Environmental Nutrition (800-829-5384)

Nutrition Action Health Letter (202-332-9110; http://www.cspinet.org)

Tufts University Health and Nutrition Letter (800-274-7581; http://www.healthletter.tufts.edu)

Organizations, Hotlines, and Web Sites

American Dietetic Association. Provides a wide variety of educational materials on nutrition.
800-366-1655
http://www.eatright.org

American Heart Association: Delicious Decisions. Provides basic information about nutrition, tips for shopping and eating out, and heart-healthy recipes.
http://www.deliciousdecisions.org

Ask the Dietitian. Questions and answers on many topics relating to nutrition.
http://www.dietitian.com

Consumer Information Center: Food. Provides government publications about dietary fat, fiber, food safety, and other nutrition issues.
http://www.pueblo.gsa.gov/food.htm

CyberDiet. Provides a variety of resources, including a profile that calculates calorie and nutrient needs and a database that provides nutrition information in food label format.
http://www.CyberDiet.com

FDA Center for Food Safety and Applied Nutrition. Offers information about topics such as food labeling, food additives, and foodborne illness.
http://vm.cfsan.fda.gov

Food Safety Hotlines. Provide information on the safe purchase, handling, cooking, and storage of food.
888-SAFEFOOD (FDA)
800-535-4555 (USDA)

Gateways to Government Nutrition Information. Provides access to government resources relating to food safety, including consumer advice and information on specific pathogens.

For Further Exploration 239

Introduction to Wellness, Fitness, and Lifestyle Management

1

LOOKING AHEAD

After reading this chapter, you should be able to

- Describe the dimensions of wellness
- Identify the major health problems in the United States today, and discuss their causes
- Describe the behaviors that are part of a fit and well lifestyle
- Explain the steps in creating a behavior management plan to change a wellness-related behavior
- Discuss the available sources of wellness information and how to think critically about them

TEST YOUR KNOWLEDGE

1. The leading cause of death among Americans age 15–34 years is unintentional injuries (accidents).
   True or false?
2. Which of the following lifestyle factors is the leading preventable cause of death for Americans?
   a. excess alcohol consumption
   b. cigarette smoking
   c. poor dietary habits and lack of exercise
3. More than two-thirds of all college students make which of the following positive lifestyle choices?
   a. using safety belts
   b. not drinking and driving
   c. eating two or fewer high-fat foods per day
   d. not smoking cigarettes

TEST YOUR KNOWLEDGE ANSWERS

1. TRUE. Homicide and suicide round out the top three leading causes of death for 15–34-year olds; in this age group, the death rate for males is more than twice that for females.

2. B. Smoking causes more than 400,000 deaths per year; poor diet and inactivity are responsible for more than 300,000; and alcohol, more than 100,000.

3. ALL FOUR. However, the majority of students do not exercise regularly, do not wear bicycle helmets, and eat few fruits and vegetables. There are many areas in which college students can change their behavior to improve their health.

Fit and Well Online Learning Center

www.mhhe.com/fahey5e

Visit the *Fit and Well* Online Learning Center for study aids, additional information about wellness, links, Internet activities that explore the importance of a wellness lifestyle, and much more.

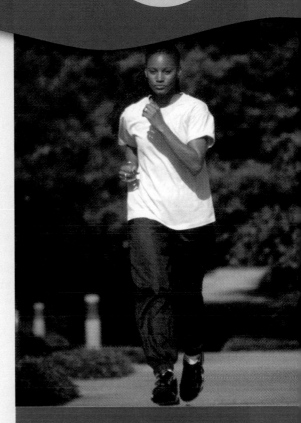

A first-year college student resolves to meet the challenge of making new friends. A long-sedentary senior starts riding her bike to school every day instead of taking the bus. A busy graduate student volunteers to plant trees in a blighted inner-city neighborhood. What do these people have in common? Each is striving for optimal health and well-being. Not satisfied to be merely free of major illness, these individuals want more. They want to live life actively, energetically, and fully, in a state of optimal personal, interpersonal, and environmental well-being. They have taken charge of their health and are on the path to wellness.

WELLNESS: THE NEW HEALTH GOAL

Wellness is an expanded idea of health. In the past, many people thought of health as being just the absence of physical disease. But wellness transcends this concept of health, as when individuals with serious illnesses or disabilities rise above their physical or mental limitations to live rich, meaningful, vital lives. Some aspects of health are determined by your genes, your age, and other factors that may be beyond your control. But true wellness is largely determined by the decisions you make about how to live your life. In this book, we will use the terms "health" and "wellness" interchangeably to mean the ability to live life fully—with vitality and meaning.

The Dimensions of Wellness

No matter what your age or health status, you can optimize your health in each of the following six interrelated dimensions. Wellness in any dimension is not a static goal but a dynamic process of change and growth (Figure 1.1).

Physical Wellness Optimal physical health requires eating well, exercising, avoiding harmful habits, making responsible decisions about sex, learning about and recognizing the symptoms of disease, getting regular medical and dental checkups, and taking steps to prevent injuries at home, on the road, and on the job. The habits you develop and the decisions you make today will largely determine not only how many years you will live, but the quality of your life during those years.

Emotional Wellness Optimism, trust, self-esteem, self-acceptance, self-confidence, self-control, satisfying relationships, and an ability to share feelings are just some of the qualities and aspects of emotional wellness. Emotional wellness is a dynamic state that fluctuates with your physical, intellectual, spiritual, interpersonal and social, and environmental wellness. Maintaining emotional wellness requires monitoring and exploring your thoughts and feelings, identifying obstacles to emotional well-being, and finding solutions to emotional problems, with the help of a therapist if necessary.

Intellectual Wellness The hallmarks of intellectual health include an openness to new ideas, a capacity to question and think critically, and the motivation to master new skills, as well as a sense of humor, creativity, and curiosity. An active mind is essential to wellness; it detects problems, finds solutions, and directs behavior. People who enjoy intellectual wellness never stop learning. They seek out and relish new experiences and challenges.

Spiritual Wellness To enjoy spiritual health is to possess a set of guiding beliefs, principles, or values that give meaning and purpose to your life, especially during difficult times. Spiritual wellness involves the capacity for love, compassion, forgiveness, altruism, joy, and fulfillment. It is an antidote to cynicism, anger, fear, anxiety, self-absorption, and pessimism. Spirituality transcends the individual and can be a common bond among people. Organized religions help many people develop spiritual

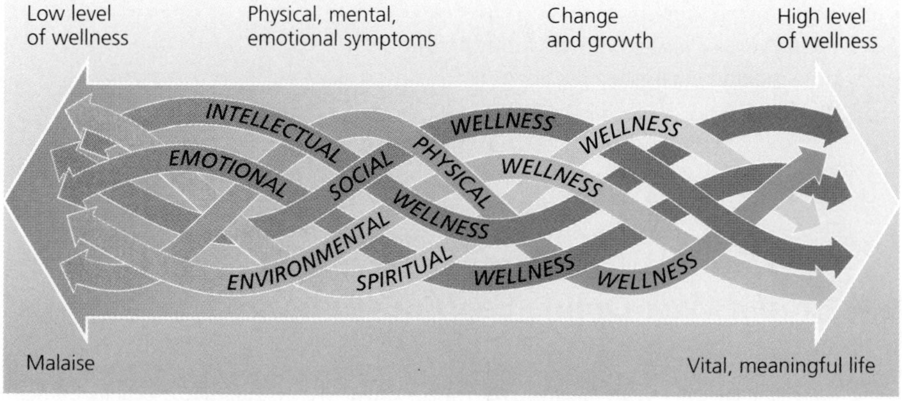

Figure 1.1 The wellness continuum. Wellness is composed of six interrelated dimensions, all of which must be developed in order to achieve overall wellness.

Paths to Spiritual Wellness

Spiritual wellness means different things to different people. For many, it involves developing a set of guiding beliefs, principles, or values that give purpose and meaning to life. It helps people achieve a sense of wholeness within themselves and in their relationships with others. Spiritual wellness influences people on an individual level, as well as on a community level, where it can bond people together through compassion, love, forgiveness, and self-sacrifice.

Regardless of how spiritual wellness is defined, its development is critical for overall well-being. Spiritual wellness is closely tied to the other components of wellness, particularly psychological wellness. And although difficult to study, spiritual wellness, researchers have found, is associated with greater self-esteem, social support, coping skills, positive health outcomes, and overall feelings of well-being. In general, people seem to feel better if they have beliefs about the ultimate purpose of life and their own place in the universe.

There are many paths to spiritual wellness. One of the most common in our society is organized religion. The major religions provide paths for transforming the self in ways that can lead to greater happiness and serenity and reduce feelings of anxiety and hopelessness. In Christianity, salvation follows turning away from the selfish ego to God's sovereignty and grace, where a joy is found that frees the believer from anxious self-concern and despair. Islam is the word for a kind of self-surrender leading to peace with God. Buddhism teaches how to detach oneself from selfish desire, leading to compassion for the suffering of others and freedom from fear-engendering illusions. Judaism emphasizes the social and ethical redemption the Jewish community can experience if it follows the laws of God. Religions teach specific techniques for achieving these transformations of the self: prayer, both in groups and in private; meditation; the performance of rituals and ceremonies symbolizing religious truths; and good works and service to others. Religious organizations also usually offer social and material support to members who might otherwise be isolated.

Spiritual wellness does not require participation in organized religion. Many people find meaning and purpose in other ways. By spending time in nature or working on environmental issues, people can experience continuity with the natural world. Spiritual wellness can come through helping others in one's community or by promoting human rights, peace and harmony among people, and opportunities for human development on a global level. Other people develop spiritual wellness through art or through their personal relationships.

How would you define spiritual wellness and its role in your life? What beliefs and practices do you associate with your sense of spiritual wellness? To achieve overall well-being, it is important to take time out to consider what you can do to help your spiritual side grow and flourish.

health, while many others find meaning and purpose in their lives on their own—through nature, art, meditation, political action, or good works (see the box "Paths to Spiritual Wellness").

Interpersonal and Social Wellness Satisfying relationships are basic to both physical and emotional health. We need to have mutually loving, supportive people in our lives. Developing interpersonal wellness means learning good communication skills, developing the capacity for intimacy, and cultivating a support network of caring friends and/or family members. Social wellness requires participating in and contributing to your community, country, and world.

Environmental, or Planetary, Wellness Increasingly, personal health depends on the health of the planet—from the safety of the food supply to the degree of violence in a society. Other examples of environmental threats to health are ultraviolet radiation in sunlight, air and water pollution, lead in old house paint, and secondhand tobacco smoke in indoor air. Wellness requires learning about and protecting yourself against such hazards—and doing what you can to reduce or eliminate them, either on your own or with others.

The six dimensions of wellness interact continuously, influencing and being influenced by one another. For example, spiritual wellness is associated with social skills, which can help build interpersonal relationships, which are in turn linked to better health and a longer life expectancy. The self-esteem that comes with emotional wellness is associated with increased physical activity and healthier eating habits, which support physical wellness. Individually and collectively, the wellness dimensions are associated with increased quality and quantity of life. Maintaining good health is a dynamic process, and increasing your level of wellness in one area of life often influences many others. For example, regular exercise (developing the physical dimension of wellness) can increase feelings of well-being and self-esteem (emotional wellness), which in turn can increase feelings of confidence in social interactions and achievements at work or school (interpersonal and social wellness). Some of the key links among different dimensions of wellness are highlighted in this text in boxes labeled Wellness Connection.

To help discover what wellness means to you and where you currently fall on the wellness continuum, complete Lab 1.1.

Terms

wellness Optimal health and vitality, encompassing physical, emotional, intellectual, spiritual, interpersonal and social, and environmental well-being.

VITAL STATISTICS

Table 1.1 *Leading Causes of Death in the United States*

Rank	Cause of Death	Number of Deaths	Percent of Total Deaths	Female/Male Ratio*	Lifestyle Factors
1	Heart disease	709,894	29.5	52/48	D I S A
2	Cancer	551,833	22.9	48/52	D I S A
3	Stroke	166,028	6.9	61/39	D I S A
4	Chronic lower respiratory diseases	123,550	5.1	50/50	S
5	Unintentional injuries (accidents)	93,592	3.9	35/65	I S A
6	Diabetes mellitus	68,662	2.9	54/46	D I S
7	Influenza and pneumonia	67,024	2.8	57/43	S
8	Alzheimer's disease	49,044	2.0	70/30	
9	Kidney disease	37,672	1.6	52/48	D I S A
10	Septicemia (systemic blood infection)	31,613	1.3	56/44	A
11	Intentional self-harm (suicide)	28,332	1.2	20/80	A
12	Chronic liver disease and cirrhosis	26,219	1.1	35/65	A
13	Hypertension (high blood pressure)	17,964	0.7	62/38	D I S A
14	Pneumonia due to aspiration	16,659	0.7	49/51	
15	Assault (homicide)	16,137	0.7	24/76	A
	All causes	2,404,624			

Key
- D Cause of death in which diet plays a part
- I Cause of death in which an inactive lifestyle plays a part
- S Cause of death in which smoking plays a part
- A Cause of death in which excessive alcohol consumption plays a part

*Ratio of females to males who died of each cause. For example, about the same number of women and men died of heart disease, but only about half as many women as men died of unintentional injuries and four times as many men as women committed suicide.

Note: Although deaths from HIV/AIDS have declined in recent years, HIV/AIDS remains a serious public health problem, causing more than 13,000 deaths per year in the United States. It is one of the 10 leading causes of death among people between the ages of 15 and 64.

SOURCE: National Center for Health Statistics. 2001. Deaths: Preliminary data for 2000. *National Vital Statistics Report* 49(12). National Center for Health Statistics. 2001. Deaths: Final data for 1999. *National Vital Statistics Report* 49(8).

New Opportunities, New Responsibilities

Wellness is a relatively recent concept. A century ago, people considered themselves lucky just to survive to adulthood. A child born in 1900, for example, could expect to live only about 47 years. Many people died as a result of common **infectious diseases** and poor environmental conditions (unrefrigerated food, poor sanitation, air and water pollution). However, over the past 100 years, the average life expectancy has nearly doubled, thanks largely to the development of vaccines and antibiotics to prevent and fight infectious diseases and to public health campaigns to improve environmental conditions.

Terms

infectious disease A disease that is communicable from one person to another; caused by invading microorganisms such as bacteria and viruses.

chronic disease A disease that develops and continues over a long period of time; usually caused by a variety of factors, including lifestyle factors.

physical fitness A set of physical attributes that allows the body to respond or adapt to the demands and stress of physical effort.

But a different set of diseases has emerged as our major health threat, and heart disease, cancer, and stroke are the three leading causes of death for Americans today (Table 1.1). Treating these and other **chronic diseases** is enormously expensive and extremely difficult. The best treatment for these diseases is prevention—people having a greater awareness about their own health and about taking care of their bodies.

The good news is that people do have some control over whether they develop cardiovascular disease (CVD), cancer, and other chronic diseases. People make choices every day that either increase or decrease their risks for these diseases—lifestyle choices involving such behaviors as exercise, diet, smoking, and drinking. When researchers look at the lifestyle factors that contribute to death in the United States (see the last column in Table 1.1), it becomes clear that individuals can profoundly influence their own health risks. For example, one large-scale study found that women who engaged in five healthy behaviors had a risk of heart disease that was more than 80% lower than the rest of the population (Figure 1.2). Wellness cannot be prescribed; physicians and other health care professionals can provide information, advice, and encouragement—but the rest is up to each of us.

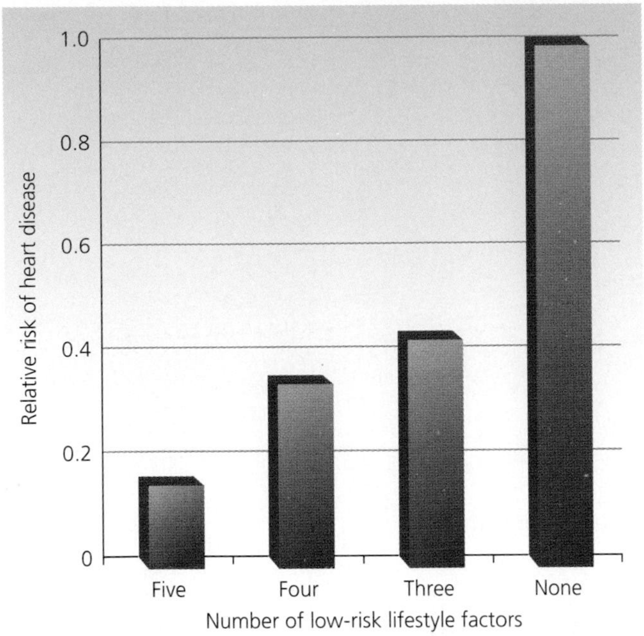

Figure 1.2 Lifestyle and risk of heart disease. Most cases of heart disease, the leading cause of death among Americans, can be prevented through low-risk behaviors such as not smoking, engaging in regular physical activity, and maintaining a healthy diet, body weight, and level of alcohol consumption. In this study of more than 80,000 nurses, those who were low-risk in all five areas had an incidence of heart disease 82% lower than the other women in the study. SOURCE: Stampfer, M. J., et al. 2000. Primary prevention of coronary heart disease in women through diet and lifestyle. *New England Journal of Medicine* 343(1): 16–22.

This chapter provides an overview of a lifestyle that contributes to wellness and describes a method that can help you make lasting changes in your life to promote good health. The chapters that follow provide more detailed information about physical activity, healthy eating habits, and other components of a wellness lifestyle. The book as a whole is designed to be used to help you take charge of your behavior and improve the quality of your life—to become fit and well.

Behaviors That Contribute to Wellness

A lifestyle based on good choices and healthy behaviors maximizes the quality of life. It helps people avoid disease, remain strong and fit, and maintain their physical and mental health as long as they live. The most important behaviors and habits are described in the following sections.

Be Physically Active The human body is designed to work best when it is active. It readily adapts to nearly any level of activity and exertion; in fact, **physical fitness** is defined as a set of physical attributes that allow the body to respond or adapt to the demands and stress of physical effort. The more we ask of our bodies—our muscles, bones, heart, lungs—the stronger and more fit they become. However, the reverse is also true: The less we ask of them, the less they can do. When our bodies are not kept active, they begin to deteriorate. Bones lose their density, joints stiffen, muscles become weak, and cellular energy systems begin to degenerate. To be truly well, human beings must be active. Unfortunately, a sedentary lifestyle is common among Americans today: More than 60% of Americans are not regularly physically active, and 25% are not active at all.

The benefits of physical activity are both physical and mental, immediate and long term (Figure 1.3, p. 6). In the short term, being physically fit makes it easier to do everyday tasks, such as lifting; it provides reserve strength for emergencies; and it helps people look and feel good. In the long term, being physically fit confers protection against chronic diseases and lowers the risk of dying prematurely. Physically active individuals are less likely to develop or die from heart disease, respiratory disease, high blood pressure, cancer, diabetes, and osteoporosis. Their cardiorespiratory systems tend to resemble those of people 10 or more years younger than themselves. As they get older, they may be able to avoid weight gain, muscle and bone loss, fatigue, and other problems associated with aging. With healthy hearts, strong muscles, lean bodies, and a repertoire of physical skills they can call on for recreation and enjoyment, fit people can maintain their physical and mental well-being throughout their lives.

Choose a Healthy Diet In addition to being sedentary, many Americans have a diet that is too high in calories, fat, and added sugars and too low in fiber and complex carbohydrates. This diet is linked to a number of chronic diseases, including heart disease, stroke, and certain kinds of cancer. It has been estimated that 15% of deaths in the United States can be attributed to poor diet combined with lack of exercise. A healthy diet promotes wellness in both the short and long term. It provides necessary nutrients and sufficient energy without also providing too much of the dietary substances linked to diseases.

Maintain a Healthy Body Weight Overweight and obesity are associated with a number of disabling and potentially fatal conditions and diseases, including heart disease, cancer, and diabetes. Healthy body weight is an important part of wellness—but short-term dieting is not part of a fit and well lifestyle. Maintaining a healthy body weight requires a lifelong commitment to regular exercise, a healthy diet, and effective stress management.

Manage Stress Effectively Many people cope with stress by eating, drinking, or smoking too much. Others don't deal with it at all. In the short term, inappropriate stress management can lead to fatigue, sleep disturbances, and other unpleasant symptoms. Over longer periods of time, poor management of stress can lead to less efficient functioning of the immune system and increased susceptibility to disease. There *are* effective ways to handle stress, and learning to incorporate them into daily life is an important part of a fit and well lifestyle.

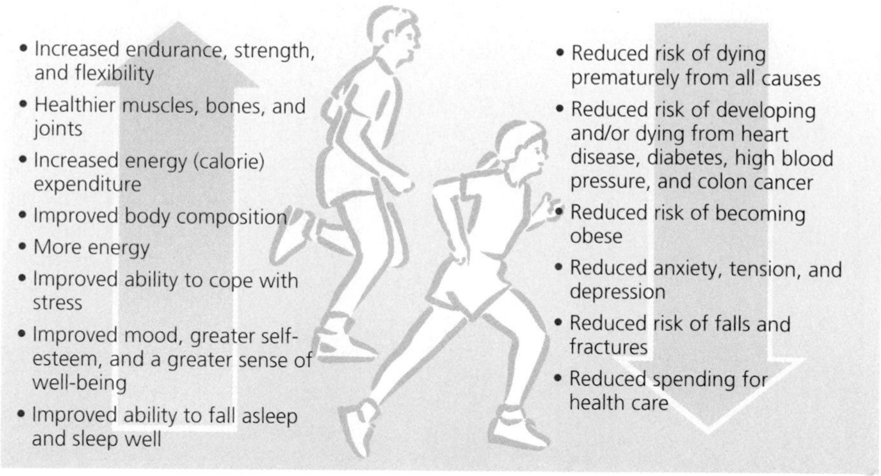

• Increased endurance, strength, and flexibility
• Healthier muscles, bones, and joints
• Increased energy (calorie) expenditure
• Improved body composition
• More energy
• Improved ability to cope with stress
• Improved mood, greater self-esteem, and a greater sense of well-being
• Improved ability to fall asleep and sleep well
• Reduced risk of dying prematurely from all causes
• Reduced risk of developing and/or dying from heart disease, diabetes, high blood pressure, and colon cancer
• Reduced risk of becoming obese
• Reduced anxiety, tension, and depression
• Reduced risk of falls and fractures
• Reduced spending for health care

Figure 1.3 Benefits of regular physical activity.

Avoid Use of Tobacco and Use Alcohol Wisely, If at All Tobacco use is associated with 8 of the top 10 causes of death in the United States; it kills more than 400,000 Americans each year, more than any other behavioral or environmental factor. A hundred years ago, before cigarette smoking was widespread, lung cancer was considered a rare disease. Today, with nearly 25% of the American population smoking, lung cancer is the most common cause of cancer death among both men and women and one of the leading causes of death overall.

Excessive alcohol consumption is linked to 6 of the top 10 causes of death and results in more than 100,000 deaths a year in the United States. It is an especially notable factor in the death and disability of young people, particularly through **unintentional injuries** (such as drownings and car crashes caused by drunken driving) and violence.

Protect Yourself from Disease and Injury The most effective way of dealing with disease and injury is to prevent them. Many of the lifestyle strategies discussed here—being physically active, managing body weight, and so on—help protect you against chronic illnesses. In addition, you can take specific steps to avoid infectious diseases, particularly those that are sexually transmitted. These diseases are preventable through responsible sexual behavior, another component of a fit and well lifestyle.

Unintentional injuries are the leading cause of death for people age 45 and under, but they, too, can be prevented. Learning and adopting safe, responsible behaviors is also part of a fit and well lifestyle.

Terms
Ww

unintentional injury An injury that occurs without harm being intended.

Other important behaviors in a fit and well lifestyle include developing meaningful relationships, planning ahead for successful aging, becoming knowledgeable about the health care system, and acting responsibly in relation to the environment. Lab 1.2 will help you evaluate your behaviors as they relate to wellness.

The Role of Other Factors in Wellness

Of course, behavior isn't the only factor involved in good health. Heredity, the environment, and access to adequate health care are other important influences. These factors can interact in ways that raise or lower the quality of a person's life and the risk of developing particular diseases. For example, a sedentary lifestyle combined with a genetic predisposition for diabetes can greatly increase a person's risk for developing the disease. If this person also lacks adequate health care, he or she is much more likely to suffer dangerous complications from diabetes and to have a lower quality of life.

But in many cases, behavior can tip the balance toward health even if heredity or environment is a negative factor. Breast cancer, for example, can run in families, but it also may be associated with overweight and a sedentary lifestyle. A woman with a family history of breast cancer is less likely to die from the disease if she controls her weight, exercises, performs regular breast self-exams, and consults with her physician about mammograms. By taking appropriate action, this woman can influence the effects of heredity on her health.

Ww National Wellness Goals

You may think of health and wellness as personal concerns, goals that you strive for on your own for your own benefit. But the U.S. government also has a vital interest in the health of all Americans. A healthy population is the nation's greatest resource, the source of its vigor and wealth. Poor health, in contrast, drains the nation's resources and raises national health care costs. As the embodiment of our society's values, the federal government also has a humane interest in people's health.

The U.S. government's national Healthy People initiative seeks to prevent unnecessary disease and disability and to achieve a better quality of life for all Americans. Healthy People reports, published first in 1980 and revised every decade, set national health goals based on 10-year agendas. Each report includes both broad goals and specific targets in many different areas of wellness. The latest report, *Healthy People 2010*, proposes two broad national goals:

- *Increase quality and years of healthy life.* The life expectancy of Americans has increased significantly in the past century; however, people can expect poor health to limit their activities and cause distress during the last 15% of their lives (Figure 1.4). Health-related quality of life calls for a full range of functional capacity to enable people to work, play, and maintain satisfying relationships.
- *Eliminate health disparities among Americans.* Many health problems today disproportionately affect certain American populations (see the box "Wellness Issues for Diverse Populations," p. 8). *Healthy People 2010* calls for eliminating disparities in health status, health risks, and use of preventive services among all population groups within the next decade.

Examples of individual health promotion objectives from *Healthy People 2010,* as well as estimates of how we are tracking toward the goals, appear in Table 1.2 (p. 9). As you can see, the objectives are tied closely to the wellness lifestyle described in this chapter. The principal topics covered in this book parallel the priority concerns of the Healthy People initiative, and the approach of *Fit and Well* is based on the initiative's premise that personal responsibility is a key to achieving wellness.

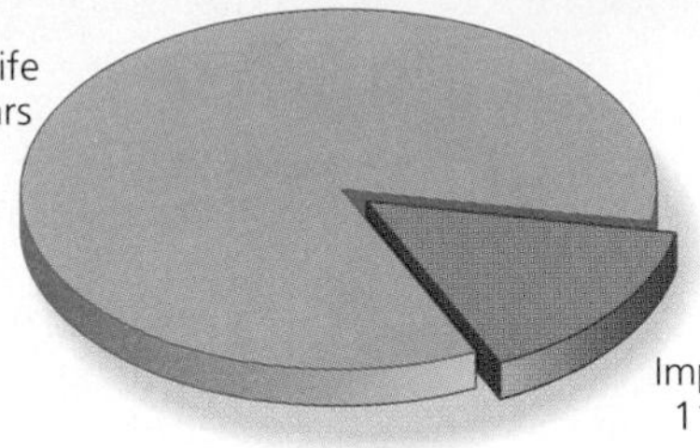

VITAL STATISTICS

Figure 1.4 Quantity of life versus quality of life. Years of healthy life as a proportion of life expectancy in the U.S. population.
SOURCES: National Center for Health Statistics. 2001. *Healthy People 2000 Final Review.* Hyattsville, Md.: Public Health Service. National Center for Health Statistics. 2001. Deaths: Preliminary data for 2000. *National Vital Statistics Reports* 49(12).

REACHING WELLNESS THROUGH LIFESTYLE MANAGEMENT

Your life may not resemble the picture drawn here of a fit and well lifestyle at all. You probably have a number of healthy habits and some others that place your health at risk. Taking big steps toward a wellness lifestyle may at first seem like too much work, but as you make progress, it gets easier. At first, you'll be rewarded with a greater sense of control over your life, a feeling of empowerment, higher self-esteem, and more joy. These benefits will encourage you to make further improvements. Over time, you'll come to know what wellness feels like—more energy, greater vitality; deeper feelings of curiosity, interest, and enjoyment; and a higher quality of life.

This section introduces the general process of behavior change and highlights the decisions and challenges you'll face at each stage. For additional help and advice, work through the activities in the Behavior Change Workbook at the end of the text.

Getting Serious About Your Health

Before you can start changing a wellness-related behavior, you have to know that the behavior is problematic and that you *can* change it. To make good decisions, you need information about relevant topics and issues, including what resources are available to help you change.

Examining Your Current Health Habits Have you considered how your current lifestyle is affecting your health today and how it will affect your health in the future? Do you know which of your current habits enhance your health and which detract from it? Begin your journey toward wellness with self-assessment: Think about your own behavior, complete the self-assessment in Lab 1.2, and talk with friends and family members about what they've noticed about your lifestyle and your health.

Many people start to consider changing a behavior when they get help from others. An observation from a friend, family member, or physician can help you see yourself as others do and may get you thinking about your behavior in a new way. For example, Jason has been getting a lot of stomachaches lately. His girlfriend, Anna, notices other changes as well and suggests that the stress of classes plus a part-time job and serving as president of the school radio station might be causing some of Jason's problems. Jason never thought much about trying to control the stressors in his life, but with encouragement from Anna he starts noticing what events trigger stress for him.

Landmark events such as a birthday, the birth of a child, or the death of someone close to you, can get you thinking about behavior change. New information can also help you get started. As you read this text, you may find yourself reevaluating some of your wellness-related

DIMENSIONS OF DIVERSITY Wellness Issues for Diverse Populations

When it comes to striving for wellness, most differences among people are insignificant. We all need to exercise, eat well, and manage stress. We need to know how to protect ourselves from heart disease, cancer, sexually transmitted diseases, and injuries.

But some of our differences—differences among us both as individuals and as members of groups—do have implications for wellness. Some of us, for example, have grown up eating foods that increase our risk of obesity or heart disease. Some of us have inherited predispositions for certain health problems, such as osteoporosis or high cholesterol levels. These health-related differences among individuals and groups can be biological—determined genetically—or cultural—acquired as patterns of behavior through daily interactions with our family, community, and society. Many health conditions are a function of biology and culture combined.

When we talk about wellness issues as they relate to diverse populations, we face two related dangers. The first is the danger of stereotyping, of talking about people as groups rather than as individuals. The second is that of overgeneralizing, of ignoring the extensive biological and cultural diversity that exists among people who may be grouped together because of their gender, socioeconomic status, or ethnicity. Every person is an individual with her or his own unique genetic endowment as well as unique experiences in life. However, many of these influences are shared with others of similar genetic and cultural backgrounds. Information about group similarities relating to wellness issues can be useful; for example, it can alert people to areas that may be of special concern for them and their families.

Wellness-related differences among groups can be identified and described along several different dimensions, including the following:

- *Gender.* Men and women have different life expectancies and different incidences of many diseases, including heart disease, cancer, and osteoporosis. Men have higher rates of death from injuries, suicide, and homicide; women are at greater risk for Alzheimer's disease and for depression. Men and women also differ in body composition and certain aspects of physical performance.
- *Ethnicity.* A genetic predisposition for a particular health problem can be linked to ethnicity as a result of each ethnic group's relatively distinct history. Diabetes is more prevalent among individuals of Native American or Latino heritage, for example, and African Americans have higher rates of hypertension. Ethnic groups may also vary in other ways that relate to wellness: traditional diets; patterns of family and interpersonal relationships; and attitudes toward using tobacco, alcohol, and other drugs, to name just a few.
- *Income and education.* Inequalities in income and education are closely related and underlie many of the health disparities among Americans. People with low incomes and less education have higher rates of injury and many diseases, are more likely to engage in unhealthy behaviors such as smoking, and have less access to health care services. Poverty and low educational attainment are far more important predictors of poor health than any ethnic factor.

These are just some of the "dimensions of diversity"—differences among people and groups that are associated with different wellness concerns. Other factors, too, such as age, geographic location, sexual orientation, and disability, can present challenges as an individual strives for wellness. In this book, topics and issues relating to wellness that affect different American populations are given special consideration in boxes labeled Dimensions of Diversity. These discussions are designed to deepen our understanding of the concepts of wellness and vitality in the context of ever-growing diversity.

behaviors. This could be a great opportunity to make healthful changes that will stay with you for the rest of your life.

Choosing a Target Behavior To maximize your chances of success, don't try to change all your problem behaviors at once—start exercising, quit smoking, give up high-fat foods, avoid drugs, get more sleep. Working on just one behavior will make high demands on your energy. Concentrate on one behavior that you want to change, your **target behavior,** and work on it systematically. Start with something simple, like snacking on candy between afternoon classes or always driving to a particular class instead of walking or biking.

Terms

Ww

target behavior An isolated behavior selected as the object for a behavior change program.

Obtaining Information About Your Target Behavior Once you've chosen a target behavior, you need to find out more about it. You need to know its risks and benefits for you—both now and in the future. How is your target behavior affecting your level of wellness today? What diseases or conditions does this behavior place you at risk for? What effect would changing your behavior have on your health? As a starting point, use material from this text and from the resources listed in the For Further Exploration section at the end of each chapter; refer to the box "Evaluating Sources of Health Information" on p. 10 for additional guidelines.

Finding Outside Help Have you identified a particularly challenging target behavior, something like alcohol addiction, binge eating, or depression, that interferes with your ability to function or places you at a serious health risk? Outside help is often needed to change behaviors or conditions that may be too deeply rooted or too serious

Table 1.2 *Selected* Healthy People 2010 *Objectives*

Objective	Estimate of Current Status (%)	Goal (%)
Increase the proportion of people age 18 and older who engage regularly, preferably daily, in moderate physical activity for at least 30 minutes per day.	15	30
Increase the proportion of people age 2 and older who consume at least 3 daily servings of vegetables, with at least one-third being dark-green or orange vegetables.	3	50
Increase the prevalence of healthy weight among all people age 20 and older.	42	60
Reduce the proportion of adults 18 and older who use cigarettes.	24	12
Reduce the proportion of college students reporting binge drinking during the past 2 weeks.	39	20
Increase the proportion of sexually active persons who use condoms.	23	50
Increase the proportion of adults who take protective measures to reduce the risk of skin cancer (sunscreens, sun-protective clothing, and so on).	47	75
Increase the use of safety belts by motor vehicle occupants.	69	92
Increase the number of residences with a functioning smoke alarm on every floor.	87	100
Increase the proportion of persons with health insurance.	83	100

SOURCE: U.S. Department of Health and Human Services. 2000. *Healthy People 2010*, 2nd ed. Washington, D.C.: DHHS.

for a self-management approach. If this is the case, don't be stopped by the seriousness of the problem—there are many resources available to help you solve it. On campus, the student health center or campus counseling center can provide assistance. To locate community resources, consult the yellow pages, your physician, your local health department, or the United Way.

Building Motivation to Change

Knowledge is a necessary ingredient for behavior change, but it isn't usually enough to make people act. Millions of people smoke or have sedentary lifestyles, for example, even though they know it's bad for their health. This is particularly true of young adults, who may not be motivated to change because they feel well despite engaging in unhealthy behaviors (see the box "Lifestyle Matters for Young Adults," p. 11). To succeed at behavior change, you need strong motivation.

Examining the Pros and Cons of Change Health behaviors have short-term and long-term benefits and costs. For example, in the short term, an inactive lifestyle allows more time to watch TV and hang out with friends but leaves a person less able to participate in recreational activities. In the long term, it increases risk of heart disease, cancer, stroke, and premature death. For successful behavior change, you must believe that the benefits of changing outweigh the costs.

Do a careful analysis of the short-term and long-term benefits and costs of continuing your current (target) behavior and of changing to a new, healthier behavior. Focus on the effects that are most meaningful to you, including those that are tied to your personal identity and values. For example, if you see yourself as an active person who is a good role model for others, then adopting behaviors such as regular physical activity and getting adequate sleep would support your personal identity. If you value independence and control over your life, then quitting smoking would be consistent with your values and goals. To complete your analysis, ask friends and family members about the effects of your behavior on them. For example, a younger sister may tell you that your smoking habit influenced her decision to take up smoking.

Pay special attention to the short-term benefits of behavior change, as these can be an important motivating force. Although some people are motivated by long-term goals, such as avoiding a disease that may hit them in 30 years, most are more likely to be moved to action by shorter-term, more personal goals. Feeling better, doing better in school, improving at a sport, reducing stress, and increasing self-esteem are common short-term benefits of health behavior change. Many wellness behaviors are associated with immediate improvements in quality of life. For example, surveys of Americans have found that nonsmokers feel healthy and full of energy more days each month than do smokers, and they report fewer days of sadness and troubled sleep; the same is true when physically active people are compared with sedentary people (Table 1.3, p. 12). Over time, these types of differences

General Strategies

A key first step in sharpening your critical thinking skills is to look carefully at your sources of wellness information. Critical thinking involves knowing where and how to find relevant information, how to separate fact from opinion, how to recognize faulty reasoning, how to evaluate information, and how to assess the credibility of sources.

- *Go to the original source.* Media reports often simplify the results of medical research. Find out for yourself what a study really reported, and determine whether it was based on good science. What type of study was it? Was it published in a recognized medical journal? Was it an animal study or did it involve people? Did the study include a large number of people? What did the authors of the study actually report in their findings? (You'll find additional strategies for evaluating research studies in Chapter 11.)
- *Watch for misleading language.* Reports that feature "breakthroughs" or "dramatic proof" are probably hype. Some studies will find that a behavior "contributes to" or is "associated with" an outcome; this does not imply a proven cause-and-effect relationship.
- *Distinguish between research reports and public health advice.* If a study finds a link between a particular vitamin and cancer, that should not necessarily lead you to change your behavior. But if the Surgeon General or the American Cancer Society advises you to eat less fat or quit smoking, you can assume that many studies point in this direction and that this is advice you should follow.
- *Remember that anecdotes are not facts.* Sometimes we do get helpful health information from our friends and family. But just because your cousin Bertha lost 10 pounds on Dr. Amazing's new protein diet doesn't mean it's a safe, effective way for you to lose weight. Before you make a big change in your lifestyle, verify the information with your physician, this text, or other reliable sources.
- *Be skeptical and use your common sense.* If a report seems too good to be true, it probably is. Be especially wary of information contained in advertisements. The goal of an ad is to sell you something, to create a feeling of need for a product where no real need exists.
- *Make choices that are right for you.* Your roommate swears by swimming; you prefer aerobics. Your sister takes a yoga class to help her manage stress; your brother unwinds by walking in the woods. Friends and family members can be a great source of ideas and inspiration, but each of us needs to find a wellness lifestyle that works for us.

Internet Resources

Evaluating health information from online sources poses special challenges; when reviewing a health-related Web site, ask the following questions:

- *What is the source of the information? Who is the author or sponsor of the Web page?* Web sites maintained by government agencies, professional associations, or established academic or medical institutions are likely to present trustworthy information. Many other groups and individuals post accurate information, but it is important to look at the qualifications of the people who are behind the site. (Check the home page or click on an "about us" or "who we are" link.)
- *How often is the site updated?* Look for sites that are updated frequently. Also check the "last modified" date of any specific Web page on a site.
- *What is the purpose of the page? Does the site promote particular products or procedures? Are there obvious reasons for bias?* Be wary of information from sites that sell specific products, use testimonials as evidence, appear to have a social or political agenda, or ask for money.
- *What do other sources say about a topic?* Be cautious of claims or information that appear at only one site or come from a chat room or bulletin board.
- *Does the site conform to any set of guidelines or criteria for quality and accuracy?* Look for sites that identify themselves as conforming to some code or set of principles, such as those set forth by the Health on the Net Foundation or the American Medical Association. These codes include criteria such as use of information from respected sources and disclosure of the site's sponsors.

add up to a substantially greater quality of life for people who engage in healthy behaviors.

You can further strengthen your motivation by raising your consciousness about your problem behavior. This will enable you to focus on the negatives of the behavior and imagine the consequences if you don't make a change. At the same time, you can visualize the positive results of changing your behavior. Ask yourself: What do I want for myself, now and in the future?

For example, Ruby has never worried much about her smoking because the problems associated with it seem so far away. But lately she's noticed her performance on the volleyball team isn't as good as it used to be. Over the summer she visited her aunt, who has chronic emphysema from smoking and can barely leave her bed. Ruby knows she wants to have children and a career as a teacher someday, and seeing her aunt makes her wonder if her smoking habit could make it difficult for her to reach these goals. She starts to wonder whether her smoking habit is worth the short- and long-term sacrifices.

Social pressures can also increase the motivation to make changes. In Ruby's case, anti-smoking ordinances

IN FOCUS Lifestyle Matters for Young Adults

Take a good look at the next group of college students you see. Chances are, they all look pretty healthy. But if you could look inside their cells and vital organs, you would see that the external appearance of health can be deceiving. Some students would have noticeable layers of fat and scar tissue lining blood vessels, including the crucial arteries that supply blood to the heart and brain. You can safely predict that a number of these students will have heart attacks or strokes when they hit middle age. Nearly all the students would have microscopic evidence of sun damage on their skin, and a few would have the early cellular changes associated with skin cancer. If you could train your super vision on their skeletons, you would detect that some students have weaker, thinner bones—not noticeable to them now but likely to result in osteoporosis and the potential for serious fractures later in life. In some students, you would also detect something slightly amiss in the balance of sugar and insulin in their blood and tissue. Students in this group are more likely to later develop diabetes.

You might think that this group of college students—with so many impending health problems—is unusual, but unfortunately, these students are similar to the majority of young adults in the United States. Most apparently healthy young people harbor early signs of serious chronic diseases that will become obvious later in life. However, the good news is that if you make some changes now in your daily habits, you can prevent or delay the onset of nearly all of these common diseases.

What does it take to stave off the typical illnesses of middle and old age? As described in the section on behaviors that contribute to wellness, the answer is less complicated than you might have thought. Lifestyle choices you make daily throughout your life can make a tremendous difference. You can choose to be a nonsmoker, to eat a healthy diet, to keep your weight under control, to wear sunscreen and protective clothing when out in the sun, and so on. If you are successful in following the guidelines for wellness behaviors most of the time, your odds for a long and vigorous life will increase dramatically.

Unfortunately, knowing what we should do to protect our health in later years is often not enough to get us to change our habits. Most of us need a more immediate payoff to get motivated. So consider all the reasons why healthy behaviors are a plus for you today as well as for your future self. For example, if you've felt tired and blue lately, being physically active is almost certain to provide you with an infusion of energy and feelings of well-being. Keeping fit will also allow you to fully enjoy your favorite activities. If you love to ski, remember that if you are in shape when you hit the slopes, you will ski better, have more fun, experience less fatigue and soreness, and be less likely to get injured. What if you want to take a hike in the mountains or learn to windsurf? Being regularly active will make it much more likely that these experiences will be exhilarating rather than merely exhausting. Everyday chores, such as hauling your books around, cleaning, and carrying groceries or children, are much easier if you are active. Life's daily activities are more satisfying when you have the strength, energy, and confidence to handle them with ease.

Think about what might motivate you to make healthy changes in your life. Have you seen the quality of life of members of your family affected by chronic diseases? Knowing that a particular disease runs in your family can help guide your priorities and motivate you to make healthy changes. You might also find motivation from thinking about the benefits for your loved ones. Consider the examples of a pregnant smoker who is finally able to quit for good when she becomes aware that smoking is harmful to her baby, and a couch potato who becomes inspired to increase his activity level in order to keep up with his kids.

Don't feel overwhelmed by the description of a wellness lifestyle and think that you must change all your bad habits at once or overhaul your lifestyle completely. Studies show that even small improvements in your lifestyle can make a big difference in your health. Start by making a few positive changes. Your efforts will be rewarded—you'll feel better now, and you will continue to reap the benefits throughout your life.

make it impossible for her to smoke in her dorm and in many public places. The inconvenience of finding a place to smoke—and pressure from her roommate, who doesn't like the smoky smell of Ruby's clothes in their room—add to Ruby's motivation to quit.

Boosting Self-Efficacy When you start thinking about changing a health behavior, a big factor in your eventual success is whether you have confidence in yourself and in your ability to change. **Self-efficacy** refers to your belief in your ability to successfully take action and perform a specific task. Strategies for boosting self-efficacy include developing an internal locus of control, using visualization and self-talk, and obtaining encouragement from supportive people.

LOCUS OF CONTROL Who do you believe is controlling your life? Is it your parents, friends, or school? Is it "fate"? Or is it you? **Locus of control** refers to the figurative "place" a person designates as the source of responsibility for the events in his or her life. People who believe they are in control of their own lives are said to have an internal locus of control. Those who believe that factors beyond

Terms

self-efficacy The belief in one's ability to take action and perform a specific behavior.

locus of control The figurative "place" a person designates as the source of responsibility for the events in his or her life.

VITAL STATISTICS

Table 1.3 *Lifestyle and Quality of Life*

	NUMBER OF DAYS IN PAST 30 DAYS			
	Felt generally healthy	Felt full of energy	Felt sad, blue, depressed	Had trouble sleeping
Nonsmoker	25.5	19.5	2.6	7.3
Smoker	22.9	17.0	4.8	9.9
Physically active	25.5	20.2	2.7	7.4
Sedentary	23.2	17.1	3.9	8.1

SOURCE: Centers for Disease Control and Prevention. 2000. *Measuring Healthy Days: Population Assessment of Health-Related Quality of Life.* Atlanta, Ga.: Centers for Disease Control and Prevention.

their control—heredity, friends and family, the environment, fate, luck, or other outside forces—are more important in determining the events of their lives are said to have an external locus of control.

For lifestyle management, an internal locus of control is an advantage because it reinforces motivation and commitment. An external locus of control can sabotage efforts to change behavior. For example, if you believe you are destined to die of breast cancer because your mother died from the disease, you may view monthly breast self-exams and regular checkups as a waste of time. In contrast, if you believe you can take action to reduce your hereditary risk of breast cancer, you will be motivated to follow guidelines for early detection of the disease.

If you find yourself attributing too much influence to outside forces, gather more information about your wellness-related behaviors. List all the ways that making lifestyle changes will improve your health. If you believe you'll succeed, and if you recognize and accept that you are in charge of your life, you're on your way to wellness.

VISUALIZATION AND SELF-TALK One of the best ways to boost your confidence and self-efficacy is to visualize yourself successfully engaging in a new, healthier behavior. Imagine yourself going for a regular after-dinner walk or choosing healthier snacks. Also visualize yourself enjoying all the short-term and long-term benefits that your lifestyle change will bring. Create a new self-image: What will you and your life be like when you become a regular exerciser or a healthy eater?

You can also use self-talk, the internal dialogue you carry on with yourself, to increase your confidence in your ability to change. Counter any self-defeating patterns of thought with more positive or realistic thoughts: "I am a strong, capable person, and I can maintain my commitment to change." Refer to Chapter 10 for more on self-talk.

ROLE MODELS AND OTHER SUPPORTIVE INDIVIDUALS Social support can make a big difference in your level of motivation and your chances of success. Perhaps you know people who have reached the goal you are striving for; they could be role models or mentors for you, providing information and support for your efforts. Gain strength from their experiences, and tell yourself, "If they can do it, so can I." In addition, find a buddy who wants to make the same changes you do and who can take an active role in your behavior change program. For example, an exercise buddy can provide companionship and encouragement for times when you might be tempted to skip your workout.

Identifying and Overcoming Key Barriers to Change

Don't let past failures at behavior change discourage you; they can be a great source of information you can use to boost your chances of future success. Make a list of the problems and challenges you faced in your previous behavior change attempts; to this, add the short-term costs of behavior change that you identified in your analysis of the pros and cons of change. Once you've listed these key barriers to change, develop a practical plan for overcoming each one. For example, if you always smoke when you're with certain friends, practice in advance how you will turn down the next cigarette you are offered.

Self-talk can also help overcome barriers. Make behavior change a priority in your life and plan to commit the necessary time and effort. Ask yourself: How much time and energy will behavior change *really* require? Isn't the effort worth the short- and long-term benefits?

Enhancing Your Readiness to Change

The transtheoretical, or "stages of change," model has been shown to be an effective approach to lifestyle self-management. According to this model, you move through distinct stages as you work to change your target behavior. Try to identify your current stage, and then adopt appropriate strategies to move forward in the cycle of change.

- *Precontemplation: No intention of changing behavior.* If you're at this stage, try raising your consciousness of your target behavior and its effects on you and those around you. Ask yourself what has prevented you from changing in the past. Get the facts about your target behavior and the resources available to help you with change.

- *Contemplation: Intending to take action within 6 months.* Begin keeping a written record of your target behavior and work on your analysis of the pros and cons of change. Try to boost self-efficacy through visualization, self-talk, and the support of other people.

- *Preparation: Planning to take action within a month.* At this stage, your next step is to create a specific plan for change (see the following section of the chapter).

Date November 5 Day M (TU) W TH F SA SU

Time of day	M/S	Food eaten	Cals.	H	Where did you eat?	What else were you doing?	How did someone else influence you?	What made you want to eat what you did?	Emotions and feelings?	Thoughts and concerns?
7:30	M	1 C Crispix cereal 1/2 C skim milk coffee, black 1 C orange juice	110 40 — 120	3	dorm cafeteria	reading newspaper	eating w/ friends, but I ate what I usually eat	I always eat cereal in the morning	a little keyed up & worried	thinking about quiz in class today
10:30	S	1 apple	90	1	library	studying	alone	felt tired & wanted to wake up	tired	worried about next class
12:30	M	1 C chili 1 roll 1 pat butter 1 orange 2 oatmeal cookies 1 soda	290 120 35 60 120 150	2	cafeteria terrace	talking	eating w/ friends; we decided to eat at the cafeteria	wanted to be part of group	excited and happy	interested in hearing everyone's plans for the weekend

M/S = Meal or snack H = Hunger rating (0–3)

Figure 1.5 Sample health journal entries.

- *Action: Outwardly changing behavior.* This stage requires the greatest commitment of time and energy to keep from reverting to old, unhealthy patterns of behavior. You'll need to use all the plans and strategies that you developed to this point.
- *Maintenance: Successful behavior change 6 or more months earlier.* To guard against slips and relapses during the maintenance stage, continue with the positive strategies you used in earlier stages.

For some behaviors, such as addictions, you may reach the sixth and final stage, *termination*. At this point, you are no longer tempted to lapse back into your old habits; you have a new self-image and total self-efficacy with regard to your target behavior.

Lapses are a natural part of the process at all stages of change. Many people lapse and must recycle through earlier stages, although most don't go back to the first stage. If you lapse, use what you learn about yourself and the process of change to help you in your next attempt.

Developing Skills for Change: Creating a Personalized Plan

Once you are committed to making a change, it's time to put together a plan of action. Your key to success is a well-thought-out plan that sets goals, anticipates problems, and includes rewards.

1. Monitor Your Behavior and Gather Data Begin by keeping careful records of the behavior you wish to change (your target behavior) and the circumstances surrounding it. Keep these records in a health journal, a notebook in which you write the details of your behavior along with observations and comments. Note exactly what the activity was, when and where it happened, what you were doing, and what your feelings were at the time (see the sample journal in Figure 1.5). If your goal is to start an exercise program, use your journal to track your daily activities to determine how best to make time for your workouts. Keep your journal for a week or two to get some solid information about the behavior you want to change.

2. Analyze the Data and Identify Patterns After you have collected data on the behavior, analyze the data to identify patterns. When are you most likely to overeat? What events trigger your appetite? Perhaps you are especially hungry at midmorning or when you put off eating dinner until 9:00. Perhaps you overindulge in food and drink when you go to a particular restaurant or when you're with certain friends. Note the connections between your feelings and such external cues as time of day, location, situation, and the actions of others around you. Do you always think of having a cigarette when you read the newspaper? Do you always bite your fingernails when you're studying?

3. Set Realistic, Specific Goals Don't set an impossibly difficult overall goal for your program—going from a sedentary lifestyle to running a marathon within 2 months, for example. Working toward more realistic, achievable goals will greatly increase your chances of success. Your goal should also be specific and measurable, something you can easily track. Instead of a vague general goal such as improving eating habits or being more physically active, set a specific target—eating 5 servings of fruits and vegetables each day or walking or biking for 30 minutes at least 5 days per week.

It's a good idea to break your ultimate goal down into a few small steps. Your plan will seem less overwhelming and more manageable, increasing the chances that you'll stick to it. You'll also build in more opportunities to reward yourself (discussed in step 4), as well as milestones you can use to measure your progress.

If you plan to lose 15 pounds, for example, you'll find it easier to take off 3 pounds at a time. If you want to start an exercise program, begin by taking 10- to 15-minute walks a few times a week. Take easier steps first and work up to harder steps. With each small success, you'll build your confidence and self-efficacy.

4. Devise a Strategy or Plan of Action Next, you need to develop specific strategies and techniques that will support your day-to-day efforts at behavior change.

OBTAIN INFORMATION AND SUPPLIES Identify campus and community resources that can provide practical help—for example, a stop-smoking course or a walking club. Take any necessary preparatory steps, such as signing up for a stress-management workshop or purchasing walking shoes, nicotine replacement patches, or a special calendar to track your progress.

MODIFY YOUR ENVIRONMENT You can be more effective in changing behavior if you control the environmental cues that provoke it. This might mean not having cigarettes or certain foods or drinks in the house, not going to parties where you're tempted to overindulge, or not spending time with particular people, at least for a while. Use the data you collected in your health journal to identify patterns. If you always get a candy bar at a certain vending machine, change your route so you don't pass by it. If you always end up taking a coffee break and chatting with friends when you go to the library to study, choose a different place to study, such as your room.

It's also helpful to control other behaviors or habits that are linked to the target behavior. You may give in to an urge to eat when you have a beer (alcohol increases the appetite) or watch TV. Try substituting other activities for habits that are linked with your target behavior, such as exercising to music instead of plopping down in front of the TV. Or put an exercise bicycle in front of the set and burn calories while watching your favorite show.

You can change the cues in your environment so they trigger the new behavior you want instead of the old one. Tape a picture of a cyclist speeding down a hill on your TV screen. Leave your exercise shoes in plain view. Put a chart of your progress in a special place at home to make your goals highly visible and inspire you to keep going.

REWARD YOURSELF Another powerful way to affect your target behavior is to set up a reward system that will reinforce your efforts. Most people find it difficult to change longstanding habits for rewards they can't see right away. Giving yourself instant, real rewards for good behavior along the way will help you stick with a plan to change your behavior.

Carefully plan your reward payoffs and what they will be. In most cases, rewards should be collected when you reach specific objectives or subgoals in your plan. For example, you might treat yourself to a movie after a week of avoiding extra snacks. Don't forget to reward yourself for good behavior that is consistent and persistent—such as simply sticking with your program week after week. Decide on a reward after you reach a certain goal or mark off the sixth week or month of a valiant effort. Write it down in your health journal and remember it as you follow your plan—especially when the going gets rough.

Make a list of your activities and favorite events to use as rewards. They should be special, inexpensive, and preferably unrelated to food or alcohol. You might treat yourself to a concert, a ball game, a new CD, a long-distance phone call to a friend, a day off from studying for a long hike in the woods—whatever is rewarding to you.

INVOLVE THE PEOPLE AROUND YOU Rewards and support can also come from family and friends. Tell them about your plan and ask for their help. Encourage them to be active, interested participants. Ask them to support you when you set aside time to go running or avoid second helpings at Thanksgiving dinner. To help friends and family members respond appropriately, you may want to create a specific list of dos and don'ts.

PLAN AHEAD FOR CHALLENGING SITUATIONS Take time out now to list situations and people that have the potential to derail your program and to develop possible coping mechanisms. For example, if you think you'll have trouble exercising during finals week, schedule short bouts of physical activity as stress-reducing study breaks. If a visit to a friend who smokes is likely to tempt you to lapse, plan to bring nicotine patches, chewing gum, and a copy of your behavior change contract to strengthen your resolve.

5. Make a Personal Contract A serious personal contract—one that commits your word—can result in a higher chance of follow-through than a casual, offhand promise. Your contract can help prevent procrastination by specifying the important dates and can also serve as a reminder of your personal commitment to change. Your contract should include a statement of your goal and your commitment to reaching it. Include details of your plan: the date you'll begin, the steps you'll use to measure your progress, the concrete strategies you've developed for promoting change, and the date you expect to reach your final goal. Have someone—preferably someone who will be actively helping you with your program—sign your contract as a witness.

My Personal Contract for Eating Three Servings of Fruit per Day

I agree to increase my consumption of fruit from one serving per week to three servings per day. I will begin my program on 10/5 and plan to reach my final goal by 12/7. I have divided my program into three parts, with three separate goals. For each step in my program, I will give myself the reward listed.

1. I will begin to have a serving of fruit with breakfast on 10/5.
   (Reward: baseball game)
2. I will begin to have a serving of fruit with lunch on 10/26.
   (Reward: music CD)
3. I will begin to substitute fruit juice for soda for one snack each day on 11/16.
   (Reward: Concert)

My plan for increasing fruit consumption includes the following strategies:

1. Keeping my dorm room refrigerator stocked with easy-to-carry fruit and fruit juice.
2. Packing fruit in my book backpack every day.
3. Placing reminders to buy, carry, and eat fruit in my dorm room, backpack, and wallet.
4. Buying lunch at a place that serves fruit or fruit juice.

I understand that it is important for me to make a strong personal effort to make the change in my behavior. I sign this contract as an indication of my personal commitment to reach my goal.

Michael Cook 9/28

Witness: Katie Lim 9/28

Figure 1.6 A sample behavior change contract.

A Sample Behavior Change Plan Let's take the example of Michael, who wants to improve his diet. By monitoring his eating habits in his health journal for several weeks, he gets a good sense of his typical diet—what he eats and where he eats it. Through self-assessment and investigation, he discovers that he currently consumes only about one serving of fruit per week, much less than the recommended two to four servings per day. He also finds out that fruit is a major source of fiber, vitamins, minerals, and other substances important for good health. He sets the target of eating three servings of fruit per day as the overall goal for his behavior change plan. Then Michael develops a specific plan for change that involves several changes in his behavior and his environment, which he describes in a contract that commits him to reaching his goal (Figure 1.6).

Putting Your Plan into Action

The starting date has arrived, and you are ready to put your plan into action. This stage requires commitment, the resolve to stick with the plan no matter what temptations you encounter. Remember all the reasons you have to make the change—and remember that *you* are the boss. Use all your strategies to make your plan work. Make sure your environment is change-friendly, and obtain as much support and encouragement from others as possible. Keep track of your progress in your health journal, and give yourself regular rewards. And don't forget to give yourself a pat on the back—congratulate yourself, notice how much better you look or feel, and feel good about how far you've come and how you've gained control of your behavior.

Staying with It

As you continue with your program, don't be surprised when you run up against obstacles; they're inevitable. In fact, it's a good idea to expect problems and give yourself time to step back, see how you're doing, and make some changes before going on. If your program is grinding to a halt, identify what is blocking your progress. It may come from one of these sources.

Social Influences Take a hard look at the reactions of the people you're counting on, and see if they're really supporting you. If they come up short, connect and network with others who will be more supportive.

A related trap is trying to get your friends or family members to change *their* behaviors. The decision to make a major behavior change is something people come to only after intensive self-examination. You may be able to influence someone by tactfully providing facts or support,

A beautiful setting and a friendly companion help make exercise a satisfying and pleasurable experience. Choosing the right activity and doing it the right way are important elements in a successful behavior change program.

but that's all. Focus on yourself. If you succeed, you may become a role model for others.

Levels of Motivation and Commitment You won't make real progress until an inner drive leads you to the stage of change at which you are ready to make a personal commitment to the goal. If commitment is your problem, you may need to wait until the behavior you're dealing with makes your life more unhappy or unhealthy; then your desire to change it will be stronger. Or you may find that changing your goal will inspire you to keep going. For more ideas, refer to the box "Motivation Boosters" and to Activity 9 in the Behavior Change Workbook at the end of the text.

Choice of Techniques and Level of Effort If your plan is not working as well as you thought it would, make changes where you're having the most trouble. If you've lagged on your running schedule, for example, maybe it's because you don't like running. An aerobics class might suit you better. There are many ways to move toward your goal. Or you may not be trying hard enough. You do have to push toward your goal. If it were easy, you wouldn't need to have a plan.

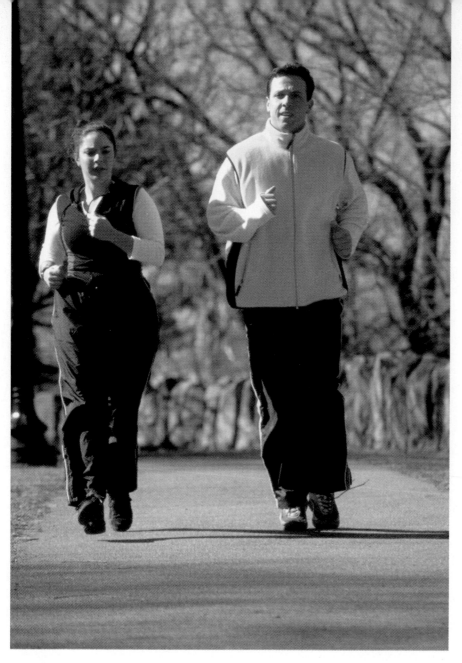

TAKE CHARGE Motivation Boosters

- Write down the potential benefits of the change. If you want to lose weight, your list might include increased ease of movement, energy, and self-confidence.
- Now write down the costs of not changing.
- Frequently visualize yourself achieving your goal and enjoying its benefits. If you want to manage time more effectively, picture yourself as a confident, organized person who systematically tackles important tasks and sets aside time each day for relaxation, exercise, and friends.
- Discount obstacles to change. Counter thoughts such as "I'll never have time to exercise" with thoughts such as "Lots of other people have done it and so can I."
- Bombard yourself with propaganda. Take a class dealing with the change you want to make. Read books and watch talk shows on the subject. Post motivational phrases or pictures on your refrigerator or over your desk. Talk to people who have already made the change you want to make.
- Build up your confidence. Remind yourself of other goals you've achieved. At the end of each day, mentally review your good decisions and actions. See yourself as a capable person, one who is in charge of his or her health.
- Create choices. You will be more likely to exercise every day if you have two or three types of exercise to choose from and more likely to quit smoking if you've identified more than one way to distract yourself when you crave a cigarette. Get ideas from people who have been successful and adapt some of their strategies to suit you.
- If you slip, keep trying. Research suggests that four out of five people will experience some degree of backsliding when they try to change a behavior. Only one in four succeeds the first time around. If you retain your commitment to change even when you lapse, you are still farther along the path to change than before you made the commitment. Try again. And again, if necessary.

Stress Barrier If you've hit a wall in your program, look at the sources of stress in your life. If the stress is temporary, such as catching a cold or having a term paper due, you may want to wait until it passes before strengthening your efforts. If the stress is ongoing, find healthy ways to manage it, such as taking a half-hour walk after lunch or beginning a yoga class. You may even want to make stress management your highest priority for behavior change (see Chapter 10).

Procrastinating, Rationalizing, and Blaming Try to detect the games you might be playing with yourself so that you can stop them. If you're procrastinating ("It's Friday already; I might as well wait until Monday to begin"), break your plan down into still smaller steps that you can accomplish one day at a time. If you're rationalizing or making excuses ("I wanted to go swimming today, but I wouldn't have had time to wash my hair afterward"), remember that when you "win" by deceiving yourself, it's not much of a victory. If you're wasting time blaming yourself or others ("Everyone in that class talks so much that I don't get a chance to speak"), recognize that blaming is a way of taking your focus off the real problem and denying responsibility for your actions. Try refocusing by taking a positive attitude and renewing your determination to succeed.

Being Fit and Well for Life

Your first attempts at making behavior changes may never go beyond the project stage. Those that do may not all succeed. But as you experience some success, you'll start to have more positive feelings about yourself. You may discover new physical activities and sports you enjoy; you may encounter new situations and meet new people. Perhaps you'll surprise yourself by accomplishing things you didn't think were possible—breaking a longstanding nicotine habit, competing in a race, climbing a mountain, developing a lean, muscular body. Most of all, you'll discover the feeling of empowerment that comes from taking charge of your health (see the box "Signs of Wellness"). Being healthy takes extra effort, but the paybacks in energy and vitality are priceless.

Once you've started, don't stop. Assume that health improvement is forever. Take on the easier problems first, and then use what you learn to tackle more difficult problems later. Periodically review what you've accomplished to make sure you don't fall into old habits. And keep informed about the latest health news and trends. Research is constantly providing new information that directly affects daily choices and habits.

This book will introduce you to the main components of a fit and well lifestyle, show you how to assess your current health status, and help you put together a program that will lead to wellness. You can't control every aspect of your health—there are too many unknowns in life for that to be possible. But you can create a lifestyle that minimizes your health risks and maximizes your enjoyment of life and well-being. You can take charge of your health in a dramatic and meaningful way. *Fit and Well* will show you how.

IN FOCUS Signs of Wellness

1. The persistent presence of a support network.
2. Chronic positive expectations; the tendency to frame events in a constructive light.
3. Episodic outbreaks of joyful, happy experiences.
4. A sense of spiritual involvement.
5. A tendency to adapt to changing conditions.
6. Rapid response and recovery of stress response systems to repeated challenges.
7. An increased appetite for physical activity.
8. A tendency to identify and communicate feelings.
9. Repeated episodes of gratitude and generosity.
10. A persistent sense of humor.

SOURCE: Ten warning signs of good health. 1996. *Mind/Body Health Newsletter* 5(1). Reprinted by permission.

Tips for Today

You are in charge of your health! Many of the decisions you make every day have an impact on the quality of your life, both now and in the future. By making positive choices, large and small, you help ensure a lifetime of wellness.

Right now you can

- Go for a 15-minute walk.
- Have an orange, a nectarine, or a plum for a snack.
- Call a friend and arrange for a time to catch up with each other.
- Start thinking about whether you have a health behavior you'd like to change. If you do, consider the elements of a behavior change strategy. For example,
  - Begin a mental list of the pros and cons of the behavior.
  - Create a format for a log to monitor your target behavior.
  - Think of someone who can support you in your attempts to make a behavior change and talk to that person about your plan.

SUMMARY

- Wellness is the ability to live life fully, with vitality and meaning. Wellness is dynamic and multidimensional; it incorporates physical, emotional, intellectual, spiritual, interpersonal and social, and environmental dimensions.
- People today have greater control over, and greater responsibility for, their health than ever before.
- Behaviors that promote wellness include being physically active; choosing a healthy diet; maintaining a healthy body weight; managing stress effectively; avoiding use of tobacco and using alcohol wisely, if at all; and protecting oneself from disease and injury.
- Although heredity, environment, and health care all play roles in wellness and disease, behavior can mitigate their effects.
- To make lifestyle changes, you need information about yourself, your health habits, and resources available to help you change.
- You can increase your motivation for behavior change by examining the benefits and costs of change, boosting self-efficacy, and identifying and overcoming key barriers to change.
- The stages of change model describes six stages that people may move through as they try to change their behavior: precontemplation, contemplation, preparation, action, maintenance, and termination.
- A specific plan for change can be developed by (1) monitoring behavior by keeping a journal; (2) analyzing the recorded data; (3) setting specific goals; (4) devising strategies for modifying the environment, rewarding yourself, involving others, and planning ahead; and (5) making a personal contract.
- To start and maintain a behavior change program you need commitment, a well-developed and manageable plan, social support, and strong stress management techniques. It is also important to monitor the progress of your program, revising it as necessary.

FOR FURTHER EXPLORATION

WW *Fit and Well* Online Learning Center (www.mhhe.com/fahey5e)

Visit the *Fit and Well* Online Learning Center and familiarize yourself with the resources available at the site. You can use the learning objectives, study guide questions, and glossary flashcards to review key terms and concepts for this chapter and prepare for exams. You can extend your knowledge of wellness and gain experience in using the Internet as a resource by completing the activities and checking out the Web links for the topics in Chapter 1 marked with the World Wide Web icon. For this chapter, there are activities relating to *Healthy People 2010* objectives, online assessments, and evaluation of online resources; there are Web links for the Vital Statistics tables and figures, the Critical Consumer box, and the chapter as a whole. Behavior change resources and tools include an online version of the Behavior Change Workbook, sample logs for a variety of target behaviors, and sample behavior change plans.

Daily Fitness and Nutrition Journal

Have you chosen a target behavior related to physical activity or diet? If so, begin reviewing the behavior change planning and monitoring tools available in the log. If you've chosen a target behavior in another area, the fitness and nutrition examples can provide a good model for the type of program plan and log you should create for your behavior change program. Visit the Online Learning Center for some blank sample logs that you can print and use.

Health*Quest*

Take a closer look at your health risks and current lifestyle by completing the Wellboard activity on the Health*Quest* CD-ROM. In addition to estimating your life expectancy based on your family and personal health history and your lifestyle, this assessment will also give you scores in eight areas and provide tips for improvement. Your scores may help you identify a target behavior for behavior change. You may also want to print and save your complete Wellboard report for later comparison—you can improve your scores and your estimated life expectancy by adopting a wellness lifestyle.

Books

Columbia University's Health Education Program. 1998. *The "Go Ask Alice" Book of Answers*. New York: Henry Holt. *Presents answers to a variety of student-oriented health questions from the popular "Go Ask Alice" Web site.*

Prochaska, J. O., J. C. Norcross, and C. C. DiClemente. 1994. *Changing for Good: The Revolutionary Program That Explains the Six Stages of Change and Teaches You How to Free Yourself from Bad Habits*. New York: Morrow. *Outlines the authors' model of behavior change and offers suggestions and advice for each stage of change.*

Smith P. B., M. MacFarlane, and E. Kalnitsky. 2002. *The Complete Idiot's Guide to Wellness*. Indianapolis, In.: Alpha Books. *A concise guide to healthy habits, including physical activity, nutrition, and stress management.*

Newsletters

Consumer Reports on Health (800-234-2188; http://www.ConsumerReports.org)
Harvard Health Letter (800-829-9045; http://www.health.harvard.edu)
Harvard Men's Health Watch (800-829-3341)
Harvard Women's Health Watch (800-829-5921)
HealthNews (781-893-3800)
Mayo Clinic Health Letter (800-333-9037)
University of California at Berkeley Wellness Letter (386-447-6328; http://www.wellnessletter.com)

WW Organizations, Hotlines, and Web Sites

The Internet addresses (also called uniform resource locators, or URLs) listed here were accurate at the time of publication. Up-to-date links to these and many other wellness-oriented Web sites are provided on the links page of the *Fit and Well* Online Learning Center (http://www.mhhe.com/fahey5e).

Centers for Disease Control and Prevention. Through phone, fax, and the Internet, the CDC provides a wide variety of health information.
800-311-3435; 888-CDC-FAXX (CDC FAX)
http://www.cdc.gov

Many other government Web sites provide access to health-related materials:
Federal Trade Commission: http://www.ftc.gov
National Institutes of Health: http://www.nih.gov
National Library of Medicine, MedlinePlus: http://www.medlineplus.gov
U.S. Consumer Gateway—Health: http://www.consumer.gov/health.htm

Go Ask Alice. Sponsored by the Columbia University Health Service, this site provides answers to student questions about stress, sexuality, fitness, and many other wellness topics.
http://www.goaskalice.columbia.edu

Healthfinder. A gateway to online publications, Web sites, support and self-help groups, and agencies and organizations that produce reliable health information.
http://www.healthfinder.gov

Healthy People 2010. Provides information on Healthy People objectives and priority areas.
202-205-8583; 301-468-5960
http://web.health.gov/healthypeople

JAMA Patient Pages. Provides consumer-oriented health information from *JAMA (Journal of the American Medical Association).*
http://www.ama-assn.org/public/journals/patient/index.htm

National Health Information Center (NHIC). Puts consumers in touch with the organizations that are best able to provide answers to health-related questions.
800-336-4797
http://www.health.gov/nhic

National Women's Health Information Center. Provides information and answers to frequently asked questions.
800-994-WOMAN
http://www.4woman.org

NOAH: New York Online Access to Health. Provides consumer health information in both English and Spanish.
http://www.noah-health.org

Nutrition.Gov. Gateway to online nutrition information from the U.S. government. http://www.nutrition.gov

Student Counseling Virtual Pamphlet Collection. Provides links to more than 400 pamphlets produced by different student counseling centers; topics include relationships, family issues, substance abuse, anger management, and study skills.
http://counseling.uchicago.edu/vpc/virtulets.html.

World Health Organization (WHO). Provides information about WHO activities and about many health topics and issues affecting people around the world; presents materials about annual reports and events, including the World Health Report, World Health Day, and World No-Tobacco Day.
http://www.who.int

The following are just a few of the many sites that provide consumer-oriented information on a variety of health issues:

InteliHealth: http://www.intelihealth.com
Mayo Health Oasis: http://www.mayohealth.org
Medscape Healthwatch: http://healthwatch.medscape.com
WebMD: http://webmd.com

The following sites provide daily health news updates:

HealthScout: http://www.healthscout.com
Yahoo Health News: http://dailynews.yahoo.com/h/hl
Your Health Daily: http://www.yourhealthdaily.com

SELECTED BIBLIOGRAPHY

American Cancer Society. 2001. *Cancer Facts and Figures 2001.* Atlanta: American Cancer Society.

American Heart Association. 2001. *2001 Heart and Stroke Statistical Update.* Dallas, Tex.: American Heart Association.

Centers for Disease Control and Prevention. 2001. Physical activity trends. *Morbidity and Mortality Weekly Report* 50(9): 166–169.

Centers for Disease Control and Prevention. 2001. Prevalence of healthy lifestyle characteristics. *Morbidity and Mortality Weekly Report* 50(34): 758–761.

Centers for Disease Control and Prevention. 1999. Ten great public health achievements—United States, 1900–1999. *Morbidity and Mortality Weekly Report* 48(50): 1141.

Centers for Disease Control and Prevention, Division of Nutrition and Physical Activity. 1999. *Promoting Physical Activity: A Guide for Community Action.* Champaign, Ill.: Human Kinetics.

Department of Health and Human Services. 2000. *Healthy People 2010,* 2nd ed. Washington, D.C.: DHHS.

Department of Health and Human Services. 1996. *Physical Activity and Health: A Report of the Surgeon General.* Atlanta, Ga.: DHHS.

Douglas, K. A., et al. 1997. Results from the 1995 National College Health Risk Behavior Survey. *Journal of American College Health* 46(2): 55–56.

Glanz, K., F. M. Lewis, and B. K. Rimer, ed. 1997. *Health Behavior and Health Education: Theory, Research, and Practice,* 2nd ed. San Francisco: Jossey-Bass.

Hu, F. B., et al. 2001. Diet, lifestyle, and the risk of type 2 diabetes mellitus in women. *New England Journal of Medicine* 345(11): 790–797.

Institute of Medicine. 2001. *Health Behavior: The Interplay of Biological, Behavioral, and Societal Influences.* Washington, D.C.: National Academy Press.

Lee, C. D., and S. N. Blair. 2002. Cardiorespiratory fitness and stroke mortality in men. *Medicine and Science in Sports and Exercise* 34(4): 592–595.

Lee, I. M., and P. J. Skerrett. 2001. Physical activity and all-cause mortality: What is the dose-response relation? *Medicine and Science in Sports and Exercise* 33(6 Suppl): S459–S471.

McClure, J. B. 2002. Are biomarkers useful treatment aids for promoting health behavior change? An empirical review. *American Journal of Preventive Medicine* 22(3): 200–207.

Muller, A. 2002. Education, income inequality, and mortality: A multiple regression analysis. *British Medical Journal* 324(7328): 23–25.

National Center for Health Statistics. 2002. Leisure-time physical activity among adults: United States, 1997–1998. *Advance Data from Vital and Health Statistics,* No. 325.

National Center for Health Statistics. 2002. United States Life Tables, 1999. *National Vital Statistics Reports* 50(6).

National Center for Health Statistics. 2001. *Early Release of Selected Estimates from the 2000 and Early 2001 National Health Interview Surveys* (http://www.cdc.gov/nchs/nhis.htm; retrieved September 25, 2001).

National Center for Health Statistics. 2001. *Health, United States, 2001.* Hyattsville, Md.: Public Health Service.

National Center for Health Statistics. 2001. Summary measures of population health: Addressing the first goal of *Healthy People 2010,* improving health expectancy. *Healthy People 2010 Statistical Notes* No. 22.

Nieman, D. C. 2001. *Exercise Testing and Prescription: A Health-Related Approach,* 5th ed. New York: McGraw-Hill.

Sesso, H. D., R. S. Paffenbarger, and I. M. Lee. 2000. Physical activity and coronary heart disease in men: The Harvard Alumni Health Study. *Circulation* 102(9): 975–980.

Stampfer, M. J., et al. 2000. Primary prevention of coronary heart disease in women through diet and lifestyle. *New England Journal of Medicine* 343(1): 16–22.

U.S. Department of Health and Human Services. 2000. *Healthy People 2010,* 2nd ed. Washington, D.C.: DHHS.

Whelton, S. P., et al. 2002. Effect of aerobic exercise on blood pressure: A meta-analysis of randomized, controlled trials. *Annals of Internal Medicine* 136(7): 493–503.

World Health Organization. 2002. *World Health Day 2002: Move for Health* (http://www.who.int/world-health-day; retrieved April 19, 2002).

World Health Organization. 2001. *What Is the WHO Definition of Health?* (http://www.who.int/aboutwho/en/qal.htm; retrieved July 26, 2001).

Zimmerman, G. L., C. G. Olsen, and M. F. Bosworth. 2000. A "stages of change" approach to helping patients change behavior. *American Family Physician* 61(5): 1409–1416.

Name ______________________ Section ____________ Date ______________

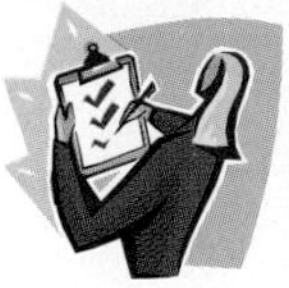

LAB 1.1 *Your Wellness Profile*

Consider how your lifestyle, attitudes, and characteristics relate to each of the six dimensions of wellness. Fill in your strengths for each dimension (examples of strengths are listed with each dimension). Once you've completed your lists, choose what you believe are your five most important strengths and circle them.

Physical wellness: To maintain overall physical health and engage in appropriate physical activity (e.g., stamina, strength, flexibility, healthy body composition).

Emotional wellness: To have a positive self-concept, deal constructively with your feelings, and develop positive qualities (e.g., optimism, trust, self-confidence, determination, persistence, dedication).

Intellectual wellness: To pursue and retain knowledge, think critically about issues, make sound decisions, identify problems, and find solutions (e.g., common sense, creativity, curiosity).

Spiritual wellness: To develop a set of beliefs, principles, or values that gives meaning or purpose to one's life; to develop faith in something beyond oneself (e.g., religious faith, service to others).

Interpersonal/social wellness: To develop and maintain meaningful relationships with a network of friends and family members, and to contribute to the community (e.g., friendly, good-natured, compassionate, supportive, good listener).

Environmental wellness: To protect yourself from environmental hazards, and to minimize the negative impact of your behavior on the environment (e.g., carpooling, recycling).

Next, think about where you fall on the wellness continuum for each of the dimensions of wellness. Indicate your placement for each—physical, emotional, intellectual, spiritual, interpersonal/social, and environmental—on the continuum below.

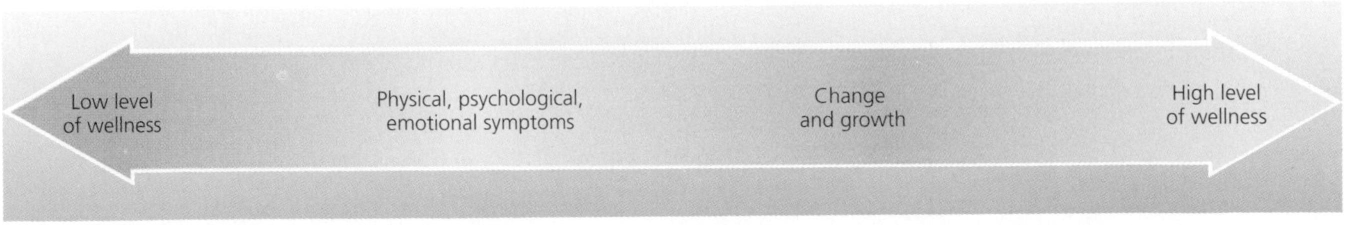

LABORATORY ACTIVITIES

Based on both your current lifestyle and your goals for the future, what do you think your placement on the wellness continuum will be in 10 years? What new health behaviors would you have to adopt to achieve your goals? Which of your current behaviors would you need to change to maintain or improve your level of wellness in the future?

Does the description of wellness given in this chapter encompass everything you believe is part of wellness for you? Write your own definition of wellness, and include any additional dimensions that are important to you. Then rate your level of wellness based on your own definition.

Using Your Results

How did you score? Are you satisfied with your current level of wellness—overall and in each dimension? In which dimension(s) would you most like to increase your level of wellness?

What should you do next? As you consider possible target behaviors for a behavior change program, choose things that will maintain or increase your level of wellness in one of the dimensions you listed as an area of concern. Remember to consider health behaviors such as smoking or eating a high-fat diet that may threaten your level of wellness in the future. Below, list several possible target behaviors and the wellness dimensions that they influence.

For additional guidance in choosing a target behavior, complete the lifestyle self-assessment in Lab 1.2.

Name ______________________ Section ______________ Date ______________

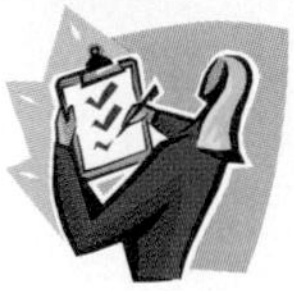

LAB 1.2 *Lifestyle Evaluation*

How does your current lifestyle compare with the lifestyle recommended for wellness? For each question, choose the answer that best describes your behavior; then add up your score for each section.

Exercise/Fitness

	Almost Always	Sometimes	Never
1. I engage in moderate exercise, such as brisk walking or swimming, for 20–60 minutes, three to five times a week.	4	1	0
2. I do exercises to develop muscular strength and endurance at least twice a week.	2	1	0
3. I spend some of my leisure time participating in individual, family, or team activities, such as gardening, bowling, or softball.	2	1	0
4. I maintain a healthy body weight, avoiding overweight and underweight.	2	1	0

Exercise/Fitness Score: 10

Nutrition

	Almost Always	Sometimes	Never
1. I eat a variety of foods each day, including five or more servings of fruits and/or vegetables.	3	1	0
2. I limit the amount of fat and saturated fat in my diet.	3	1	0
3. I avoid skipping meals.	2	1	0
4. I limit the amount of salt and sugar I eat.	2	1	0

Nutrition Score: 6

Tobacco Use

If you never use tobacco, enter a score of 10 for this section and go to the next section.

	Almost Always	Sometimes	Never
1. I avoid using tobacco.	2	1	0
2. I smoke only low-tar-and-nicotine cigarettes, or I smoke a pipe or cigars, or I use smokeless tobacco.	2	1	0

Tobacco Use Score: 10

Alcohol and Drugs

	Almost Always	Sometimes	Never
1. I avoid alcohol, or I drink no more than 1 (women) or 2 (men) drinks a day.	4	1	0
2. I avoid using alcohol or other drugs as a way of handling stressful situations or the problems in my life.	2	1	0
3. I am careful not to drink alcohol when taking medications (such as cold or allergy medications) or when pregnant.	2	1	0
4. I read and follow the label directions when using prescribed and over-the-counter drugs.	2	1	0

Alcohol and Drugs Score: 10

Emotional Health

	Almost Always	Sometimes	Never
1. I enjoy being a student, and I have a job or do other work that I enjoy.	2	1	0
2. I find it easy to relax and express my feelings freely.	2	1	0
3. I manage stress well.	2	1	0
4. I have close friends, relatives, or others whom I can talk to about personal matters and call on for help when needed.	2	1	0
5. I participate in group activities (such as community or church organizations) or hobbies that I enjoy.	2	1	0

Emotional Health Score: 5

Safety

1. I wear a safety belt while riding in a car.	2	1	0
2. I avoid driving while under the influence of alcohol or other drugs.	2	1	0
3. I obey traffic rules and the speed limit when driving.	2	1	0
4. I read and follow instructions on the labels of potentially harmful products or substances, such as household cleaners, poisons, and electrical appliances.	2	1	0
5. I avoid smoking in bed.	2	1	0

Safety Score: 8

Disease Prevention

1. I know the warning signs of cancer, heart attack, and stroke.	2	1	0
2. I avoid overexposure to the sun and use sunscreen.	2	1	0
3. I get recommended medical screening tests (such as blood pressure checks and Pap tests), immunizations, and booster shots.	2	1	0
4. I practice monthly breast/testicle self-exams.	2	1	0
5. I am not sexually active *or* I have sex with only one mutually faithful, uninfected partner *or* I always engage in "safer sex" (using condoms), *and* I do not share needles to inject drugs.	2	1	0

Disease Prevention Score: 6

Scores of 9 and 10 Excellent! Your answers show that you are aware of the importance of this area to your health. More important, you are putting your knowledge to work for you by practicing good health habits. As long as you continue to do so, this area should not pose a serious health risk.

Scores of 6 to 8 Your health practices in this area are good, but there is room for improvement.

Scores of 3 to 5 Your health risks are showing!

Scores of 0 to 2 You may be taking serious and unnecessary risks with your health.

Using Your Results

How did you score? In which areas did you score the lowest? Are you satisfied with your scores in each area? In which areas would you most like to improve your scores?

What should you do next? To improve your scores, look closely at any item to which you answered "sometimes" or "never." Identify and list at least three possible targets for a health behavior change program. (If you are aware of other risky health behaviors you currently engage in, but which were not covered by this assessment, you may include those in your list.) For each item on your list, identify your current "stage of change" and one strategy you could adopt to move forward (see pp. 12–13 in Chapter 1). Possible strategies might be obtaining information about the behavior, completing an analysis of the pros and cons of change, or beginning a written record.

Behavior	Stage	Strategy
1. ______	______	______
2. ______	______	______
3. ______	______	______

SOURCE: Adapted from *Healthstyle: A Self-Test,* developed by the U.S. Public Health Service. The behaviors covered in this test are recommended for most Americans, but some may not apply to people with certain chronic diseases or disabilities or to pregnant women, who may require special advice from their physician.

Basic Principles of Physical Fitness

2

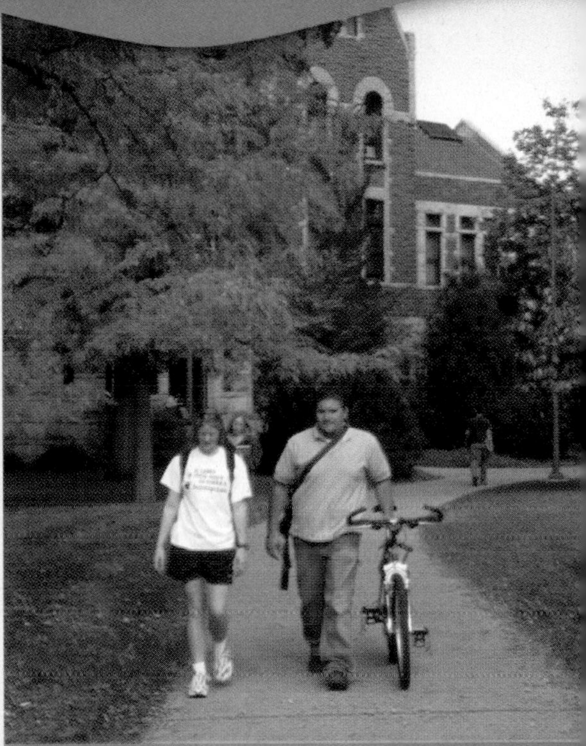

LOOKING AHEAD

After reading this chapter, you should be able to

- Describe how much exercise is recommended for developing health and fitness
- Identify the components of physical fitness and how each component affects wellness
- Explain the goal of physical training and the basic principles of training
- Describe the principles involved in designing a well-rounded exercise program
- Discuss the steps that can be taken to make an exercise program safe, effective, and successful

TEST YOUR KNOWLEDGE

1. To improve your health, you must do high-intensity exercise. True or false?
2. Among American adults, about what percentage of trips of less than 1 mile long are made by walking?
   a. 15%
   b. 25%
   c. 50%
3. If all inactive American adults became physically active, the savings in direct costs for medical care would be about ______ per year.
   a. $75 million
   b. $7.5 billion
   c. $75 billion

TEST YOUR KNOWLEDGE ANSWERS

1. FALSE. Even moderate physical activity—walking the dog, taking the stairs, or doing yard work—has significant health benefits.

2. A. The vast majority of short trips are made in automobiles. Most people have many opportunities to incorporate more moderate physical activity into their daily routine.

3. C. People who engage in regular physical activity make fewer physician visits, use less medication, and have fewer hospital stays than physically inactive people.

Fit and Well Online Learning Center

www.mhhe.com/fahey5e

Visit the *Fit and Well* Online Learning Center for study aids, additional information about physical activity, links, Internet activities that explore the importance of physical activity, consumer resources, and much more.

Hundreds of studies show that exercise gives people both a longer life and a healthier life. Most of us want to live longer and avoid heart disease, cancer, and other chronic diseases, but many people choose to be active for other reasons. Some get a kick out of hitting a game-winning cross-court backhand, backpacking through a wilderness area, or completing a difficult skateboard move. Others enjoy the friends they make in group exercise classes; the way their fitness program gives them more energy; or the satisfaction they get from walking farther, running faster, or lifting more weight.

Samantha is a single 28-year-old junior executive from Boston who has a busy work and social schedule. Her fast-paced life makes it essential that she stay in shape. She attends an exercise class at a health club three times a week and lifts weights after the class. "The gym is an oasis in my incredibly busy day. I finish my exercise class refreshed and invigorated. I feel healthy, and I like the way my clothes fit. Being fit gives me the energy and self-confidence I need to compete in the business world. It's given my social life a boost, too."

Max is a 22-year-old college student who lives in Salt Lake City and loves to ski. "I came to Salt Lake because the surrounding mountains have the best snow in the world. I love the feeling of plunging down a steep chute and feeling the fresh powder surround me. The solitude and the beauty of the mountains are a spiritual experience for me. I stay in shape and eat right so that I can better enjoy the high I get from skiing."

Nora is a 42-year-old mother of three children who lives in a small town outside Austin, Texas. She gets plenty of physical activity in her daily routine, which includes biking to her part-time job and helping out with after-school youth programs at the local community center. However, her passion is throwing the javelin in masters track and field competitions. "I developed a love for the sport in college. I enjoy the competition and striving to improve in a very difficult event. I have friends all over the world who share my passion. I like testing myself in competition—when I win or perform up to my personal best, the feeling is indescribable."

Bill is an 18-year-old college student at a small Midwest college who loves to run. "I run almost every day to forget my problems and relieve stress. Going away to college has been a big shock—I've gone from being part of a tight family to being on my own. Running helps me sort things out. I get lost in myself while I run through the woods and fields around the college. I do some of my best and most creative thinking when I run. I can't imagine my life without running."

The benefits of exercise go far beyond its disease-preventive effects. The enjoyment you get from physical activity enriches your life and makes you a more complete person.

Any list of the benefits of physical activity is impressive. A physically active lifestyle helps you generate more energy, control your weight, manage stress, and boost your immune system. It provides psychological and emotional benefits, contributing to your sense of competence and well-being. It offers protection against heart disease, diabetes, high blood pressure, depression, anxiety, osteoporosis, some types of cancer, and even premature death. Exercise increases your physical capacity so that you are better able to meet the challenges of daily life with energy and vigor. Although people vary greatly in the levels of physical fitness and performance they can ultimately achieve, the benefits of regular physical activity are available to everyone. (For more on the benefits of exercise, see the box "Exercise and Total Wellness.")

This chapter provides an overview of physical fitness. It explains how lifestyle physical activity and more formal exercise programs contribute to wellness. It describes the components of fitness, the basic principles of physical training, and the essential elements of a well-rounded exercise program. Chapters 3–6 provide an in-depth look at each of the elements of a fitness program; Chapter 7 will help you put all these elements together into a complete, personalized program.

Terms

physical activity Any body movement carried out by the skeletal muscles and requiring energy.

exercise Planned, structured, repetitive movement of the body designed to improve or maintain physical fitness.

PHYSICAL ACTIVITY AND EXERCISE FOR HEALTH AND FITNESS

Despite the many benefits of an active lifestyle, levels of physical activity have declined in recent years and remain low for all populations of Americans (Figure 2.1). According to *Healthy People 2010,* more than 60% of U.S. adults do not engage in recommended amounts of physical activity; 25% are not active at all. In the summer of 1996, the U.S. Surgeon General published *Physical Activity and Health,* a landmark report designed to reverse these trends and get Americans moving. Here is a summary of its findings:

- People of all ages benefit from regular physical activity.
- People can obtain significant health benefits by including a moderate amount of physical activity on most, if not all, days of the week. Through a modest increase in daily activity, most Americans can improve their health and quality of life.
- Additional health benefits can be gained through greater amounts of physical activity. People who can

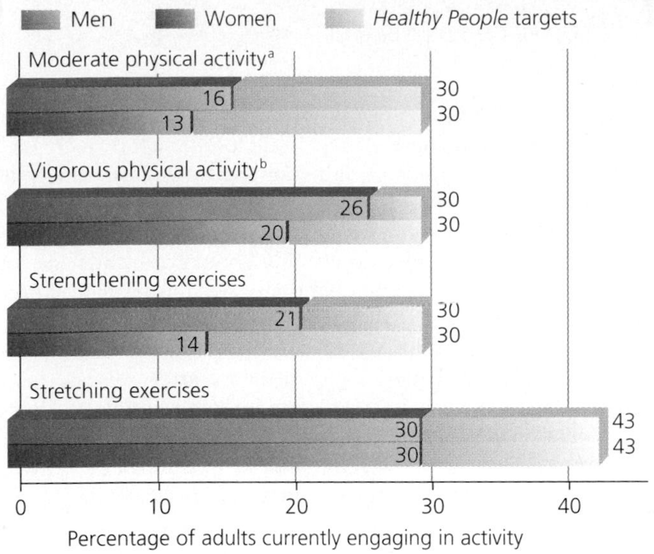

[a]Moderate physical activity for 30 or more minutes on 5 or more days per week
[b]Vigorous physical activity for 20 or more minutes on 3 or more days per week

VITAL STATISTICS

Figure 2.1 Current levels of physical activity among American adults. SOURCE: U.S. Department of Health and Human Services. 2000. *Healthy People 2010*, 2d ed. Washington, D.C.: DHHS.

maintain a regular regimen of more vigorous or longer-duration activity are likely to obtain even greater benefits.

Why aren't more Americans active? Possible barriers include lack of time and resources, social and environmental influences, and lack of motivation and commitment. Some people also fear serious injury. Although physical activity does carry some risks, the risks of inactivity are far greater (see the box "Is Exercise Safe?" on p. 28). Evidence is growing that for most Americans, simply becoming more physically active may be the single most important lifestyle change for promoting health and well-being.

Physical Activity on a Continuum

Physical activity can be defined as any body movement carried out by the skeletal muscles and requiring energy. Different types of physical activity can be arranged on a continuum based on the amount of energy they require. Quick, easy movements such as standing up or walking down a hallway require little energy or effort; more intense, sustained activities such as cycling 5 miles or running in a race require considerably more.

Exercise refers to a subset of physical activity—planned, structured, repetitive movement of the body designed specifically to improve or maintain physical fitness. As discussed in Chapter 1, physical fitness is a set of physical attributes that allows the body to respond or adapt to the demands and stress of physical effort—to perform moderate-to-vigorous levels of physical activity without becoming overly tired. Levels of fitness depend on such physiological factors as the heart's ability to pump blood and the size of muscle fibers. To develop fitness, a person must perform enough physical activity to stress the body and cause long-term physiological changes. Only exercise will significantly improve fitness. Knowing this is important for setting goals and developing a program.

Less Vigorous, More Time

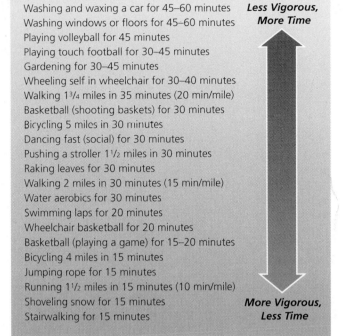

Washing and waxing a car for 45–60 minutes
Washing windows or floors for 45–60 minutes
Playing volleyball for 45 minutes
Playing touch football for 30–45 minutes
Gardening for 30–45 minutes
Wheeling self in wheelchair for 30–40 minutes
Walking 1¾ miles in 35 minutes (20 min/mile)
Basketball (shooting baskets) for 30 minutes
Bicycling 5 miles in 30 minutes
Dancing fast (social) for 30 minutes
Pushing a stroller 1½ miles in 30 minutes
Raking leaves for 30 minutes
Walking 2 miles in 30 minutes (15 min/mile)
Water aerobics for 30 minutes
Swimming laps for 20 minutes
Wheelchair basketball for 20 minutes
Basketball (playing a game) for 15–20 minutes
Bicycling 4 miles in 15 minutes
Jumping rope for 15 minutes
Running 1½ miles in 15 minutes (10 min/mile)
Shoveling snow for 15 minutes
Stairwalking for 15 minutes

More Vigorous, Less Time

Figure 2.2 Examples of moderate amounts of physical activity. A moderate amount is roughly equivalent to physical activity that uses approximately 150 calories of energy a day, or 1000 calories a week. Some activities can be performed at various intensities; the suggested durations correspond to expected intensity of effort. SOURCE: Department of Health and Human Services. 1996. *Physical Activity and Health: A Report of the Surgeon General.* Atlanta, Ga.: DHHS.

Lifestyle Physical Activity for Health Promotion The Surgeon General's report recommends that all Americans include a moderate amount of physical activity on most, preferably all, days of the week. The report suggests a goal of expending 150 calories a day, or about 1000 calories a week, in physical activity. The same amount of activity can be obtained in longer sessions of moderately intense activities as in shorter sessions of more strenuous activities. Thus, 30 minutes of brisk walking or leaf raking is equivalent to 15 minutes of running or snow shoveling. Examples of moderate physical activities are given in Figure 2.2.

In this lifestyle approach to physical activity, the daily total of activity can be accumulated in multiple short bouts—for example, two 10-minute bicycle rides to and

IN FOCUS Is Exercise Safe?

Participating in exercise and sports is usually a wonderful experience that improves wellness in both the short and long term. Occasionally, though, vigorous exertion is associated with sudden death. It may seem difficult to understand that although regular exercise protects people from heart disease, it also increases the risk of sudden death.

What causes sudden death during or immediately following exercise? In nearly all cases, coronary artery disease is responsible. In this condition, fat and other substances build up in the arteries that supply blood to the heart. Death can result if an artery becomes blocked or if the heart's rhythm and pumping action are disrupted. Exercise, particularly intense exercise, may trigger a heart attack in someone with underlying heart disease. (In the very rare cases of death among young athletes, the cause may be a congenital or genetic cardiovascular disorder rather than coronary artery disease.)

How great is the risk of dying suddenly during exercise? A study of jogging deaths in Rhode Island found that there was one death per 396,000 hours of jogging, or about one death per 7620 joggers per year—an extremely low risk for each individual jogger. A more recent study of men involved in a variety of physical activities found one death per 1.51 million hours of exercise. This 12-year study of more than 21,000 men found that those who didn't exercise vigorously were 74 times more likely to die suddenly from cardiac arrest during or shortly after exercise. It is also important to note that people are much safer exercising than engaging in many other common activities, including driving a car.

Although quite small, the risk does exist and may lead some people to wonder why exercise is considered such an important part of a wellness lifestyle. Exercise causes many positive changes in the body—in healthy people as well as those with heart disease—that more than make up for the slightly increased short-term risk of sudden death. Training slows or reverses the fatty buildup in arteries and helps protect people from deadly heart rhythm abnormalities. People who exercise regularly have an overall risk of sudden death only about two-thirds that of nonexercisers. Active people who stop exercising can expect their heart attack risk to increase by 300%.

Who is most at risk for sudden death during exercise? Obviously, someone with underlying coronary artery disease is at greater risk than someone who is free from the condition. However, many cases of heart disease may go undiagnosed. The riskiest scenario may be when a middle-aged or older individual suddenly begins participating in a vigorous sport or activity after a long period of a sedentary lifestyle. This finding provides strong evidence for the recommendation that people increase their level of physical activity gradually and engage in regular, rather than sporadic, activity.

Specific guidelines for determining who should check with a physician before engaging in an exercise program are provided later in this chapter, along with an exercise safety self-assessment. For the vast majority of people, exercise is a safe and effective way to increase both life expectancy and quality of life. If you decide you don't want to exercise, you might want to see your physician to determine if you can resist the deadly effects of a sedentary lifestyle.

SOURCES: Thompson, P. D. 2001. Cardiovascular risks of exercise. *The Physician and Sportsmedicine* 29(4). Albert, C. M., et al. 2000. Trigger of sudden death from cardiac causes by vigorous exertion. *New England Journal of Medicine* 343(19): 1355–1361.

from class and a brisk 15-minute walk to the post office. People can choose activities that they find enjoyable and that fit into their daily routine; everyday tasks at school, work, and home can be structured to contribute to the daily activity total (see the box "Becoming More Active"). In addition to recommending moderate-intensity physical activity, the Surgeon General's report recommends that people perform resistance training (exercising against an opposing force such as a weight) at least twice a week to build and maintain muscular strength.

By increasing lifestyle physical activity in accordance with the guidelines given in the Surgeon General's report, people can expect to significantly improve their health and well-being. If all the Americans who are now completely sedentary were to adopt a more active lifestyle, there would be enormous benefit to the public's health and to individual well-being. Such a program may not, however, significantly increase physical fitness.

Exercise Programs to Develop Physical Fitness The Surgeon General's report also summarizes the benefits of more formal exercise programs. It concludes that people can obtain even greater health benefits by increasing the duration and intensity of activity. Thus, a person who engages in a structured, formal exercise program designed to measurably improve physical fitness will obtain even greater improvements in quality of life and greater reductions in disease and mortality risk.

How Much Physical Activity Is Enough?

Some experts feel that people get most of the health benefits of an exercise program simply by becoming more active over the course of the day. Others feel that the activity goal set by the lifestyle approach is too low; they argue that people should exercise long enough and intensely enough to improve their body's capacity for exercise—that is, to improve physical fitness. More research is needed to clarify the health effects of moderate-intensity vs. high-intensity exercise and continuous vs. intermittent exercise. However, there is probably truth in both of these positions.

Regular physical activity, regardless of intensity, makes you healthier and can help protect you from many chronic

TAKE CHARGE Becoming More Active

"Too little time" is a common excuse for not being physically active. Learning to manage your time successfully is crucial if you are to maintain a wellness lifestyle. You can begin by keeping a record of how you are currently spending your time; in your health journal, use a grid broken into blocks of 15, 20, or 30 minutes to track your daily activities. Then analyze your record: List each type of activity and the total time you engaged in it on a given day—for example, sleeping, 7 hours; eating, 1.5 hours, studying, 3 hours; and so on. Take a close look at your list of activities and prioritize them according to how important they are to you, from essential to somewhat important to not important at all.

Based on the priorities you set, make changes in your daily schedule by subtracting time from some activities in order to make time for physical activity. Look particularly carefully at your leisure time activities and your methods of transportation; these are areas where it is easy to build in physical activity. Make changes using a system of tradeoffs. For example, you may choose to reduce the total amount of time you spend playing computer games, listening to the radio, and chatting on the telephone in order to make time for an after-dinner bike ride or walk with a friend. You may decide to watch 10 fewer minutes of television in the morning in order to change your 5-minute drive to class into a 15-minute walk. In making these kinds of changes in your schedule, don't feel that you have to miss out on anything you enjoy. You can get more from less time by focusing on what you are doing and by combining activities.

The following are just a few ways to become more active:

- Take the stairs instead of the elevator or escalator.
- Walk to the mailbox, post office, store, bank, or library whenever possible.
- Park your car a mile or even just a few blocks from your destination, and walk briskly.
- Do at least one chore every day that requires physical activity: wash the windows or your car, clean your room or house, mow the lawn, rake the leaves.
- Take study or work breaks to avoid sitting for more than 30 minutes at a time. Get up and walk around the library, your office, or your home or dorm; go up and down a flight of stairs.
- Stretch when you stand in line or watch TV.
- When you take public transportation, get off one stop down the line and walk to your destination.
- Go dancing instead of to a movie.
- Walk to visit a neighbor or friend rather than calling him or her on the phone. Go for a walk while you chat.
- Put your remote controls in storage; when you want to change TV or radio stations, get up and do it by hand.
- Take the dog for a walk (or an extra walk) every day.
- Play actively with children or go for a walk pushing a stroller.
- Seize every opportunity to get up and walk around. Move more and sit less.

diseases (Figure 2.3, p. 30). However, exercising at low intensities does little to improve physical fitness. Although you get many of the health benefits of exercise by simply being more active, you obtain even more benefits when you are physically fit. In addition to long-term health benefits, fitness also significantly contributes to quality of life. Fitness can give you freedom—freedom to move your body the way you want. Fit people have more energy and better body control. They can enjoy a more active lifestyle—cycling, hiking, skiing, and so on—than their more sedentary counterparts. Even if you don't like sports, you need physical energy and stamina in your daily life and for many nonsport leisure activities—visiting museums, playing with children, gardening, and so on.

Where does this leave you? Most experts agree that some physical activity is better than none, but that more—as long as it does not result in injury—is probably better than some. At the very least, strive to become more active and meet the goal set by the Surgeon General's report of using about 150 calories a day in physical activity. Choose to be active whenever you can. For even better health and well-being, participate in a structured exercise program that develops physical fitness. Any increase in physical activity will contribute to your health and well-being, now and in the future.

Next, let's take a closer look at the components of physical fitness and the basic principles of fitness training.

HEALTH-RELATED COMPONENTS OF PHYSICAL FITNESS

Physical fitness has many components, some related to general health and others related more specifically to particular sports or activities. The five components of fitness most important for health are cardiorespiratory endurance, muscular strength, muscular endurance, flexibility, and body composition. **Health-related fitness** contributes to your capacity to enjoy life, helps your body withstand physical and psychological challenges, and protects you from chronic disease.

Terms

health-related fitness Physical capacities that contribute to health: cardiorespiratory endurance, muscular strength, muscular endurance, flexibility, and body composition.

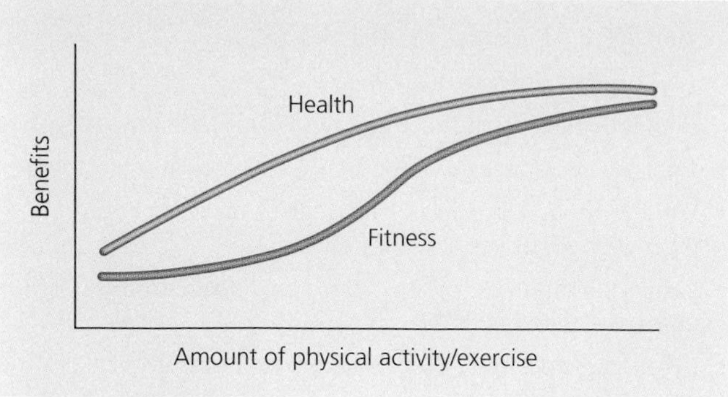

Figure 2.3 Relationship between amount of activity and health and fitness benefits. The health benefits of physical activity and exercise exist along a continuum. A fairly low level of physical activity can provide substantial health benefits, although it does little to increase fitness. Engaging in exercise that is more intense or of longer duration leads to greater health benefits and significant increases in fitness. SOURCE: American College of Sports Medicine. 2001. *ACSM's Resource Manual for Guidelines for Exercise Testing and Prescription,* 4th ed. Philadelphia: Williams & Wilkins, p. 452.

Cardiorespiratory Endurance

Cardiorespiratory endurance is the ability to perform prolonged, large-muscle, dynamic exercise at moderate-to-high levels of intensity. It depends on such factors as the ability of the lungs to deliver oxygen from the environment to the bloodstream, the heart's capacity to pump blood, the ability of the nervous system and blood vessels to regulate blood flow, and the capability of the body's chemical systems to use oxygen and process fuels for exercise.

When levels of cardiorespiratory fitness are low, the heart has to work very hard during normal daily activities and may not be able to work hard enough to sustain high-intensity physical activity in an emergency. As cardiorespiratory fitness improves, the heart begins to function more efficiently. It doesn't have to work as hard at rest or during low levels of exercise. The heart pumps more blood per heartbeat, resting heart rate slows, blood volume increases, blood supply to the tissues improves, the body is better able to cool itself, and resting blood pressure decreases. A healthy heart can better withstand the strains of everyday life, the stress of occasional emergencies, and the wear and tear of time. Endurance training also improves the functioning of the chemical systems, particularly in the muscles and liver, thereby enhancing the body's ability to use energy supplied by food and to do more exercise with less effort from the oxygen transport system.

Cardiorespiratory endurance is a central component of health-related fitness because the functioning of the heart and lungs is so essential to overall good health. A person can't live very long or very well without a healthy heart. Low levels of cardiorespiratory fitness are linked with heart disease, the leading cause of death in the United States. In addition to protecting against heart disease, cardiorespiratory fitness also reduces the risk of diabetes, colon cancer, stroke, depression, and anxiety. It further benefits quality of life by improving self-image, mood, cognitive functioning, and the ability to manage stress. Exercising to improve cardiorespiratory endurance also provides opportunities to have fun and to socialize.

Muscular Strength

Muscular strength is the amount of force a muscle can produce with a single maximum effort. It depends on such factors as the size of muscle cells and the ability of nerves to activate muscle cells. Strong muscles are important for the smooth and easy performance of everyday activities, such as carrying groceries, lifting boxes, and climbing stairs, as well as for emergency situations. They help keep the skeleton in proper alignment, preventing back and leg pain and providing the support necessary for good posture. Muscular strength has obvious importance in recreational activities. Strong people can hit a tennis ball harder, kick a soccer ball farther, and ride a bicycle uphill more easily. Muscle tissue is an important element of overall body composition. Greater muscle mass means a higher rate of **metabolism** and faster energy use. Training to build muscular strength can also help people manage stress and boost their self-confidence.

Maintaining strength and muscle mass is vital for healthy aging. Older people tend to lose both number and size of muscle cells. Many of the muscle cells that remain become slower, and some become nonfunctional because they lose their attachment to the nervous system.

Terms

Vw

cardiorespiratory endurance The ability of the body to perform prolonged, large-muscle, dynamic exercise at moderate-to-high levels of intensity.

muscular strength The amount of force a muscle can produce with a single maximum effort.

metabolism The sum of all the vital processes by which food energy and nutrients are made available to and used by the body.

muscular endurance The ability of a muscle or group of muscles to remain contracted or to contract repeatedly for a long period of time.

flexibility The range of motion in a joint or group of joints; flexibility is related to muscle length.

body composition The proportion of fat and fat-free mass (muscle, bone, and water) in the body.

fat-free mass The nonfat component of the human body, consisting of skeletal muscle, bone, and water.

skill-related fitness Physical capacities that contribute to performance in a sport or activity: speed, power, agility, balance, coordination, and reaction time.

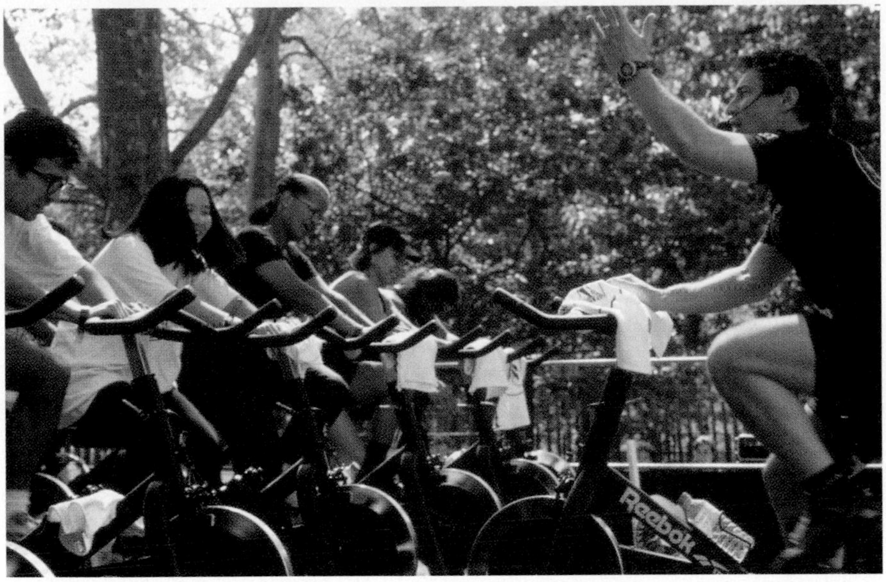

Cardiorespiratory endurance is a key component of health-related fitness. These participants in a group cycling (spinning) class are conditioning their hearts and lungs as well as gaining many other health benefits.

Strength training helps maintain muscle mass and function and possibly helps decrease the risk of osteoporosis in older people, which greatly enhances their quality of life and prevents life-threatening injuries.

Muscular Endurance

Muscular endurance is the ability to resist fatigue and sustain a given level of muscle tension—that is, to hold a muscle contraction for a long period of time or to contract a muscle over and over again. It depends on such factors as the size of muscle cells, the ability of muscles to store fuel, and the blood supply to muscles. Muscular endurance is important for good posture and for injury prevention. For example, if abdominal and back muscles can't hold the spine correctly, the chances of low-back pain and back injury are increased. Recent research suggests that good muscular endurance in the trunk muscles is more important than muscular strength for preventing back pain. Muscular endurance helps people cope with the physical demands of everyday life and enhances performance in sports and work. It is also important for most leisure and fitness activities.

Flexibility

Flexibility is the ability to move the joints through their full range of motion. It depends on joint structure, the length and elasticity of connective tissue, and nervous system activity. Although range of motion isn't a significant factor in everyday activities for most people, inactivity causes the joints to become stiffer with age. Stiffness often causes older people to assume unnatural body postures that can stress joints and muscles. Stretching exercises can help ensure a healthy range of motion for all major joints.

Body Composition

Body composition refers to the proportion of fat and **fat-free mass** (muscle, bone, and water) in the body. Healthy body composition involves a high proportion of fat-free mass and an acceptably low level of body fat, adjusted for age and gender. A person with excessive body fat is more likely to experience a variety of health problems, including heart disease, high blood pressure, stroke, joint problems, diabetes, gallbladder disease, some types of cancer, and back pain. However, recent studies suggest that cardiorespiratory fitness is more important than body composition in determining health status. People who are lean but who have low cardiorespiratory fitness have been found to have higher death rates than people with higher levels of body fat who are otherwise fit. It appears that regular exercise and a moderate level of fitness may help compensate for some of the health risks of extra body fat.

The best way to lose fat is through a lifestyle that includes a sensible diet and exercise. The best way to add muscle mass is through resistance training, also known as strength training or, when weights are used, weight training.

Skill-Related Components of Fitness

In addition to the five health-related components of physical fitness, the ability to perform a particular sport or activity may depend on **skill-related fitness** components such as the following:

DIMENSIONS OF DIVERSITY Fitness and Disability

Physical fitness and athletic achievement are not limited to the able-bodied. People with disabilities can also attain high levels of fitness and performance, as shown by the elite athletes who compete in the Paralympics. The premier event for athletes with disabilities, the Paralympics are held in the same year and city as the Olympics. The performance of these skilled athletes makes it clear that people with disabilities can be active, healthy, and extraordinarily fit; just like able-bodied athletes, athletes with disabilities strive for excellence and can serve as role models.

Currently, some 50 million Americans are estimated to have chronic, significant disabilities. Some disabilities are the result of injury, such as spinal cord injuries sustained in car crashes. Other disabilities result from illness, such as the blindness that sometimes occurs as a complication of diabetes or the joint stiffness that accompanies arthritis. And some disabilities are present at birth, as in the case of congenital limb deformities or cerebral palsy.

Exercise and physical activity are as important for people with disabilities as for able-bodied individuals—if not *more* important. Being active helps prevent secondary conditions that may result from prolonged inactivity, such as circulatory or muscular problems. It provides an emotional boost that helps support a positive attitude as well as opportunities to make new friends, increase self-confidence, and gain a sense of accomplishment. Currently, about 12% of people with disabilities engage in regular moderate activity.

People with disabilities don't have to be elite athletes to participate in sports and lead an active life. Some health clubs and fitness centers offer activities and events geared for people of all ages and types of disabilities. They may have modified aerobics classes, special weight training machines, classes involving mild exercise in warm water, and other activities adapted for people with disabilities. Popular sports and recreational activities include adapted horseback riding, golf, swimming, and skiing. Competitive sports are also available—for example, there are wheelchair versions of billiards, tennis, hockey, and basketball, as well as sports for people with hearing, visual, or mental impairments. For those who prefer to get their exercise at home, special videos are available geared to individuals who use wheelchairs or who have arthritis, hearing impairments, or many other disabilities.

If you have a disability and want to be more active, check with your physician about what's appropriate for you. Call your local community center, YMCA/YWCA, independent living center, or fitness center to locate potential facilities; look for a facility with experienced personnel and appropriate adaptive equipment. For specialized videos, check with hospitals and health associations that are geared to specific disabilities, such as the Arthritis Foundation. Remember that no matter what your level of ability or disability, it's possible to make physical activity an integral part of your life.

SOURCES: U.S. Department of Health and Human Services. 2000. *Healthy People 2010,* 2d ed. Washington, D.C.: DHHS. National Center on Physical Activity and Disability. 2000. *White Paper: Spinal Cord Injury and Fitness.* Chicago: National Center on Physical Activity and Disability. U.S. Department of Health and Human Services. 1996. *Physical Activity and Health: A Report of the Surgeon General.* Atlanta. Ga.: DHHS.

- *Speed:* The ability to perform a movement in a short period of time.
- *Power:* The ability to exert force rapidly, based on a combination of strength and speed.
- *Agility:* The ability to change the position of the body quickly and accurately.
- *Balance:* The ability to maintain equilibrium while moving or while stationary.
- *Coordination:* The ability to perform motor tasks accurately and smoothly using body movements and the senses.
- *Reaction time:* The ability to respond or react quickly to a stimulus.

Skill-related fitness tends to be sport-specific and is best developed through practice. For example, the speed, coordination, and agility needed to play basketball can be developed by playing basketball. Many fitness experts downplay sports participation because some sports don't contribute to all the health-related components of physical fitness. However, engaging in sports can help you build fitness and contribute to other areas of wellness. You can get immense satisfaction from hitting a well-executed cross-court backhand in tennis, climbing a challenging rock wall, hitting the green from 150 yards out in golf, or spiking a ball past an opponent in volleyball. Sports can be an important and fun part of an active wellness lifestyle.

Ww PRINCIPLES OF PHYSICAL TRAINING: ADAPTATION TO STRESS

The human body is very adaptable. The greater the demands made on it, the more it adjusts to meet those demands. Over time, immediate, short-term adjustments translate into long-term changes and improvements. When breathing and heart rate increase during exercise, for example, the heart gradually develops the ability to pump more blood with each beat. Then, during exercise, it doesn't have to beat as fast to meet the cells' demands for oxygen. The goal of **physical training** is to produce these long-term changes and improvements in the body's functioning. Although people differ in the maximum levels of physical fitness and performance they can achieve through training, the wellness benefits of exercise are available to everyone (see the box "Fitness and Disability").

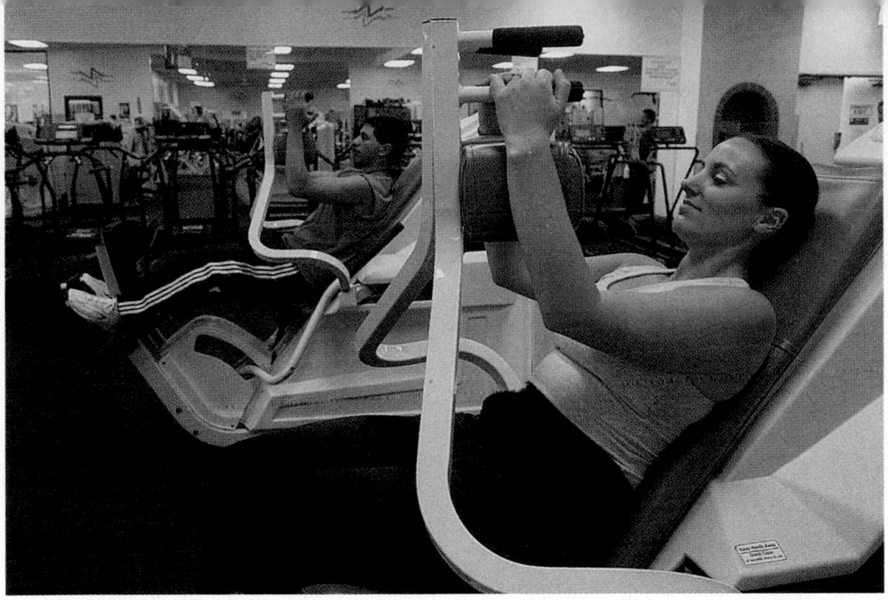

When stressed by the demands of lifting more than the usual amount of weight, the body responds by building muscular strength and endurance. To safely and effectively develop strength, these exercisers must overload their muscles with enough weight to improve their bodies' functioning but not so much weight that they become injured.

Particular types and amounts of exercise are most effective in developing the various components of fitness. To put together an effective exercise program, a person should first understand the basic principles of physical training. Important principles are specificity, progressive overload, reversibility, and individual differences. All of these rest on the larger principle of adaptation.

Specificity—Adapting to Type of Training

To develop a particular fitness component, exercises must be performed that are specifically designed for that component. This is the principle of **specificity.** Weight training, for example, develops muscular strength, not cardiorespiratory endurance or flexibility. Specificity also applies to the skill-related fitness components—to improve at tennis, you must practice tennis—and to the different parts of the body—to develop stronger arms, you must exercise your arms. A well-rounded exercise program includes exercises geared to each component of fitness, to different parts of the body, and to specific activities or sports.

Progressive Overload—Adapting to Amount of Training

The body adapts to the demands of exercise by improving its functioning. When the amount of exercise (also called overload or stress) is progressively increased, fitness continues to improve. This is the principle of **progressive overload.**

The amount of overload is very important. Too little exercise will have no effect on fitness (although it may improve health); too much may cause injury and problems with the body's immune system and hormone levels. The point at which exercise becomes excessive is highly individual—it occurs at a much higher level in an Olympic athlete than in a sedentary person. For every type of exercise, there is a training threshold at which fitness benefits begin to occur, a zone within which maximum fitness benefits occur, and an upper limit of safe training. The amount of exercise needed depends on the individual's current level of fitness, his or her fitness goals, and the component being developed. A novice, for example, might experience fitness benefits from jogging a mile in 10 minutes, but this level of exercise would cause no physical adaptations in a trained distance runner. Beginners should start at the lower end of the fitness benefit zone; fitter individuals will make more rapid gains by exercising at the higher end of the fitness benefit zone.

The amount of overload needed to maintain or improve a particular level of fitness is determined in terms of three dimensions: exercise frequency (how often), intensity (how hard), and duration (how long).

Frequency Developing fitness requires regular exercise. Optimum exercise frequency, expressed in number of days per week, varies with the component being developed and the individual's fitness goals. For most people, a frequency of 3–5 days per week for cardiorespiratory

Terms

physical training The performance of different types of activities that cause the body to adapt and improve its level of fitness.

specificity The training principle that the body adapts to the particular type and amount of stress placed on it.

progressive overload The training principle that placing increasing amounts of stress on the body causes adaptations that improve fitness.

endurance exercise and 2–3 days per week for resistance and flexibility training is appropriate for a general fitness program.

Intensity Fitness benefits occur when a person exercises harder than his or her normal level of activity. The appropriate exercise intensity varies with each fitness component. To develop cardiorespiratory endurance, for example, a person must raise his or her heart rate above normal; to develop muscular strength, a person must lift a heavier weight than normal; to develop flexibility, a person must stretch muscles beyond their normal length.

Duration Fitness benefits occur when you exercise for an extended period of time. For cardiorespiratory endurance exercise, 20–60 minutes is recommended; exercise can take place in a single session or in several sessions of 10 or more minutes. The greater the intensity of exercise, the less time needed to obtain fitness benefits. For high-intensity exercise, such as running, for example, 20–30 minutes is appropriate. For more moderate-intensity exercise, such as walking, 45–60 minutes may be needed. High-intensity exercise poses a greater risk of injury than lower-intensity exercise, so if you are a nonathletic adult, it's probably best to emphasize lower-to-moderate-intensity activity of longer duration.

To build muscular strength, muscular endurance, and flexibility, similar amounts of time are advisable, but these exercises are more commonly organized in terms of a specific number of repetitions of particular exercises. For resistance training, for example, a recommended program includes 1 or more sets of 8–12 repetitions of 8–10 different exercises that work the major muscle groups.

Reversibility—Adapting to a Reduction in Training

Fitness is a reversible adaptation. The body adjusts to lower levels of physical activity the same way it adjusts to higher levels. This is the principle of **reversibility.** When a person stops exercising, up to 50% of fitness improvements are lost within 2 months. If a training schedule must be curtailed temporarily, fitness improvements are best maintained if exercise intensity is kept constant and frequency and/or duration is reduced.

Individual Differences—Limits on Adaptability

Anyone watching the Olympics, a professional football game, or a tennis championship match can readily see that, from a physical standpoint, we are not all created equal. There are large individual differences in our ability to improve fitness, achieve a desirable body composition, perform and learn sports skills. Some people are able to run longer distances, or lift more weight, or kick a soccer ball more skillfully than others will ever be able to, no matter how much they train. There are limits on the adaptability—the potential for improvement—of any human body. The body's ability to transport and use oxygen, for example, can be improved by only about 15–30% through training. An endurance athlete must therefore inherit a large metabolic capacity in order to reach competitive performance levels. In the past few years, scientists have identified specific genes that influence body fat, strength, and endurance.

However, a person doesn't have to be an Olympic sprinter to experience health benefits from running. Physical training improves fitness regardless of heredity. For the average person, the body's adaptability is enough to achieve reasonable fitness goals.

Terms Ww

reversibility The training principle that fitness improvements are lost when demands on the body are lowered.

Ww DESIGNING YOUR OWN EXERCISE PROGRAM

Physical training works best when you have a plan. A plan helps you make gradual but steady progress toward your goals. Planning for physical fitness consists of assessing how fit you are now, determining where you want to be, and choosing the right activities to help you get there. These activities are discussed next, along with some general guidelines for training.

Assessment

The first step in creating a successful fitness program is to assess your current level of physical activity and fitness for each of the five health-related fitness components. The results of the assessment tests will help you set specific fitness goals and plan your fitness program. Lab 2.1 gives you the opportunity to assess your current overall level of activity and determine if it is appropriate. Assessment tests in Chapters 3, 4, 5, and 6 will help you evaluate your cardiorespiratory endurance, muscular strength, muscular endurance, flexibility, and body composition.

Setting Goals

The ultimate general goal of every health-related fitness program is the same—wellness that lasts a lifetime. Whatever your specific goals, they must be important enough to you to keep you motivated. Studies have shown that exercising for yourself, rather than for the impression you think you'll make on others, is more likely to lead to long-lasting commitment. After you complete the assessment tests in Chapters 3–6, you will be able to set goals directly related to each fitness component, such as working toward a 3-mile jog or doing 20 push-ups. First,

Figure 2.4 Physical activity pyramid. Similar to the Food Guide Pyramid, this physical activity pyramid is designed to help people become more active. If you are currently sedentary, begin at the bottom of the pyramid and gradually increase the amount of moderate-intensity physical activity in your life. If you are already moderately active, begin a formal exercise program that includes cardiorespiratory endurance exercise, flexibility training, and strength training to help you develop all the health-related components of fitness.

though, think carefully about your overall goals, and be clear about why you are starting a program.

Choosing Activities for a Balanced Program

An ideal fitness program combines a physically active lifestyle with a systematic exercise program to develop and maintain physical fitness. This overall program is shown in the physical activity pyramid in Figure 2.4. If you are currently sedentary, your goal is to start at the bottom of the pyramid and gradually increase the amount of moderate-intensity physical activity in your daily life. Appropriate activities include brisk walking, climbing stairs, yard work, and washing your car. You don't have to exercise vigorously, but you should experience a moderate increase in your heart and breathing rates. As described earlier, your activity time can be broken up into small blocks over the course of a day.

The next two levels of the pyramid illustrate parts of a formal exercise program. The principles of this program are consistent with those of the American College of Sports Medicine (ACSM), the professional organization for people involved in sports medicine and exercise science. The ACSM has established guidelines for creating an exercise program that will develop physical fitness (Table 2.1, p. 36). A balanced program includes activities to develop all the health-related components of fitness.

- *Cardiorespiratory endurance* is developed by continuous rhythmic movements of large-muscle groups in activities such as walking, jogging, cycling, swimming, and aerobic dance and other forms of group exercise. Choose activities that you enjoy and that are convenient. Other popular choices are in-line skating, dancing, and backpacking. Start-and-stop activities such as tennis, racquetball, and soccer can also develop endurance if one's skill level is sufficient to enable periods of continuous play. Training for cardiorespiratory endurance is discussed in Chapter 3.

- *Muscular strength and endurance* can be developed through resistance training—training with weights or performing calisthenic exercises such as push-ups and curl-ups. Training for muscular strength and endurance is discussed in Chapter 4.

- *Flexibility* is developed by stretching the major muscle groups, regularly and with proper technique. Flexibility is discussed in Chapter 5.

- *Healthy body composition* can be developed through a sensible diet and a program of regular exercise. Endurance exercise is best for reducing body fat;

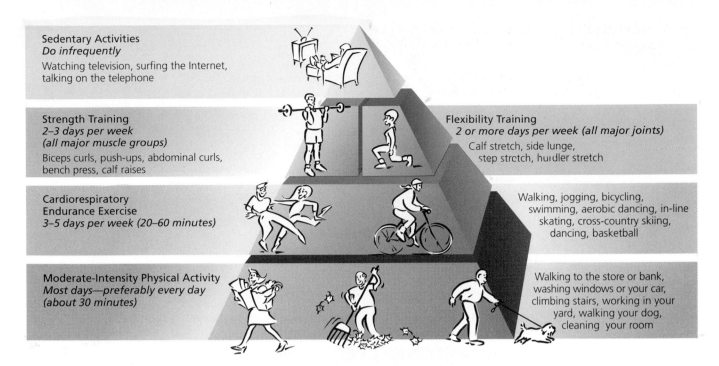

Table 2.1 *Exercise Recommendations for Healthy Adults*

Exercise to Develop and Maintain Cardiorespiratory Endurance and Body Composition	
Mode of activity	Any activity that uses large-muscle groups, can be maintained continuously, and is rhythmic and aerobic in nature, for example, walking-hiking, running-jogging, cycling-bicycling, cross-country skiing, aerobic dance and other forms of group exercise, rope skipping, rowing stair climbing, swimming, skating, and endurance game activities.
Frequency of training	3–5 days per week.
Intensity of training	55/65–90% of maximum heart rate or 40/50–85% of maximum oxygen uptake reserve.* The lower intensity values (55–64% of maximum heart rate and 40–49% of maximum oxygen uptake reserve) are most applicable to individuals who are quite unfit. For average individuals, intensities of 70–85% of maximum heart rate are appropriate.
Duration of training	20–60 total minutes of continuous, or intermittent (in sessions lasting 10 or more minutes) aerobic activity. Duration is dependent on the intensity of activity; thus, lower-intensity activity should be conducted over a longer period of time (30 minutes or more). Lower-to-moderate-intensity activity of longer duration is recommended for the nonathletic adult.
Exercise to Develop and Maintain Muscular Strength and Endurance, Flexibility, and Body Composition	
Resistance training	One set of 8–10 exercises that condition the major muscle groups should be performed 2–3 days per week. Most people should complete 8–12 repetitions of each exercise; for older and more frail people (approximately 50–60 years of age and above), 10–15 repetitions with a lighter weight may be more appropriate. Multiple-set regimens will provide greater benefits if time allows.
Flexibility training	Stretches for the major muscle groups should be performed a minimum of 2–3 days per week; at least 4 repetitions, held for 10–30 seconds should be completed.

*Instructions for calculating target heart rate intensity for cardiorespiratory endurance exercise are presented in Chapter 3.

SOURCE: American College of Sports Medicine. 1998. Position stand: The recommended quantity and quality of exercise for developing and maintaining cardiorespiratory and muscular fitness, and flexibility in healthy adults. *Medicine and Science in Sports and Exercise* 30(6): 975–991.

resistance training builds muscle mass, which, to a small extent, helps increase metabolism. Body composition is discussed in Chapter 6.

There are as many different fitness programs as there are individuals. Consider the following examples:

• Maggie is a person whose life revolves around sports. She's been on softball teams and swim teams, and now she's on her college varsity soccer team. She follows a rigorous exercise regimen established by her soccer coach. Soccer practice is from four to six afternoons a week. It begins with warm-ups, drills, and practice in specific skills, and it ends with a scrimmage and then a jog around the soccer field. Games are every Saturday. Maggie likes team sports, but she also enjoys exercising alone, so she goes on long bicycle rides whenever she can fit them in. She can't imagine what it would be like not to be physically active every day.

• Maria is a busy young mother of twins. To keep in shape, she joined a health club with a weight room, exercise classes, and child care. Every Monday, Wednesday, and Friday morning, she takes the twins to the club and attends the 7:00 "wake-up" low-impact aerobics class. The instructor leads the class through warm-ups; a 20-minute aerobic workout; exercises for the arms, abdomen, buttocks, and legs; stretches; and a relaxation exercise. Maria is exhilarated and ready for the rest of the day before 9:00 A.M.

• Tom is an engineering student with a lot of studying to do and an active social life as well. For exercise, he plays tennis three times a week. He likes to head for the courts around 6:00 P.M., when most people are eating dinner. He warms up for 10 minutes by practicing his forehand and backhand against a backboard and then plays a hard, fast game with his regular partner for 45 minutes to an hour. Afterwards, he does some stretching exercises while his muscles are still warm and then cools down with an easy 5-minute walk. Then he showers and gets ready for dinner. Twice a week he works out at the gym, with particular attention to keeping his arms strong and his shoulders limber. On Saturday nights, he goes dancing with friends.

• Ruben started a new job as a financial advisor in a large city. He spends 3 hours a day commuting on the train and has a new family, so he has no time for a structured exercise program. However, he manages to stay active during his busy work week by engaging in short bouts of physical activity. He parks some distance from the train station and walks briskly to and from his car—15 minutes each way. At work, he takes the stairs to his sixth-floor office. During several breaks during the day,

	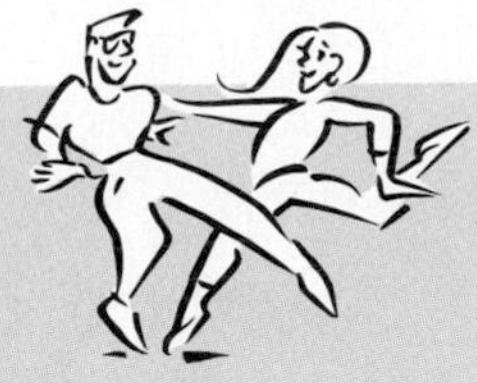 **Lifestyle physical activity**	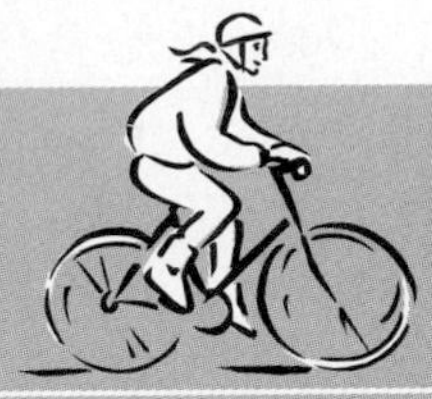 **Moderate exercise program**	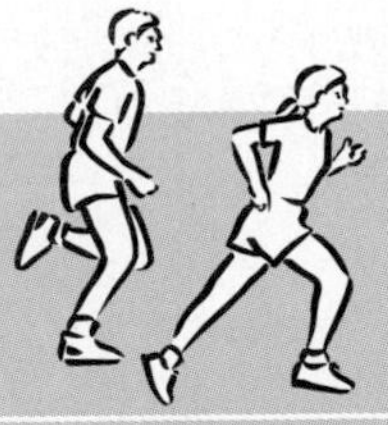 **Vigorous exercise program**
Description	Moderate physical activity—an amount of activity that uses about 150 calories per day	Cardiorespiratory endurance exercise (20–60 minutes, 3–5 days per week); strength training and stretching exercises (2–3 days per week)	Cardiorespiratory endurance exercise (20–60 minutes, 3–5 days per week); interval training; strength training (3–4 days per week); and stretching exercises (3–5 days per week)
Sample activities or program	*One of the following:* • Walking to and from work, 15 minutes each way • Cycling to and from class, 10 minutes each way • Raking leaves for 30 minutes • Dancing (fast) for 30 minutes • Playing basketball for 20 minutes	• Jogging for 30 minutes, 3 days per week • Weight training, 1 set of 8 exercises, 2 days per week • Stretching exercises, 3 days per week	• Running for 45 minutes, 3 days per week • Intervals: running 400 m at high effort, 4 sets, 2 days per week • Weight training, 3 sets of 10 exercises, 3 days per week • Stretching exercises, 5 days per week
Health and fitness benefits	Better blood cholesterol levels, reduced body fat, better control of blood pressure, improved metabolic health, and enhanced glucose metabolism; improved quality of life; reduced risk of some chronic diseases	All the benefits of lifestyle physical activity, plus improved physical fitness (increased cardiorespiratory endurance, muscular strength and endurance, and flexibility) and even greater improvements in health and quality of life and reductions in chronic disease risk	All the benefits of lifestyle physical activity and a moderate exercise program, with greater increases in fitness and somewhat greater reductions in chronic disease risk Participating in a vigorous exercise program may increase risk of injury and overtraining

Figure 2.5 Health and fitness benefits of different amounts of physical activity and exercise.

he does isometric exercises and stretches; these breaks help him maintain fitness and reduce the physical and mental stress of his high-pressure, sedentary job. Twice a week, he does calisthenic exercises at home in the evening, and he goes for a 30-minute jog on Saturday mornings.

Each of these people has worked an adequate or more-than-adequate fitness program into a busy daily routine. Chapter 7 contains guidelines to help you choose activities and put together a complete exercise program that suits your goals and preferences. (Refer to Figure 2.5 for a summary of the health and fitness benefits of different levels of physical activity.)

What about the tip of the activity pyramid? Although sedentary activities are often unavoidable—attending class, studying, working in an office, and so on—many people choose inactivity over activity during their leisure time. Change sedentary patterns by becoming more active whenever you can. Move more and sit less.

Guidelines for Training

The following guidelines will make your exercise program more effective and successful.

• *Train the way you want your body to change.* Stress your body such that it adapts in the desired direction. To have a more muscular build, lift weights. To be more flexible, do stretching exercises. To improve performance in a particular sport, practice that sport or the movements used in it.

• *Train regularly.* Consistency is the key to improving fitness. Fitness improvements are lost if too much time is allowed to pass between exercise sessions.

• *Get in shape gradually.* An exercise program can be divided into three phases: the beginning phase, during which the body adjusts to the new type and level of activity; the progress phase, during which fitness is increased; and the maintenance phase, in which the targeted level of fitness is maintained over the long term (Figure 2.6, p. 38). When beginning a program, start slowly to give your body time to adapt to the stress of exercise. As you progress, increase duration and frequency before increasing intensity. If you train too much or too intensely, you are more likely to suffer injuries or become **overtrained,** a condition characterized by lack of energy, aching muscles and joints, and decreased physical performance. Injuries and

overtraining A condition caused by training too much or too intensely, characterized by lack of energy, decreased physical performance, fatigue, depression, aching muscles and joints, and susceptibility to injury.

Terms

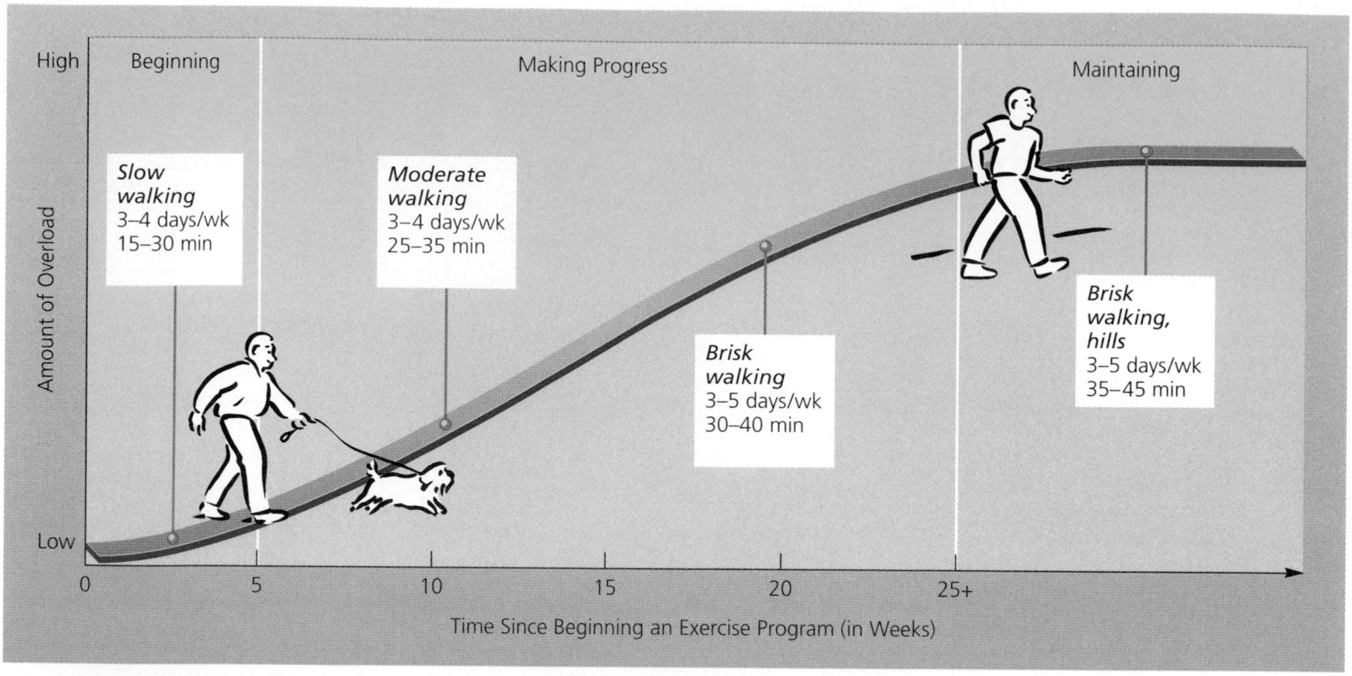

Figure 2.6 Progression of an exercise program. This figure shows how the amount of overload is increased gradually over time in a sample walking program. Regardless of the activity chosen, it is important that an exercise program begin slowly and progress gradually. Once a person achieves the desired level of fitness, she or he can maintain it by exercising 3 to 5 days a week. SOURCE: Progression data from American College of Sports Medicine. 2000. *ACSM's Guidelines for Exercise Testing and Prescription,* 6th ed. Baltimore, Md.: Lippincott Williams & Wilkins.

overtraining slow down an exercise program and impede motivation. The goal is not to get in shape as quickly as possible but to gradually become and remain physically fit.

• *Warm up before exercising and cool down afterward.* Warming up decreases the chances of injury by helping the body gradually progress from rest to activity. A warm-up should include low-intensity movements similar to those used in the activity that will follow. Stretching exercises are also often recommended. Cooling down after exercise is important for restoring circulation to its normal resting condition. Cool down by continuing to exercise but at a lower level of intensity.

• *Listen to your body.* Don't exercise if it doesn't feel right. Sometimes you need a few days of rest to recover enough to train with the intensity required for improving fitness. On the other hand, you can't train sporadically either. If you listen to your body and it always tells you to rest, you won't make any progress.

• *Try training with a partner.* Training partners can motivate and encourage each other through hard spots and help each other develop proper exercise techniques. Training with a partner can make exercising seem easier and more fun.

• *Train your mind.* This is one of the most difficult skills to acquire, but it is critical for achieving and maintaining fitness. Becoming fit requires commitment, discipline, and patience. These qualities come from understanding the importance of exercise and having clear and reachable goals. Use the lifestyle management techniques discussed in Chapter 1 to keep your program on track. Believe in yourself and your potential—and you *will* achieve your goals!

• *Add variety and have fun.* You are more likely to stick with an exercise program if it's fun. Choose a variety of activities that you enjoy. Change your exercise program occasionally to keep things fresh and help develop a higher degree of fitness. The body adapts more quickly to new activities than to familiar ones. Changing activities may also help reduce your risk of injury.

• *Keep your exercise program in perspective.* As important as physical fitness is, it is only part of a well-rounded life. You have to have time for work and school, family and friends, relaxation and hobbies. Some people become overinvolved in exercise and neglect other parts of their lives. They think of themselves as runners, dancers, swimmers, or triathletes rather than as people

Terms

exercise stress test A test usually administered on a treadmill or cycle ergometer that involves analysis of the changes in electrical activity in the heart from an electrocardiogram (EKG or ECG) taken during exercise. Used to determine if any heart disease is present and to assess current fitness level.

graded exercise test (GXT) An exercise test that starts at an easy intensity and progresses to maximum capacity.

who participate in those activities. Balance and moderation are the key ingredients of a fit and well life.

Tips for Today

Physical activity and exercise offer benefits in nearly every area of wellness, helping you generate energy, manage stress, improve your mood, and, of course, become physically stronger and healthier. Even a low-to-moderate level of activity provides valuable health benefits. The important thing is to get moving!

Right now you can

- Go outside and take a brisk 15-minute walk.
- Look at your calendar for the rest of the week and write in some physical activity—such as walking, running, biking, skating, swimming, hiking, or playing Frisbee—on as many days as you can. Schedule the activity for a specific time and stick to it.
- If you don't yet use the gym or fitness center on your campus, go there now and begin planning how to use it.
- Call a friend and invite her or him to start planning a regular exercise program with you.

SUMMARY

- Exercising daily in moderation contributes substantially to good health. Even without a formal, vigorous exercise program, you can get many of the same health benefits by becoming more physically active.
- If you are already active, you benefit even more by increasing the intensity or duration of your activity.
- The five components of physical fitness most important for health are cardiorespiratory endurance, muscular strength, muscular endurance, flexibility, and body composition.
- Physical training is the process of producing long-term improvements in the body's functioning through exercise. All training is based on the fact that the body adapts to physical stress.
- According to the principle of *specificity,* bodies change specifically in response to the type of training received.
- Bodies also adapt to *progressive overload*. Therefore, when we progressively increase our amount of exercise—its frequency, intensity, and duration—we become increasingly fit.
- Bodies adjust to lower levels of activity by losing fitness, a principle known as *reversibility*. To counter the effects of reversibility we should keep training at the same intensity, even if we reduce the number or length of sessions.
- According to the principle of *individual differences,* people vary in the maximum level of fitness they can achieve.
- When designing an exercise program, assess your current level of fitness, set realistic goals, and choose activities that develop all components of fitness.
- In addition, train regularly, get in shape gradually, warm up and cool down, maintain a structured but flexible program, consider training with a partner, train your mind, have fun, and keep exercise in perspective.

COMMON QUESTIONS ANSWERED

Is exercise safe for me? People of any age who are not at high risk for serious health problems can safely exercise at a moderate intensity (60% or less of maximum heart rate) without a prior medical evaluation. (See Chapter 3 for a discussion of maximum heart rate.) Likewise, if you are male and under 40 or female and under 50 and in good health, exercise is probably safe for you. If you are over these ages or have health problems (especially high blood pressure, heart disease, muscle or joint problems, or obesity), see your physician before starting a vigorous exercise program. The Canadian Society for Exercise Physiology has developed the Physical Activity Readiness Questionnaire (PAR-Q) to help determine exercise safety. This questionnaire is included in Lab 2.2. Completing it should alert you to any potential problems you may have. If a physician isn't sure whether exercise is safe for you, he or she may recommend an **exercise stress test** or a **graded exercise test (GXT)** to see whether you show symptoms of heart disease during exercise. For most people, however, it's far safer to exercise than to remain sedentary.

You must also consider your physical safety when exercising. If you ride a bicycle or run on public streets, wear clothing that can be seen easily. Bicyclists should always wear helmets. Even though you may have the right-of-way, give cars plenty of leeway; in a collision, a car will sustain less damage than a bicycle or your unprotected body. Don't train in isolated areas unless you're with a friend. Exercising alone, you could be injured or become a crime victim. (See Appendix A for more information on personal safety.)

Where can I get help and advice about exercise? Because fitness is essential to a wellness lifestyle, you need to learn as much as you can about exercise. One of the best places to get help is an exercise class. There, expert instructors can help you learn the basics of training and answer your questions. Make sure the instructor is certified by ACSM or has formal training in exercise physiology. Read articles by credible experts in fitness magazines. Because of competition among publications,

(continued)

COMMON QUESTIONS ANSWERED (continued)

many of these magazines include articles by leading experts in exercise science written at a layperson's level.

A qualified personal trainer can also be helpful in getting you started in an exercise program or a new form of training. Make sure this person has proper qualifications, such as a college degree in exercise physiology or physical education or ACSM, National Strength and Conditioning Association (NSCA), or American Council on Exercise (ACE) certification. Don't seek out a person for advice simply because he or she looks fit.

Where can I work out? Identify accessible and pleasant places to work out. For running, find a field or park with a soft surface. For swimming, find a pool that's open at times convenient for you. For cycling, find an area with minimal traffic and air pollution. Make sure the place you exercise is safe and convenient. If you join a health club or fitness center, follow the guidelines in the box "Choosing a Fitness Center."

Should I follow my exercise program if I'm sick? If you have a mild head cold or feel one coming on, it is probably OK to exercise moderately. Just begin slowly and see how you feel. However, if you have symptoms of a more serious illness—fever, swollen glands, nausea, extreme tiredness, muscle aches—wait until you have fully recovered before resuming your exercise program, Continuing to exercise while suffering from an illness more serious than a cold can compromise your recovery and may even be dangerous.

How can I fit my exercise program into my day? Good time management is an important skill in creating and maintaining an exercise program. Choose a regular time to exercise, preferably the same time every day. Don't tell yourself you'll exercise "sometime during the day" when you have free time—that free time may never come. Schedule your workout, and make it a priority. Include alternative plans in your program to account for circumstances like bad weather or vacations.

You don't have to work on all fitness components in the same exercise session. The important thing is to have a regular schedule. (You'll have the chance to develop strategies for successful time management in the Behavior Change Workbook at the end of the text.)

FOR FURTHER EXPLORATION

WW *Fit and Well* Online Learning Center (www.mhhe.com/fahey5e)

Use the learning objectives, study guide questions, and glossary flashcards to review key terms and concepts and prepare for exams. You can extend your knowledge of physical activity and gain experience in using the Internet as a resource by completing the activities and checking out the Web links for the topics in Chapter 2 marked with the World Wide Web icon. For this chapter, Internet activities explore common fitness terms, your current level of fitness, and a variety of physical activities that you can incorporate into your life; there are Web links for the Vital Statistics figure, the Critical Consumer box on fitness centers, and the chapter as a whole.

Daily Fitness and Nutrition Journal

Start completing the fitness program planning portion of the log by beginning an analysis of the costs and benefits of increasing physical activity, setting some general fitness goals, and thinking about your current activity and exercise habits. If you need to track your daily activities in order to identify ways to incorporate more lifestyle physical activity into your daily life, visit the Online Learning Center for some blank sample logs that you can print and use; also refer to the time management section (Activity 10) in the Behavior Change Workbook at the end of the text.

Health*Quest*

Are you ready to become more active? You can find out by completing the Stages of Change activity on the Health*Quest* CD-ROM (select Stages of Change from the Wellness Activities menu in the Fitness module). You'll receive an assessment of your stage plus advice on moving forward toward the action and maintenance stages.

Books

American College of Sports Medicine. 2000. *ACSM's Guidelines for Exercise Testing and Prescription,* 6th ed. Baltimore, Md.: Lippincott Williams & Wilkins. *Includes the ACSM guidelines for safety of exercising, a basic discussion of exercise physiology, and information about fitness testing and prescription.*

Department of Health and Human Services. 1996. *Physical Activity and Health: A Report of the Surgeon General.* Atlanta, Ga.: DHHS (also available online: http://www.cdc.gov/nccdphp/sgr/sgr.htm). *Summarizes evidence for the benefits of physical activity and makes recommendations.*

Fahey, T. D. 2000. *Super Fitness for Sports, Conditioning, and Health.* Boston: Allyn & Bacon. *A brief guide to developing fitness that emphasizes training techniques for improving sports performance.*

Manson, J., and P. Amend. 2001. *The 30-Minute Fitness Solution.* Cambridge, Mass.: Harvard University Press. *Provides an easy four-step plan for implementing an exercise program as well as many tips for incorporating physical activity into one's daily routine.*

National Center for Chronic Disease Prevention and Health Promotion. 1999. *Promoting Physical Activity: A Guide for Community Action.* Champaign Ill.: Human Kinetics. *Although designed for professionals, this guide provides a wealth of helpful advice for overcoming barriers to physical activity.*

Nieman, D. C. 2003. *Exercise Testing and Prescription: A Health-Related Approach,* 5th ed. New York: McGraw-Hill. *Comprehensive discussions of fitness testing, exercise and disease, nutrition and physical performance, and exercise prescription.*

Fitness centers can provide you with many benefits—motivation and companionship are among the most important. A fitness center may also offer expert instruction and supervision as well as access to better equipment than you could afford on your own. If you're thinking of joining a fitness center, here are some guidelines to help you choose a club that's right for you.

Convenience

- Look for an established facility that's within 10–15 minutes of your home or work. If it's farther away, your chances of sticking to an exercise regimen start to diminish.
- Check out the facility's hours, then visit it at the time you would normally exercise. Will you have easy access to the equipment and exercise classes you want at that time?

Atmosphere

- Look around to see if there are other members who are your age and at about your fitness level. (If everyone seems close in age or fitness level, then the club may cater to a certain age group or lifestyle—for example, hard-core bodybuilders.)
- If you like to exercise to music, make sure you like the music played there, both its type and loudness.
- Observe how the members dress. Will you fit in, or will you be uncomfortable?
- Check to see that the facility is clean, including showers and lockers. Make sure the facility is climate controlled and well ventilated.

Safety

- Find out if the facility offers basic fitness testing that includes cardiovascular screening.
- Determine if there is emergency equipment on the premises and if personnel are trained in CPR.
- Ask if at least one staff member on each shift is trained in first aid.
- Find out if the club has an emergency plan in the event that a member has a heart attack or serious injury (many clubs do not).

Trained Personnel

- Determine if the personal trainers and fitness instructors are certified by a recognized professional association such as the American College of Sports Medicine (ACSM), National Strength and Conditioning Association (NSCA), or American Council on Exercise (ACE). All personal trainers are not equal—more than 100 organizations certify trainers and few of these require much formal training.
- Find out if the club has a trained exercise physiologist on staff, someone with a degree in exercise physiology, kinesiology, or exercise science. If the facility offers nutritional counseling, it should employ someone who is a registered dietitian (R.D.) or who has other formal training.
- Ask how much experience the instructors have. Clubs may employ people because they were good athletes or look fit; by themselves, these are not good reasons to hire someone. Ideally, trainers should have both academic preparation and practical experience.

Cost

- Buy only what you need and can afford. If you want to use only workout equipment, you may not need a club that has racquetball courts and saunas.
- Check the contract. Choose the one that covers the shortest period of time possible, especially if it's your first fitness club experience.
- Make sure the contract permits you to extend your membership if you have a prolonged illness or go on vacation.
- Try out the club. Ask for a free trial workout, or a 1-day pass, or an inexpensive 1- or 2-week trial membership.
- Find out whether there is an extra charge for the particular services you want.

Effectiveness

- Tour the facility. Does it offer what the brochure says it does?
- Check the equipment. A good club will have treadmills, bikes, stair-climbers, resistance machines, and weights. Make sure these machines are up-to-date and well maintained.
- Make sure the facility is certified. Look for the displayed names American College of Sports Medicine (ACSM), American Council on Exercise (ACE), Aerobics and Fitness Association of America (AFAA), or International Health, Racquet, and Sportsclub Association (IHRSA).
- Don't get cheated. Check with your Better Business Bureau or Consumer Affairs office to see if others have complained.

Journals

ACSM Health and Fitness Journal (401 West Michigan Street, Indianapolis, IN 46202; http://www.health-fitjrnl.com)

Physician and Sportsmedicine (4530 W. 77th Street, Minneapolis, MN 55435; many of the articles are also available online at http://www.physsportsmed.com)

Organizations, Hotlines, and Web Sites

American Alliance for Health, Physical Education, Recreation, and Dance (AAHPERD). A professional organization dedicated to promoting quality health and education programs.
800-213-7193
http://www.aahperd.org

American College of Sports Medicine (ACSM). The principal professional organization for sports medicine and exercise science. Provides brochures, publications, and audio- and videotapes.
317-637-9200
http://www.acsm.org
American Council on Exercise (ACE). Promotes exercise and fitness; the Web site features fact sheets on many consumer topics, including choosing shoes, cross-training, and steroids.
800-529-8227 (Consumer Fitness Hotline)
http:/www.acefitness.org
American Heart Association: Just Move. Provides practical advice for people of all fitness levels plus an online fitness diary.
http://www.justmove.org
Canada's Physical Activity Guide. Offers many suggestions for incorporating physical activity into everyday life; also includes the Physical Activity Readiness Questionnaire (PAR-Q).
http://www.hc-sc.gc.ca/hppb/paguide
CDC Physical Activity Information. Provides information on the benefits of physical activity and suggestions for incorporating moderate physical activity into daily life.
http://www.cdc.gov/nccdphp/phyactiv.htm
Disabled Sports USA. Provides sports and recreation services to people with physical or mobility disorders.
http://www.dsusa.org
Georgia State University: Exercise and Physical Fitness Page. Provides information about the benefits of exercise and how to get started on a fitness program.
http://www.gsu.edu/~wwwfit
International Health, Racquet, and Sportsclub Association (IHRSA): Health Clubs. Provides guidelines for choosing a health or fitness facility and links to clubs that belong to IHRSA.
http://www.healthclubs.com
MedlinePlus: Exercise and Physical Fitness. Provides links to news and reliable information about fitness and exercise from government agencies and professional associations.
http://www.nlm.nih.gov/medlineplus/exercisephysicalfitness.html
President's Council on Physical Fitness and Sports (PCPFS). Provides information on PCPFS programs and publications, including fitness guides and fact sheets.
http://www.fitness.gov
Shape Up America! Fitness Center. Provides information on the benefits of fitness, assessment tests, and tips on overcoming barriers to physical activity.
http://shapeup.org/fitness

The following provide links to sites with information on a wide variety of activities and fitness issues:

Fitness Partner Connection Jumpsite: http//www.primusweb.com/fitnesspartner
NetSweat: The Internet's Fitness Resource: http//www.sickbay.com/netsweat
Yahoo! Recreation and Sports: http//dir.yahoo.com/Recreation/Sports
Yahoo!Fitness: dir.yahoo.com/Health/Fitness

SELECTED BIBLIOGRAPHY

American College of Sports Medicine. 2000. *ACSM's Guidelines for Exercise Testing and Prescription,* 6th ed. Baltimore, Md.: Lippincott Williams & Wilkins.

American College of Sports Medicine. 1998. ACSM position stand: The recommended quantity and quality of exercise for developing and maintaining cardiorespiratory and muscular fitness, and flexibility in healthy adults. *Medicine and Science in Sports and Exercise* 30(6): 975–991.

Balady, G. J. 2002. Survival of the fittest—more evidence. *New England Journal of Medicine* 346(11): 852–854.

Blair, S. N., Y. Cheng, and J. S. Holder. 2001. Is physical activity or physical fitness more important in defining health benefits? *Medicine and Science in Sports and Exercise* 33(6 Suppl): S379–S399.

Boreham, C. A., W. F. Wallace, and A. Nevill. 2000. Training effects of accumulated daily stair-climbing exercise in previously sedentary young women. *Preventive Medicine* 30(4): 277–281.

Bouchard, C., and T. Rankinen. 2001. Individual differences in response to regular physical activity. *Medicine and Science in Sports and Exercise* 33(6 Suppl): S446–S451.

Byers, T., et al. 2002. American Cancer Society guidelines on nutrition and physical activity for cancer prevention: Reducing the risk of cancer with healthy food choices and physical activity. *CA: A Cancer Journal for Clinicians* 52(2): 92–119.

Centers for Disease Control and Prevention. 2001. Physical activity trends—United States, 1990–1998. *Morbidity and Mortality Weekly Report* 50(9): 166–169.

Centers for Disease Control and Prevention. 2001. *Lower Direct Medical Costs Associated with Physical Activity* (http://www.cdc.gov/nccdphp/ndpa/pr-cost.htm; retrieved October 9, 2001).

Department of Health and Human Services. 1996. *Physical Activity and Health: A Report of the Surgeon General.* Atlanta, Ga.: DHHS.

Hale, B. S., and J. S. Raglin. 2002. State anxiety responses to acute resistance training and step aerobic exercise across eight weeks of training. *Journal of Sports Medicine and Physical Fitness* 42(1): 108–112.

Hansen, C. J., L. C. Stevens, and J. R. Coast. 2001. Exercise duration and mood state: How much is enough to feel better? *Health Psychology* 20(4): 267–275.

Laukkanen, J. A., et al. 2001. Cardiovascular fitness as a predictor of mortality in men. *Archives of Internal Medicine* 161(6): 825–831.

Lee, C. D., S. N. Blair, and A. S. Jackson. 1999. Cardiorespiratory fitness, body composition, and all-cause and cardiovascular disease mortality in men. *American Journal of Clinical Nutrition* 69(3): 373–380.

Lee, I. M., and P. J. Skerrett. 2001. Physical activity and all-cause mortality: What is the dose-response relation? *Medicine and Science in Sports and Exercise* 33(6 Suppl): S459–S471.

Pescatello, L. S. 2001. Exercising for health: The merits of lifestyle physical activity. *Western Journal of Medicine* 174(2): 114–118.

President's Council on Physical Fitness and Sports. 2000. Definitions: Health, fitness, and physical activity. *Research Digest* 3(9).

Van, V., J. Buckworth, and C. Mattern. 2002. Physical self-concept and strength changes in college weight classes. *Research Quarterly for Exercise and Sport* 73(1): 113–117.

Whelton, S. P., et al. 2002. Effect of aerobic exercise on blood pressure: A meta-analysis of randomized, controlled trials. *Annals of Internal Medicine* 136(7): 493–503.

Williams, P. T. 2001. Health effects resulting from exercises versus those from body fat loss. *Medicine and Science in Sports and Exercise* 33(6 Suppl): S611–S621.

Name ______________________ Section ______________ Date ______________

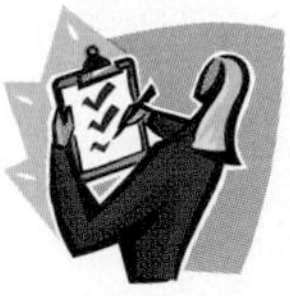

LAB 2.1 *Your Physical Activity Profile*

Ww

Complete this lab to assess your overall level of activity on a typical day. The amount of time you spend on sleep and on light, moderate, and vigorous activity should total 24 hours. To complete the chart below, fill in your activities and the amount of time you spend on each one; in addition, keep track of the number of flights of stairs you climb. Classify each activity as light, moderate, or vigorous according to the following guidelines:

Light activities—most sitting and standing activities: Attending class; studying; using a computer; watching TV; listening to music; talking on the phone; eating meals; walking slowly; driving; most child-care activities; light housework such as ironing, cooking, dusting, vacuuming; light yard work or home repair such as pruning, weeding, plumbing; office work, sales, or another occupational activity involving sitting or standing and movement of little more than hands.

Moderate activities—breathing rate increases but comfortable conversation is possible: Walking moderately or briskly; cycling moderately; active play with children or pushing a stroller; moderate housework such as scrubbing floors, washing windows; moderate yard work or home repair such as planting, raking, painting, wallpapering; hand-washing a car; waiting tables, washing dishes, or another occupational activity involving extended periods of moderate effort; social dancing; fitness activities requiring moderate effort such as low-impact aerobic dance, Frisbee, recreational swimming, hitting a punching bag.

Vigorous activities—too out of breath to talk easily: Walking briskly uphill; heavy housework such as moving furniture or carrying heavy items upstairs; vigorous yard work or home activities such as shoveling snow, trimming trees, hand-sawing; heavy construction work or digging; fitness activities requiring vigorous effort, such as jogging or running, high-impact aerobic dance; circuit weight training, swimming laps, most competitive sports.

Activity	Duration	Classification

Number of flights of stairs: ______________ flights

LABORATORY ACTIVITIES

Physical Activity Summary (should total 24 hours)

Sleep: ______________ hours

Light activity: ______________ hours

Moderate activity: ______________ hours

Vigorous activity: ______________ hours

Number of flights of stairs: ______________ flights

Using Your Results

How did you score? Are you at all surprised by the amount of time you spend in light, moderate, and vigorous activity? Do you spend at least 30 minutes each day—the recommended minimum—in moderate or vigorous activity? Are you satisfied with the amount of moderate and vigorous physical activity in your daily life?

What should you do next? Enter the results of this lab in the Preprogram Assessment column in Appendix D. If you want to increase the amount of moderate or vigorous physical activity in your life, begin by analyzing the amount of time in each intensity category according to the type of activity:

	Light activity (hours)	Moderate activity (hours)	Vigorous activity (hours)
Home and child-care activities			
School- or job-related activities			
Transportation-related activities			
Leisure activities			
Exercise/sport activities			

How much of your time in transportation-related activities and leisure activities is classified as light activity? Transportation and leisure activities are often the areas where it is easiest to substitute moderate activities for light activities. Examples include walking or biking rather than driving for short errands and going for a walk with a friend rather than chatting on the phone; see p. 29 for additional suggestions. Below, identify three strategies for boosting physical activity in your daily life.

1. ______________________________

2. ______________________________

3. ______________________________

Can you also identify additional opportunities to climb stairs each day?

Begin to adopt the strategies you've identified to increase physical activity. After several weeks of a program to become more physically active, do this lab again, and enter the results in the Postprogram Assessment column of Appendix D. How do the results compare?

SOURCE: Activity classifications from CDC Division of Nutrition and Physical Activity. 1999. *Promoting Physical Activity: A Guide for Community Action.* Champaign, Ill.: Human Kinetics.

Name ______________________ Section ______________ Date ______________

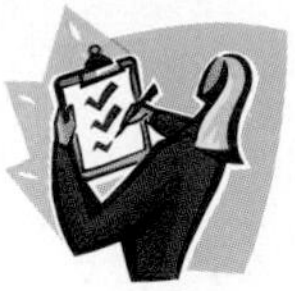

LAB 2.2 *Safety of Exercise Participation*

PAR-Q & YOU

(A Questionnaire for People Age 15 to 69)

Part I Regular physical activity is fun and healthy, and increasingly more people are starting to become more active every day. Being more active is very safe for most people. However, some people should check with their doctor before they start becoming much more physically active.

If you are planning to become much more physically active than you are now, start by answering the seven questions in the box below. If you are between the ages of 15 and 69, the PAR-Q will tell you if you should check with your doctor before you start. If you are over 69 years of age, and you are not used to being very active, check with your doctor.

Common sense is your best guide when you answer these questions. Please read the questions carefully and answer each one honestly: check YES or NO.

YES	NO	
☐	☐	1. Has your doctor ever said that you have a heart condition and that you should only do physical activity recommended by a doctor?
☐	☐	2. Do you feel pain in your chest when you do physical activity?
☐	☐	3. In the past month, have you had chest pain when you were not doing physical activity?
☐	☐	4. Do you lose your balance because of dizziness or do you ever lose consciousness?
☐	☐	5. Do you have a bone or joint problem that could be made worse by a change in your physical activity?
☐	☐	6. Is your doctor currently prescribing drugs (for example, water pills) for your blood pressure or heart condition?
☐	☐	7. Do you know of <u>any other reason</u> why you should not do physical activity?

If you answered

YES to one or more questions

Talk with your doctor by phone or in person BEFORE you start becoming much more physically active or BEFORE you have a fitness appraisal. Tell your doctor about the PAR-Q and which questions you answered YES.

- You may be able to do any activity you want—as long as you start slowly and build up gradually. Or, you may need to restrict your activities to those which are safe for you. Talk with your doctor about the kinds of activities you wish to participate in and follow his/her advice.
- Find out which community programs are safe and helpful for you.

NO to all questions

If you answered NO honestly to <u>all</u> PAR-Q questions, you can be reasonably sure that you can:

- start becoming much more physically active—begin slowly and build up gradually. This is the safest and easiest way to go.
- take part in a fitness appraisal—this is an excellent way to determine your basic fitness so that you can plan the best way for you to live actively.

DELAY BECOMING MUCH MORE ACTIVE:

- if you are not feeling well because of a temporary illness such as a cold or a fever—wait until you feel better; or
- if you are or may be pregnant—talk to your doctor before you start becoming more active

Please note: If your health changes so that you then answer YES to any of the above questions, tell your fitness or health professional. Ask whether you should change your physical activity plan.

<u>Informed Use of the PAR-Q:</u> The Canadian Society for Exercise Physiology, Health Canada, and their agents assume no liability for persons who undertake physical activity, and if in doubt after completing this questionnaire, consult your doctor prior to physical activity.

You are encouraged to copy the PAR-Q but only if you use the entire form.

Note: If the PAR-Q is being given to a person before he or she participates in a physical activity program or a fitness appraisal, this section may be used for legal or administrative purposes.

I have read, understood and completed this questionnaire. Any questions I had were answered to my full satisfaction.

NAME ______________________________

SIGNATURE ______________________________ DATE ______________

SIGNATURE OF PARENT ______________________ WITNESS ______________
or GUARDIAN (for participants under the age of majority)

Supported by: Health Canada Santé Canada

Part II General Health Profile

To help further assess the safety of exercise for you, complete as much of this health profile as possible.

General Information

Age: ________ Total cholesterol: ________ Blood pressure: _____ /_____

Height: ________ HDL: ________ Triglycerides: ________

Weight: ________ LDL: ________ Blood glucose level: ________

Are you currently trying to _____ gain or _____ lose weight? (check one if appropriate)

Medical Conditions/Treatments

Check any of the following that apply to you and add any other conditions that might affect your ability to exercise safely.

_____ heart disease

_____ lung disease

_____ diabetes

_____ allergies

_____ asthma

_____ depression, anxiety, or another psychological disorder

_____ eating disorder

_____ back pain

_____ arthritis

_____ other injury or joint problem: ____________

_____ substance abuse problem

_____ other: ____________

_____ other: ____________

_____ other: ____________

_____ Do you have a family history of cardiovascular disease (CVD) (a parent, sibling, or child who had a heart attack or stroke before age 55 for men or 65 for women)?

List any medications or supplements you are taking or any medical treatments you are undergoing. Include the name of the substance or treatment and its purpose. Include both prescription and over-the-counter drugs and supplements.

____________________ ____________________

____________________ ____________________

Lifestyle Information

Check any of the following that is true for you, and fill in the requested information.

_____ I usually eat high-fat foods (fatty meats, cheese, fried foods, butter, full-fat dairy products) every day.

_____ I consume fewer than 5 servings of fruits and vegetables on most days.

_____ I smoke cigarettes or use other tobacco products. If true, describe your use of tobacco (type and frequency): ____________________

_____ I regularly drink alcohol. If true, describe your typical weekly consumption pattern: ____________________

____

_____ I often feel as if I need more sleep. (I need about _____ hours per day; I get about _____ hours per day.)

_____ I feel as though stress has adversely affected my level of wellness during the past year.

Describe your current activity pattern. What types of moderate physical activity do you engage in on a daily basis? Are you involved in a formal exercise program or do you regularly participate in sports or recreational activities?

____

____

Using Your Results

How did you score? Did the PAR-Q indicate that exercise is likely to be safe for you? Is there anything in your Health Profile that you think may affect your ability to exercise safely? Have you had any problems with exercise in the past?

What should you do next? If the assessments in this lab indicate that you should see your physician before beginning an exercise program, or if you have any questions about the safety of exercise for you, make an appointment to talk with your health care provider to address your concerns.

Cardiorespiratory Endurance

3

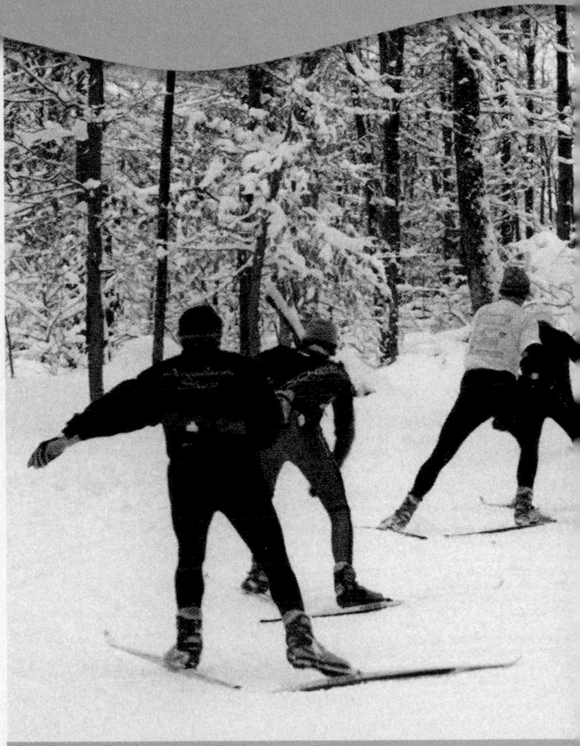

LOOKING AHEAD

After reading this chapter, you should be able to

- Describe how the body produces the energy it needs for exercise
- List the major effects and benefits of cardiorespiratory endurance exercise
- Explain how cardiorespiratory endurance is measured and assessed
- Describe how type, intensity, duration, and frequency of exercise affect the development of cardiorespiratory endurance
- Explain the best ways to prevent and treat common exercise injuries

TEST YOUR KNOWLEDGE

1. Compared to sedentary people, those who engage in regular moderate endurance exercise are likely to
   a. have fewer colds.
   b. be less anxious and depressed.
   c. fall asleep more quickly and sleep better.
   d. be more alert and creative.
2. About what percentage of home exercise equipment purchased in the last five years is still in use?
   a. 25%
   b. 50%
   c. 75%
3. To stay appropriately hydrated during exercise, you should drink only if thirsty. True or false?

TEST YOUR KNOWLEDGE ANSWERS

1. ALL FOUR. Endurance exercise has many immediate benefits that affect all the dimensions of wellness and improve overall quality of life.

2. A. Before you buy a piece of equipment, make sure that it will help you achieve your fitness goals, that you enjoy using it regularly, and that it functions as promised.

3. FALSE. Thirst is a poor indicator of fluid needs. Drink about 2 cups of fluid 2 hours before exercise and then 1 cup about every 20–30 minutes during exercise—more if it's hot or you sweat heavily.

Fit and Well Online Learning Center

www.mhhe.com/fahey5e

Visit the *Fit and Well* Online Learning Center for study aids, additional information about cardiorespiratory endurance, links, Internet activities that explore the development of cardiorespiratory fitness, consumer resources, and much more.

Cardiorespiratory endurance—the ability of the body to perform prolonged, large-muscle, dynamic exercise at moderate-to-high levels of intensity—is a key health-related component of fitness. As explained in Chapter 2, a healthy cardiorespiratory system is essential to high levels of fitness and wellness.

This chapter reviews the short- and long-term effects and benefits of cardiorespiratory endurance exercise. It then describes several tests that are commonly used to assess cardiorespiratory fitness. Finally, it provides guidelines for creating your own cardiorespiratory endurance program, one that is geared to your current level of fitness and built around activities you enjoy.

BASIC PHYSIOLOGY OF CARDIORESPIRATORY ENDURANCE EXERCISE

A basic understanding of the body processes involved in cardiorespiratory endurance exercise can help you design a safe and effective fitness program. In this section, we'll take a brief look at how the cardiorespiratory system functions and how the body produces the energy it needs to respond to the challenge of physical activity.

The Cardiorespiratory System

The cardiorespiratory system picks up and transports oxygen, nutrients, and other key substances to the organs and tissues that need them; it also picks up waste products and carries them to where they can be used or expelled. The cardiorespiratory system consists of the heart, the blood vessels, and the respiratory system (Figure 3.1).

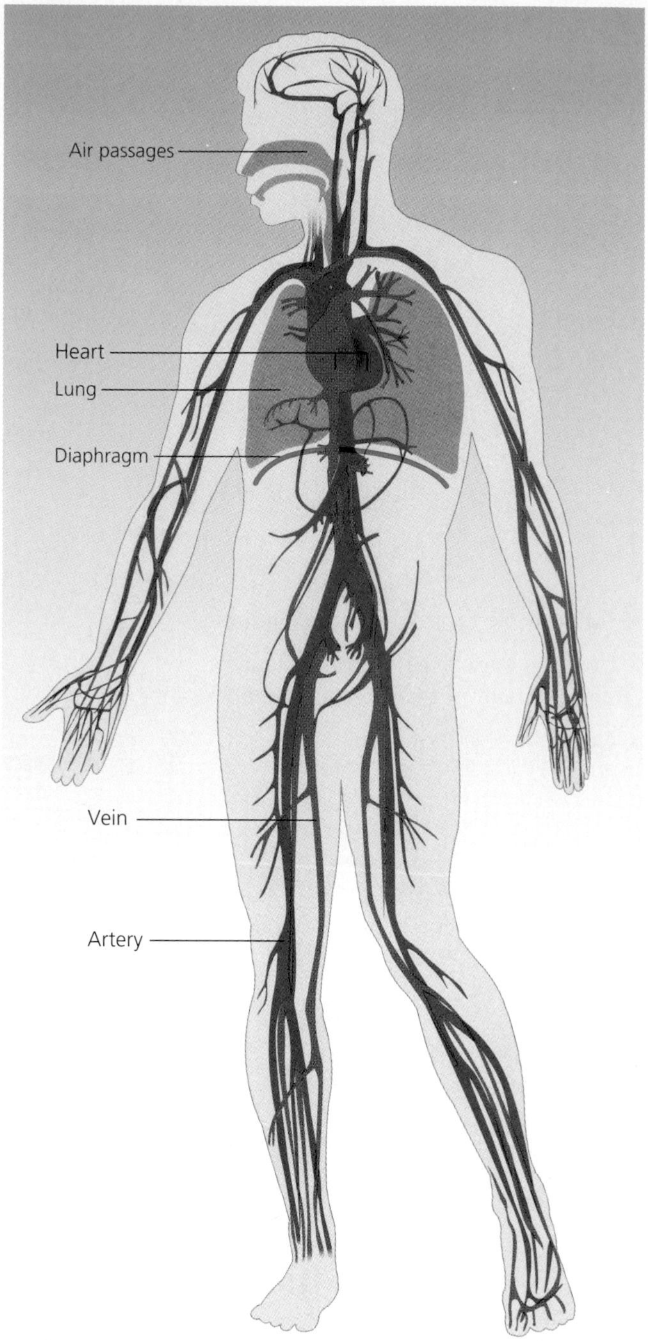

Figure 3.1 The cardiorespiratory system.

The Heart The heart is a four-chambered, fist-sized muscle located just beneath the ribs under the sternum (breastbone). Its role is to pump oxygen-poor blood to the lungs and oxygenated (oxygen-rich) blood to the rest of the body. Blood actually travels through two separate circulatory systems: The right side of the heart pumps blood to the lungs in what is called **pulmonary circulation,** and the left side pumps blood through the rest of the body in **systemic circulation.**

Waste-carrying, oxygen-poor blood enters the right upper chamber, or **atrium,** of the heart through the **venae cavae,** the largest veins in the body (Figure 3.2). As the right atrium fills, it contracts and pumps blood into the right lower chamber, or **ventricle,** which, when it contracts, pumps blood through the pulmonary artery into the lungs. There, blood picks up oxygen and discards carbon dioxide. Cleaned, oxygenated blood then flows from the lungs through the pulmonary veins into the left atrium. As this chamber fills, it contracts and pumps blood into the powerful left ventricle, which pumps it through the **aorta,** the body's largest artery, to be fed into the rest of the body's blood vessels.

The period of the heart's contraction is called **systole;** the period of relaxation is called **diastole.** During systole, the atria contract first, pumping blood into the ventricles; a fraction of a second later, the ventricles contract, pumping blood to the lungs and the body. During diastole, blood flows into the heart. **Blood pressure,** the force exerted by blood on the walls of the blood vessels, is created by the pumping action of the heart; blood pressure is greater during systole than during diastole. A person weighing 150 pounds has about 5 quarts of blood, which are circulated about once every minute.

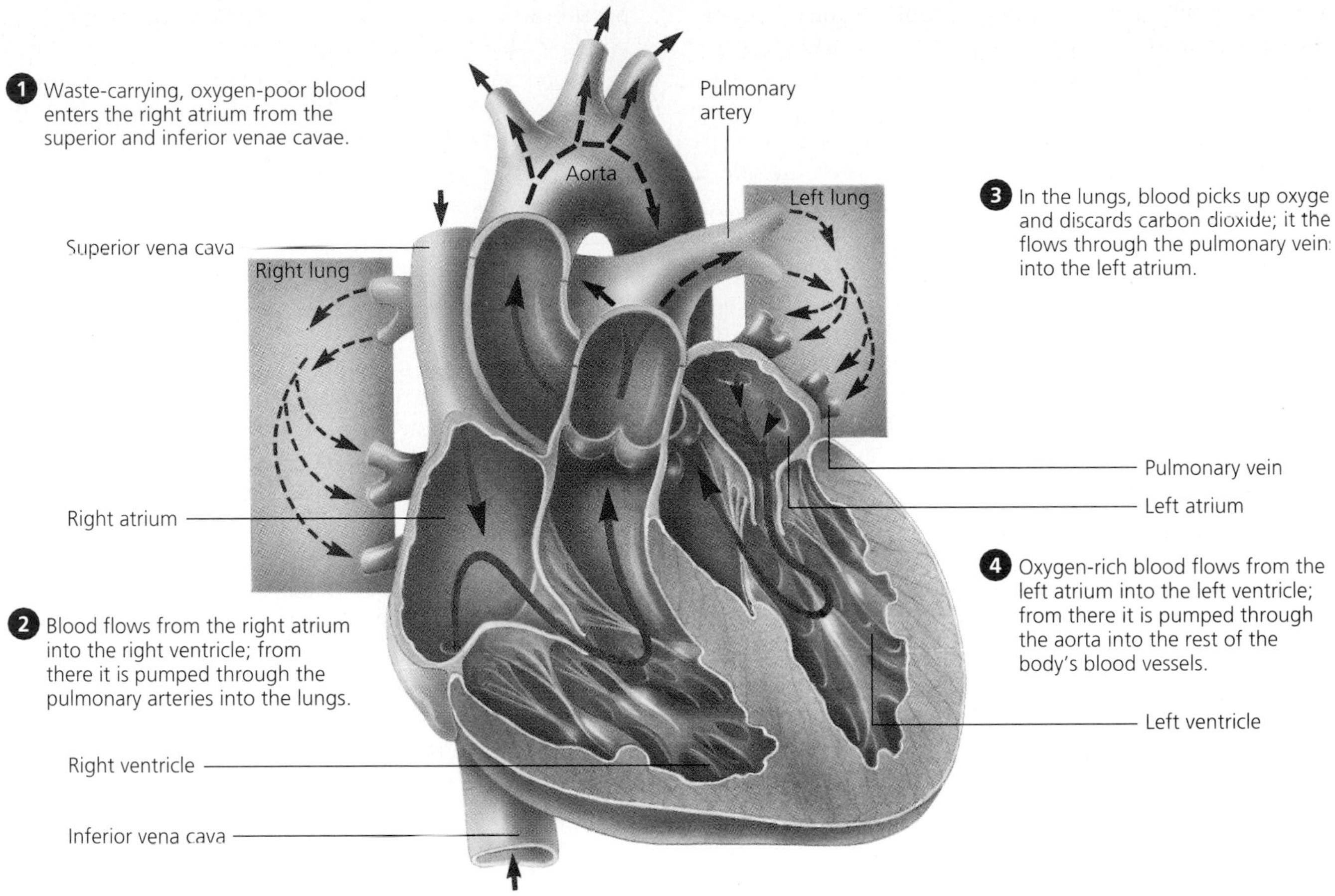

1 Waste-carrying, oxygen-poor blood enters the right atrium from the superior and inferior venae cavae.
Pulmonary artery
Aorta
Left lung
3 In the lungs, blood picks up oxyge and discards carbon dioxide; it the flows through the pulmonary vein into the left atrium.
Superior vena cava
Right lung
Pulmonary vein
Left atrium
Right atrium
4 Oxygen-rich blood flows from the left atrium into the left ventricle; from there it is pumped through the aorta into the rest of the body's blood vessels.
2 Blood flows from the right atrium into the right ventricle; from there it is pumped through the pulmonary arteries into the lungs.
Left ventricle
Right ventricle
Inferior vena cava

Figure 3.2 Circulation in the heart.

The heartbeat—the split-second sequence of contractions of the heart's four chambers—is controlled by nerve impulses. These signals originate in a bundle of specialized cells in the right atrium called the pacemaker or sinoatrial (SA) node. Unless it is speeded up or slowed down by the brain in response to such stimuli as danger or the tissues' need for more oxygen, the heart produces nerve impulses at a steady rate.

The Blood Vessels Blood vessels are classified by size and function. **Veins** carry blood to the heart; **arteries** carry it away from the heart. Veins have thin walls, but arteries have thick elastic walls that enable them to expand and relax with the volume of blood being pumped through them. After leaving the heart, the aorta branches into smaller and smaller vessels. The smallest arteries branch still further into **capillaries,** tiny vessels only one cell thick. The capillaries deliver oxygen and nutrient-rich blood to the tissues and pass on oxygen-poor, waste-carrying blood. From the capillaries, this blood empties into small veins (venules) and then into larger veins that return it to the heart to repeat the cycle.

Blood pumped through the heart doesn't reach its cells, so the heart has its own network of arteries, veins, and capillaries. Two large vessels, the right and left coronary

Terms

pulmonary circulation The part of the circulatory system that moves blood between the heart and the lungs; controlled by the right side of the heart.

systemic circulation The part of the circulatory system that moves blood between the heart and the rest of the body; controlled by the left side of the heart.

atria The two upper chambers of the heart in which blood collects before passing to the ventricles; also called *auricles.*

venae cavae The large veins through which blood is returned to the right atrium of the heart.

ventricles The two lower chambers of the heart from which blood flows through arteries to the lungs and other parts of the body.

aorta The large artery that receives blood from the left ventricle and distributes it to the body.

systole Contraction of the heart.

diastole Relaxation of the heart.

blood pressure The force exerted by the blood on the walls of the blood vessels; created by the pumping action of the heart. Blood pressure increases during systole and decreases during diastole.

veins Vessels that carry blood to the heart.

arteries Vessels that carry blood away from the heart.

capillaries Very small blood vessels that distribute blood to all parts of the body.

arteries, branch off the aorta and supply the heart muscle with oxygenated blood. Blockage of a coronary artery is a leading cause of heart attacks (see Chapter 11).

The Respiratory System The **respiratory system** supplies oxygen to the body and carries off carbon dioxide, a waste product of body processes. Air passes in and out of the lungs as a result of pressure changes brought about by the contraction and relaxation of the diaphragm and rib muscles; the lungs expand and contract about 12–20 times a minute. As air is inhaled, it passes through the nasal passages, the throat, larynx, trachea (windpipe), and bronchi into the lungs. The lungs consist of many branching tubes that end in tiny, thin-walled air sacs called **alveoli.**

Carbon dioxide and oxygen are exchanged between alveoli and capillaries in the lungs. Carbon dioxide passes from blood cells into the alveoli, where it is carried up and out of the lungs (exhaled). Oxygen from inhaled air is passed from the alveoli into blood cells; these oxygen-rich blood cells then return to the heart and are pumped throughout the body. Oxygen is an important component of the body's energy-producing system, so the cardiorespiratory system's ability to pick up and deliver oxygen is critical for the functioning of the body—at rest and during exercise.

The Cardiorespiratory System at Rest and During Exercise At rest and during light activity, the cardiorespiratory system functions at a fairly steady pace. Your heart beats at a rate of about 50–90 beats per minute, and you take about 12–20 breaths per minute. A typical resting blood pressure, measured in millimeters of mercury, is 120 systolic and 80 diastolic (120/80); as described earlier, blood pressure is higher when the heart contracts (systole) than when the heart relaxes (diastole).

During exercise, the demands on the cardiorespiratory system increase. Body cells, particularly working muscles, need to obtain more oxygen and fuel and to eliminate more waste products. In order to meet this increased demand, your heart rate increases, up to 170–210 beats per minute during intense exercise; the heart also pumps out more blood with each beat (stroke volume). The combination of faster heart rate and greater stroke volume means the heart pumps and circulates more blood per minute—a **cardiac output** of 20 or more quarts per minute, compared to about 5 quarts per minute at rest. Blood flow also changes: At rest, about 15–20% of blood is distributed to the skeletal muscles; during exercise, as much as 85–90% may be delivered to working muscles. Systolic blood pressure increases, while diastolic pressure holds steady or declines slightly; a typical exercise blood pressure might be 175/70. You will take deeper breaths and breathe more quickly, up to 40–60 breaths per minute. All of these changes are controlled and coordinated by special centers in the brain, which use the nervous system and chemical messengers to control the process.

Later in this chapter you'll learn more about the short- and long-term effects of exercise on the body.

Energy Production

Metabolism is the sum of all the chemical processes necessary to maintain the body. Energy is required to fuel vital body functions—to build and break down tissue, contract muscles, conduct nerve impulses, regulate body temperature, and so on. The rate at which your body uses energy—its metabolic rate—depends on your level of activity. At rest, you have a low metabolic rate; if you stand up and begin to walk, your metabolic rate increases. If you jog, your metabolic rate may increase more than 800% above its resting level. Olympic-caliber distance runners can increase their metabolic rate by a whopping 2000% or more.

Energy from Food The body converts chemical energy from food into substances that cells can use as fuel. These fuels can be used immediately or stored for later use. The body's ability to store fuel is critical, because if all the energy from food were released immediately, much of it would be wasted.

The three classes of energy-containing nutrients in food are carbohydrates, fats, and proteins. During digestion, most carbohydrates are broken down into the simple sugar **glucose.** Some glucose remains circulating in the blood ("blood sugar"), where it can be used as a quick source of fuel to produce energy. Glucose may also be

Terms

Ww

respiratory system The lungs, air passages, and breathing muscles; supplies oxygen to the body and carries off carbon dioxide.

alveoli Tiny air sacs in the lungs through whose walls gases such as oxygen and carbon dioxide diffuse in and out of blood.

cardiac output The amount of blood pumped by the heart each minute; a function of heart rate and stroke volume (the amount of blood pumped during each beat).

glucose A simple sugar that circulates in the blood and can be used by cells to fuel adenosine triphosphate (ATP) production.

glycogen A complex carbohydrate stored principally in the liver and skeletal muscles; the major fuel source during most forms of intense exercise. Glycogen is the storage form of glucose.

adenosine triphosphate (ATP) Energy source for cellular processes.

immediate energy system Energy system that supplies energy to muscle cells through the breakdown of cellular stores of ATP and creatine phosphate (CP).

nonoxidative (anaerobic) energy system Energy system that supplies energy to muscle cells through the breakdown of muscle stores of glucose and glycogen; also called the *anaerobic system* or the *lactic acid system* because chemical reactions take place without oxygen and produce lactic acid.

anaerobic Occurring in the absence of oxygen.

Table 3.1 *Characteristics of the Body's Energy Systems*

	ENERGY SYSTEM*		
	Immediate	**Nonoxidative**	**Oxidative**
Duration of activity for which system predominates	0–10 seconds	10 seconds–2 minutes	>2 minutes
Intensity of activity for which system predominates	High	High	Low to moderately high
Rate of ATP production	Immediate, very rapid	Rapid	Slower but prolonged
Fuel	Adenosine triphosphate (ATP), creatine phosphate (CP)	Muscle stores of glycogen and glucose	Body stores of glycogen, glucose, fat, and protein
Oxygen used?	No	No	Yes
Sample activities	Weight lifting, picking up a bag of groceries	400-meter run, running up several flights of stairs	1500-meter run, 30-minute walk, standing in line for a long time

*For most activities, all three systems contribute to energy production; the duration and intensity of the activity determine which system predominates.

SOURCE: Adapted from Brooks, G. A., et. al. 2000. *Exercise Physiology. Human Bioenergetics and its Applications,* 3d ed. Mountain View, Calif.: Mayfield. Copyright © 2002 Mayfield Publishing Co. Reproduced with permission of The McGraw-Hill Companies.

converted to **glycogen** and stored in the liver, muscles, and kidneys. If glycogen stores are full and the body's immediate need for energy is met, the remaining glucose is converted to fat and stored in the body's fatty tissues. Excess energy from dietary fat is also stored as body fat. Protein in the diet is used primarily to build new tissue, but it can be broken down for energy or incorporated into fat stores. Glucose, glycogen, and fat are important fuels for the production of energy in the cells; protein is a significant energy source only when other fuels are lacking. (See Chapter 8 for more on the other roles of carbohydrate, fat, and protein in the body.)

ATP: The Energy "Currency" of Cells The basic form of energy used by cells is **adenosine triphosphate,** or **ATP.** When a cell needs energy, it breaks down ATP, a process that releases energy in the only form the cell can use directly. Cells store a small amount of ATP; when they need more, they create it through chemical reactions that utilize the body's stored fuels—glucose, glycogen, and fat. When you exercise, your cells need to produce more energy. Consequently, your body mobilizes its stores of fuel to increase ATP production.

Exercise and the Three Energy Systems

The muscles in your body use three energy systems to create ATP and fuel cellular activity. These systems use different fuels and chemical processes and perform different, specific functions during exercise (Table 3.1).

The Immediate Energy System The **immediate energy system** provides energy rapidly but for only a short period of time. It is used to fuel activities that last for about 10 or fewer seconds—examples in sports include weight lifting and shot-putting; examples in daily life include rising from a chair or picking up a bag of groceries. The components of this energy system include existing cellular ATP stores and creatine phosphate (CP), a chemical that cells can use to make ATP. CP levels are depleted rapidly during exercise, so the maximum capacity of this energy system is reached within a few seconds. Cells must then switch to the other energy systems to restore levels of ATP and CP. (Without adequate ATP, muscles will stiffen and become unusable.)

The Nonoxidative (Anaerobic) Energy System The **nonoxidative energy system** is used at the start of an exercise session and for high-intensity activities lasting for about 10 seconds to 2 minutes, such as the 400-meter run. During daily activities, this system may be called on to help you run to catch a bus or dash up several flights of stairs. The nonoxidative energy system creates ATP by breaking down glucose and glycogen. This system doesn't require oxygen, which is why it is sometimes referred to as the **anaerobic** system. The capacity of this system to produce energy is limited, but it can generate a great deal of ATP in a short period of time. For this reason, it is the most important energy system for very intense exercise.

There are two key limiting factors for the nonoxidative energy system. First, the body's supply of glucose and glycogen is limited. Once these are depleted, a person may experience fatigue and dizziness, and judgment may be impaired. (The brain and nervous system rely on carbohydrates as fuel and must have a continuous supply to function properly.) Second, the nonoxidative system results in the production of **lactic acid.** Although lactic acid is an important fuel for the body, it releases substances called hydrogen ions that are thought to interfere with metabolism and muscle contraction, thereby causing fatigue. During heavy exercise, such as sprinting, the body produces large amounts of lactic acid and hydrogen ions, and muscles become fatigued rapidly. Fortunately, exercise training increases the body's ability to cope with these substances.

The Oxidative (Aerobic) Energy System The **oxidative energy system** is used during any physical activity that lasts longer than about 2 minutes, such as distance running, swimming, hiking, or even standing in line for a long time. The oxidative system requires oxygen to generate ATP, which is why it is considered an **aerobic** process. The oxidative system cannot produce energy as quickly as the other two systems, but it can supply energy for much longer periods of time. It provides energy during most daily activities.

In the oxidative energy system, ATP production takes place in cellular structures called **mitochondria.** Because mitochondria can use carbohydrates (glucose and glycogen) or fats to produce ATP, the body's stores of fuel for this system are much greater than those for the other two energy systems. The actual fuel used depends on the intensity and duration of exercise and on the fitness status of the individual. Carbohydrates are favored during more intense exercise (over 65% of maximum capacity); fats, for mild, low-intensity activities. During a prolonged exercise session, carbohydrates are the predominant fuel at the start of the workout, but fat utilization increases over time. Fit individuals use a greater proportion of fat as fuel because increased fitness allows people to do activities at lower intensities. This is an important adaptation because glycogen depletion is one of the limiting factors for the oxidative energy system. Thus, by being able to use more fat as fuel, a fit individual can exercise for a longer time before glycogen is depleted and muscles become fatigued.

Oxygen is another limiting factor. The oxygen requirement of this energy system is proportional to the intensity of exercise—as intensity increases, so does oxygen consumption. There is a limit to the body's ability to increase the transport and use of oxygen; this limit is referred to as **maximal oxygen consumption,** or $\dot{V}O_{2max}$. $\dot{V}O_{2max}$ is determined partly by genetics and partly by fitness status (the muscles' power-generating capacity and fatigue resistance). It depends on many factors, including the capacity of blood to carry oxygen, the rate at which oxygen is transported to the tissues, and the amount of oxygen that cells extract from the blood. $\dot{V}O_{2max}$ determines how intensely a person can perform endurance exercise and for how long, and it is considered the best overall measure of the capacity of the cardiorespiratory system. (The assessment tests described later in the chapter are designed to help you predict your $\dot{V}O_{2max}$.)

The Energy Systems in Combination Your body typically uses all three energy systems when you exercise. The intensity and duration of the activity determine which system predominates. For example, when you play tennis, you use the immediate energy system when hitting the ball, but you replenish cellular energy stores using the nonoxidative and oxidative systems. When cycling, the oxidative system predominates. However, if you must suddenly exercise very intensely—ride up a steep hill, for example—the other systems become important because the oxidative system is unable to supply ATP fast enough to sustain high-intensity effort.

Physical Fitness and Energy Production Physically fit people can increase their metabolic rate substantially, generating the energy needed for powerful or sustained exercise. People with lower levels of fitness cannot respond to exercise in the same way. Their bodies are less capable of delivering oxygen and fuel to exercising muscles; they are also less able to cope with lactic acid and other substances produced during intense physical activity that contribute to fatigue. Because of this, they become fatigued more rapidly—their legs hurt and they breathe heavily walking up a flight of stairs, for example. Regular physical training can substantially improve the body's ability to produce energy and meet the challenges of increased physical activity.

For many sports, one energy system will be most important. For weight lifters, for example, it is the immediate energy system; for sprinters, the nonoxidative system; and for endurance runners, the oxidative system. In designing an exercise program, focus on the energy sys-

Terms

Vw

lactic acid A metabolic acid resulting from the metabolism of glucose and glycogen; an important source of fuel for many tissues of the body, its accumulation may produce fatigue.

oxidative (aerobic) energy system Energy system that supplies energy to cells through the breakdown of glucose, glycogen, fats, and amino acids; also called the *aerobic system* because chemical reactions require oxygen.

aerobic Dependent on the presence of oxygen.

mitochondria Intracellular structures containing enzymes used in the chemical reactions that convert the energy in food to a form the body can use.

maximal oxygen consumption ($\dot{V}O_{2max}$) The highest rate of oxygen consumption an individual is capable of during maximum physical effort, reflecting the body's ability to transport and use oxygen; measured in milliliters used per minute per kilogram of body weight.

Exercise offers both long-term health benefits and immediate pleasures. Many popular sports and activities develop cardiorespiratory endurance.

tem most important to your goals. Because improving the functioning of the cardiorespiratory system is critical to overall wellness, endurance exercise that utilizes the oxidative energy system—activities performed at moderate to high intensities for a prolonged duration—is a key component of any health-related fitness program.

BENEFITS OF CARDIORESPIRATORY ENDURANCE EXERCISE

Cardiorespiratory endurance exercise helps the body become more efficient and better able to cope with physical challenges. It also lowers risk for many chronic diseases. Let's take a closer look at the physiological adaptations and long-term benefits of regular endurance exercise.

Improved Cardiorespiratory Functioning

At rest, a healthy cardiorespiratory system has little difficulty keeping pace with the body's need for oxygen, fuel, and waste removal. During exercise, however, the demands on the system increase dramatically as metabolic rate goes up. The principal cardiorespiratory responses to exercise include the following:

- Increased cardiac output and blood pressure. More blood is pumped by the heart each minute because both heart rate and stroke volume (the amount of blood pumped with each beat) go up. Increased cardiac output and blood pressure speed the delivery of oxygen and fuel and the removal of waste products.
- Increased ventilation (rate and depth of breathing).
- Increased blood flow to active skeletal muscles and to the heart; constant or slightly increased blood flow to the brain. The body controls blood pressure and blood flow by adjusting cardiac output and regulating the size of the blood vessels feeding different tissues.
- Increased blood flow to the skin and increased sweating. The chemical reactions that produce energy for exercise release heat, which must be dissipated to maintain a safe body temperature.
- Decreased blood flow to the stomach, intestines, liver, and kidneys, resulting in reduced activity in the gastrointestinal tract and reduced urine output.

All of these changes help the body respond to the challenge of exercise in the short term. When performed regularly, endurance exercise also causes more permanent adaptations. It improves the functioning of the heart, the ability of the cardiorespiratory system to carry oxygen to the body's tissues, and the capacity of the cells to take up and use oxygen. These improvements reduce the effort required to carry out everyday activities and make the body better able to respond to physical challenges.

Endurance training enhances the health of the heart by maintaining or increasing its blood and oxygen supply, decreasing work and oxygen demand of the heart, and increasing the function of the heart muscle. The trained heart is more efficient and subject to less stress. It pumps more blood per beat, so heart rate is lower at rest and during exercise. The resting heart rate of a fit person is often 10–20 beats per minute lower than that of a sedentary person; this translates into as many as 10 million fewer beats in the course of one year. Improved heart efficiency results because endurance training improves heart contraction strength, increases heart cavity size (in young adults), and increases blood volume so that the heart pushes more blood into the circulation system during each of its contractions. Training also tends to reduce blood pressure, so the heart does not have to work as hard when it contracts.

Improved Cellular Metabolism

Regular endurance exercise also improves metabolism at the cellular level. It increases the number of capillaries in the muscles so that they can be supplied with more oxygen and fuel. It also trains the muscles to make the most

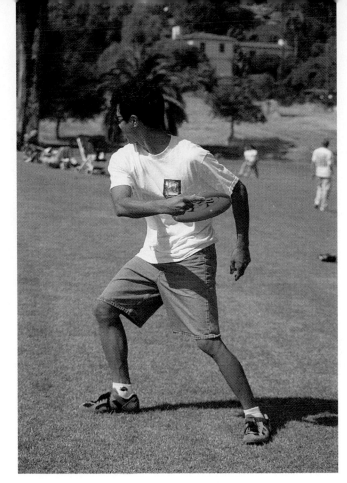

DIMENSIONS OF DIVERSITY Benefits of Exercise for Older Adults

Research has shown that most aspects of physiological functioning peak when people are about 30 years old and then decline at a rate of about 0.5–1.0% a year. This decline in physical capacity is characterized by a decrease in maximal oxygen consumption, cardiac output, muscular strength, fat-free mass, joint mobility, and other factors. However regular exercise can substantially alter the rate of decline in functional status, and it is associated with both longevity and improved quality of life.

Regular endurance exercise can improve maximal oxygen consumption in older people by up to 15–30%—the same degree of improvement seen in younger individuals. In fact, studies have shown that Masters athletes in their 70s have $\dot{V}O_{2max}$ values equivalent to those of sedentary 20-year-olds: At any age, endurance training can improve cardiorespiratory functioning, cellular metabolism, body composition, and psychological and emotional well-being. Older people who exercise regularly have better balance and greater bone density and are less likely than their sedentary peers to suffer injuries as a result of falls. Regular endurance training also substantially reduces the risk of many chronic and disabling diseases including heart disease, cancer, diabetes, and osteoporosis.

Other forms of exercise training are also beneficial for older adults. Resistance training is a safe and effective way to build strength and fat-free mass and can help people remain independent as they age. Lifting weights has also been shown to boost spirits in older people, perhaps because improvements in strength appear quickly and are easily applied to everyday tasks such as climbing stairs and carrying groceries. Flexibility exercises can improve the range of motion in joints and also help people maintain functional independence as they age.

Life expectancy in the United States has increased dramatically over the past century, and about 70% of Americans now live to at least age 70. A lifetime of regular exercise is one of the best age-proofing strategies available however, it's never too late to start. Even in people over 80, beginning an exercise program can improve physical functioning and quality of life. Most older adults are able to participate in a program that includes moderate walking and strengthening and stretching exercises, and modified programs can be created for people with chronic conditions and other special health concerns (see Chapter 7). The wellness benefits of exercise are available to people of all ages and levels of ability.

SOURCES Brooks, G. A., et al. 2000. *Exercise Physiology Human Bioenergetics and Its Applications,* 3d ed. Mountain View, Calif.: Mayfield. American College of Sports Medicine. 2001. *ACSM's Resource Manual for Guidelines for Exercise Testing and Prescription,* 4th ed. Philadelphia: Williams & Wilkins.

of available oxygen and fuel so that they work more efficiently. Exercise increases the size and number of mitochondria in muscle cells, thereby increasing the energy capacity of the cells. Endurance training also helps in energy production by preventing glycogen depletion and increasing the muscles' ability to use lactic acid and fat as fuels.

Fitness programs that best develop metabolic efficiency include both long-duration, moderately intense endurance exercise and brief periods of more intense effort. For example, climbing a small hill while jogging or cycling introduces the kind of intense exercise that leads to more efficient use of lactic acid and fats.

Regular exercise may also help protect your cells from chemical damage. Many scientists believe that aging and some chronic diseases are linked to cellular damage caused by **free radicals.** Training activates antioxidant enzymes that prevent free radical damage to cell structures, thereby enhancing health. (See Chapter 8 for more on free radicals and antioxidants.) Training also improves the functional stability of cells and tissues by improving the regulation of salts and fluids in the cells. This is particularly important in the heart, where instability can lead to cardiac arrest and death.

Reduced Risk of Chronic Disease

Regular endurance exercise lowers your risk of many chronic, disabling diseases. It can also help people with those diseases improve their health (see the box "Benefits of Exercise for Older Adults").

Cardiovascular Disease A sedentary lifestyle is one of the six major risk factors for **cardiovascular disease (CVD)** (see Chapter 11). The other primary factors are smoking, unhealthy cholesterol levels, high blood pressure, diabetes, and obesity. People who are sedentary have CVD death rates significantly higher than those of fit individuals. Cardiovascular disease usually begins to develop in childhood and adolescence; it progresses slowly over many years before producing any symptoms. Adopting healthy habits while young can help many people prevent or delay a heart attack or other serious form of CVD.

Endurance exercise has a positive effect on levels of fats in the blood. High concentrations of blood fats such as cholesterol and triglycerides are linked to cardiovascular disease because they contribute to the formation of fatty deposits on the lining of arteries. If one of the coronary arteries, which supply oxygenated blood to the heart, becomes blocked by such a deposit, the result is a heart attack; blockage of a cerebral artery can cause a stroke.

Cholesterol is carried in the blood by **lipoproteins,** which are classified according to size and density. Cholesterol carried by low-density lipoproteins (LDLs) tends to stick to the walls of arteries. High-density lipoproteins (HDLs), on the other hand, pick up excess cholesterol in the bloodstream and carry it back to the liver for excretion from the body. High LDL levels and low HDL levels are associated with a high risk of CVD. High levels of HDL and low levels of LDL are associated with lower risk. More information about cholesterol and heart disease is provided in Chapter 11. For our purposes in this chapter, it is important to know only that endurance exercise influences blood fat levels in a positive way—by increasing HDL and decreasing triglycerides (and possibly LDL)—thereby reducing the risk of CVD.

Regular exercise tends to reduce high blood pressure, a contributing factor in diseases such as **coronary heart disease,** stroke, kidney failure, and blindness. It also helps prevent obesity and diabetes, both of which contribute to CVD.

Cancer Some studies have shown a relationship between increased physical activity and a reduction in a person's risk of all types of cancer, but these findings are not conclusive. There is strong evidence that exercise reduces the risk of colon cancer and promising data that it reduces the risk of cancer of the breast and reproductive organs in women. Exercise may decrease the risk of colon cancer by speeding the movement of food through the gastrointestinal tract (quickly eliminating potential carcinogens), enhancing immune function, and reducing blood fats. The protective mechanism in the case of reproductive system cancers is less clear, but physical activity during the high school and college years may be particularly important for preventing breast cancer later in life. Some preliminary evidence also suggests that regular physical activity reduces the risk of pancreatic cancer and prostate cancer.

Diabetes Recent studies have shown that regular exercise helps prevent the development of the most common form of diabetes (see Chapter 6 for more on diabetes). Exercise burns excess sugar and makes cells more sensitive to the hormone insulin, which is involved in the regulation of blood sugar levels. Obesity is a key risk factor for diabetes, and exercise helps keep body fat at healthy levels. But even without fat loss, exercise improves control of blood sugar levels in many people with diabetes, and physical activity is an important part of treatment.

Osteoporosis A special benefit of exercise, especially for women, is protection against osteoporosis, a disease that results in loss of bone density and poor bone strength. Weight-bearing exercise helps build bone during the teens and twenties. People with denser bones can better endure the bone loss that occurs with aging. With stronger bones and muscles and better balance, fit people are less likely to experience debilitating falls and bone fractures. (See Chapter 8 for more on osteoporosis.)

Deaths from All Causes Studies of adults in the United States and Europe have found that physically fit people have a reduced risk of dying from all causes, with the greatest benefits found for people with the highest levels of fitness. These studies suggest that poor fitness is a good predictor of premature death and is as important a risk factor as smoking, high blood pressure, obesity, and diabetes.

Better Control of Body Fat

Too much body fat is linked to a variety of health problems, including CVD, cancer, and diabetes. Healthy body composition can be difficult to achieve and maintain because a diet that contains all essential nutrients can be relatively high in calories, especially for someone who is sedentary. Excess calories are stored in the body as fat. Regular exercise increases daily calorie expenditure so that a healthy diet is less likely to lead to weight gain. Endurance exercise burns calories directly and, if intense enough, continues to do so by raising resting metabolic rate for several hours following an exercise session. A higher metabolic rate means that a person can consume more calories without gaining weight.

Endurance exercise can also help maintain or increase metabolic rate slightly by helping people maintain a high proportion of fat-free mass. Strength training, discussed in Chapter 4, is even more effective at building muscle mass than endurance training. (Energy balance and the role of exercise in improving body composition are discussed in detail in Chapter 6.) However, even if regular exercise doesn't lead to significant changes in body composition, it is still extremely beneficial for wellness and has been found to help compensate for the harmful health effects of excess body fat. People with excess body fat can significantly improve health and well-being by including moderate physical activity in their daily routine.

Improved Immune Function

Exercise can have either positive or negative effects on the immune system, the physiological processes that protect us from disease. Moderate endurance exercise boosts immune function, whereas excessive training (overtraining) depresses it. Physically fit people get fewer colds and upper respiratory tract infections than people who are not fit. Exercise affects immune function by influencing levels of specialized cells and chemicals involved in the immune

Terms

Ww

free radicals Highly reactive compounds that can damage cells by taking electrons from key cellular components such as DNA or the cell membrane; produced by normal metabolic processes and through exposure to environmental factors, including sunlight.

cardiovascular disease (CVD) Disease of the heart and blood vessels.

lipoproteins Substances in blood, classified according to size, density, and chemical composition, that transport fats.

coronary heart disease Heart disease caused by the buildup of fatty deposits on the arteries that supply oxygen to the heart; also called *coronary artery disease*.

Although much of the discussion of the benefits of exercise focuses on improvements to physical wellness, many people discover that the best reason to become and stay active is the boost that regular exercise provides to the nonphysical dimensions of wellness. The following are just some of the effects of regular physical activity.

- *Reduced anxiety.* Exercise reduces symptoms of anxiety such as worry and self-doubt both in people who are anxious most of the time (trait anxiety) and in people who become anxious in response to a particular experience (state anxiety).
- *Reduced depression and improved mood.* Exercise relieves feelings of sadness and hopelessness and can be as effective as psychotherapy in treating mild-to-moderate cases of depression. Exercise improves mood and increases feelings of well-being in both depressed and nondepressed people.
- *Improved sleep.* Regular physical activity helps people fall asleep more easily; it also improves the quality of sleep, making it more restful.
- *Reduced stress.* Exercise reduces the body's overall response to all forms of stressors and helps people deal more effectively with the stress they do experience.
- *Enhanced self-esteem, self-confidence, and self-efficacy.* Exercise can boost self-esteem and self-confidence by providing opportunities for people to succeed and excel; it also improves body image (see Chapters 6 and 9). Sticking with an exercise program increases people's belief in their ability to be active, thereby increasing self-efficacy.
- *Enhanced creativity and intellectual functioning.* In studies of college students, physically active students score higher on tests of creativity than sedentary students. Exercise improves alertness and memory in the short term, and over time, exercise helps maintain reaction time, short-term memory, and nonverbal reasoning skills.
- *Increased opportunities for social interaction.* Exercise provides many opportunities for positive interaction with others.

How does exercise cause all these positive changes? A variety of mechanisms has been proposed. Physical activity stimulates the thought and emotion centers of the brain, producing improvements in mood and cognitive functioning. It increases alpha brain-wave activity, which is associated with a highly relaxed state. Exercise stimulates the release of chemicals such as **endorphins,** which may suppress fatigue, decrease pain, and produce euphoria; and phenylethylamine, which may boost energy, mood, and attention. Exercise decreases the secretion of hormones triggered by emotional stress and alters the levels of many other **neurotransmitters,** including serotonin, a brain chemical linked to mood.

Exercise also provides a distraction from stressful stimuli and an emotional outlet for feelings of stress, hostility and aggression. It relaxes and warms the body, which may improve both mood and sleep. And exercise is a fun way to spend time!

The message from all this research is that exercise is a critical factor in developing all the dimensions of wellness. A lifetime of physical activity can leave you with a healthier body and a sharper, happier, more creative mind.

response. In addition to regular moderate exercise, the immune system can be strengthened by eating a well-balanced diet, managing stress, and getting 7–8 hours of sleep every night.

Improved Psychological and Emotional Well-Being

Most people who participate in regular endurance exercise experience social, psychological, and emotional benefits. Performing physical activities provides proof of skill mastery and self-control, thus enhancing self-image. Recreational sports provide an opportunity to socialize, have fun, and strive to excel. Endurance exercise lessens anxiety, depression, stress, anger, and hostility, thereby improving mood and boosting cardiovascular health. Regular exercise also improves sleep. For more on the wellness benefits of regular endurance exercise, see the box "Exercise and the Mind."

Refer to Figure 3.3 for a summary of specific physiological benefits of cardiorespiratory endurance exercise. As cardiorespiratory fitness is developed, these benefits translate into both physical and emotional well-being and a much lower risk of chronic disease.

ASSESSING CARDIORESPIRATORY FITNESS

The body's ability to maintain a level of exertion (exercise) for an extended period of time is a direct reflection of cardiorespiratory fitness. It is determined by the body's ability to take up, distribute, and use oxygen during physical activity. As explained earlier, the best quantitative measure of cardiorespiratory endurance is maximal oxygen consumption, expressed as $\dot{V}O_{2max}$, the amount of oxygen the body uses when a person reaches maximum ability to supply oxygen during exercise (measured in milliliters of oxygen used per minute for each kilogram of body weight). Maximal oxygen consumption can be

Terms

endorphins Substances resembling morphine that are secreted by the brain and that decrease pain, suppress fatigue, and produce euphoria.

neurotransmitters Brain chemicals that transmit nerve impulses.

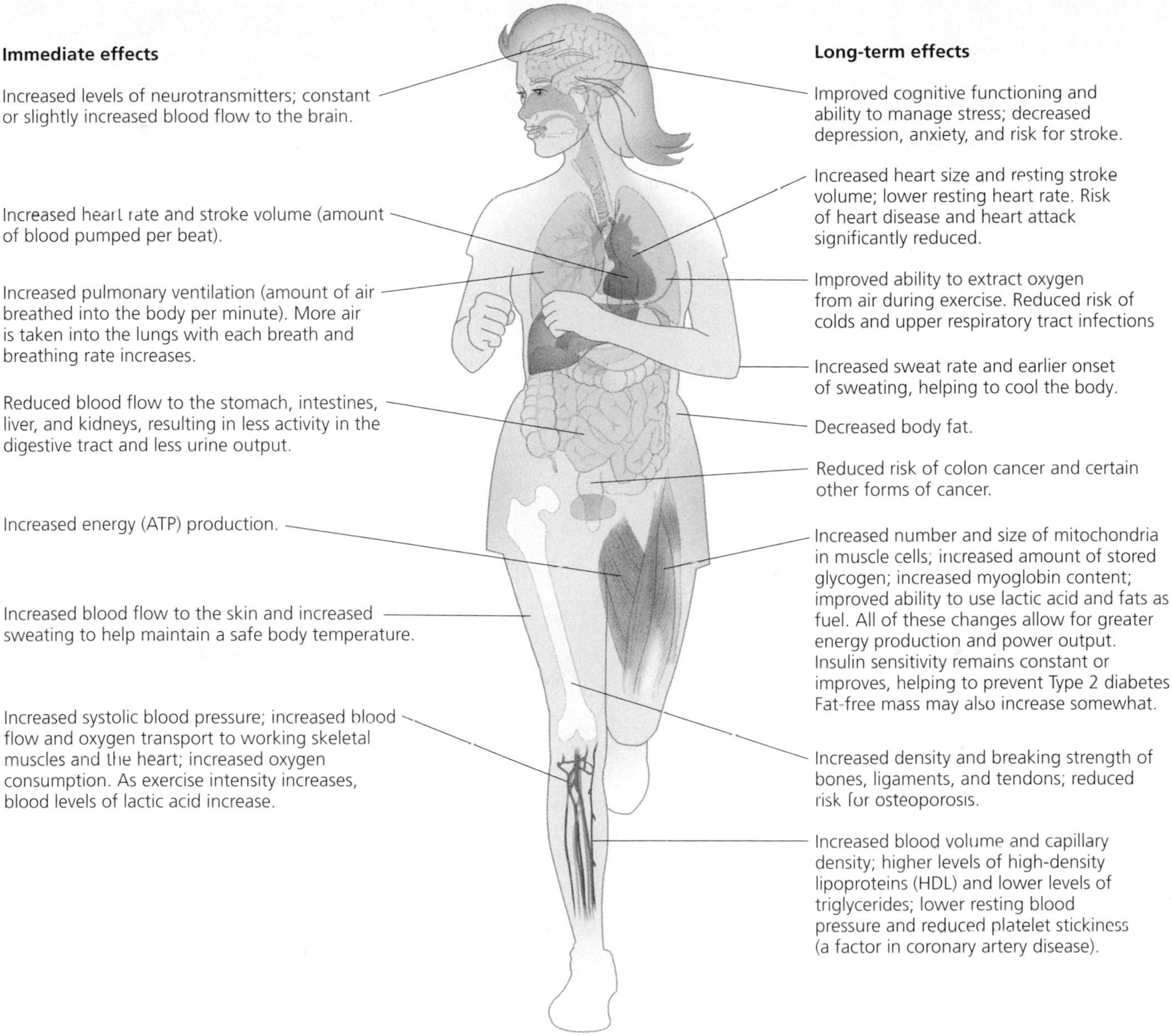

Immediate effects
Increased levels of neurotransmitters; constant or slightly increased blood flow to the brain.
Increased heart rate and stroke volume (amount of blood pumped per beat).
Increased pulmonary ventilation (amount of air breathed into the body per minute). More air is taken into the lungs with each breath and breathing rate increases.
Reduced blood flow to the stomach, intestines, liver, and kidneys, resulting in less activity in the digestive tract and less urine output.
Increased energy (ATP) production.
Increased blood flow to the skin and increased sweating to help maintain a safe body temperature.
Increased systolic blood pressure; increased blood flow and oxygen transport to working skeletal muscles and the heart; increased oxygen consumption. As exercise intensity increases, blood levels of lactic acid increase.
Long-term effects
Improved cognitive functioning and ability to manage stress; decreased depression, anxiety, and risk for stroke.
Increased heart size and resting stroke volume; lower resting heart rate. Risk of heart disease and heart attack significantly reduced.
Improved ability to extract oxygen from air during exercise. Reduced risk of colds and upper respiratory tract infections
Increased sweat rate and earlier onset of sweating, helping to cool the body.
Decreased body fat.
Reduced risk of colon cancer and certain other forms of cancer.
Increased number and size of mitochondria in muscle cells; increased amount of stored glycogen; increased myoglobin content; improved ability to use lactic acid and fats as fuel. All of these changes allow for greater energy production and power output. Insulin sensitivity remains constant or improves, helping to prevent Type 2 diabetes Fat-free mass may also increase somewhat.
Increased density and breaking strength of bones, ligaments, and tendons; reduced risk for osteoporosis.
Increased blood volume and capillary density; higher levels of high-density lipoproteins (HDL) and lower levels of triglycerides; lower resting blood pressure and reduced platelet stickiness (a factor in coronary artery disease).

Figure 3.3 Immediate and long-term effects of regular cardiorespiratory endurance exercise. When endurance exercise is performed regularly, short-term changes in the body develop into more permanent adaptations; these include improved ability to exercise, reduced risk of many chronic diseases, and improved psychological and emotional well-being.

measured precisely in an exercise physiology laboratory through analysis of the air a person inhales and exhales when exercising to a level of exhaustion (maximum intensity). This procedure can be expensive and time-consuming, making it impractical for the average person.

Four Assessment Tests

Fortunately, several simple assessment tests provide reasonably good estimates of maximal oxygen consumption (within $\pm$10–15% of the results of a laboratory test). Four methods are described here and presented in Lab 3.1: a 1-mile walk test, a 3-minute step test, a 1.5-mile run-walk test, and the Åstrand-Rhyming cycle ergometer test. To assess yourself, choose among these methods based on your access to equipment, your current physical condition, and your own preference. Don't take any of these tests without checking with your physician if you are ill or have any of the risk factors for exercise discussed in Chapter 2 and Lab 2.2. Table 3.2 on p. 58 lists the fitness prerequisites and cautions recommended for each test.

- *The 1-Mile Walk Test.* The 1-mile walk test estimates your level of cardiorespiratory fitness (maximal oxygen consumption) based on the amount of time it takes you to complete 1 mile of brisk walking and your exercise heart rate at the end of your walk. A fast time and a

Table 3.2 *Fitness Prerequisites and Cautions for the Cardiorespiratory Endurance Assessment Tests*

Note: The conditions for exercise safety given in Chapter 2 apply to all fitness assessment tests. If you answered yes to any question on the PAR-Q in Lab 2.2, see your physician before taking any assessment test. If you experience any unusual symptoms while taking a test, stop exercising and discuss your condition with your instructor.

Test	Fitness Prerequisites/Cautions
1-mile walk test	Recommended for anyone who meets the criteria for safe exercise. Can be used by individuals who cannot perform other tests because of low fitness level or injury.
3-minute step test	If you suffer from joint problems in your ankles, knees, or hips or you are significantly overweight, check with your physician before taking this test.
1.5-mile run-walk test	Recommended for people who are healthy and at least moderately active. If you have been sedentary, you should participate in a 4- to 8-week walk-run program before taking the test. Don't take this test in extremely hot or cold weather if you aren't used to exercising under those conditions.
Åstrand-Rhyming test	Recommended for people who are healthy and at least moderately active. It can be taken by people with some joint problems because body weight is supported by the cycle.

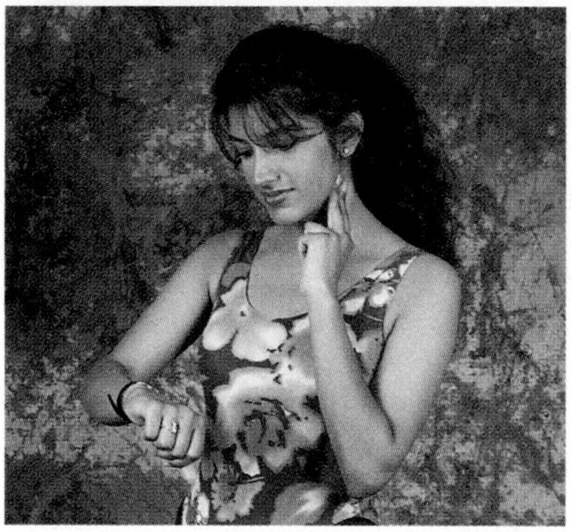

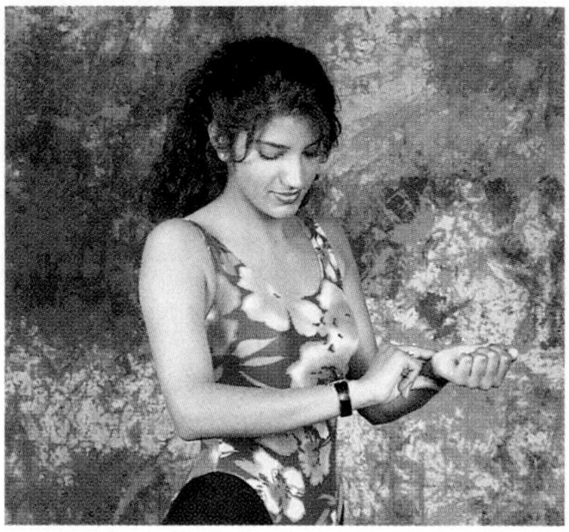

A pulse count can be used to determine exercise heart rate. The pulse can be taken at the carotid artery in the neck (left) or at the radial artery in the wrist (right).

low heart rate indicate a high level of cardiorespiratory endurance.

- *The 3-Minute Step Test.* The rate at which the pulse returns to normal after exercise is also a good measure of cardiorespiratory capacity; heart rate remains lower and recovers faster in people who are more physically fit. For the step test, you step continually at a steady rate and then monitor your heart rate during recovery.
- *The 1.5-Mile Run-Walk Test.* Oxygen consumption increases with speed in distance running, so a fast time on this test indicates high maximal oxygen consumption.
- *The Åstrand-Rhyming Cycle Ergometer Test.* This test estimates maximal oxygen consumption from the exercise heart rate reached after pedaling a cycle ergometer for 6 minutes at a constant rate and resistance (power output). A low exercise heart rate after pedaling at a high power output indicates a high maximal oxygen consumption.

Monitoring Your Heart Rate

Each time your heart beats, it pumps blood into your arteries; this surge of blood causes a pulse that you can feel by holding your fingers against an artery. Counting your pulse to determine your exercise heart rate is a key part of most assessment tests for maximal oxygen consumption. Heart rate can also be used to monitor exercise intensity during a workout. (Intensity is described in more detail in the next section.)

The two most common sites for monitoring heart rate are the carotid artery in the neck and the radial artery in the wrist. To take your pulse, press your index and middle fingers gently on the correct site. You may have to shift position several times to find the best place to feel your pulse. Don't use your thumb to check your pulse; it has a pulse of its own that can confuse your count. Be careful not to push too hard, particularly when taking your pulse in the carotid artery (strong pressure on this artery may cause a reflex that slows the heart rate).

Heart rates are usually assessed in beats per minute (bpm). But counting your pulse for an entire minute isn't practical when you're exercising. And because heart rate slows rapidly when you stop exercising, it can give inaccurate results. It's best to do a shorter count—10 seconds—and then multiply the result by 6 to get your heart rate in beats per minute. The same procedure can be used to take someone else's pulse, as in the cycle ergometer test.

Interpreting Your Score

Once you've completed one or more of the assessment tests, use the table under "Rating Your Cardiovascular Fitness" at the end of Lab 3.1 to determine your current level of cardiorespiratory fitness. As you interpret your score, remember that field tests of cardiorespiratory fitness are not precise scientific measurements and do have a 10–15% margin of error.

You can use the assessment tests to monitor the progress of your fitness program by retesting yourself from time to time. Always compare scores for the *same* test: Your scores on different tests may vary considerably because of differences in skill and motivation and weaknesses in the tests themselves.

Ww DEVELOPING A CARDIORESPIRATORY ENDURANCE PROGRAM

Cardiorespiratory endurance exercises are best for developing the type of fitness associated with good health, so they should serve as the focus of your exercise program. To create a successful endurance exercise program, you must set realistic goals; choose suitable activities; set your starting frequency, intensity, and duration of exercise at appropriate levels; remember to warm up and cool down; and adjust your program as your fitness improves.

Setting Goals

You can use the results of cardiorespiratory fitness assessment tests to set a specific oxygen consumption goal for your cardiorespiratory endurance program. Your goal should be high enough to ensure a healthy cardiorespiratory system, but not so high that it will be impossible to achieve. Scores in the fair and good ranges for maximal oxygen consumption suggest good fitness; scores in the excellent and superior ranges indicate a high standard of physical performance.

Through endurance training, an individual may be able to improve maximal oxygen consumption ($\dot{V}O_{2max}$) by about 10–30%. The amount of improvement possible depends on age, health status, and initial fitness level; people who start at a very low fitness level can improve by a greater percentage than elite athletes because the latter are already at a much higher fitness level, a level that may approach their genetic physical limits. If you are tracking $\dot{V}O_{2max}$ using the field tests described in this chapter, you may be able to increase your score by more than 30% due to improvements in other physical factors, such as muscle power, which can affect your performance on the tests.

Another physical factor you can track to monitor progress is resting heart rate—your heart rate at complete rest, measured in the morning before you get out of bed and move around. Resting heart rate may decrease by as much as 10–15 beats per minute in response to endurance training. Changes in resting heart rate may be noticeable after only about 4–6 weeks of training.

You may want to set other types of goals for your fitness program. For example, if you walk, jog, or cycle as part of your fitness program, you may want to set a time or distance goal—working up to walking 5 miles in one session, completing a 4-mile run in 28 minutes, or cycling a total of 35 miles per week. A more modest goal might be to achieve the Surgeon General's minimum activity level of doing at least 30 minutes of moderate activity on most days. Although it's best to base your program on measurable goals, you may also want to set some more qualitative goals, such as becoming more energetic, sleeping better, and improving the fit of your clothes.

Choosing Sports and Activities

Cardiorespiratory endurance exercises include activities that involve the rhythmic use of large-muscle groups for an extended period of time, such as jogging, walking, cycling, aerobic dancing and other forms of group exercise, cross-country skiing, and swimming. Start-and-stop sports, such as tennis and racquetball, also qualify, as long as you have enough skill to play continuously and intensely enough to raise your heart rate to target levels.

Having fun is a strong motivator; select a physical activity that you enjoy, and it will be easier to stay with your program. Exercising with a friend can also be helpful as a motivator. Consider whether you prefer competitive or individual sports, or whether starting something new would be best. Other important considerations are access to facilities, expense, equipment, and the time required to achieve an adequate skill level and workout (see the box "Evaluating Home Exercise Equipment," p. 60).

Determining Frequency of Training

To build cardiorespiratory endurance, you should exercise 3–5 days per week. Beginners should start with 3 and work up to 5 days per week. Training more than 5 days per week can lead to injury and isn't necessary for

CRITICAL CONSUMER Evaluating Home Exercise Equipment

Does your exercise program include a piece of home fitness equipment such as a treadmill or stationary cycle? Good equipment can enhance your enjoyment of your fitness program and decrease your risk of injury. Before considering any piece of equipment, ask yourself the following questions:

- *Will the equipment help me achieve my fitness goals?* Make sure the piece of equipment you're considering works your target fitness components. Don't be fooled by outrageous advertising claims, and be sure to check the fine print of any advertisement. Exercise is not "easy" or "effortless," and it is impossible for any equipment to make you lose fat in a particular area (spot reduce). The Federal Trade Commission provides good general advice for people shopping for exercise equipment (http://www.ftc.gov).
- *Will I really use the equipment regularly?* Before you invest money in a piece of equipment, try it out for a time at a fitness center or health club. Make sure it is something you can use safely and comfortably over the long term.
- *Is the equipment well made?* Before you buy, do some research. Ask coaches and fitness instructors, and check consumer publications. If you intend to push the equipment to the limit, look for a heavy-duty model.
- *Is the equipment easy to use?* You will be more likely to use a piece of equipment regularly if it is easy to set up and use. Any instructions should be easy to follow.
- *Do I have room for the equipment?* A good treadmill or home gym may be large and require significant space to use and store. Make sure you have a place to use it that is pleasant and well ventilated and where any noise produced by the equipment will not be a problem.
- *Can I afford a quality piece of equipment?* Shop around to find the best deal; try discount stores, specialty shops, and catalogs. However, be aware of deals that seem too good to be true; an exceptionally low price may indicate poor quality. In addition, get the details on warranties, guarantees, and return policies before you buy.

The following are among the most popular types of home exercise equipment:

Treadmills: Choose a motorized treadmill with a platform or surface that is large enough to fit your stride, stable enough to accommodate your weight, and cushioned enough to absorb the impact of your feet. The handrails should be able to support your weight if you lose your balance.

Stationary cycles: Try both upright and recumbent (reclining) models to see which type suits you best. Check to make sure the seat and handlebars of the cycle can be adjusted to comfortably fit your height and leg extension. Look for a model whose resistance can be changed easily.

Cross-country ski machines: Although learning to coordinate the movements needed to use a cross-country ski machine may take time, this type of equipment typically provides a full-body workout. Look for a model that allows separate adjustment of the lower-body sliding footpads and the upper-body rope-and-pulley device.

Stair climbers: Check to be sure that you can work the pedals securely and smoothly while maintaining good posture; machines with independent foot action usually allow a more natural rhythm. For greater durability, choose a machine with hydraulic rather than air-filled shock absorbers.

Another key piece of equipment for many fitness activities and sports is proper footwear; refer to Chapter 7 for advice on shopping for athletic shoes.

the typical person on an exercise program designed to promote wellness. Training fewer than 3 days per week makes it difficult to improve your fitness (unless exercise intensity is very high) or to use exercise to lose weight. In addition, you risk injury because your body never gets a chance to fully adapt to regular exercise training.

Terms

target heart rate zone The range of heart rates that should be reached and maintained during cardiorespiratory endurance exercise to obtain training effects.

heart rate reserve The difference between maximum heart rate and resting heart rate; used in one method for calculating target heart rate range.

ratings of perceived exertion (RPE) A system of monitoring exercise intensity based on assigning a number to the subjective perception of target intensity.

Determining Intensity of Training

Intensity is the most important factor in achieving training effects. You must exercise intensely enough to stress your body so that fitness improves. Two methods of monitoring exercise intensity are described below; choose the method that works best for you. Be sure to make adjustments in your intensity levels for environmental or individual factors. For example, on a hot and humid day or on your first day back to your program after an illness, you should decrease your intensity level.

Target Heart Rate Zone One of the best ways to monitor the intensity of cardiorespiratory endurance exercise is to measure your heart rate. It isn't necessary to exercise at your maximum heart rate to improve maximal oxygen consumption. Fitness adaptations occur at lower heart rates with a much lower risk of injury.

According to the American College of Sports Medicine, your **target heart rate zone**—rates at which you should exercise to experience cardiorespiratory benefits—is between 65% and 90% of your maximum heart rate. To calculate your target heart rate zone, follow these steps:

1. Estimate your maximum heart rate (MHR) by subtracting your age from 220, or have it measured precisely by undergoing an exercise stress test in a doctor's office, hospital, or sports medicine lab.
2. Multiply your MHR by 65% and 90% to calculate your target heart rate zone. (Note: Very unfit people should use 55% of MHR for their training threshold.)

For example, a 19-year-old would calculate her target heart rate zone as follows:

MHR = 220 − 19 = 201

65% training intensity = 0.65 × 201 = 131 bpm

90% training intensity = 0.90 × 201 = 181 bpm

To gain fitness benefits, the young woman in our example would have to exercise at an intensity that raises her heart rate to between 131 and 181 bpm.

An alternative method for calculating target heart rate range uses **heart rate reserve,** the difference between maximum heart rate and resting heart rate. Using this method, target heart rate is equal to resting heart rate plus between 50% (40% for very unfit people) and 85% of heart rate reserve. Although some people will obtain more accurate results using this more complex method, both methods provide reasonable estimates of an appropriate target heart rate zone. Formulas for both methods of calculating target heart rate are given in Lab 3.2.

If you have been sedentary, start by exercising at the lower end of your target heart rate range (65% of maximum heart rate or 50% of heart rate reserve) for at least 4–6 weeks. Fast and significant gains in maximal oxygen consumption can be made by exercising closer to the top of the range, but you may increase your risk of injury and overtraining. You *can* achieve significant health benefits by exercising at the bottom of your target range, so don't feel pressured into exercising at an unnecessarily intense level. If you exercise at a lower intensity, you can increase the duration or frequency of training to obtain as much benefit to your health, as long as you are above the 65% training threshold. (For people with a very low initial level of fitness, a lower training intensity, 55–64% of maximum heart rate or 40–49% of heart rate reserve, may be sufficient to achieve improvements in maximal oxygen consumption, especially at the start of an exercise program. Intensities of 70–85% of maximum heart rate are appropriate for average individuals.)

By monitoring your heart rate, you will always know if you are working hard enough to improve, not hard enough, or too hard. To monitor your heart rate during exercise, count your pulse while you're still moving or immediately after you stop exercising. Count beats for 10 seconds, and then multiply that number by 6 to see if your heart rate is in your target zone. If the young woman in our example were aiming for 144 bpm, she would want a 10-second count of 24 beats.

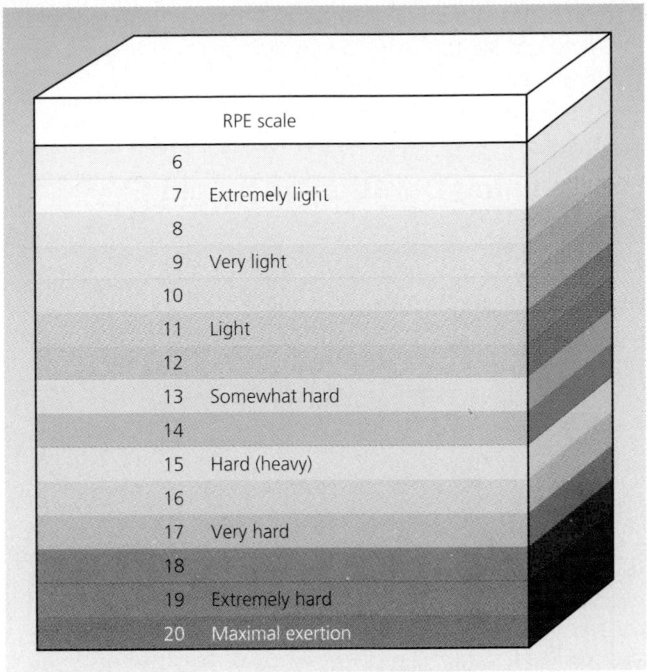

Figure 3.4 Ratings of perceived exertion (RPE). Experienced exercisers may use this subjective scale to estimate how near they are to their target heart rate zone. The scale was developed in the 1950s by Swedish exercise physiologist Gunnar Borg and is also known as the Borg scale. SOURCE: From *Psychology from Research to Practice,* edited by H. L. Pick. Reprinted with permission from Kluwer Academic/Plenum Publishing Corporation.

Ratings of Perceived Exertion Another way to monitor intensity is to monitor your perceived level of exertion. Repeated pulse counting during exercise can become a nuisance if it interferes with the activity. As your exercise program progresses, you will probably become familiar with the amount of exertion required to raise your heart rate to target levels. In other words, you will know how you feel when you have exercised intensely enough. If this is the case, you can use the scale of **ratings of perceived exertion (RPE)** shown in Figure 3.4 to monitor the intensity of your exercise session without checking your pulse.

To use the RPE scale, select a rating that corresponds to your subjective perception of how hard you are exercising when you are training in your target heart rate zone. If your target zone is about 135–155 bpm, exercise intensely enough to raise your heart rate to that level, and then associate a rating—for example, "somewhat hard" or "hard" (14 or 15)—with how hard you feel you are working. To reach and maintain intensity in future workouts, exercise hard enough to reach what you feel is the same level of exertion. You should periodically check your RPE against your target heart rate zone to make sure it's correct.

Research has shown RPE to be an accurate means of monitoring exercise intensity, and you may find it more convenient than pulse counting.

Determining Duration of Training

A total duration of 20–60 minutes is recommended; exercise can take place in a single session or in multiple sessions lasting 10 or more minutes. The total duration of exercise depends on its intensity. To improve cardiorespiratory endurance during a low-to-moderate-intensity activity such as walking or slow swimming, you should exercise for 45–60 minutes. For high-intensity exercise performed at the top of your target heart rate zone, a duration of 20 minutes is sufficient. Some studies have shown that 5–10 minutes of extremely intense exercise (greater than 90% of maximal oxygen consumption) improves cardiorespiratory endurance. However, training at this intensity, particularly during high-impact activities, increases the risk of injury. Also, because of the discomfort of high-intensity exercise, you are more likely to discontinue your exercise program. Longer-duration, low-to-moderate-intensity activities generally result in more gradual gains in maximal oxygen consumption. In planning your program, start with less vigorous activities and gradually increase intensity.

Warming Up and Cooling Down

It's important to warm up before every session of cardiorespiratory endurance exercise and to cool down afterward. Because the body's muscles work better when their temperature is slightly above resting level, warming up enhances performance and decreases the chance of injury. It gives the body time to redirect blood to active muscles and the heart time to adapt to increased demands. Warming up also helps spread **synovial fluid** throughout the joints, which helps protect their surfaces from injury.

As mentioned in Chapter 2, a warm-up session should include low-intensity movements similar to those in the activity that will follow. Low-intensity movements include walking slowly before beginning a brisk walk, hitting forehands and backhands before a tennis match, and running a 12-minute mile before progressing to an 8-minute one. An active warm-up of 5–10 minutes is adequate for most types of exercise. Some experts also recommend including stretching exercises in your warm-up; however, it's best to stretch after your body temperature has been elevated by the active part of the warm-up (see Chapter 5).

Terms
Ww

synovial fluid Fluid found within many joints that provides lubrication and nutrition to the cells of the joint surface.

Cooling down after exercise is important for returning the body to a nonexercising state. A cool-down helps maintain blood flow to the heart and brain and redirects blood from working muscles to other areas of the body; it helps prevent a large drop in blood pressure, dizziness, and other potential cardiovascular complications. A cool-down, consisting of 5–10 minutes of reduced activity, should follow every workout to allow heart rate, breathing, and circulation to return to normal. Stretching exercise can be part of a cool-down.

The general pattern of a safe and successful workout for cardiorespiratory fitness is illustrated in Figure 3.5.

Building Cardiorespiratory Fitness

Building fitness is as much an art as a science. Your rate of progress will depend on your age, health status, initial level of fitness, and motivation. Your fitness improves when you overload your body. However, you must increase the intensity, frequency, and duration of exercise carefully to avoid injury and overtraining.

For the initial phase of your program, which may last anywhere from 3 to 6 weeks, exercise at the low end of your target heart rate zone. Begin with a frequency of 3–4 days per week, and choose a duration appropriate for your fitness level: 12–15 minutes if you are very unfit, 20 minutes if you are sedentary but otherwise healthy, and 30–40 minutes if you are an experienced exerciser. Use this phase of your program to allow both your body and your schedule to adjust to your new exercise routine. Once you can exercise at the upper levels of frequency (4–5 days per week) and duration (30–40 minutes) without excessive fatigue or muscle soreness, you are ready to progress.

The next phase of your program is the improvement phase, lasting from 4 to 6 months. During this phase, slowly and gradually increase the amount of overload until you reach your target level of fitness (see the sample training progression in Table 3.3). Take care not to increase overload too quickly. It is usually best to avoid increasing intensity and duration during the same session or all three training variables in one week. Increasing duration in increments of 5–10 minutes every 2–3 weeks is usually appropriate. Signs of a too rapid progression in overload include muscles aches and pains, lack of usual interest in exercise, extreme fatigue, and inability to complete a workout. Keep an exercise log or training diary to help monitor your workouts and progress.

Maintaining Cardiorespiratory Fitness

You will not improve your fitness indefinitely. The more fit you become, the harder you have to work to improve. There are limits to the level of fitness you can achieve, and if you increase intensity and duration indefinitely, you are

Table 3.3 *Sample Progression for an Endurance Program*

Stage/Week	Frequency (days/week)	Duration (minutes)	Intensity* (beats/minute)
Initial stage			
1	3	20	120–135
2	3	25	120–135
3	4	25	135–150
4	4	30	135–150
Improvement stage			
5–7	3–4	25–30	150–160
8–10	3–4	30–35	150–160
11–13	3–4	30–35	155–170
14–16	4–5	30–35	155–170
17–20	4–5	35–40	155–170
21–24	4–5	35–40	160–180
Maintenance stage			
25+	3–5	30–45	160–180

*The target heart rates shown here are based on calculations for a healthy 20-year-old; the program progresses from an initial target heart rate of 60% to a maintenance range of 80–90% of maximum heart rate.

SOURCE: Adapted from American College of Sports Medicine. 2000. *ACSM's Guidelines for Exercise Testing and Prescription,* 6th. ed. Philadelphia: Lippincott Williams & Wilkins. Reprinted with permission from the publisher.

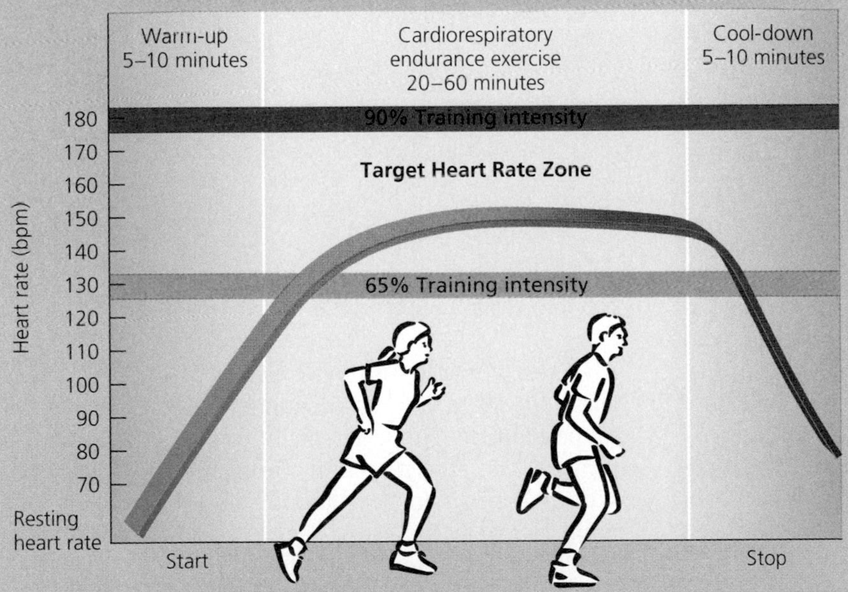

Type of activity: Cardiorespiratory endurance exercises, such as walking, jogging, biking, swimming, cross-country skiing, and rope skipping

Frequency: 3–5 days per week

Intensity: 55/65–90% of maximum heart rate, 40/50–85% of heart rate reserve plus resting heart rate, or an RPE rating of about 12–17 (lower intensities—55–64% of maximum heart rate and 40–49% of heart rate reserve—are applicable to people who are quite unfit; for average individuals, intensities of 70–85% of maximum heart rate are appropriate)

Duration: 20–60 minutes (one session or multiple sessions lasting 10 or more minutes)

Figure 3.5 A cardiorespiratory endurance workout. Longer-duration exercise at lower intensities can often be as beneficial for promoting health as shorter-duration, high-intensity exercise.

Table 3.4 Care of Common Exercise Injuries and Discomforts

Injury	Symptoms	Treatment
Blister	Accumulation of fluid in one spot under the skin	Don't pop or drain it unless it interferes too much with your daily activities. If it does pop, clean the area with antiseptic and cover with a bandage. Do not remove the skin covering the blister.
Bruise (contusion)	Pain, swelling, and discoloration	R-I-C-E: rest, ice, compression, elevation.
Fractures and dislocations	Pain, swelling, tenderness, loss of function, and deformity	Seek medical attention, immobilize the affected area, and apply cold.
Joint sprain	Pain, tenderness, swelling, discoloration, and loss of function	R-I-C-E. Apply heat when swelling has disappeared. Stretch and strengthen affected area.
Muscle cramp	Painful, spasmodic muscle contractions	Gently stretch for 15–30 seconds at a time and/or massage the cramped area. Drink fluids and increase dietary salt intake if exercising in hot weather.
Muscle soreness or stiffness	Pain and tenderness in the affected muscle	Stretch the affected muscle gently; exercise at a low intensity; apply heat. Nonsteroidal anti-inflammatory drugs, such as ibuprofen, help some people.
Muscle strain	Pain, tenderness, swelling, and loss of strength in the affected muscle	R-I-C-E; apply heat when swelling has disappeared. Stretch and strengthen the affected area.
Shin splints	Pain and tenderness on the front of the lower leg; sometimes also pain in the calf muscle	Rest; apply ice to the affected area several times a day and before exercise; wrap with tape for support. Stretch and strengthen muscles in the lower legs. Purchase good-quality footwear and run on soft surfaces.
Side stitch	Pain on the side of the abdomen	Stretch the arm on the affected side as high as possible; if that doesn't help, try bending forward while tightening the abdominal muscles.
Tendinitis	Pain, swelling, and tenderness of the affected area	R-I-C-E; apply heat when swelling has disappeared. Stretch and strengthen the affected area.

likely to become injured or overtrained. After a progression phase of 4–6 months, you may reach your goal of an acceptable level of fitness. You can then maintain fitness by continuing to exercise at the same intensity at least 3 nonconsecutive days every week. If you stop exercising, you lose your gains in fitness fairly rapidly. If you take time off for any reason, start your program again at a lower level and rebuild your fitness in a slow and systematic way.

When you reach the maintenance phase, you may want to set new goals for your program and make some adjustments to maintain your motivation. Adding variety to your program can be a helpful strategy. Engaging in multiple types of endurance activities, an approach known as cross-training, can help boost enjoyment and prevent some types of injuries. For example, someone who has been jogging 5 days a week may change her program so that she jogs 3 days a week, plays tennis 1 day a week, and goes for a bike ride 1 day a week.

EXERCISE INJURIES

Even the most careful physically active person can suffer an injury. Most injuries are annoying rather than serious or permanent. However, an injury that isn't cared for properly can escalate into a chronic problem, sometimes serious enough to permanently curtail the activity. It's important to learn how to deal with injuries so they don't derail your fitness program. Strategies for the care of common exercise injuries and discomforts appear in Table 3.4; some general guidelines are given below.

When to Call a Physician

Some injuries require medical attention. Consult a physician for head and eye injuries, possible ligament injuries, broken bones, and internal disorders such as chest pain, fainting, elevated body temperature, and intolerance to hot weather. Also seek medical attention for ostensibly

TAKE CHARGE Rehabilitation Following a Minor Athletic Injury

1. Reduce the initial inflammation using the R-I-C-E principle:

Rest: Stop using the injured area as soon as you experience pain. Avoid any activity that causes pain.

Ice: Apply ice to the injured area to reduce swelling and alleviate pain. Apply ice immediately for 10–20 minutes and repeat every few hours until the swelling disappears. Let the injured part return to normal temperature between icings, and do not apply ice to one area for more than 20 minutes. An easy method for applying ice is to freeze water in a paper cup, peel some of the paper away, and rub the exposed ice on the injured area. If the injured area is large, you can surround it with several bags of crushed ice or ice cubes, or bags of frozen vegetables. Place a thin towel between the bag and your skin. If you use a cold gel pack, limit application time to 10 minutes.

Compression: Wrap the injured area firmly with an elastic or compression bandage between icings. If the area starts throbbing or begins to change color, the bandage may be wrapped too tightly. Do not sleep with the wrap on.

Elevation: Raise the injured area above heart level to decrease the blood supply and reduce swelling. Use pillows, books, or a low chair or stool to raise the injured area.

2. After 36–48 hours, apply heat *if the swelling has completely disappeared.* Immerse the affected area in warm water or apply warm compresses, a hot water bottle, or a heating pad. As soon as it's comfortable, begin moving the affected joints slowly. If you feel pain, or if the injured area begins to swell again, reduce the amount of movement. Continue stretching and moving the affected area until you have regained normal range of motion.

3. Gradually begin exercising the injured area to build strength and endurance. Depending on the type of injury, weight training, walking, and resistance training with a partner can all be effective.

4. Gradually reintroduce the stress of an activity until you can return to full intensity. Don't progress too rapidly or you'll reinjure yourself. Before returning to full exercise participation, you should have a full range of motion in your joints, normal strength and balance among your muscles, normal coordinated patterns of movement (with no injury compensation movements, such as limping), and little or no pain.

minor injuries that do not get better within a reasonable amount of time. You may need to modify your exercise program for a few weeks to allow an injury to heal.

Managing Minor Exercise Injuries

For minor cuts and scrapes, stop the bleeding and clean the wound. Treat injuries to soft tissue (muscles and joints) immediately with rest and ice packs. Elevate the affected part of the body, and compress it with an elastic bandage to minimize swelling. Apply ice regularly for 36–48 hours after an injury occurs or until all the swelling is gone. (Don't leave ice on one spot for more than 20 minutes.) Some experts also recommend taking an over-the-counter medication such as aspirin, ibuprofen, or naproxen to decrease inflammation.

Don't apply heat to an injury at first, because heat draws blood to the area and increases swelling. After the swelling has subsided, apply either moist heat (hot towels, heat packs, warm water immersion) or dry heat (heating pads) to speed up healing.

To rehabilitate your body, follow the steps listed in the box "Rehabilitation Following a Minor Athletic Injury."

Preventing Injuries

The best method for dealing with exercise injuries is to prevent them. If you choose activities for your program carefully and follow the training guidelines described here and in Chapter 2, you should be able to avoid most types of injuries. Important guidelines for preventing athletic injuries include the following:

- Train regularly and stay in condition.
- Gradually increase the intensity, duration, or frequency of your workouts.
- Avoid or minimize high-impact activities; alternate them with low-impact activities.
- Get proper rest between exercise sessions.
- Drink plenty of fluids.
- Warm up thoroughly before you exercise and cool down afterward.
- Achieve and maintain a good level of flexibility.
- Use proper body mechanics when lifting objects or executing sports skills.
- Don't exercise when you are ill or overtrained.
- Use proper equipment, particularly shoes, and choose an appropriate exercise surface. If you exercise on a grass field, soft track, or wooden floor, you are less likely to be injured than on concrete or a hard track.
- Don't return to your normal exercise program until your athletic injuries have healed. Restart your program at a lower intensity and gradually increase the amount of overload.

COMMON QUESTIONS ANSWERED

What kind of clothing should I wear during exercise? Exercise clothing should be comfortable, let you move freely, and allow your body to cool itself. Avoid clothing that constricts normal blood flow or is made from nylon or rubberized fabrics that prevent evaporation of perspiration. Cotton is an excellent material for facilitating the evaporation of sweat. If you sweat heavily when you exercise and find that too much moisture accumulates in cotton clothing, try fabrics containing synthetic materials such as polypropylene that wick moisture away from the skin. Socks made with moisture-wicking compounds may be particularly helpful for people whose feet sweat heavily.

Do I need a special diet for my endurance exercise program? No. For most people, a nutritionally balanced diet contains all the energy and nutrients needed to sustain an exercise program. Don't waste your money on unnecessary vitamins, minerals, and protein supplements, (Chapter 8 has information about putting together a healthy diet.)

Should I drink extra fluids before or during exercise? Yes. Your body depends on water to carry out many chemical reactions and to regulate body temperature. Sweating during exercise depletes your body's water supply and can lead to dehydration if fluids aren't replaced. Serious dehydration can cause reduced blood volume, increased heart rate, elevated body temperature, muscle cramps, heat stroke, and even death. Drinking water before and during exercise is important to prevent dehydration and enhance your performance.

Thirst alone isn't a good indication of how much you need to drink because one's sense of thirst is quickly depressed by drinking even small amounts of water. As a rule of thumb, drink 2 cups (16 ounces) of fluid 2 hours before exercise and then drink enough during exercise to match fluid losses in sweat. Drink at least 1 cup of fluid for every 20–30 minutes of exercise, more in hot weather or if you sweat heavily. To determine if you're drinking enough fluid, weigh yourself before and after an exercise session; any weight loss is due to fluid loss that needs to be replaced. Bring a water bottle when you exercise so you can replace your fluids while they're being depleted. Water, preferably cold, and diluted carbohydrate drinks are the best fluid replacements. (See Chapter 8 for more on diet and fluid recommendations for active people.)

Should I use a heart rate monitor to keep track of exercise intensity? Electronic heart rate monitors, which are relatively accurate and inexpensive, can help you stay within your target heart rate range. If very close tracking of heart rate is important in your program, you may find a monitor to be helpful. However, other measures of exercise intensity also work well, including pulse taking and RPE. An even simpler, although less accurate, method is the talk test: If you can comfortably carry on a conversation, you are probably exercising at a low to moderate intensity; if you can't finish a sentence without taking a breath, you are probably exercising at a moderate to high intensity (about 70% of maximum heart rate for most people).

Will interval training develop cardiorespiratory endurance (CRE)? Interval training refers to short bouts of high-intensity exercise alternated with short periods of rest or light activity. An example of a workout based on interval training is a 400-meter run followed by a 200-meter walk, with the cycle repeated two to ten times. You will develop CRE more quickly doing interval training. However, intervals are also more uncomfortable and increase your risk of injury and overtraining. Don't perform interval training more than 2–3 days per week.

Is it all right to participate in cardiorespiratory endurance exercise while menstruating? Yes. There is no evidence that exercise during menstruation is unhealthy or that it has negative effects on performance. If you have headaches, backaches,

(continued)

Tips for Today

Good cardiorespiratory fitness is essential for a long and healthy life. It also provides many immediate benefits that span all the dimensions of wellness—improved mood, better sleep, greater creativity, and fewer colds, to name just a few. The good news is that you don't have to be an elite athlete to enjoy these benefits. Regular, moderate exercise, even in short bouts spread through the day, can build and maintain cardiorespiratory fitness.

Right now you can

- Make a list of five benefits of endurance exercise that are particularly meaningful to you. Put the list on your mirror and use it as motivational tool for beginning and maintaining your fitness program.
- If you have physical activity planned for later in the day, drink some fluids now to make sure you are fully hydrated for your workout.
- Consider the exercise equipment, including shoes, you currently have on hand. If you'll need new equipment to begin your program, check the phone book, campus store, Internet, and other resources to start gathering the information you'll need to get the best equipment you can afford.
- Think of someone you know who engages in regular endurance exercise. Call or e-mail that person and ask what strategies she or he uses to find time for exercise and to stay motivated.
- Do a short bout of endurance exercise: 10–15 minutes of walking, jogging, cycling, or another endurance activity.

COMMON QUESTIONS ANSWERED (continued)

and abdominal pain during menstruation, you may not feel like exercising; for some women, exercise helps relieve these symptoms. Listen to your body, and exercise at whatever intensity is comfortable for you.

What causes muscle cramps and what can I do about them? Muscle cramps are caused by local muscle fatigue that triggers the nervous system to overstimulate the muscles. Until recently, muscle cramps were thought to be caused by dehydration or salt depletion in the muscles, but scientists have found little evidence for this. Muscle cramps can occur during or after exercise performed either in heat or in cold. You can prevent cramps by improving your fitness and making sure you consume enough fluid and electrolytes during exercise and in your diet. When cramps do occur, gently stretch the cramping muscle for 15–30 seconds. Do not overstretch the cramping muscle because this can lead to serious injury.

Is it safe to exercise in hot weather? Prolonged, vigorous exercise can be dangerous in hot and humid weather. Heat from exercise is released in the form of sweat, which cools the skin and the blood circulating near the body surface as it evaporates. The hotter the weather, the more water the body loses through sweat; the more humid the weather, the less efficient the sweating mechanism is at lowering body temperature. If you lose too much water or if your body temperature rises too high, you may suffer from a heat disorder such as heat exhaustion or heat stroke. Use caution when exercising if the temperature is above 80°F or if the humidity is above 60%. To exercise safely, watch for the signals of heat disorder, regardless of the weather, and follow the tips given in the box "Exercising in Hot Weather on p. 68."

Is it safe to exercise in cold weather? If you dress warmly in layers and don't stay out in very cold temperatures for too long, exercise can be safe even in subfreezing temperatures. Take both the temperature and the wind-chill factor into account when choosing clothing. Dress in layers so you can subtract them as you warm up and add them if you get cold. A substantial amount of heat loss comes from the head and neck, so keep these areas covered. In subfreezing temperatures, protect the areas of your body most susceptible to frost-bite—fingers, toes, ears, nose, and cheeks—with warm socks, mittens or gloves, and a cap, hood, or ski mask. Wear clothing that "breathes" and will wick moisture away from your skin to avoid being overheated by trapped perspiration. Warm up thoroughly and drink plenty of fluids.

Is it safe to exercise in a smoggy city? Do not exercise outdoors during a smog alert or if air quality is very poor (symptoms of poor air quality include eye and throat irritations and respiratory discomfort). If you have any type of cardiorespiratory difficulty, avoid exertion outdoors when air quality is poor. You can avoid smog and air pollution by exercising in parks, near water (riverbanks, lakeshores, and ocean beaches), or in residential areas with less traffic (areas with stop-and-go traffic will have lower air quality than areas where traffic moves quickly). Air quality is usually better in the early morning and late evening.

Will high altitude affect my ability to exercise? At high altitudes (above 1500 meters or about 4900 feet) there is less oxygen available in the air than at lower altitudes. High altitude doesn't affect anaerobic exercise, such as stretching and weight lifting, but it does affect aerobic activities—that is, any type of cardiovascular endurance exercise. The reason is that the heart and lungs have to work harder, even when the body is at rest, to deliver enough oxygen to body cells. The increased cardiovascular strain of exercise reduces endurance. To play it safe when at high altitudes, avoid heavy exercise—at least for the first few days—and drink plenty of water. And don't expect to reach your normal lower altitude exercise capacity.

SUMMARY

- The cardiorespiratory system consists of the heart, blood vessels, and respiratory system; it picks up and transports oxygen, nutrients, and waste products.
- The body takes chemical energy from food and uses it to produce ATP and fuel cellular activities. ATP is stored in the body's cells as the basic form of energy.
- During exercise, the body supplies ATP and fuels cellular activities by combining three energy systems: *immediate,* for short periods of energy; *nonoxidative (anaerobic),* for intense activity; and *oxidative (aerobic),* for prolonged activity. Which energy system predominates depends on the duration and intensity of the activity.
- Cardiorespiratory endurance exercise improves cardiorespiratory functioning and cellular metabolism; it reduces the risk of chronic disease such as heart disease, cancer, Type 2 diabetes, obesity, and osteoporosis; and it improves immune function and psychological and emotional well-being.
- Cardiorespiratory fitness is measured by seeing how well the cardiorespiratory system transports and uses oxygen. The upper limit of this measure is called maximal oxygen consumption, or $\dot{V}O_{2max}$.
- $\dot{V}O_{2max}$ can be measured precisely in a laboratory, or it can be estimated reasonably well through less expensive assessment tests.
- To have a successful exercise program, set realistic goals; choose suitable activities; begin slowly; always warm up and cool down; and as fitness improves, exercise more often, longer, and/or harder.

TAKE CHARGE Exercising in Hot Weather

- Use caution when exercising in extreme heat or humidity (over 80°F and/or 60% humidity).
- Slow exercise or add rest breaks to maintain your prescribed target heart rate; as you become acclimatized, you can gradually increase intensity and duration.
- Exercise in the early morning or evening, when temperatures are lowest.
- Drink 2 cups of fluids 2 hours before you begin exercising, and drink 4–8 ounces of fluid every 10–15 minutes during exercise (more frequently during high-intensity activities).
- Wear clothing that "breathes," allowing air to circulate and cool the body. Wearing white or light colors will help by reflecting rather than absorbing, heat. A hat can help keep direct sun off your face. Do not wear rubber, plastic, or other nonporous clothing.
- Rest frequently in the shade.
- Keep a record of your morning body weight to track whether weight lost through sweating is restored.
- Slow down or stop if you begin to feel uncomfortable. Watch for the signs of heat disorders listed below; if they occur, act appropriately.

Problem	Symptoms	Treatment
Heat cramps	Muscle cramps, usually in the muscles most used during exercise.	Stop exercising, drink fluids, and massage or stretch cramped muscles.
Heat exhaustion	Weakness, dizziness, headache, rapid pulse, profuse sweating, pale face, normal or slightly elevated temperature.	Cool the body. Stop exercising, get out of the heat, remove excess clothing, drink cold fluids, and apply cool and/or damp towels to the body.
Heat stroke	Hot, flushed skin (may be dry or sweaty), red face, chills, shivering, disorientation, erratic behavior, high body temperature, unconsciousness, convulsions.	*Get immediate medical attention,* and try to lower body temperature. Get out of the heat, remove excess clothing, drink cold fluids, and apply cool and/or damp towels to the body or immerse it in cold water.

- Intensity of training can be measured through target heart rate zone and ratings of perceived exertion.
- Serious injuries require medical attention. Application of the R-I-C-E principle (rest, ice, compression, elevation) is appropriate for treating many types of muscle or joint injuries.

FOR FURTHER EXPLORATION

WW *Fit and Well* Online Learning Center (www.mhhe.com/fahey5e)

Use the learning objectives, study guide questions, and glossary flashcards to review key terms and concepts and prepare for exams. You can extend your knowledge of cardiorespiratory endurance and gain experience in using the Internet as a resource by completing the activities and checking out the Web links for the topics in Chapter 3 marked with the World Wide Web icon. For this chapter, Internet activities explore the benefits of endurance exercise, target heart rate zone, and activities to improve cardiorespiratory fitness; there are Web links for the Critical Consumer box on exercise equipment and the chapter as a whole.

Daily Fitness and Nutrition Journal

Complete the cardiorespiratory endurance portion of the program plan by setting goals and selecting activities that will build endurance. Also calculate and record your current resting heart rate and your target heart rate zone or RPE value.

Health*Quest*

Learn more about the functioning of the cardiovascular system by completing the Cardiovascular Tutorial on the Health*Quest* CD-ROM; it is found in the Cardiovascular Health module (select Cardiovascular Exploration from the Wellness Activities menu). For further help in choosing activities for your cardiorespiratory endurance program, complete the Exercise Interest Inventory in the Fitness module (select Fitness Planner from the Wellness Activities menu). You'll receive activity suggestions based on your personal exercise preferences.

Books

Bingham, J. 2002. *No Need for Speed: A Beginner's Guide to the Joy of Running.* Emmaus, Pa.: Rodale Press. A practical, nonintimidating, and inspirational guide for the beginning runner.

Brennfleck, J. 2002. *Sports Injuries Sourcebook.* Detroit, Mich.: Omnigraphics. Provides information about the prevention and care of exercise injuries, with specific sections on different age groups and popular activities.

Burfoot, A. 2001. *Runner's World Complete Book of Running.* Philadelphia: Running Press. *Includes basic information about training, nutrition, and avoiding injury.*

Fenton, M. 2001. *Walking Magazine: Complete Guide to Walking for Health, Weight Loss, and Fitness.* New York: Lyons Press. *A 52-week walking program (including distances and time) plus information on footwear, clothing, and motivation.*

Garrick, J., and P. Radetsky. 2000. *Anybody's Sports Medicine Book: The Complete Guide to Quick Recovery from Injuries.* Berkeley, Calif.: Ten Speed. *Includes information for fitness exercisers and recreational athletes about emergency care, when to see a physician, and how to rehabilitate an injury.*

Heyward, V. 2002. *Advanced Fitness Assessment and Exercise Prescription.* 4th ed. Champaign, Ill.: Human Kinetics. Provides information and ratings for a large number of fitness tests as well as guidelines for putting together a successful program.

Hines, E. W. 1999. *Fitness Swimming.* Champaign, Ill.: Human Kinetics. *Provides step-by-step instructions for setting up a swimming fitness program.*

Juba, K. 2002. *Swimming for Fitness.* New York: Lyons Press. Provides step-by-step instructions for setting up a swimming fitness program, including advice on technique and avoiding injury and overtraining.

Ledeboer, S. 2001. *A Basic Guide to Cycling.* Torrance, Calif.: Griffin Pub. *Includes information on buying and caring for a bicycle as well as increasing fitness.*

Nieman, D. C. 2003. *Exercise Testing and Prescription: A Health-Related Approach,* 5th ed. New York: McGraw-Hill. *A comprehensive discussion of the effect of exercise and exercise testing and prescription.*

Pryor, E., and M. Kraines. 2000. *Keep Moving! Fitness through Aerobics and Step,* 4th ed. Mountain View, Calif.: Mayfield. *The fitness principles and techniques every aerobic dancer should know.*

WW Organizations and Web Sites

American Academy of Orthopaedic Surgeons. Provides fact sheets on many fitness and sports topics, including how to begin a program, how to choose equipment, and how to prevent and treat many types of injuries.
http://orthinfo.aaos.org

American Heart Association. Provides information on cardiovascular health and disease, including the role of exercise in maintaining heart health and exercise tips for people of all ages.
800-AHA-USA1
http://www.americanheart.org
http://www.justmove.org

Canada's Physical Activity Guide. Provides information on adding physical activity to your life; includes extensive material for older adults.
http://www.hc-sc.gc.ca/hppb/paguide

Dr. Pribut's Running Injuries Page. Provides information about running and many types of running injuries.
http://www.drpribut.com/sports/spsport.html

Federal Trade Commission: Consumer Protection—Diet, Health, and Fitness. Provides several brochures with consumer advice about purchasing exercise equipment.
http://www.ftc.gov/bcp/menu-health.htm

Franklin Institute Science Museum/The Heart: An Online Exploration. An online museum exhibit with information on the structure and function of the heart, blood vessels, and respiratory system.
http://www.fi.edu/biosci/heart.html

Georgia State University: Exercise and Physical Fitness Page. Provides information about the benefits of exercise and how to get started on a fitness program.
http://www.gsu.edu/~wwwfit

MedlinePlus: Exercise and Physical Fitness. Provides links to news and reliable information about fitness from government agencies and professional associations.
http://www.nlm.nih.gov/medlineplus/exercisephysicalfitness.html

Physician and Sportsmedicine. Provides many articles with easy-to-understand advice about exercise injuries.
http://www.physsportsmed.com

Runner's World Online. Contains a wide variety of information about running, including tips for beginning runners, advice about training, and a shoe buyer's guide.
http://www.runnersworld.com

Shape Up America! Fitness Center. Includes fitness assessments, information on the benefits of exercise, tips for overcoming barriers, and tracking forms.
http://shapeup.org/fitness

University of Florida: Keeping Fit. Provides useful information about fitness in a question-and-answer format; an extensive set of links is also provided.
http://www.hhp.ufl.edu/keepingfit
http://www.hhp.ufl.edu/personalfitness.htm

Women's Sports Foundation. Provides information and links about training and about many specific sports activities.
http://www.womenssportsfoundation.org/cgi-bin/iowa/sports/index.html

Yahoo/Recreation. Contains links to many sites with practical advice on many sports and activities.
http://dir.yahoo.com/recreation/sports

See also the listings in Chapter 2.

SELECTED BIBLIOGRAPHY

American Academy of Orthopaedic Surgeons. 2001. *Selecting Home Exercise Equipment* (http://orthoinfo.aaos.org/fact/ thr_report.cfm; retrieved October 17, 2001).

American College of Sports Medicine. 2000. *ACSM's Guidelines for Exercise Testing and Prescription,* 6th ed. Baltimore, Md.: Lippincott Williams & Wilkins.

American College of Sports Medicine. 1998. ACSM position stand: The recommended quantity and quality of exercise for developing and maintaining cardiorespiratory and muscular fitness, flexibility in healthy adults. *Medicine and Science in Sports and Exercise* 30(6): 975–991.

American College of Sports Medicine. 2001. *ACSM's Resource Manual for Guidelines for Exercise Testing and Prescription,* 4th ed. Philadelphia: Williams & Wilkins.

Blair, S. N., and A. S. Jackson. 2001. Physical fitness and activity as separate heart disease risk factors: A meta-analysis. *Medicine and Science in Sports and Exercise* 33(5): 762–764.

Branch, J. D., et al. 2000. Moderate intensity exercise training improves cardiorespiratory fitness in women. *Journal of Women's Health and Gender-Based Medicine* 9(1): 65–73.

Brehm, B. A. 2000. Maximizing the psychological benefits of physical activity. *ACSM's Health and Fitness Journal* 4(6): 7–11.

Brooks, G. A., et al. 2000. *Exercise Physiology: Human Bioenergetics and Its Applications,* 3d ed. Mountain View, Calif.: Mayfield.

Carroll, J. F., and C. K. Kyser. 2002. Exercise training in obesity lowers blood pressure independent of weight change. *Medicine and Science in Sports and Exercise* 34(4): 596–601.

Erikssen, G. 2001. Physical fitness and changes in mortality: The survival of the fittest. *Sports Medicine* 31(8): 571–576.

Faulkner, G., and S. Biddle. 2001. Exercise and mental health: It's just not psychology! *Journal of Sports Science* 19(6): 433–444.

Finch, C. F., and N. Owen. 2001. Injury prevention and the promotion of physical activity: What is the nexus? *Journal of Science and Medicine in Sports* 4(1): 77–87.

Gutin, B. et al. 2002. Effects of exercise intensity on cardiovascular fitness, total body composition, and visceral adiposity of obese adolescents. *American Journal of Clinical Nutrition* 75(5): 818–826.

Haennel, R. G., and F. Lemire. 2002. Physical activity to prevent cardiovascular disease. How much is enough? *Canadian Family Physician* 48: 65–71.

Houde, S. C., and K. D. Melillo. 2002. Cardiovascular health and physical activity in older adults: An integrative review of research methodology and results. *Journal of Advanced Nursing* 38(3): 219–234.

Humpel, N., N. Owen, and E. Leslie. 2002. Environmental factors associated with adults' participation in physical activity. A review. *American Journal of Preventive Medicine* 22(3): 188–199.

Keteyian, S. J., and I. Kolokouri. 2001. Guidelines for selecting home exercise equipment. *ACSM's Fit Society Page,* January/February.

Kohl, H. W. 2001. Physical activity and cardiovascular disease: Evidence for a dose response. *Medicine and Science in Sports and Exercise* 33(6 Suppl): S472–S483.

Laukkanen, J. A., et al. 2001. Cardiovascular fitness as a predictor of mortality in men. *Archives of Internal Medicine* 161(6): 825–831.

Maltby, J., and L. Day. 2001. The relationship between exercise motives and psychological well-being. *Journal of Psychology.* 135(6): 651–660.

Mayers, J. N. 2001. The physiology behind exercise testing. *Primary Care* 28(1): 5–28.

Michaud, D. S. 2001. Physical activity, obesity, height, and the risk of pancreatic cancer. *Journal of the American Medical Association* 286(8): 921–929.

Morimoto, K., et al. 2001. Lifestyles and mental health status are associated with natural killer cell and lymphokine-activated killer cell activities. *The Science of the Total Environment* 270(1–3): 3–11.

Nieman, D. C. 2001. Does exercise alter immune function and respiratory infections? *President's Council on Physical Fitness and Sports Research Digest* 3(13).

Orleans, C. T. 2000. Promoting the maintenance of health behavior change. *Health Psychology* 19(1 Suppl.): 76–83.

PBS Healthweek. 2001. *Home Exercise Equipment* (http://www.pbs.org/healthweek/featurep4_339.htm; retrieved October 18, 2001).

Perini, R., et al. 2002. Aerobic training and cardiovascular responses at rest and during exercise in older men and women. *Medicine and Science in Sports and Exercise* 34(40): 700–708.

Szabo, A. E. Billett, and J. Turner. 2001. Phenylethylamine, a possible link to the antidepressant effects of exercise? *British Journal of Sports Medicine* 35(5): 342–343.

Talbot, L. A., E. J. Metter, and J. L. Fleg. 2000. Leisure-time physical activities and their relationship to cardiorespiratory fitness in healthy men and women 18–95 years old. *Medicine and Science in Sports and Exercise* 32(2): 417–425.

Thompson, P. D., et al. 2001. The acute versus the chronic response to exercise. *Medicine and Science in Sports and Exercise* 33(6 Suppl): S438–S445.

Tolfrey, K., A. M. Jones, and I. G. Campbell. 2000. The effect of aerobic exercise training on the lipid-lipoprotein profile of children and adolescents. *Sports Medicine* 29(2): 99–112.

Uusi-Rasi, K., et al. 2002. Associations of calcium intake and physical activity with bone density and size in premenopausal and postmenopausal women. *Journal of Bone Mineral Research* 17(3): 544–552.

Whelton, S. P., et al. 2002. Effect of aerobic exercise on blood pressure: A meta-analysis of randomized, controlled trials. *Annals of Internal Medicine* 136(7): 493–503.

Williams, P. T. 2001. Health effects resulting from exercise versus those from body fat loss. *Medicine and Science in Sports and Exercise* 33(6 Suppl): S611–S621.

Woods, J. A., T. W. Lowder, and K. T. Keylock. 2002. Can exercise training improve immune function in the aged? *Annals of the New York Academy of Science* 959: 117–127.

Name ______________________ Section ______________ Date ______________

LAB 3.1 *Assessing Your Current Level of Cardiorespiratory Endurance*

Before taking any of the cardiorespiratory endurance assessment tests, refer to the fitness prerequisites and cautions given in Table 3.2. For best results, don't exercise strenuously or consume caffeine the day of the test, and don't smoke or eat a heavy meal within about 3 hours of the test.

The 1-Mile Walk Test

Equipment

1. A track or course that provides a measurement of 1 mile
2. A stopwatch, clock, or watch with a second hand
3. A weight scale

Preparation

Measure your body weight (in pounds) before taking the test.

Body weight: 138 lb

Instructions

1. Warm up before taking the test. Do some walking, easy jogging, or calisthenics and some stretching exercises.
2. Cover the 1-mile course as quickly as possible. Walk at a pace that is brisk but comfortable. You must raise your heart rate above 120 beats per minute (bpm).
3. As soon as you complete the distance, note your time and take your pulse for 10 seconds.

   Running ~~Walking~~ time: ~~10:08~~ 11 min 32 sec

   10-second pulse count: __________ beats — While running averaged 160 bpm
4. Cool down after the test by walking slowly for several minutes.

Determining Maximal Oxygen Consumption

1. Convert your 10-second pulse count into a value for exercise heart rate by multiplying it by 6.

   Exercise heart rate: __________ (10-sec pulse count) × 6 = __________ bpm
2. Convert your walking time from minutes and seconds to a decimal figure. For example, a time of 14 minutes and 45 seconds would be 14 + (45/60), or 14.75 minutes.

   Walking time: __________ min + (__________ sec ÷ 60 sec/min) = __________ min
3. Insert values for your age, gender, weight, walking time, and exercise heart rate in the following equation, where

   W = your weight (in pounds)

   A = your age (in years)

   G = your gender (male = 1; female = 0)

   T = your time to complete the 1-mile course (in minutes)

   H = your exercise heart rate (in beats per minute)

   $\dot{V}O_{2max} = 132.853 - (0.0769 \times W) - (0.3877 \times A) + (6.315 \times G) - (3.2649 \times T) - (0.1565 \times H)$

For example, a 20-year-old, 190-pound male with a time of 14.75 minutes and an exercise heart rate of 152 bpm would calculate maximal oxygen consumption as follows:

$$\dot{V}O_{2max} = 132.853 - (0.0769 \times 190) - (0.3877 \times 20) + (6.315 \times 1) - (3.2649 \times 14.75) - (0.1565 \times 152)$$
$$= 45 \text{ ml/kg/min}$$

$\dot{V}O_{2max}$ = 132.853 − (0.0769 × ________ [weight (lb)]) − (0.3877 × ________ [age (years)]) + (6.315 × ________ [gender]) − (3.2649 × ________ [walking time (min)]) − (0.1565 × ________ [exercise heart rate (bpm)]) = ________ ml/kg/min

4. Copy this value for $\dot{V}O_{2max}$ into the appropriate place in the chart on the final page of this lab.

The 3-Minute Step Test

Equipment

1. A step, bench, or bleacher step that is 16.25 inches from ground level
2. A stopwatch, clock, or watch with a second hand
3. A metronome

Preparation

Practice stepping up onto and down from the step before you begin the test. Each step has four beats: up-up-down-down. Males should perform the test with the metronome set for a rate of 96 beats per minute, or 24 steps per minute. Females should set the metronome at 88 beats per minute, or 22 steps per minute.

Instructions

1. Warm up before taking the test. Do some walking, easy jogging, and stretching exercises.
2. Set the metronome at the proper rate. Your instructor or a partner can call out starting and stopping times; otherwise, have a clock or watch within easy viewing during the test.
3. Begin the test and continue to step at the correct pace for 3 minutes.
4. Stop after 3 minutes. Remain standing and count your pulse for the 15-second period from 5 to 20 seconds into recovery.

   15-second pulse count: ________ beats
5. Cool down after the test by walking slowly for several minutes.

Determining Maximal Oxygen Consumption

1. Convert your 15-second pulse count to a value for recovery heart rate by multiplying by 4.

   Recovery heart rate: ________ [15-sec pulse count] × 4 = ________ bpm
2. Insert your recovery heart rate in the equation below, where

   H = recovery heart rate (in beats per minute)

   Males: $\dot{V}O_{2max} = 111.33 - (0.42 \times H)$

   Females: $\dot{V}O_{2max} = 65.81 - (0.1847 \times H)$

   For example, a man with a recovery heart rate of 162 bpm would calculate maximal oxygen consumption as follows:

   $\dot{V}O_{2max} = 111.33 - (0.42 \times 162) = 43$ ml/kg/min

   Males: $\dot{V}O_{2max}$ = 111.33 − (0.42 × ________ [recovery heart rate (bpm)]) = ________ ml/kg/min

   Females: $\dot{V}O_{2max}$ = 65.81 − (0.1847 × ________ [recovery heart rate (bpm)]) = ________ ml/kg/min
3. Copy this value for $\dot{V}O_{2max}$ into the appropriate place in the chart on the final page of this lab.

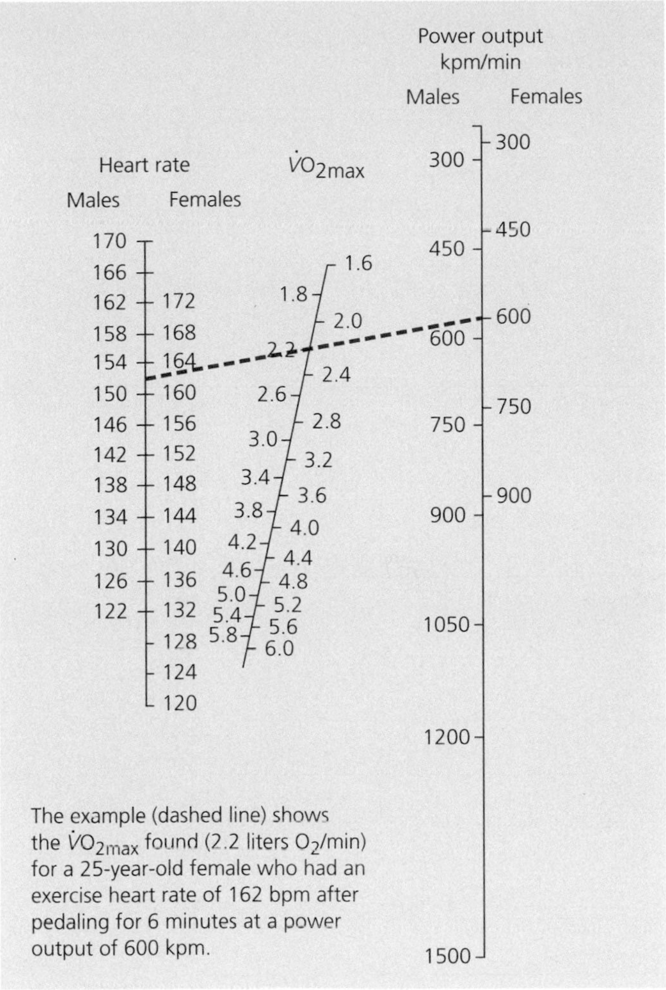
Power output
kpm/min
Males
Females
Heart rate
Males
Females
$\dot{V}O_{2max}$
The example (dashed line) shows the $\dot{V}O_{2max}$ found (2.2 liters O_2/min) for a 25-year-old female who had an exercise heart rate of 162 bpm after pedaling for 6 minutes at a power output of 600 kpm.

Nomogram for use with the Åstrand-Rhyming cycle ergometer test.

For example, a 135-pound, 25-year-old female whose 10-second count was 27 at a workload of 600 kpm would calculate maximal oxygen consumption as follows:

1. 27 beats × 6 = 162 bpm
2. Connecting 600 kpm and 162 bpm on the nomogram gives a $\dot{V}O_{2max}$ value of 2.2 l/min
3. The age-adjustment factor for a 25-year-old is 1.00.
   2.2 l/min × 1.00 = 2.2 l/min
4. To convert 135 pounds to kilograms:
   135 lb ÷ 2.2 lb/kg = 61.4 kg

   To convert liters to milliliters:

   2.2 l/min × 1000 ml/l = 2200 ml/min

   To adjust for weight:

   2200 ml/min ÷ 61.4 kg = 35.8 ml/kg/min

   Convert body weight to kg: ________ lb ÷ 2.2 lb/kg = ________ kg

   Convert from liters to milliliters: ________ (age-corrected $\dot{V}O_{2max}$) l/min × 1000 ml/l = ________ ml/min

   Adjust for weight:

   $\dot{V}O_{2max}$ = ________ ($\dot{V}O_{2max}$) ml/min ÷ ________ (body weight) kg = ________ ml/kg/min
5. Copy this value for $\dot{V}O_{2max}$max into the appropriate place in the chart on the following page.

LABORATORY ACTIVITIES

Rating Your Cardiovascular Fitness

Record your $\dot{V}O_{2max}$ score(s) and the corresponding fitness rating from the table below.

Women	*Very Poor*	*Poor*	*Fair*	*Good*	*Excellent*	*Superior*
Age: 18–29	Below 31.6	31.6–35.4	35.5–39.4	39.5–43.9	44.0–50.1	Above 50.1
30–39	Below 29.9	29.9–33.7	33.8–36.7	36.8–40.9	41.0–46.8	Above 46.8
40–49	Below 28.0	28.0–31.5	31.6–35.0	35.1–38.8	38.9–45.1	Above 45.1
50–59	Below 25.5	25.5–28.6	28.7–31.3	31.4–35.1	35.2–39.8	Above 39.8
60–69	Below 23.7	23.7–26.5	26.6–29.0	29.1–32.2	32.3–36.8	Above 36.8
Men						
Age: 18–29	Below 38.1	38.1–42.1	42.2–45.6	45.7–51.0	51.1–56.1	Above 56.1
30–39	Below 36.7	36.7–40.9	41.0–44.3	44.4–48.8	48.9–54.2	Above 54.2
40–49	Below 34.6	34.6–38.3	38.4–42.3	42.4–46.7	46.8–52.8	Above 52.8
50–59	Below 31.1	31.1–35.1	35.2–38.2	38.3–43.2	43.3–49.6	Above 49.6
60–69	Below 27.4	27.4–31.3	31.4–34.9	35.0–39.4	39.5–46.0	Above 46.0

SOURCE: Ratings based on norms from the Cooper Institute for Aerobics Research, Dallas, Texas, *The Physical Fitness Specialist Manual,* Revised 2002. Used with permission.

	$\dot{V}O_{2max}$	Cardiovascular Fitness Rating
1-mile walk test		
3-minute step test		
1.5-mile run-walk test	39.5	Good
Åstrand-Rhyming cycle ergometer test		

Using Your Results

How did you score? Are you surprised by your rating for cardiovascular fitness? Are you satisfied with your current rating?

If you're not satisfied, set a realistic goal for improvement: ____________________

Are you satisfied with your current level of cardiovascular fitness as evidenced in your daily life—your ability to walk, run, bicycle, climb stairs, do yardwork, engage in recreational activities?

If you're not satisfied, set some realistic goals for improvement, such as completing a 5K run or 25-mile bike ride:

What should you do next? Enter the results of this lab in the Preprogram Assessment column in Appendix D. If you've set goals for improvement, begin planning your cardiorespiratory endurance exercise program by completing the plan in Lab 3.2. After several weeks of your program, complete this lab again, and enter the results in the Postprogram Assessment column of Appendix D. How do the results compare? (Remember, it's best to compare $\dot{V}O_{2max}$ scores for the same test.)

SOURCES: Kline, G. M., et al. 1987. Estimation of $\dot{V}O_{2max}$ from a one-mile track walk, gender, age, and body weight. *Medicine and Science in Sports and Exercise* 19(3): 253–259. McArdle, W. D., F. I. Katch, and V. L. Katch. 1991. *Exercise Physiology: Energy, Nutrition, and Human Performance.* Philadelphia: Lea & Febiger, pp. 225–226. Brooks, G. A., and T. D. Fahey. 1987. *Fundamentals of Human Performance.* New York: Macmillan. Åstrand, P. O., and I. Rhyming. 1954. A nomogram for calculation of aerobic capacity (physical fitness) from pulse rate during submaximal work. *Journal of Applied Physiology* 7:218–221. Used with permission.

Name ______________________ **Section** ____________ **Date** ____________

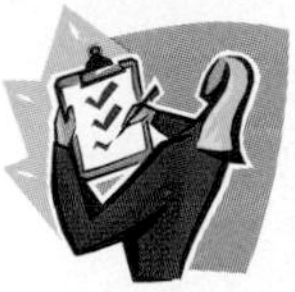

LAB 3.2 *Developing an Exercise Program for Cardiorespiratory Endurance*

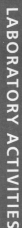

1. *Goals.* List goals for your cardiorespiratory endurance exercise program. Your goals can be specific or general, short or long term. In the first section, include specific, measurable goals that you can use to track the progress of your fitness program. These goals might be things like raising your cardiorespiratory fitness rating from fair to good or swimming laps for 30 minutes without resting. In the second section, include long-term and more qualitative goals, such as improving self-confidence and reducing your risk for chronic disease.

Specific Goals: Current Status	Final Goal
______________________	______________________
______________________	______________________
______________________	______________________

Other goals: ____

____

2. *Activities.* Next, choose one or more endurance activities for your program. These can include any activity that uses large-muscle groups, can be maintained continuously, and is rhythmic and aerobic in nature. Examples include walking, jogging, cycling, group exercise such as aerobic dance, rowing, rope skipping, stair climbing, cross-country skiing, swimming, skating, and endurance game activities such as soccer and tennis. Choose activities that are both convenient and enjoyable. Fill in the activity names on the program plan on the following page.

3. *Intensity.* Determine your exercise intensity using one of the following methods, and enter it on the program plan on the following page. You should begin your program at a lower intensity and slowly increase intensity as your fitness improves, so select a range of intensities for your program.

   a. Target heart rate zone: Calculate target heart rate zone in beats per minute and then calculate the corresponding 10-second exercise count by dividing the total count by 6. For example, the 10-second exercise counts corresponding to a target heart rate zone of 122–180 bpm would be 20–30 beats.

   Maximum heart rate: 220 − ________ (age (years)) = ________ bpm

   Maximum Heart Rate Method

   65% training intensity = ________ (maximum heart rate) bpm × 0.65 = ________ bpm

   90% training intensity = ________ (maximum heart rate) bpm × 0.90 = ________ bpm

   Target heart rate zone = ________ to ________ bpm   10-second count = ________ to ________

   Heart Rate Reserve Method

   Resting heart rate: ________ bpm (taken after 10 minutes of complete rest)

   Heart rate reserve = ________ (maximum heart rate) bpm − ________ (resting heart rate) bpm = ________ bpm

   50% training intensity = (________ (heart rate reserve) bpm × 0.50) + ________ (resting heart rate) bpm = ________ bpm

   85% training intensity = (________ (heart rate reserve) bpm × 0.85) + ________ (resting heart rate) bpm = ________ bpm

   Target heart rate zone = ________ to ________ bpm   10-second count = ________ to ________

   b. Ratings of perceived exertion (RPE): If you prefer, determine an RPE value that corresponds to your target heart rate range (see pp. 61–62 and Figure 3.4).

4. *Duration.* A total duration of 20–60 minutes is recommended; your duration of exercise will vary with intensity. For developing cardiorespiratory endurance, higher-intensity activities can be performed for a shorter duration; lower intensities require a longer duration. Enter a duration (or a range of duration) on the program plan.
5. *Frequency.* Fill in how often you plan to participate in each activity; the ACSM recommends participating in cardiorespiratory endurance exercise 3–5 days per week.

Program Plan

Activity	Duration (min)	Intensity (bpm or RPE)	Frequency (check ✓)						
			M	T	W	Th	F	Sa	Su

6. *Monitoring your program.* Complete a log like the one below to monitor your program and track your progress. Note the date on top, and fill in the intensity and duration for each workout. If you prefer, you can also track other variables such as distance. For example, if your cardiorespiratory endurance program includes walking and swimming, you may want to track miles walked and yards swum in addition to the duration of each exercise session. For more extensive sets of logs, refer to the Daily Fitness and Nutrition Journal that accompanies your text.

Activity/Date													
1	Intensity												
	Duration												
	Distance												
2	Intensity												
	Duration												
	Distance												
3	Intensity												
	Duration												
	Distance												
4	Intensity												
	Duration												
	Distance												

7. *Making progress.* Follow the guidelines in the chapter and Table 3.3 to slowly increase the amount of overload in your program. Continue keeping a log, and periodically evaluate your progress.

Progress Check-Up: Week ____ of program

Goals: Original Status   Current Status

______________________________   ______________________________

______________________________   ______________________________

______________________________   ______________________________

List each activity in your program and describe how satisfied you are with the activity and with your overall progress. List any problems you've encountered or any unexpected costs or benefits of your fitness program so far.

Muscular Strength and Endurance

4

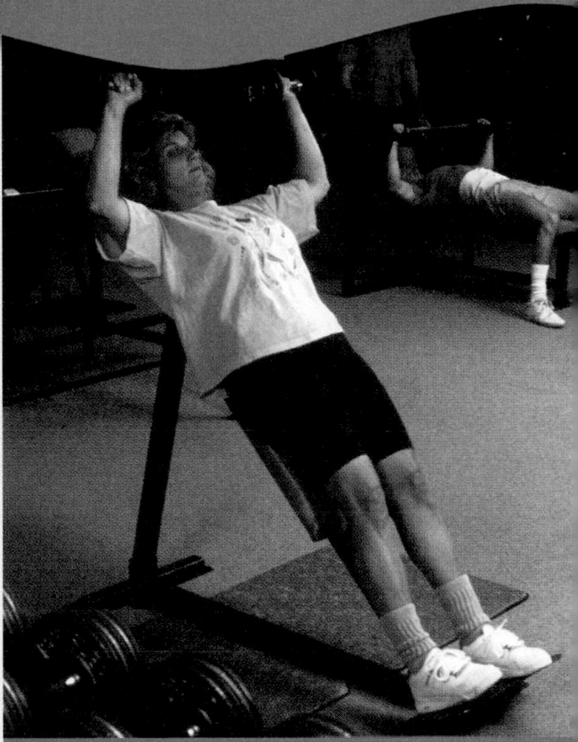

LOOKING AHEAD

After reading this chapter, you should be able to

- Define muscular strength and endurance and describe how they relate to wellness
- Explain how muscular strength and endurance can be assessed
- Describe how strength training exercises affect muscles
- List the type, frequency, and number of strength training exercises that make up a successful program
- Describe the effects of supplements and drugs that are marketed to active people and athletes
- Explain how to safely perform common strength training exercises using free weights and weight machines

TEST YOUR KNOWLEDGE

1. For women, weight training typically results in which of the following?
   a. bulky muscles
   b. significant increases in body weight
   c. improved body image
2. To maximize strength gains, it is a good idea to hold your breath as you lift a weight.
   True or false?
3. Regular strength training is associated with which of the following benefits?
   a. denser bones
   b. reduced risk of heart disease
   c. improved body composition
   d. higher grades

TEST YOUR KNOWLEDGE ANSWERS

1. C. Because the vast majority of women have low levels of testosterone, they do not develop large muscles or gain significant amounts of weight in response to a moderate weight training program. Men have higher levels of testosterone, so they can build large muscles more easily.

2. FALSE. Holding one's breath while lifting weights, called the Valsalva maneuver, can significantly (and possibly dangerously) elevate blood pressure; it also reduces blood flow to the heart and may cause faintness. You should breathe smoothly and normally while weight training.

3. ALL FOUR. Regular strength training has many benefits for lifetime wellness.

Fit and Well Online Learning Center

www.mhhe.com/fahey5e

Visit the *Fit and Well* Online Learning Center for study aids, additional information about muscular strength and endurance, links, Internet activities that explore the development of a strength training program, consumer resources, and much more.

Exercise experts have long emphasized the importance of cardiovascular fitness. Other physical fitness factors, such as muscle strength and flexibility, were mentioned almost as an afterthought. As more was learned about how the body responds to exercise, however, it became obvious that these other factors are vital to health, wellness, and overall quality of life. Muscles make up more than 40% of your body mass. You depend on them for movement, and, because of their mass, they are the site of a large portion of the energy reactions (metabolism) that take place in your body. Strong, well-developed muscles help you perform daily activities with greater ease, protect you from injury, and enhance your well-being in other ways.

This chapter explains the benefits of strength training (also called resistance training) and describes methods of assessing muscular strength and endurance. It then explains the basics of weight training and provides guidelines for setting up your own weight training program.

Ww BENEFITS OF MUSCULAR STRENGTH AND ENDURANCE

As described in Chapter 2, muscular strength is the ability to generate force during a maximal effort; muscular endurance is the ability to resist fatigue while holding or repeating a muscular contraction. Enhanced muscular strength and endurance can lead to improvements in the areas of performance, injury prevention, body composition, self-image, lifetime muscle and bone health, and chronic disease prevention.

Improved Performance of Physical Activities

A person with a moderate-to-high level of muscular strength and endurance can perform everyday tasks—such as climbing stairs and carrying books or groceries—with ease. Muscular strength and endurance are also important in recreational activities: People with poor muscle strength tire more easily and are less effective in activities like hiking, skiing, and playing tennis. Increased strength can enhance your enjoyment of recreational sports by making it possible to achieve high levels of performance and to handle advanced techniques. Strength training also results in modest improvements in maximal oxygen consumption.

Injury Prevention

Increased muscle strength provides protection against injury because it helps people maintain good posture and appropriate body mechanics when carrying out everyday activities like walking, lifting, and carrying. Strong muscles in the abdomen, hips, low back, and legs support the back in proper alignment and help prevent low-back pain, which afflicts more than 85% of all Americans at some time in their lives. (Prevention of low-back pain is discussed in Chapter 5.) Training for muscular strength also makes the **tendons, ligaments,** and cartilage cells stronger and less susceptible to injury.

Improved Body Composition

As Chapter 2 explained, healthy body composition means that the body has a high proportion of fat-free mass (primarily composed of muscle) and a relatively small proportion of fat. Strength training improves body composition by increasing muscle mass, thereby tipping the body composition ratio toward fat-free mass and away from fat. Building muscle mass through strength training also helps with losing fat because metabolic rate is related to muscle mass: The more muscle mass, the higher the metabolic rate. A high metabolic rate means that a nutritionally sound diet coupled with regular exercise will not lead to an increase in body fat.

Enhanced Self-Image and Quality of Life

Strength training leads to an enhanced self-image by providing stronger, firmer-looking muscles and a toned, healthy-looking body. Men tend to build larger, stronger muscles. Women tend to lose inches, increase strength, and develop greater muscle definition. The larger muscles in men combine with high levels of the hormone **testosterone,** the principal androgen, for a strong tissue-building effect; see the box "Gender Differences in Muscular Strength." Strength training improves body image in both men and women.

Because strength training involves measurable objectives (pounds lifted, repetitions accomplished), a person can easily recognize improved performance, leading to greater self-confidence and self-esteem. It's especially satisfying to work on improving one's personal record. Strength training also improves quality of life by increasing energy, preventing injuries, and making daily activities easier and more enjoyable.

Improved Muscle and Bone Health with Aging

Research has shown that good muscle strength helps people live healthier lives. A lifelong program of regular

Terms Ww

tendon A tough band of fibrous tissue that connects a muscle to a bone or other body part and transmits the force exerted by the muscle.

ligament A tough band of tissue that connects the ends of bones to other bones or supports organs in place.

testosterone The principal male hormone, responsible for the development of secondary sex characteristics and important in increasing muscle size.

DIMENSIONS OF DIVERSITY Gender Differences in Muscular Strength

Men are generally stronger than women because they typically have larger bodies overall and a larger proportion of their total body mass is made up of muscle. But when strength is expressed per unit of cross-sectional area of muscle tissue, men are only 1–2% stronger than women in the upper body and about equal to women in the lower body. (Men have a larger proportion of muscle tissue in the upper body, so it's easier for them to build upper-body strength than it is for women.) Individual muscle fibers are larger in men, but the metabolism of cells within those fibers is the same in both sexes.

Two factors that help explain these disparities between the sexes are androgen levels and the speed of nervous control of muscle. Androgens are naturally occurring hormones that are responsible for the development of secondary sex characteristics in males (facial hair, deep voice, and so forth). Androgens also promote the growth of muscle tissue in both males and females. Androgen levels are about 6–10 times higher in men than in women, so men tend to have larger muscles. Also, because the male nervous system can activate muscles faster, men tend to have more power.

Some women are concerned that they will develop large muscles from weight training. Because of hormonal differences, most women do not develop big muscles unless they train intensely over many years. A bigger concern for women is *losing* muscle, especially as they age. Both men and women lose muscle mass and power as they age, but because men start out with more muscle when they are young and don't lose power as quickly, older women tend to have greater impairment of muscle function than older men. This may partially account for the higher incidence of life-threatening falls in older women.

The bottom line is that both men and women can increase strength through weight training. Women may not be able to lift as much weight as men, but pound for pound of muscle, they have nearly the same capacity to gain strength as men. The lifetime wellness benefits of strength training are available to everyone. Weight training is particularly beneficial for women because it helps prevent bone and muscle loss with aging and maintains fat-free weight during weight control programs.

SOURCE: Krivickas, L. S., et al. 2001. Age and gender-related differences in maximum shortening velocity of skeletal muscle fibers. *American Journal of Physical Medicine and Rehabilitation* 80:447–455. Fahey, T. D. 2000. *Weight Training for Men and Women,* 4th ed. Mountain View, Calif.: Mayfield.

strength training prevents muscle and nerve degeneration that can compromise the quality of life and increase the risk of hip fractures and other potentially life-threatening injuries. In the general population people begin to lose muscle mass after age 30, a condition called *sarcopenia.* At first they may notice that they can't play sports as well as they could in high school. After more years of inactivity and strength loss, people may have trouble performing even the simple movements of daily life—getting out of a bathtub or automobile, walking up a flight of stairs, or doing yard work. By age 75 about 25% of men and 75% of women can't lift more than 10 pounds. Although aging contributes to decreased strength, inactivity causes most of the loss. Poor strength makes it much more likely that a person will be injured during everyday activities.

As a person ages, motor nerves can become disconnected from the portion of muscle they control. Muscle physiologists estimate that by age 70, 15% of the motor nerves in most people are no longer connected to muscle tissue. Aging and inactivity also cause muscles to become slower and therefore less able to perform quick, powerful movements. Strength training helps maintain motor nerve connections and the quickness of muscles.

Osteoporosis is common in people over age 55, particularly postmenopausal women. Osteoporosis leads to fractures that can be life-threatening. Hormonal changes from aging account for much of the bone loss that occurs, but lack of bone stress due to inactivity and a poor diet are contributing factors. Recent research indicates that strength training can lessen bone loss even if it is taken up later in life. Increased muscle strength can also help prevent falls, which are a major cause of injury in people with osteoporosis. (Additional strategies for preventing osteoporosis are described in Chapter 8.)

Prevention and Management of Chronic Disease

Strength training helps in the prevention and management of several major chronic diseases. Strength training improves glucose metabolism, an important factor in the prevention of the most common form of diabetes. It also modifies risk factors for cardiovascular disease. Regular strength training is associated with increased maximal oxygen consumption, decreased diastolic blood pressure, and, in some people, positive changes in blood fat levels (increased HDL cholesterol and decreased LDL cholesterol). Improvements in body composition and glucose metabolism are also beneficial for cardiovascular health. As described earlier, strength training also boosts bone mineral density, helping to prevent osteoporosis and associated bone fractures.

ASSESSING MUSCULAR STRENGTH AND ENDURANCE

Muscular strength and muscular endurance are distinct but related components of fitness. Muscular strength, the maximum amount of force a muscle can produce in a single

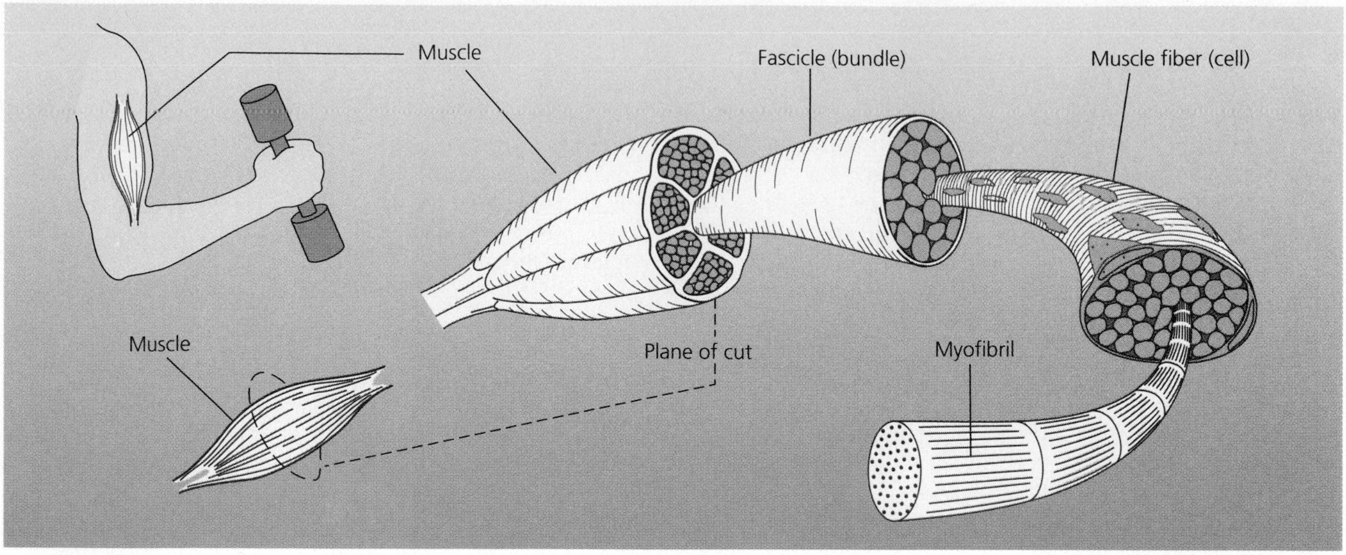

Figure 4.1 Components of skeletal muscle tissue.

effort, is usually assessed by measuring the maximum amount of weight a person can lift one time. This single maximal movement is referred to as a **repetition maximum (RM).** You can assess the strength of your major muscle groups by taking the one-repetition maximum (1 RM) tests for the bench press and the leg press. Refer to Lab 4.1 for guidelines on taking these tests. Instructions for assessing grip strength using a dynamometer are also included in Lab 4.1. For more accurate results, avoid any strenuous weight training for 48 hours beforehand.

Muscular endurance is the ability of a muscle to exert a submaximal force repeatedly or continuously over time. This ability depends on muscular strength because a certain amount of strength is required for any muscle movement. Muscular endurance is usually assessed by counting the maximum number of **repetitions** of a muscular contraction a person can do (such as in push-ups) or the maximum amount of time a person can hold a muscular contraction (such as in the flexed-arm hang). You can test the muscular endurance of major muscle groups in your body by taking the curl-up test and the push-up or bench press test. Refer to Lab 4.2 for complete instructions on taking these assessment tests.

Record your results and your fitness rating from the assessment tests in Labs 4.1 and 4.2. If the results show that improvement is needed, a weight training program will enable you to make rapid gains in muscular strength and endurance.

FUNDAMENTALS OF WEIGHT TRAINING

Weight training develops muscular strength and endurance in the same way that endurance exercise develops cardiovascular fitness: When the muscles are stressed by a greater load than they are used to, they adapt and improve their function. The type of adaptation that occurs depends on the type of stress applied.

Physiological Effects of Weight Training

Muscles move the body and enable it to exert force because they move the skeleton. When a muscle contracts (shortens), it moves a bone by pulling on the tendon that attaches the muscle to the bone. Muscles consist of individual muscle cells, or **muscle fibers,** connected in bundles (Figure 4.1). A single muscle is made up of many bundles of muscle fibers and is covered by layers of connective tissue that hold the fibers together. Muscle fibers, in turn, are made up of smaller units called **myofibrils.** When your muscles are given the signal to contract, protein filaments within the myofibrils slide across one another, causing the muscle fiber to shorten. Weight training causes the size of individual muscle fibers to increase by increasing the number of myofibrils. Larger muscle fibers mean a larger and stronger muscle. The development of large muscle fibers is called **hypertrophy.**

Muscle fibers are classified as fast-twitch or slow-twitch fibers according to their strength, speed of contraction, and energy source. **Slow-twitch fibers** are relatively fatigue resistant, but they don't contract as rapidly or strongly as fast-twitch fibers. The principal energy system that fuels slow-twitch fibers is aerobic. **Fast-twitch fibers** contract more rapidly and forcefully than slow-twitch fibers but fatigue more quickly. Although oxygen is important in the energy system that fuels fast-twitch fibers, they rely more on anaerobic metabolism than do slow-twitch fibers (see Chapter 3 for a discussion of energy systems).

Table 4.1 Physiological Changes and Benefits from Weight Training

Change	Benefits
Increased muscle mass*	Increased muscular strength Improved body composition Higher rate of metabolism Toned, healthy-looking muscles
Increased utilization of motor units during muscle contractions	Increased muscular strength and power
Improved coordination of motor units	Increased muscular strength and power
Increased strength of tendons, ligaments, and bones	Lower risk of injury to these tissues
Increased storage of fuel in muscles	Increased resistance to muscle fatigue
Increased size of fast-twitch muscle fibers (from a high-resistance program)	Increased muscular strength and power
Increased size of slow-twitch muscle fibers (from a high-repetition program)	Increased muscular endurance
Increased blood supply to muscles (from a high-repetition program)	Increased delivery of oxygen and nutrients Increased elimination of wastes
Biochemical improvements (for example, increased sensitivity to insulin)	Enhanced metabolic health
Improved blood fat levels	Reduced risk of heart disease

*Due to genetic and hormonal differences, men will build more muscle mass than women.

Most muscles contain a mixture of slow-twitch and fast-twitch fibers. The type of fiber that acts depends on the type of work required. Endurance activities like jogging tend to use slow-twitch fibers, whereas strength and **power** activities like sprinting use fast-twitch fibers. Weight training can increase the size and strength of both fast-twitch and slow-twitch fibers, although fast-twitch fibers are preferentially increased.

To exert force, the body recruits one or more motor units to contract. A **motor unit** is made up of a nerve connected to a number of muscle fibers. The number of muscle fibers in a motor unit varies from two to hundreds. When a motor nerve calls on its fibers to contract, all fibers contract to their full capacity. The number of motor units recruited depends on the amount of strength required: When a person picks up a small weight, he or she uses fewer motor units than when picking up a large weight. Weight training improves the body's ability to recruit motor units—a phenomenon called muscle learning—which increases strength even before muscle size increases.

In summary, weight training increases muscle strength because it increases the size of muscle fibers and improves the body's ability to call on motor units to exert force. The physiological changes and benefits that result from weight training are summarized in Table 4.1.

Types of Weight Training Exercises

Weight training exercises are generally classified as static or dynamic. Each involves a different way of using and strengthening muscles.

Static Exercise Also called **isometric** exercise, **static exercise** involves a muscle contraction without a change in the length of the muscle or the angle in the joint on which the muscle acts. To perform an isometric exercise, a person can use an immovable object like a wall to provide resistance, or just tighten a muscle while remaining

Terms

repetition maximum (RM) The maximum amount of resistance that can be moved a specified number of times; 1 RM is the maximum weight that can be lifted once. 5 RM is the maximum weight that can be lifted five times.

repetitions The number of times an exercise is performed during one set.

muscle fiber A single muscle cell, usually classified according to strength, speed of contraction, and energy source.

myofibrils Protein structures that make up muscle fibers.

hypertrophy An increase in the size of a muscle fiber, usually stimulated by muscular overload.

slow-twitch fibers Red muscle fibers that are fatigue-resistant but have a slow contraction speed and a lower capacity for tension; usually recruited for endurance activities.

fast-twitch fibers White muscle fibers that contract rapidly and forcefully but fatigue quickly; usually recruited for actions requiring strength and power.

power The ability to exert force rapidly.

motor unit A motor nerve (one that initiates movement) connected to one or more muscle fibers.

static (isometric) exercise Exercise involving a muscle contraction without a change in the length of the muscle.

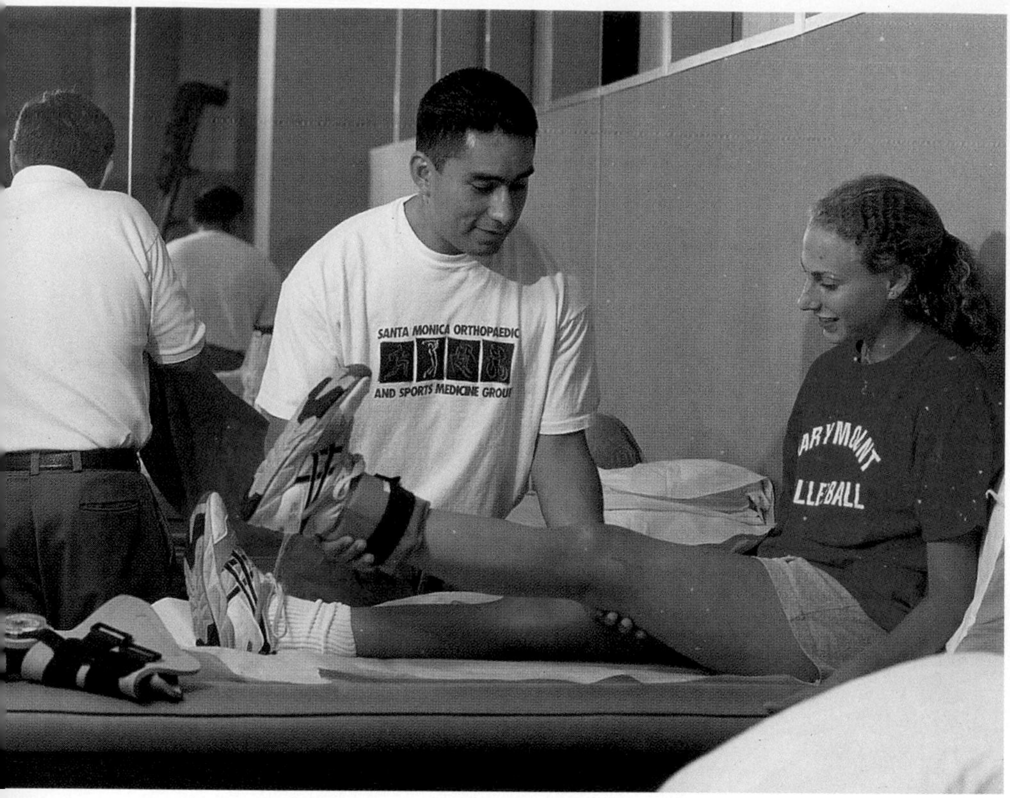

Static (isometric) exercises are often used for rehabilitation following an injury. In this exercise, gravity and an angle weight provide resistance for an isometric contraction of the upper thigh muscles (quadriceps).

still (for example, tightening the abdominal muscles while sitting at a desk). In isometrics, the muscle contracts, but there is no movement.

Isometric exercises aren't as widely used as isotonic exercises because they don't develop strength throughout a joint's entire range of motion. However, static exercises are useful in strengthening muscles after an injury or surgery, when movement of the affected joint could delay healing. Isometrics are also used to overcome weak points in an individual's range of motion. Statically strengthening a muscle at its weakest point will allow more weight to be lifted with that muscle during dynamic exercise. For maximum strength gains, hold the isometric contraction maximally for 6 seconds; do 5–10 repetitions.

Dynamic Exercise Also called **isotonic** exercise, **dynamic exercise** involves a muscle contraction with a change in the length of the muscle. Dynamic exercises are the most popular type of exercises for increasing muscle strength and seem to be most valuable for developing strength that can be transferred to other forms of physical activity. They can be performed with weight machines, free weights, or a person's own body weight (as in sit-ups or push-ups).

There are two kinds of dynamic muscle contractions: concentric and eccentric. A **concentric muscle contraction** occurs when the muscle applies enough force to overcome resistance and shortens as it contracts. An **eccentric muscle contraction** occurs when the resistance is greater than the force applied by the muscle and the muscle lengthens as it contracts. For example, in an arm curl, the biceps muscle works concentrically as the weight is raised toward the shoulder and eccentrically as the weight is lowered.

Two of the most common dynamic exercise techniques are constant resistance exercise and variable resistance exercise. Constant resistance exercise uses a constant load (weight) throughout a joint's entire range of motion. Training with free weights is a form of constant resistance exercise. A problem with this technique is that, because of differences in leverage, there are points in a joint's range of motion where the muscle controlling the movement is stronger and points where it is weaker. The amount of weight a person can lift is limited by the weakest point in the range. In variable resistance exercise, the load is changed to provide maximum load throughout the entire range of motion. This form of exercise uses machines that place more stress on muscles at the end of the range of motion, where a person has better leverage and is capable of exerting more force. The Nautilus pull-over machine is an example of a variable resistance exercise machine. Constant and variable resistance exercises are both extremely effective for building strength and endurance.

Four other kinds of isotonic techniques, used mainly by athletes for training and rehabilitation, are eccentric loading, plyometrics, speed loading, and isokinetics.

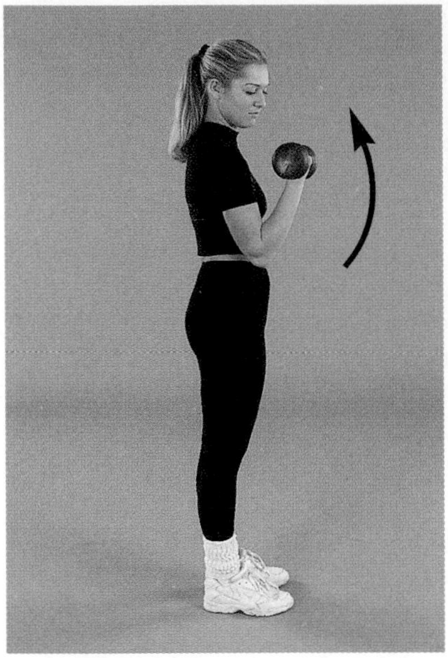

Left: A concentric contraction: The biceps muscle shortens as the arm lifts a weight toward the shoulder. **Right:** An eccentric contraction: The biceps muscle lengthens as the arm lowers a weight toward the thigh.

- **Eccentric loading** involves placing a load on a muscle as it lengthens. The muscle contracts eccentrically in order to control the weight. Eccentric loading is practiced during most types of resistance training. For example, you are performing an eccentric movement as you lower the weight to your chest during a bench press in preparation for the active movement. You can also perform exercises designed specifically to overload muscle eccentrically, a technique called negatives.
- **Plyometrics** is the sudden eccentric loading and stretching of muscles followed by a forceful concentric contraction. An example would be the action of the lower-body muscles when jumping from a bench to the ground and then jumping back onto the bench. This type of exercise is used to develop explosive strength; it also helps build and maintain bone density.
- **Speed loading** involves moving a weight as rapidly as possible in an attempt to approach the speeds used in movements like throwing a softball or sprinting. In the bench press, for example, speed loading might involve doing 5 repetitions as fast as possible using a weight that is half the maximum load you can lift. You can gauge your progress by timing how fast you can perform the repetitions.
- **Isokinetic** exercise involves exerting force at a constant speed against an equal force exerted by a special strength training machine. The isokinetic machine provides variable resistance at different points in the joint's range of motion, matching the effort applied by the individual, while keeping the speed of the movement constant. In other words, the force exerted by the individual at any point in the range of motion is resisted by an equal force from the isokinetic machine. Isokinetic exercises are excellent for building strength and endurance, but the equipment is expensive and less commonly available than other kinds of weight machines.

Comparing the Different Types of Exercise Static exercises require no equipment, so they can be done virtually anywhere. They build strength rapidly and are useful for rehabilitating injured joints. On the other hand, they have to be performed at several different angles for each joint to improve strength throughout the joint's entire range of motion. Dynamic exercises can be performed without equipment (calisthenics) or with equipment (weight lifting). They are excellent for building strength and endurance, and they tend to build strength through a joint's full range of motion.

Most people develop muscular strength and endurance using dynamic exercises. Ultimately, the type of exercise a person chooses depends on individual goals, preferences, and access to equipment.

Terms

dynamic (isotonic) exercise Exercise involving a muscle contraction with a change in the length of the muscle.

concentric muscle contraction An isotonic contraction in which the muscle gets shorter as it contracts.

eccentric muscle contraction An isotonic contraction in which the muscle lengthens as it contracts.

eccentric loading Loading the muscle while it is lengthening; sometimes called *negatives*.

plyometrics Rapid stretching of a muscle group that is undergoing eccentric stress (the muscle is exerting force while it lengthens), followed by a rapid concentric contraction.

speed loading Moving a load as rapidly as possible.

isokinetic The application of force at a constant speed against an equal force.

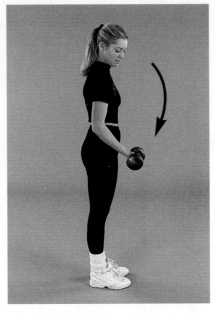

CREATING A SUCCESSFUL WEIGHT TRAINING PROGRAM

To get the most out of your weight training program, you must design it to achieve maximum fitness benefits with a low risk of injury. Before you begin, seriously consider the type and amount of training that's right for you.

Choosing Equipment: Weight Machines Versus Free Weights

Your muscles will get stronger if you make them work against a resistance. Resistance can be provided by free weights, by your own body weight, or by sophisticated exercise machines. Weight machines are preferred by many people because they are safe, convenient, and easy to use. You just set the resistance (usually by placing a pin in the weight stack), sit down at the machine, and start working. Machines make it easy to isolate and work specific muscles. You don't need a **spotter,** someone who stands by to assist when free weights are used, and you don't have to worry about dropping a weight on yourself.

Free weights require more care, balance, and coordination to use, but they strengthen your body in ways that are more adaptable to real life. Free weights are more popular with athletes for developing explosive strength for sports. Unless you are training seriously for a sport that requires a great deal of strength, training on machines is probably safer, more convenient, and just as effective as training with free weights. However, you can increase strength either way, depending on personal preference. The box "Exercise Machines Versus Free Weights" can help you make a decision.

Ww Selecting Exercises

A complete weight training program works all the major muscle groups. It usually takes about 8–10 different exercises to get a complete workout. For overall fitness, you need to include exercises for your neck, upper back, shoulders, arms, chest, abdomen, lower back, thighs, buttocks, and calves. If you are also training for a particular sport, include exercises to strengthen the muscles important for optimal performance *and* the muscles most likely to be injured. A weight training program for general fitness is presented later in this chapter.

It is important to balance exercises between **agonist** and **antagonist** muscle groups. (When a muscle contracts, it is known as the agonist; the opposing muscle, which must relax and stretch to allow contraction by the agonist, is known as the antagonist.) Whenever you do an exercise that moves a joint in one direction, also select an exercise that works the joint in the opposite direction. For example, if you do knee extensions to develop the muscles on the front of your thighs, also do leg curls to develop the antagonistic muscles on the back of your thighs.

The order of exercises can also be important. Do exercises for large-muscle groups or for more than one joint before you do exercises that use small-muscle groups or single joints. This allows for more effective overload of the larger, more powerful muscle groups. Small-muscle groups fatigue more easily than larger ones, and small-muscle fatigue limits your capacity to overload larger-muscle groups. For example, lateral raises, which work the shoulder muscles, should be performed after bench presses, which work the chest and arms in addition to the shoulders. If you fatigue your shoulder muscles by doing lateral raises first, you won't be able to lift as much weight and effectively fatigue all the key muscle groups used during the bench press.

Resistance

The amount of weight (resistance) you lift in weight training exercises is equivalent to intensity in cardiorespiratory endurance training. It determines the way your body will adapt to weight training and how quickly these adaptations will occur. Choose weights based on your current level of muscular fitness and your fitness goals. To build strength rapidly, you should lift weights as heavy as 80% of your maximum capacity (1 RM). If you're more interested in building endurance, choose a lighter weight (perhaps 40–60% of 1 RM) and do more repetitions. For example, if your maximum capacity for the leg press is 160 pounds, you might lift 130 pounds to build strength and 80 pounds to build endurance. For a general fitness program to develop both strength and endurance, choose a weight in the middle of this range, perhaps 70% of 1 RM.

Because it can be tedious and time-consuming to continually reassess your maximum capacity for each exercise, you might find it easier to choose a weight based on the number of repetitions of an exercise you can perform with a given resistance.

Repetitions and Sets

To improve fitness, you must do enough repetitions of each exercise to fatigue your muscles. The number of repetitions needed to cause fatigue depends on the amount of resistance: the heavier the weight, the fewer repetitions to reach fatigue. In general, a heavy weight and a low number of repetitions (1–5) build strength, whereas a light weight and a high number of repetitions (15–20) build endurance (Figure 4.2). For a general fitness pro-

Terms Ww

spotter A person who assists with a weight training exercise done with free weights.

agonist A muscle in a state of contraction, opposed by the action of another muscle, its *antagonist.*

antagonist A muscle that opposes the action of another muscle, its *agonist.*

set A group of repetitions followed by a rest period.

Exercise Machines

Advantages

- Safe and convenient
- Don't require spotters
- Don't require lifter to balance bar
- Provide variable resistance
- Require less skill
- Make it easy to move from one exercise to the next
- Allow easy isolation of muscles and muscle groups
- Support back (on many machines)

Disadvantages

- Limited availability
- Inappropriate for performing dynamic movements
- Allow a limited number of exercises

Free Weights

Advantages

- Allow dynamic movements
- Allow the user to develop control of the weights
- Allow a greater variety of exercises
- Widely available
- Truer to real-life situations; strength transfers to daily activities

Disadvantages

- Not as safe
- Require spotters
- Require more skill
- Cause more blisters and calluses

gram to build both strength and endurance, try to do about 8–12 repetitions of each exercise; a few exercises, such as abdominal crunches and calf raises, may require more. Choose a weight heavy enough to fatigue your muscles but light enough for you to complete the repetitions with good form. To avoid risk of injury, older (approximately 50–60 years of age and above) and more frail people should perform more repetitions (10–15) using a lighter weight.

In weight training, a **set** refers to a group of repetitions of an exercise followed by a rest period. Surprisingly, exercise scientists have not identified the optimal number of sets for increasing strength. For developing strength and endurance for general fitness, a single set of each exercise is sufficient, provided you use enough resistance to fatigue your muscles. (You should just barely be able to complete the 8–12 repetitions—using good form—for each exercise.) Doing more than 1 set of each exercise may increase strength development, and most serious weight trainers do at least 3 sets of each exercise (see below for additional guidelines for more advanced programs).

If you perform more than 1 set of an exercise, you need to rest long enough between sets to allow your muscles to work at a high enough intensity to increase fitness. The length of the rest interval depends on the amount of resistance. In a program to develop a combination of strength and endurance for wellness, a rest period of 1–3 minutes between sets is appropriate; if you are lifting heavier loads to build maximum strength, rest 3–5 minutes between sets. You can save time in your workouts if you alternate sets of different exercises. Each muscle group can rest between sets while you work on other muscles.

Overtraining—doing more exercise than your body can recover from—can occur in response to heavy resistance training. Possible signs of overtraining include lack of progress or decreased performance, chronic fatigue, decreased coordination, and chronic muscle soreness. The best remedy for overtraining is rest: Add more days of

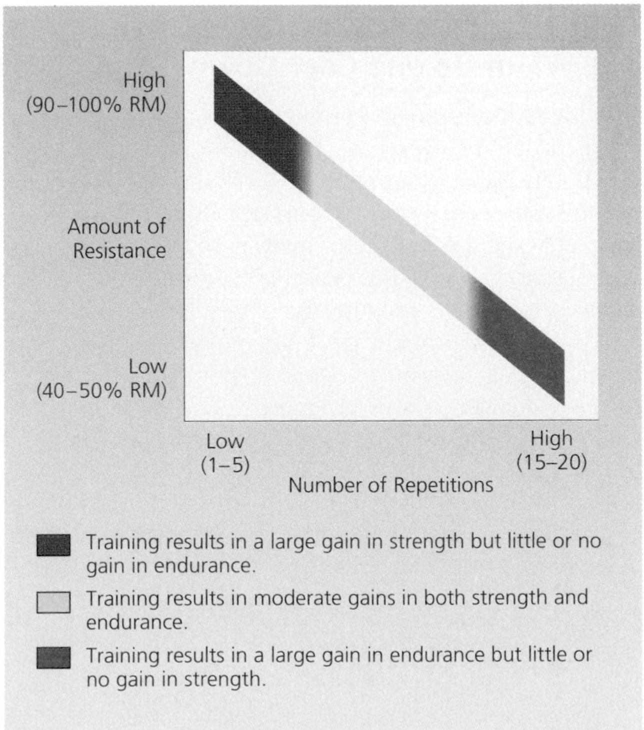
High
(90–100% RM)
Amount of
Resistance
Low
(40–50% RM)
Low
(1–5)
High
(15–20)
Number of Repetitions
Training results in a large gain in strength but little or no gain in endurance.
Training results in moderate gains in both strength and endurance.
Training results in a large gain in endurance but little or no gain in strength.

Figure 4.2 Training for strength versus training for endurance.

Warm-up 5–10 minutes	Strength training exercises for major muscle groups (8–10 exercises)		Cool-down 5–10 minutes
	Sample program		
	Exercise	*Muscle group developed*	
	Bench press	Chest, shoulders, triceps	
	Shoulder press	Shoulders, trapezius, triceps	
	Pull-ups	Lats, biceps	
	Lateral raises	Shoulders	
	Biceps curls	Biceps	
	Squats	Gluteals, quadriceps	
	Heel raises	Calves	
	Abdominal curls	Abdominals	
	Spine extensions	Low- and mid-back spine extensors	
Start	Neck flexion	Neck flexors	*Stop*

Type of activity: 8–10 strength training exercises that focus on major muscle groups

Frequency: 2–3 days per week

Resistance: Weights heavy enough to cause muscle fatigue when exercises are performed with good form for the selected number of repetitions

Repetitions: 8–12 of each exercise (10–15 with a lower weight for people over age 50–60)

Sets: 1 (doing more than 1 set per exercise may result in faster and greater strength gains)

Figure 4.3 A strength training workout.

recovery between workouts. With extra rest, chances are you'll be refreshed and ready to train again. Adding variety to your program, discussed later in the chapter, can also help with overtraining from resistance exercise.

The Warm-Up and Cool-Down

As with cardiorespiratory endurance exercise, you should warm up before every weight training session and cool down afterward (Figure 4.3). You should do both a general warm-up—several minutes of walking or easy jogging—and a warm-up for the weight training exercises you plan to perform. For example, if you plan to do 1 or more sets of 10 repetitions of bench presses with 125 pounds, you might do 1 set of 10 repetitions with 50 pounds as a warm-up. Do similar warm-up exercises for each exercise in your program.

To cool down after weight training, relax for 5–10 minutes after your workout. Although this is controversial, a few studies have suggested that including a period of postexercise stretching may help prevent muscle soreness; warmed-up muscles and joints make this a particularly good time to work on flexibility.

Frequency of Exercise

For general fitness, the American College of Sports Medicine recommends a frequency of 2–3 days per week for weight training. Allow your muscles at least 1 day of rest between workouts; if you train too often, your muscles won't be able to work at a high enough intensity to improve their fitness, and soreness and injury are more likely to result. If you enjoy weight training and would like to train more often, try working different muscle groups on alternate days. For example, work your arms and upper body one day, work your lower body the next day, and then return to upper-body exercises on the third day.

Making Progress

The first few sessions of weight training should be devoted to learning the exercises. You need to learn the movements, and your nervous system needs to practice communicating with your muscles so you can develop strength effectively. To start, choose a weight that you can move easily through 8–12 repetitions, and do only 1 set of each exercise. Gradually add weight and (if you want) sets to your program over the first few weeks until you are doing 1–3 sets of 8–12 repetitions of each exercise.

As you progress, add weight when you can do more than 12 repetitions of an exercise. If adding weight means you can do only 7 or 8 repetitions, stay with that weight until you can again complete 12 repetitions per set. If you can do only 4–6 repetitions after adding weight, or if you can't maintain good form, you've added too much and should take some off. Knowing how much resistance to

WORKOUT CARD FOR Scott Peterson

Exercise/Date		9/14	9/16	9/18	9/21	9/23	9/25	9/28	9/30	10/2	10/5	10/7	10/9	10/12	10/14	10/16									
Bench press	Wt.	70	70	70	75	75	75	80	80	80	90	90	95	105	105	105									
	Sets	1	1	1	1	1	1	1	1	1	1	1	1	1	1	1									
	Reps.	10	10	12	10	12	12	10	9	12	12	12	12	8	7	8									
Shoulder press	Wt.	40	40	40	55	55	60	60	60	70	70	75	75	75	80	85									
	Sets	1	1	1	1	1	1	1	1	1	1	1	1	1	1	1									
	Reps.	10	10	12	10	12	10	10	12	10	12	8	11	12	12	8									
Pull-ups	Wt.	—	—	—	—	—	—	—	—	—	—	—	—	—	—	—									
	Sets	1	1	1	1	1	1	1	1	1	1	1	1	1	1	1									
	Reps.	2	2	2	2	3	3	4	4	4	4	4	5	5	6	6									
Lateral raises	Wt.	5	5	5	7.5	7.5	7.5	7.5	7.5	7.5	7.5	7.5	7.5	10	10	10									
	Sets	1	1	1	1	1	1	1	1	1	1	1	1	1	1	1									
	Reps.	10	10	10	7	8	7	10	8	8	11	12	12	7	7	8									
Biceps curls	Wt.	35	35	35	40	40	40	45	45	45	50	50	50	50	50	50									
	Sets	1	1	1	1	1	1	1	1	1	1	1	1	1	1	1									
	Reps.	10	10	10	10	12	12	10	12	12	10	8	8	10	10	10									
Squats	Wt.	—	—	—	45	45	85	85	105	115	125	135	135	145	145	145									
	Sets	1	1	1	1	1	1	1	1	1	1	1	1	1	1	1									
	Reps.	10	10	10	12	15	10	12	12	15	12	10	12	9	8	9									
Heel raises	Wt.	—	—	—	45	45	85	85	105	115	125	135	135	145	145	145									
	Sets	1	1	1	1	1	1	1	1	1	1	1	1	1	1	1									
	Reps.	15	15	15	15	15	15	15	15	15	15	15	15	15	15	15									
Abdominal curls	Wt.	—	—	—	—	—	—	—	—	—	—	—	—	—	—	—									
	Sets	1	1	1	1	1	1	1	1	1	1	1	1	1	1	1									
	Reps.	20	20	20	20	20	20	25	25	25	30	30	30	30	30	30									
Spine extensions	Wt.	—	—	—	—	—	—	—	—	—	—	—	—	—	—	—									
	Sets	1	1	1	1	1	1	1	1	1	1	1	1	1	1	1									
	Reps.	5	5	5	8	8	8	10	10	10	10	10	10	10	10	10									
Neck flexion	Wt.	—	—	—	—	—	—	—	—	—	—	—	—	—	—	—									
	Sets	1	1	1	1	1	1	1	1	1	1	1	1	1	1	1									
	Reps.	5	5	5	10	10	10	10	10	10	10	10	10	10	10	10									

Figure 4.4 A sample workout card for a general fitness strength training program.

add and when to add it is as much an art as a science. You can add more resistance in large muscle exercises, such as squats and bench presses, than you can in smaller muscle exercises, such as curls. For example, when you can complete 12 repetitions of squats with good form, you may be able to add 10–20 pounds of additional resistance; for curls, on the other hand, you might add only 3–5 pounds. As a general guideline, try increases of approximately 5%, half a pound of additional weight for each 10 pounds you are currently lifting.

You can expect to improve rapidly during the first 6–10 weeks of training: a 10–30% increase in the amount of weight lifted. Gains will then come more slowly. Your rate of improvement will depend on how hard you work and how your body responds to resistance training. There will be individual differences in the rate of improvement. Factors such as age, motivation, and heredity will affect your progress.

Your ultimate goal depends on you. After you have achieved the level of strength and muscularity that you want, you can maintain your gains by training 2–3 days per week. You can monitor the progress of your program by recording the amount of resistance and the number of repetitions and sets you perform on a workout card like the one shown in Figure 4.4.

More Advanced Strength Training Programs

The weight training program described in this section—1 set of 8–12 repetitions of 8–10 exercises, performed 2–3 days per week—is sufficient to develop and maintain muscular strength and endurance for general fitness. If you have a different goal, you may need to adjust your program accordingly. As described above, performing more sets of a smaller number of repetitions with a heavier load will cause greater increases in strength. A program designed to build strength might include 3–5 sets of 4–6 repetitions each; the load used should be heavy enough to cause fatigue with the smaller number of repetitions. Rest long enough after a set to allow your muscles to recover and to work intensely during the next set.

Experienced weight trainers often engage in some form of cycle training, also called periodization, in which the exercises, number of sets and repetitions, and intensity are varied within a workout and/or between workouts. For example, you might do a particular exercise more intensely during some sets or on some days than others; you might also vary the exercises you perform for particular muscle groups. For information on these more advanced training techniques, consult a strength coach certified by the

TAKE CHARGE Safe Weight Training

- Lift weights from a stabilized body position.
- Be aware of what's going on around you. Stay away from other people when they're doing exercises. If you bump into someone, you could cause an injury.
- Don't use defective equipment. Report any equipment malfunctions immediately.
- Protect your back by maintaining control of your spine (protect your spine from dangerous positions). Observe proper lifting techniques and good form at all times. If you have to alter your technique to complete a repetition, you are probably lifting too much weight.
- Don't hold your breath while doing weight training exercises.
- Always warm up before training and cool down afterward.
- Don't exercise if you're ill, injured, or overtrained.

National Strength and Conditioning Association or another reliable source. If you decide to adopt a more advanced training regimen, start off slowly to give your body a chance to adjust and to minimize the risk of injury.

Weight Training Safety

Injuries do happen in weight training. Maximum physical effort, elaborate machinery, rapid movements, and heavy weights can combine to make the weight room a dangerous place if proper precautions aren't taken. To help ensure that your workouts are safe and productive, follow the guidelines in the box "Safe Weight Training" and the suggestions given below.

Use Proper Lifting Technique Every exercise has a proper technique that is important for obtaining maximum benefits and preventing injury. Your instructor or weight room attendant can help explain the specific techniques for performing different exercises and using different weight machines. Perform exercises smoothly and with good form. Lift or push the weight forcefully during the active phase of the lift and then lower it slowly with control. Perform all lifts through the full range of motion.

Use Spotters and Collars with Free Weights Spotters are necessary when an exercise has potential for danger: A weight that is out of control or falls can cause a serious injury. A spotter can assist you if you cannot complete a lift or if the weight tilts. A spotter can also help you move a weight into position before a lift and provide help or additional resistance during a lift. Spotting requires practice and coordination between the lifter and the spotter(s).

Collars are devices that secure weights to a barbell or dumbbell. Although people lift weights without collars, doing so is dangerous. It is easy to lose your balance or to raise one side of the weight faster than the other. Without collars, the weights on one side of the bar will slip off, and the weights on the opposite side will crash to the floor.

Proper lifting technique for free weights also includes the following:

- Keep weights as close to your body as possible.
- Do most of your lifting with your legs. Keep your hips and buttocks tucked in.
- When you pick a weight up from the ground, keep your back straight and your head level or up. Don't bend at the waist with straight legs.
- Don't twist your body while lifting.
- Lift weights smoothly and slowly; don't jerk them. Control the weight through the entire range of motion.
- Don't bounce weights against your body during an exercise.
- Never hold your breath when you lift. Exhale when exerting the greatest force, and inhale when moving the weight into position for the active phase of the lift. (Holding your breath causes a decrease in blood returning to the heart and can make you become dizzy and faint.)
- Rest between sets if you perform more than 1 set of each exercise. Fatigue hampers your ability to obtain maximum benefits from your program and is a prime cause of injury.
- When lifting barbells and dumbbells, wrap your thumbs around the bar when gripping it. You can easily drop the weight when using a "thumbless" grip.
- Gloves are not mandatory but may prevent calluses on your hands.
- When doing standing lifts, maintain a good posture so that you protect your back.
- Don't lift beyond the limits of your strength.

Use Common Sense When Exercising on Weight Machines Although notable for their safety, weight machines are not completely danger-free. The following strategies can help prevent injuries.

- Keep away from moving weight stacks. Pay attention when you're changing weights. Someone may jump on the machine ahead of you and begin an exercise while your fingers are close to the weight stack.

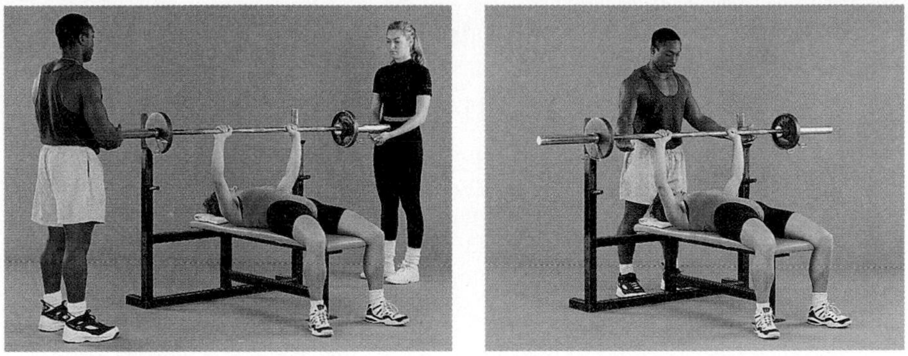

(a) (b)

Spotters should be present when a person trains with free weights. **(a)** If two spotters are used, one spotter should stand at each end of the barbell. **(b)** If one spotter is present, he or she should stand behind the lifter.

- Stay away from moving parts of the machine that could pinch your skin.
- Adjust each machine for your body so that you don't have to work in an awkward position. Lock everything in place before you begin.
- Beware of broken bolts, frayed cables, broken chains, or loose [illegible] and cause serious injury. If you notice a broken [illegible] frayed part, tell an instructor immediately.
- Make sure the machines are clean. Dirty vinyl is a breeding ground for germs that can cause skin diseases. Carry a towel around with you, and place it on the machine where you will sit or lie down.
- Be aware of what's happening around you. Talking between exercises is a great way to relax and have fun, but inattention can lead to injury.

Be Alert for Injuries Report any obvious muscle or joint injuries to your instructor or physician, and stop exercising the affected area. Training with an injured joint or muscle can lead to a more serious injury. Make sure you get the necessary first aid. Even minor injuries heal faster if you use the R-I-C-E principle of treating injuries described in Chapter 3.

Consult a physician if you're having any unusual symptoms during exercise or if you're uncertain whether weight training is a proper activity for you. Conditions such as heart disease and high blood pressure can be aggravated during weight training. Symptoms such as headaches; dizziness; labored breathing; numbness; vision disturbances; and chest, neck, or arm pains should be reported immediately.

Ww A Caution About Supplements and Drugs

Many active people use a wide variety of nutritional supplements and drugs in the quest for improved performance and appearance. Most of these substances are ineffective and expensive and many are dangerous. A selective summary of "performance aids" is given in Table 4.2, along with their potential side effects.

Supplements Taken to Increase Muscle Growth The most popular category of supplements are those taken to increase muscle growth.

- **Anabolic steroids** are a group of synthetic derivatives of testosterone. People take them in hope of gaining weight and muscle size and improving strength, power, speed, endurance, aggressiveness, and appearance. Despite drug testing, anabolic steroids are taken by some athletes in sports such as bodybuilding, track and field, and football. Use of anabolic steroids has filtered down to high school students, and about 6% of all high school students have used them.

Anabolic steroids increase protein synthesis, which enhances fat-free weight, muscle mass, and strength. Side effects include liver damage and tumors, decreased levels of high-density lipoprotein (good cholesterol), heart disease, depressed sperm and testosterone production, high blood pressure, increased risk of AIDS (through shared needles), depressed immune function, problems with sugar metabolism, psychological disturbances, masculinization in women and children, premature closure of bone growth centers, and an increased risk of cancer. Side effects are greatest in people who take high doses of drugs for prolonged periods.

- Human chorionic gonadotrophin (HCG) is sometimes taken by anabolic steroid users to boost natural testosterone production, which is suppressed by steroids, and to prevent the muscle atrophy common during withdrawal from steroids. Although HCG tends to increase testosterone levels, it sometimes interferes with normal testosterone regulation, which causes additional deterioration in health and well-being. Use of HCG is not recommended and is banned in most sports.
- Growth hormone is used to increase muscle mass and strength. Reports in the news media suggest that, as with anabolic steroids, its general use has filtered down to high school students. Although advances in genetics

anabolic steroids Synthetic male hormones taken to enhance athletic performance and body composition.

Terms Ww

Table 4.2 Performance Aids Marketed to Weight Trainers

Substance	Supposed Effects	Actual Effects	Selected Potential Side Effects
Adrenal androgens: DHEA, androstenedione	Increased testosterone, muscle mass, and strength; decreased body fat	Increased testosterone, strength, and fat-free mass and decreased fat in older subjects (more studies needed in younger people)	Gonadal suppression, prostate hypertrophy, breast development in males, masculinization in women and children. Long-term effects unknown
Amino acids	Increased muscle mass	No effects if dietary protein intake is adequate	Minimal side effects; unbalanced amino acid intake can cause problems with protein metabolism
Anabolic steroids	Increased muscle mass, strength, power, psychological aggressiveness, and endurance	Increased strength, power, fat-free mass, and aggression; no effects on endurance	Minor to severe: gonadal suppression, liver disease, acne, breast development in males, masculinization in women and children, heart disease, cancer. Steroids are controlled substances[a]
Chromium picolinate	Increased muscle mass; decreased body fat	Well-controlled studies show no significant effect on fat-free mass or on body fat	Moderate doses (50–200 μg) appear safe; higher doses may cause DNA damage and other serious effects. Long-term effects unknown
Creatine monohydrate	Increased muscle creatine phosphate, muscle mass, and capacity for high-intensity exercise	Increased muscle mass and performance in some types of high-intensity exercise	Minimal side effects; some reports of muscle cramping and exacerbation of existing kidney problems. Long-term effects unknown
Ephedrine (usually sold combined with caffeine or another stimulant)	Decreased body fat; increased training intensity due to stimulant effect	Decreased appetite, particularly when taken with caffeine; some evidence for increased training intensity	Abnormal heart rhythms, nervousness, headache, and gastrointestinal distress
Ginseng	Decreased effects of physical and emotional stress; increased oxygen consumption	Most well-controlled studies show no effect on performance	No serious side effects; high doses can cause high blood pressure, nervousness, and insomnia
Growth hormone	Increased muscle mass, strength, and power; decreased body fat	Increased muscle mass and strength	Diabetes, acromegaly (disease characterized by increased growth of bones in hands and face), enlarged heart and other organs. An extremely expensive controlled substance[a]
HMB (beta-hydroxy-beta-methylbutyrate)	Increased strength and muscle mass; decreased body fat	Some studies show increased fat-free mass and decreased fat; more research needed	No reported side effects. Long-term effects unknown
"Metabolic-optimizing" meals for athletes	Increased muscle mass; energy supply; decreased body fat	No proven effects beyond those of balanced meals	No reported side effects; extremely expensive
Protein	Increased muscle mass	No effects if dietary protein intake is adequate	Can be dangerous for people with liver or kidney disease

[a]Possession of a controlled substance is illegal without a prescription, and physicians are not allowed to prescribe controlled substances for the improvement of athletic performance. In addition, the use of anabolic steroids, growth hormone, or any of several other substances listed in this table is banned for athletic competition.

SOURCES: Brooks, G. A., et al. 2000. *Exercise Physiology: Human Bioenergetics and Its Applications*, 3d ed. Mountain View, Calif: Mayfield. Sports-supplement dangers. 2001. *Consumer Reports*, June. Williams, M. H. 1998. *The Ergogenics Edge: Pushing the Limits of Sports Performance.* Champaign, Ill.: Human Kinetics.

have made human growth hormone more widely available, it is extremely expensive and has serious side effects. Growth hormone builds muscles, but the few studies on the hormone in humans have shown no beneficial effects on muscle or exercise performance. Prolonged growth hormone administration may result in elevated blood sugar, high insulin levels, heart enlargement, and increased blood fat levels. Prolonged use could also lead to acromegaly, characterized by enlarged bones in the head, face, and hands, as well as diseases of the heart, nerves, bones, and joints.

- Dehydroepiandrosterone (DHEA) and androstenedione are two relatively weak male hormones produced in the adrenal glands of both men and women. Both are broken down into testosterone. People take these drugs to stimulate muscle growth and aid in weight control. Because they are sold as supplements, they are widely available in health food stores and supermarkets (see the box "Dietary Supplements: A Consumer Dilemma," p. 94). The few studies in humans show that they are of little value in improving athletic performance. These substances have side effects similar to those of anabolic steroids, particularly when taken in high doses.
- Insulin is used by the body to help control carbohydrate, fat, and protein metabolism. Some athletes take insulin injections to promote muscle hypertrophy, but its effectiveness in stimulating muscle growth is not known. Insulin supplementation is an extremely dangerous practice because it can cause insulin shock (characterized by extremely low blood sugar), which can lead to unconsciousness and death.
- Insulin-like growth factor (IGF-1) is produced by the pituitary gland and is stimulated by growth hormone. Although IGF-1 is a powerful anabolic agent, its effects in healthy, active people are unknown. Side effects are thought to be similar to those of growth hormone. Long-term use is known to promote cancer.
- Beta-agonists are a type of medication used to treat asthma, including exercise-induced asthma; this family of drugs includes salmeterol and terbutaline. Some athletes who do not have asthma take beta-agonists in an attempt to enhance performance. They hope to prevent muscle atrophy, increase fat-free weight, and decrease body fat. Potential side effects include insomnia, heart arrhythmias, anxiety, anorexia, and nausea. More serious side effects include heart enlargement and heart attack (particularly if used with anabolic steroids).
- Protein, amino acid, and polypeptide supplements are taken to accelerate muscle development, decrease body fat, and stimulate the release of growth hormone. By a wide margin, these products are the most popular supplements taken by active people. Still, there is little scientific proof to support their use, even in athletes on extremely heavy training routines. The protein requirements of these athletes are not much higher than those of sedentary individuals. Also, most athletes take in more than enough protein in their diets. Although there appear to be few side effects from using these products, substituting amino acid or polypeptide supplements for protein-rich food can cause deficiencies in important nutrients, such as iron and the B vitamins.
- So-called metabolic-optimizing meals contain a wide variety of individual supplemental components and are widely used by athletes and active people. Some studies suggest that these meals may increase the hormone concentrations necessary for the development of fitness, but their effects on muscle growth and performance have not been demonstrated.

Supplements Taken to Speed Recovery from Training The primary purpose of taking these agents is to replenish depleted body fuel supplies that are important during exercise and recovery.

- Creatine monohydrate is used in an effort to enhance recovery, power, strength, and muscle size. Creatine monohydrate supplements increase creatine phosphate levels in muscle. As discussed in Chapter 3, creatine phosphate is a critical fuel source in the body. Several, but not all, studies have shown that creatine monohydrate supplementation improves performance in short-term, high-intensity, repetitive exercise. It may help to enlarge muscles in people who lift weights by allowing them to train harder. On the other hand, in 2000, a panel of ACSM experts found no evidence that creatine supplements increase the aerobic power of muscle. Creatine may increase water retention in muscles, giving the feeling of increased muscularity without an actual increase in muscle size. Although this supplement appears safe, its long-term effects are unknown, so people should take this substance with caution.
- Chromium picolinate is used to enhance the action of insulin and to improve carbohydrate metabolism. Although a few studies have shown benefits, the efficacy of this supplement is extremely controversial.
- Other substances in this category include carbohydrate beverages that athletes use during and immediately following exercise to help them recover from intense training; these beverages may speed the replenishment of liver and muscle glycogen.

Substances Taken to Increase Training Intensity and Overcome Fatigue Active people often spend many hours a day training, and monotony and fatigue sometimes impede significant improvement. Some people use stimulants to help them increase training intensity and overcome fatigue.

- Amphetamines are sometimes used by athletes to prevent fatigue and to increase confidence and training intensity. These drugs stimulate the nervous system, causing increased arousal, wakefulness, confidence, and the feeling of an enhanced capability to make decisions; they mask fatigue, so users feel energized, but once the

"Builds lean muscle fast!" "Burns fat and gives you super energy!" "The most effective muscle-building product ever!" It's only human nature to want to feel, perform, and look as good as possible. But wading through advertising hype can be tricky when you are considering taking a dietary supplement. While drugs and food products undergo stringent government testing, dietary supplements can be freely marketed without testing for safety or effectiveness. There is no guarantee that advertising claims about dietary supplements are accurate or true.

What's the difference between a drug—which must be approved by the Food and Drug Administration (FDA)—and a dietary supplement? In some cases, the only real difference is in how the product is marketed. Some dietary supplements are as potentially dangerous as potent prescription drugs. For example, the male hormone testosterone, a powerful drug with many adverse affects, is closely regulated by the FDA. Androstenedione, a hormone converted in the body to testosterone (and estrogen), is readily available without a prescription as a dietary supplement. Androstenedione ("andro") is legal and can be purchased in thousands of stores and Internet sites. Andro disrupts the hormonal balance of its users and can increase the risk of heart disease. Teens who take andro are at risk for early closure of bone growth centers, which could limit their adult height. Other potential adverse effects of andro include acne, psychological disturbances, male breast development, baldness, and kidney and liver dysfunction. Advertisements for andro claim that it will increase muscle size, strength, and performance, but there are actually very few good studies of andro's effects on humans; the two best studies showed no significant difference in muscle growth and strength in andro users compared with nonusers. Most medical experts believe that andro is neither safe nor effective—yet it is used by thousands of athletes, most of whom are unaware of the risks.

Androstenedione is only one of the many popular dietary supplements that are of questionable benefit and safety. Ephedra is another common ingredient in dietary supplements, often touted as an "energy booster" and a "fat burner." Consumers might assume that ephedra is free of serious side effects since it is a natural herbal product and is available without a prescription. But ephedra has caused severe high blood pressure, heart attacks, strokes, and seizures, and has been implicated in numerous deaths. Adverse effects are much more likely when ephedra, which is a stimulant, is combined with other stimulants such as caffeine. Despite the risk, many ephedra-containing dietary supplements do contain caffeine or other stimulants—a fact that may not be clear from their labels. Many sports organizations, including the National Football League, have banned the use of ephedra because of safety concerns. However, it's estimated that more than 12 million Americans use ephedra-containing products. (Chapter 9 has more information about ephedra and other dietary supplements marketed for weight loss.)

Glowing reports about the supposed effects of dietary supplements may sound very enticing, but how can you determine if a particular supplement might be helpful? Ask yourself the following questions:

- *Do you really need a supplement at all?* Nutritional authorities agree that most athletes and young adults can obtain all the necessary ingredients for health and top athletic performance by eating a well-balanced diet and training appropriately. There is no dietary supplement that outperforms wholesome real food and a good training regimen. Remember, too, that athletic performance and appearance are not life and death issues. It's one thing to take a cancer chemotherapy drug with many known adverse effects if there is a reasonable chance that it will save your life. It's another to take a potentially dangerous dietary supplement that may not even work for you when your goal is to increase your sports performance.
- *Is the product safe and effective?* The fact that a dietary supplement is available in your local store is no guarantee of safety. As described above, the FDA doesn't regulate supplements in the same way as drugs. The only way to determine if a supplement really works is to perform carefully controlled research on human subjects. Testimonials from individuals who claim to have benefited from the product don't count. Few dietary supplements have undergone careful human testing, so it is difficult to tell which of them may actually work. Reliable resources for information on dietary supplements include the FDA Center for Food Safety and Applied Nutrition (http://www.cfsan.fda.gov/~dms/supplmnt.html) and the Nutritional Supplements for Athletes Web site from Kansas State University (http://www.oznet.ksu.edu/nutrition/supplements.htm).
- *Can you be sure that the specific product is of high quality?* There is no official agency that ensures the quality of dietary supplements. There is no guarantee that a supplement contains the desired ingredient, that dosages are appropriate, that potency is standardized, or that the product is free from contaminants (see Chapter 8 for more information on dietary supplement labeling).

A recent study of twelve over-the-counter brands of supplements containing androstenedione and related steroids found that one brand contained more and eleven brands contained less than the amount stated on the label; in addition, one brand contained a significant amount of a controlled steriod. The International Olympic Committee recently issued a warning to athletes based on a test of 634 different nutritional supplements; researchers found that 15% of the supplements tested contained unlabled substances that would cause an athlete to fail a drug test.

Many dietary supplements are ineffective and/or unsafe, but it is extremely difficult for consumers to get the information they need to make an informed decision. Once you have gathered the best information you can find, consider whether the potential benefits of the supplement appear to outweigh the risks and the cost. When in doubt, it's best not to buy or take the product. Remember that no supplement eliminates the need for proper training, and no supplement has been shown to be safe and effective in long-term weight loss. A product that is marginally effective, not proven safe, and expensive to boot is probably not worth the money or the risk.

drug wears off, depression or fatigue sets in. Because amphetamines can cause extreme confusion, they are of little use in sports requiring rapid decisions. Amphetamines can cause severe neural and psychological effects that include aggressiveness, paranoia, hallucinations, compulsive behavior, restlessness, irritability, heart arrhythmias, high blood pressure, and chest pains (see Chapter 13).

- Caffeine, found naturally in many plant species, is a favorite stimulant among many active people. Caffeine stimulates the nervous system and helps increase fat levels in the blood. Although there is some evidence that caffeine may improve endurance, the drug does not appear to enhance short-term maximal exercise capacity. Caffeine increases the incidence of abnormal heart rhythms and insomnia and is addictive. Ephedra, another naturally occurring stimulant, is described in more detail below and in the box on p. 94.

Substances Taken to Increase Endurance Erythropoietin and darbepoetin are related drugs that stimulate the growth of oxygen-carrying red blood cells. These drugs are used to help treat anemia in patients with cancer and kidney disease. Some athletes have taken these drugs in an effort to boost their performance in endurance events. By increasing the production of red blood cells, erythropoietin and darbepoetin enhance oxygen uptake and endurance. However, these supplements are extremely dangerous because they increase blood viscosity (thickness) and can cause potentially fatal blood clots.

Substances Taken to Aid Weight Control Substances used in weight control include drugs that suppress appetite, drugs that affect metabolic rate, and diuretics to control weight and increase muscle definition.

- Prescription appetite suppressants include diethylpropion and phentermine; these and related drugs can have serious side effects and are not approved for long-term use. A related drug, phenylpropanolamine (PPA), was a common ingredient in over-the-counter weight control medications until studies began linking the drug to an increased risk of stroke. Stimulants such as caffeine and ephedrine are sometimes used for weight control, and some studies have found them to be effective, at least in the short term. However, there have been reports of adverse effects from the use of ephedra, including an increased risk of heart attack or stroke in some people. An additional concern is the lack of standardization; labels may not correctly indicate the amount of stimulant that an over-the-counter supplement contains. (See Chapter 9 for more on over-the-counter diet pills and diet aids.)
- Diuretics (drugs that promote loss of body fluid) and potassium supplements are sometimes taken by people in an attempt to accentuate muscle difinition. Others take potassium supplements to promote fluid retention in their muscle cells, thus increasing muscle size. Athletes may combine these practices with very-low-calorie diets and dehydration in the quest for weight loss and leanness. There is no evidence that these unhealthy practices improve appearance or muscle size. Serious complications have developed from these practices, including muscle cell destruction, low blood pressure, blood chemistry abnormalities, and heart problems.

Supplement and Drug Use by Active People The variety and combinations of supplements and drugs used by physically active people make it extremely difficult to determine the efficacy of these practices or to predict their side effects. Many medical studies describe catastrophic side effects from use of unsafe drugs and nutritional supplements. Most supplements simply don't work.

Keep in mind that no nutritional supplement or drug will change a weak, untrained person into a strong, fit person. Those changes require regular training that stresses the muscles, heart, lungs, and metabolism and causes the body to adapt. They also require a healthy, balanced diet, as described in Chapter 8. The next section describes weight training exercises that can help you reach your goals.

Weight Training Exercises

A general book on fitness and wellness cannot include a detailed description of all weight training exercises. Here we present a basic program for developing muscular strength and endurance for general fitness using free weights and weight machines. Instructions for each exercise are accompanied by photographs and a listing of the muscles being trained. (Figure 4.5 on p. 96 is a diagram of the muscular system.) Table 4.3 on p. 97 lists alternative and additional exercises that can be performed on Cybex, Nautilus, or Universal machines or with free weights. If you are interested in learning how to do these exercises, ask your instructor or coach for assistance.

If you want to develop strength for a particular activity, your program should contain exercises for general fitness, exercises for the muscle groups most important for the activity, and exercises for muscle groups most often injured. Labs 4.2 and 4.3 will help you assess your current level of muscular endurance, design your own weight training program, and apply it in the fitness facility you plan to use. Regardless of the goals of your program or the type of equipment you use, your program should be structured so that you obtain maximum results without risking injury. You should train at least 2 days per week, and each exercise session should contain a warm-up, 1 or more sets of 8–12 repetitions of 8–10 exercises, and a period of rest.

Weight training exercises begin on p. 98.

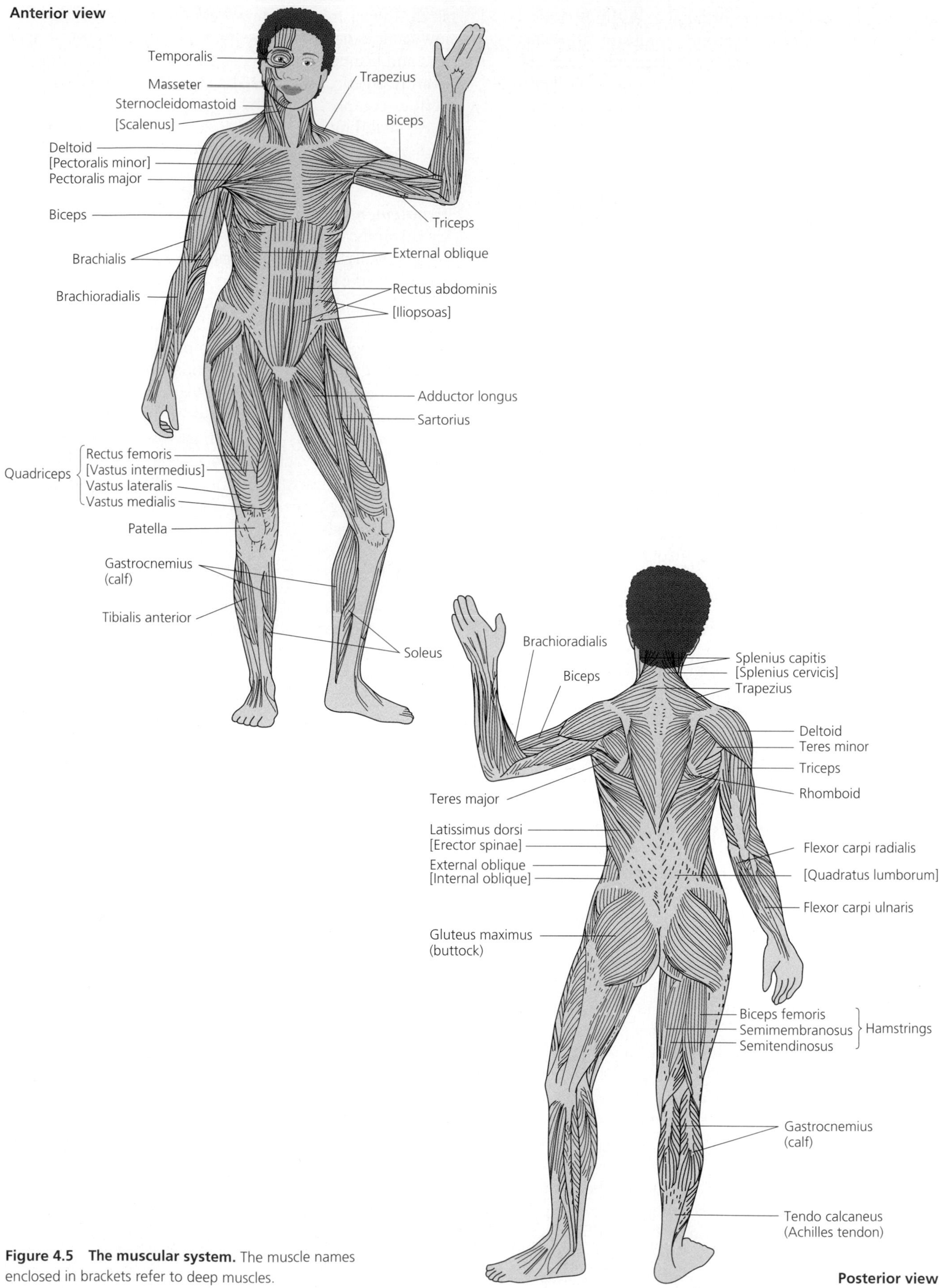

Figure 4.5 The muscular system. The muscle names enclosed in brackets refer to deep muscles.

Table 4.3 *Weight Training Exercises for Machines and Free Weights*

Body Part	Cybex	Nautilus	Universal Gym	Free Weights
Neck	4-way neck	4-way neck	Neck conditioning station	Neck harness Manual exercises
Trapezius ("traps")	Chest/incline press Incline press Overhead press	Overhead press Lateral raise Reverse pull-over Compound row Shoulder shrug Rowing back	Shoulder press Shoulder shrug Upright row Bent-over row Rip-up Front raise Pull-up	Overhead press Lateral raise Shoulder shrug Power clean Upright row
Chest (Pectoralis major)	Incline press Chest/incline press Fly Chest press	Vertical chest Incline press Bench press Pec fly 10° chest	Bench press	Bench press Incline press Dumbbell fly
Deltoids	Chest/incline press Incline press Row/rear delt Overhead press Lateral raise Chest press	Lateral raise Overhead press Reverse pull-over Double chest 10° chest 50° chest Seated dip Bench press Compound row Rotary shoulder	Bench press Shoulder shrug Shoulder press Upright row Rip-up Front raise Pull-up	Raise Bench press Shoulder press Upright row Pull-up
Biceps	Row/rear delt Pull-down Arm curl	Biceps curl Lat pull	Biceps curl Lat pull	Biceps curl Lat pull Pull-up
Triceps	Chest/incline press Chest press Incline press Overhead press Arm extension	Triceps extension Seated dip Triceps extension (lat machine) Bench press Overhead press	French curl Dip Triceps extension (lat machine) Bench press Seated press	French curl Dip Triceps extension (lat machine) Bench press Military press
Latissimus dorsi ("lats")	Row/rear delt Pull-down Lat pull-down	Pull-over Behind neck Torso arm Lat pull Seated dip Compound row	Pull-up Lat pull Bent-over row Pull-over Dip	Pull-up Pull-over Dip Bent-over row Lat pull
Abdominals	Torso rotation Ab crunch	Abdominal Rotary torso	Hip flexor Leg raise Crunch Sit-up Side-bend	Hip flexor Leg raise Crunch Sit-up Side-bend Isometric tightener
Lower back	Torso rotation Back extension	Lower back	Back extension Back leg raise	Back extension Good-morning
Thigh and buttocks	Seated leg press Leg extension Prone leg curl Seated leg curl Hip adduction Hip abduction	Leg press Leg extension Prone leg curl Seated leg curl Hip extension Hip adduction Hip abduction	Leg press Leg curl Leg extension Adductor kick Abductor kick Back hip extension	Squat Leg press Leg extension Leg curl Power clean Snatch Dead lift
Calf	Rotary calf	Seated calf Heel raise: multiexercise	Calf press	Heel raise

WEIGHT TRAINING EXERCISES
Free Weights

EXERCISE 1

BENCH PRESS

Muscles developed: Pectoralis major, triceps, deltoids

Instructions: **(a)** Lying on a bench on your back with your feet on the floor, grasp the bar with palms upward and hands shoulder-width apart. **(b)** Lower the bar to your chest. Then press it to the starting position. If your back arches too much, try doing this exercise with your feet on the bench.

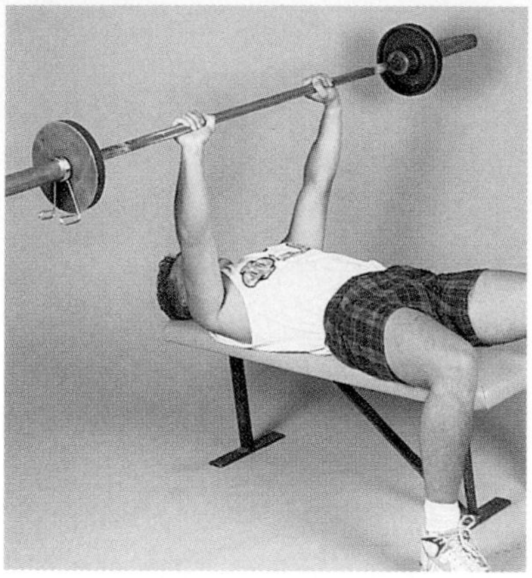

(a)

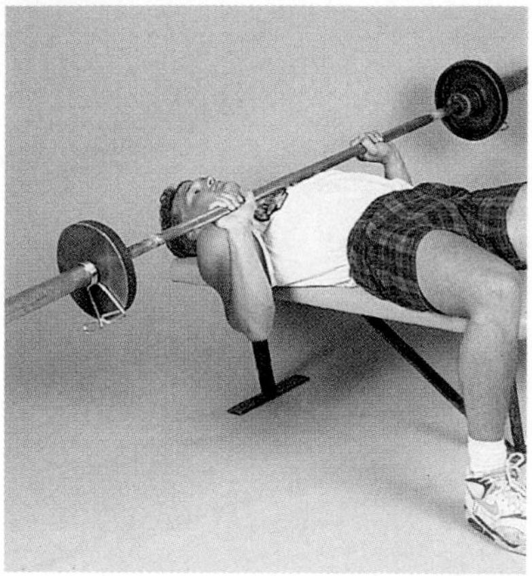

(b)

EXERCISE 2

SHOULDER PRESS
(Overhead or Military Press)

Muscles developed: Deltoids, triceps, trapezius

Instructions: This exercise can be done standing or seated, with dumbbells or a barbell. The shoulder press begins with the weight at your chest, preferably on a rack. **(a)** Grasp the weight with your palms facing away from you. **(b)** Push the weight overhead until your arms are extended. Then return to the starting position (weight at chest). Be careful not to arch your back excessively.

If you are a more advanced weight trainer, you can "clean" the weight to your chest (lift it from the floor to your chest). The clean should be attempted only after instruction from a knowledgeable coach; otherwise, it can lead to injury.

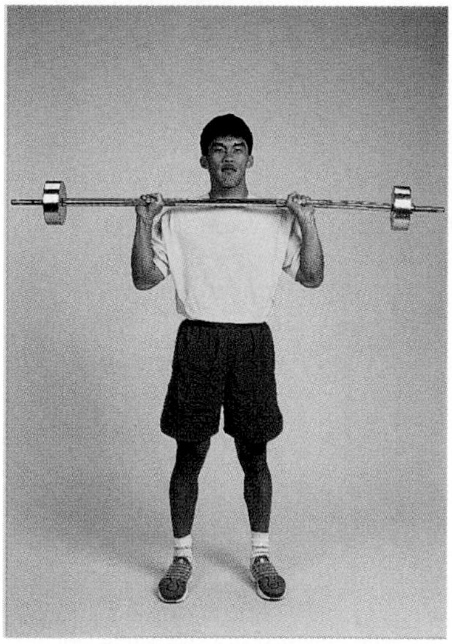

(a)

(b)

To allow an optimal view of exercise technique, a spotter does not appear in these demonstration photographs; however, spotters should be used for most exercises with free weights.

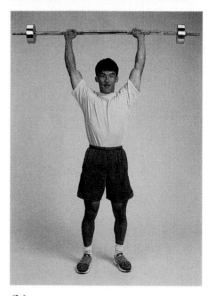

EXERCISE 3

PULL-UP

Muscles developed: Latissimus dorsi, biceps

Instructions: (a) Begin by grasping the pull-up bar with both hands, palms facing forward and elbows extended fully. **(b)** Pull yourself upward until your chin goes above the bar. Then return to the starting position.

Assisted pull-up: (c) This is done as described above for a pull-up, except that a spotter assists the person by pushing upward at the waist, hips, or legs during exercise.

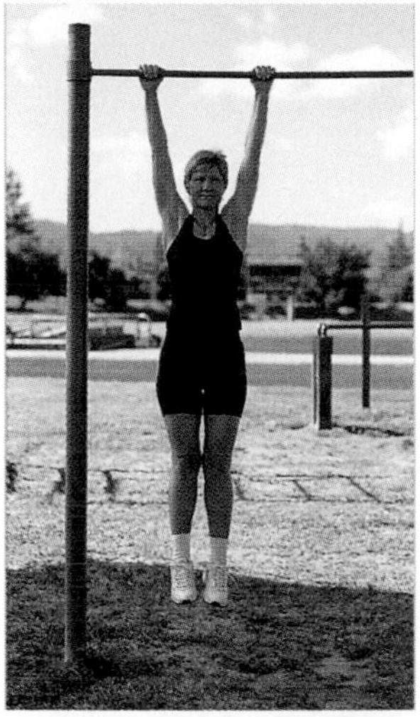

(a)

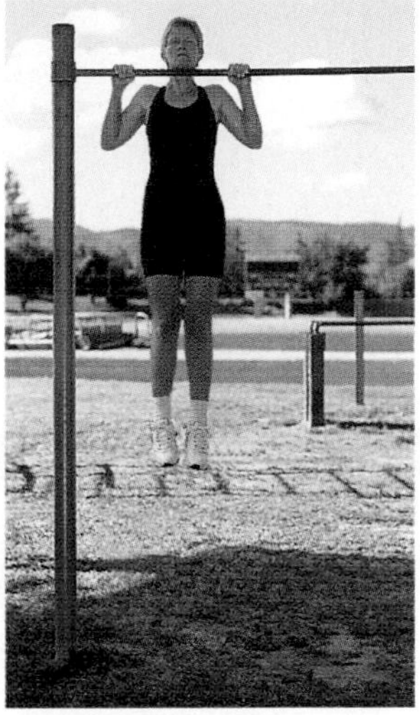

(b)

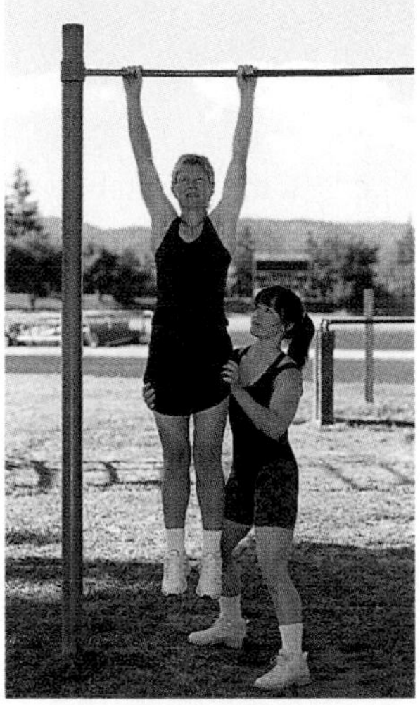

(c)

EXERCISE 4

LATERAL RAISE

Muscles developed: Deltoids

Instructions: (a) Stand with feet shoulder-width apart and a dumbbell in each hand. Hold the dumbbells parallel to each other. **(b)** With elbows slightly bent, slowly lift both weights until they reach shoulder level. Keep your wrists in a neutral position, in line with your forearms. Return to the starting position.

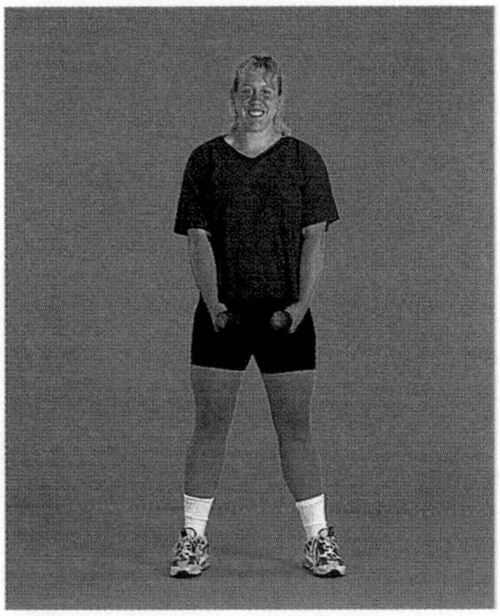

(a)

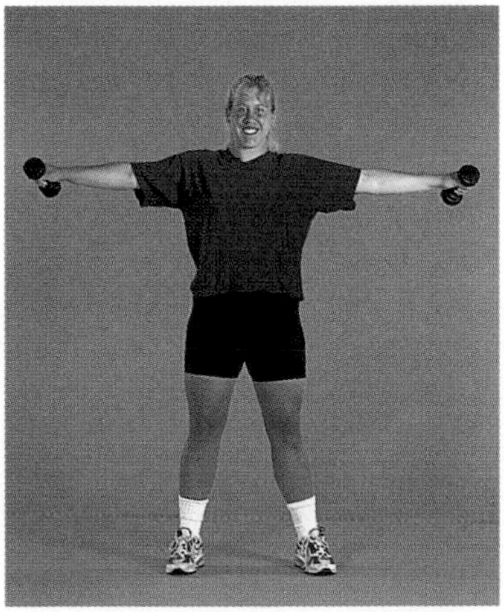

(b)

EXERCISE 5

BICEPS CURL

Muscles developed: Biceps, brachialis

Instructions: **(a)** From a standing position, grasp the bar with your palms upward and your hands shoulder-width apart. **(b)** Keeping your upper body rigid, flex (bend) your elbows until the bar reaches a level slightly below the collarbone. Return the bar to the starting position.

The exercise can be done using dumbbells, a curl bar (shown) or a straight bar; some people find that using a curl bar places less stress on the wrists.

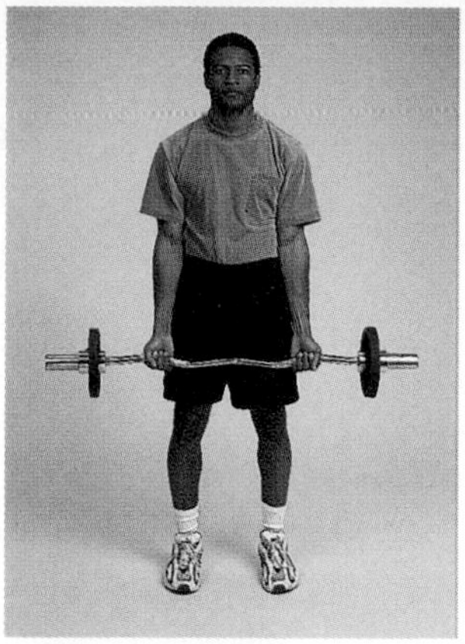

(a)

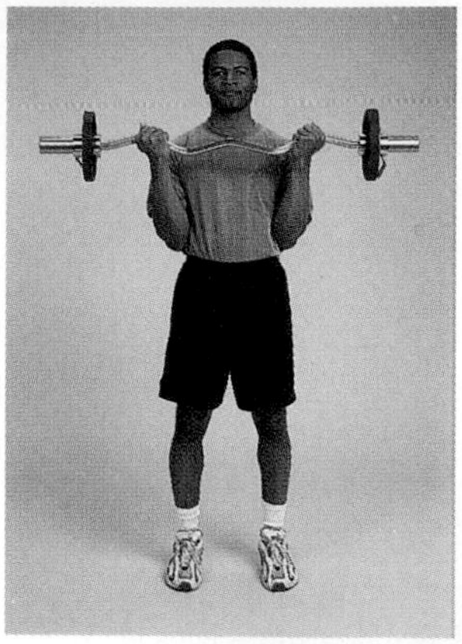

(b)

EXERCISE 6

SQUAT

Muscles developed: Quadriceps, gluteus maximus, hamstrings, gastrocnemius

Instructions: Stand with feet shoulder-width apart and toes pointed slightly outward. **(a)** Rest the bar on the back of your shoulders, holding it there with hands facing forward. **(b)** Keeping your head up and lower back straight, squat down until your thighs are almost parallel with the floor. Drive upward toward the starting position, keeping your back in a fixed position throughout the exercise.

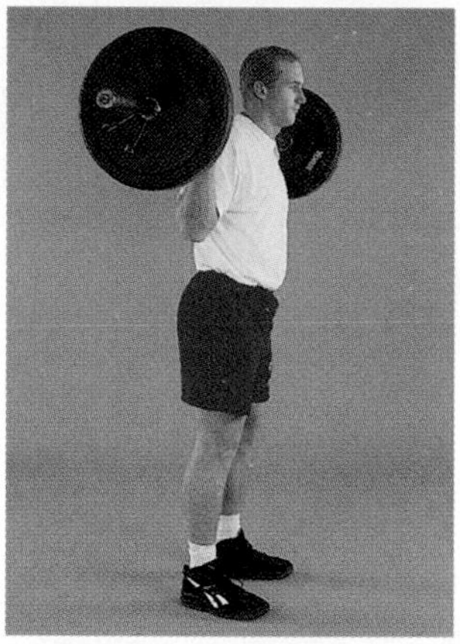

(a)

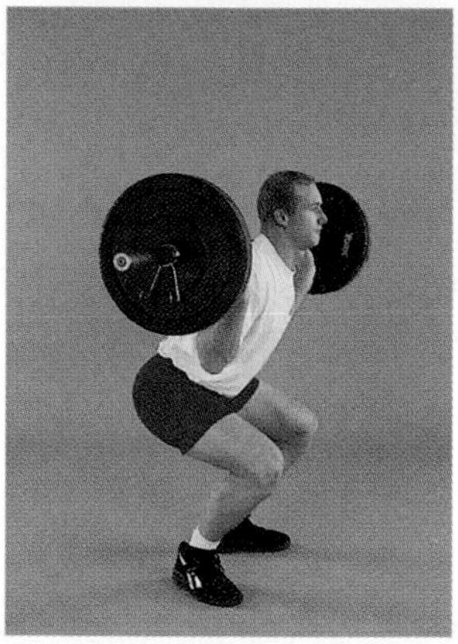

(b)

EXERCISE 7

HEEL RAISE

Muscles developed: Gastrocnemius, soleus

Instructions: Stand with feet shoulder-width apart and toes pointed straight ahead. **(a)** Rest the bar on the back of your shoulders, holding it there with hands facing forward. **(b)** Press down with your toes while lifting your heels. Return to the starting position.

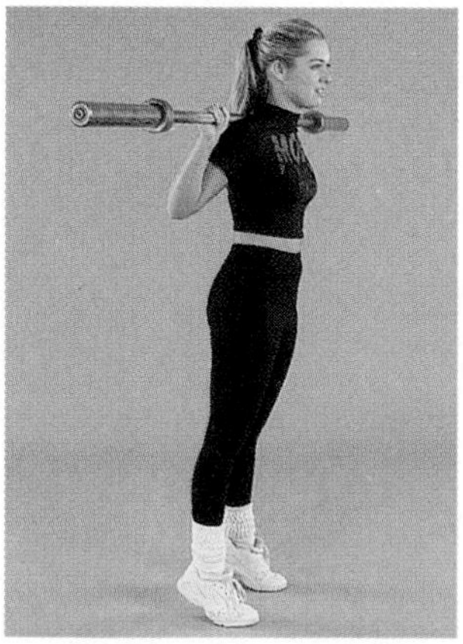

(a)

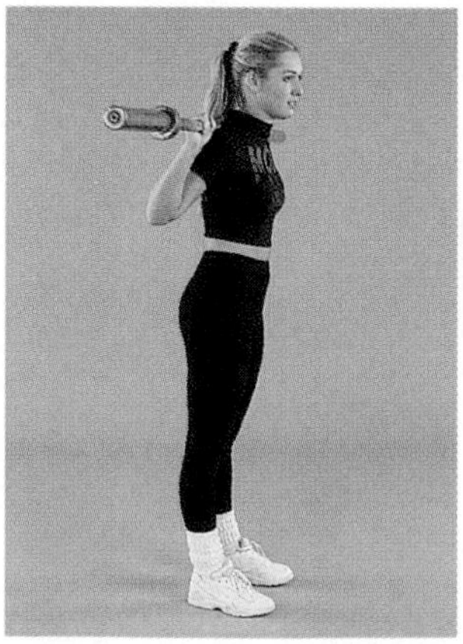

(b)

To allow an optimal view of exercise technique, a spotter does not appear in these demonstration photographs; however, spotters should be used for most exercises with free weights.

EXERCISE 8

CURL-UP OR CRUNCH

Muscles developed: Rectus abdominis, obliques

Instructions: **(a)** Lie on your back on the floor with your arms folded across your chest and your feet on the floor or on a bench. **(b)** Curl your trunk up and forward by raising your head and shoulders from the ground. Lower to the starting position.

This exercise can also be done using an exercise ball (see p. 142).

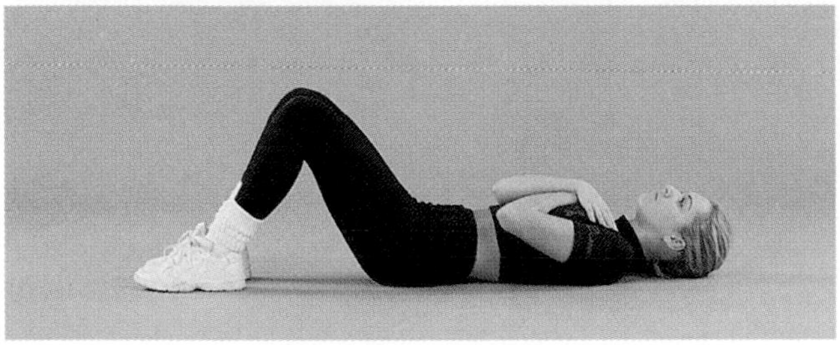

(a)

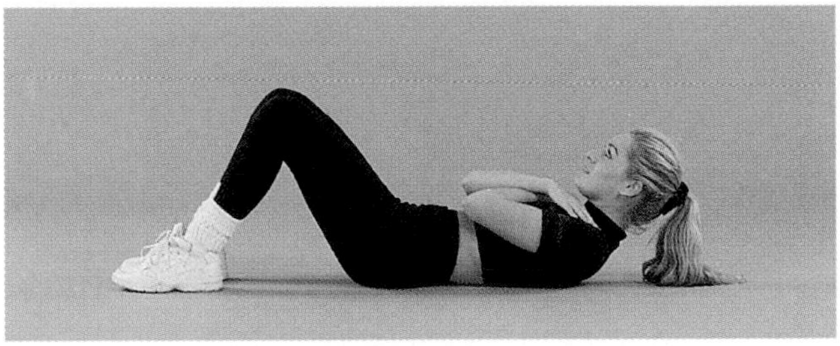

(b)

EXERCISE 9

SPINE EXTENSION (Isometric Exercises)

Muscles developed: Erector spinae, gluteus maximus, hamstrings, deltoids

Instructions: Begin on all fours with your knees below your hips and your hands below your shoulders.

Unilateral spine extension: **(a)** Extend your right leg to the rear and reach forward with your right arm. Keep your neck neutral and your raised arm and leg in line with your torso. Don't arch your back or let your hip or shoulder sag. Hold this position for 10–30 seconds. Repeat with your left leg and left arm.

Bilateral spine extension: **(b)** Extend your left leg to the rear and reach forward with your right arm. Keep your neck neutral and your raised leg in line with your torso. Don't arch your back or let your hip or shoulder sag. Hold this position for 10–30 seconds. Repeat with your right leg and left arm.

You can make this exercise more difficult by attaching weights to your ankles and wrists.

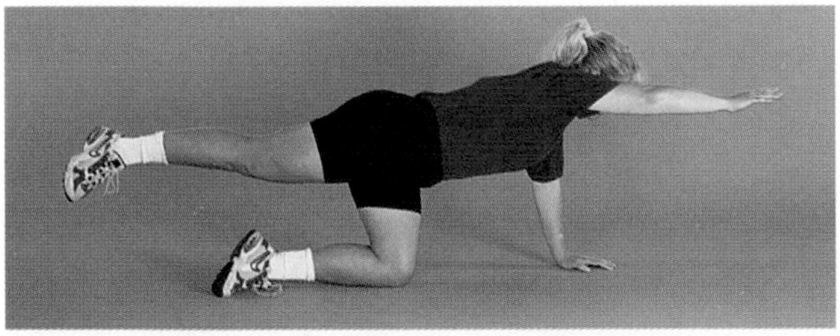

(a)

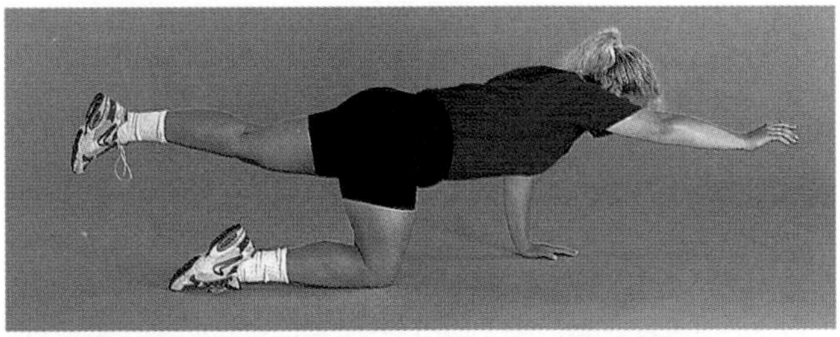

(b)

EXERCISE 10

NECK FLEXION AND LATERAL FLEXION (Isometric Exercises)

Muscles developed: Sternocleidomastoids, scaleni

Instructions:

Neck flexion: (a) Place your hand on your forehead with fingertips pointed up. Using the muscles at the back of your neck, press your head forward and resist the pressure with the palm of your hand.

Lateral flexion: (b) Place your hand on the right side of your face, fingertips pointed up. Using the muscles on the left side of your neck, press your head to the right and resist the pressure with the palm of your hand. Repeat on the left side.

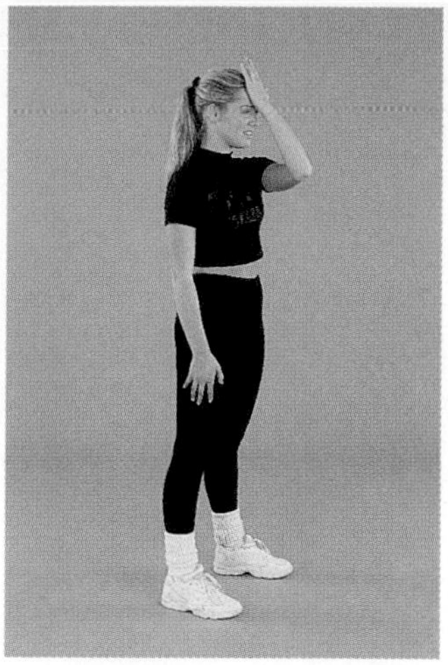

(a)

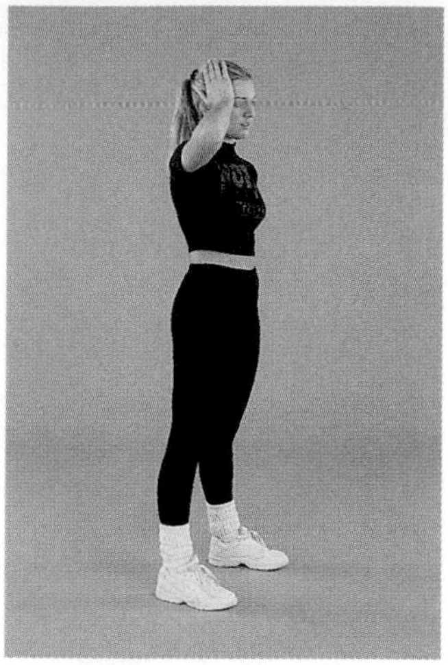

(b)

Weight Machines

EXERCISE 1

BENCH PRESS

Muscles developed: Pectoralis major, anterior deltoids, triceps

Instructions: Lie on the bench so the tops of the handles are aligned with the tops of your armpits. Place your feet flat on the floor; if they don't reach, place them on the bench. **(a)** Grasp the handles with your palms facing away from you. **(b)** Push the bars until your arms are fully extended. Return to the starting position.

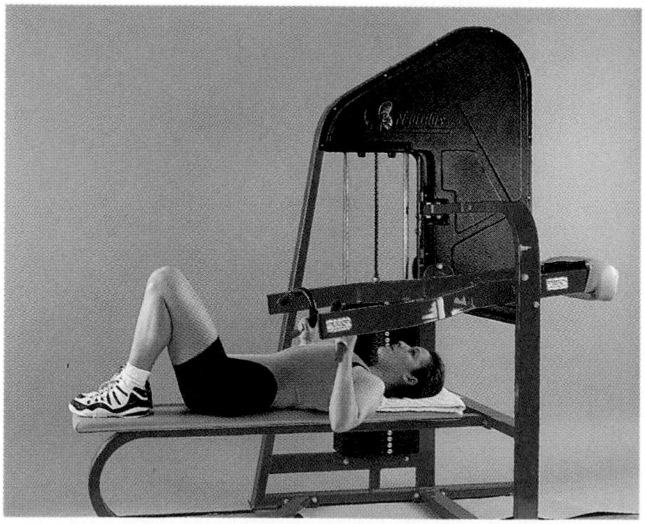

(a)

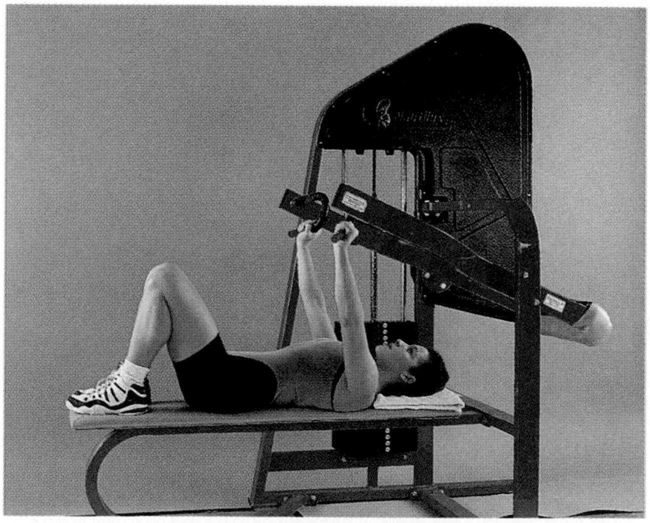

(b)

EXERCISE 2

OVERHEAD PRESS (Shoulder Press)

Muscles developed: Deltoids, trapezius, triceps

Instructions: Adjust the seat so that your feet are flat on the ground and the hand grips are slightly above your shoulders. **(a)** Sit down, facing away from the machine, and grasp the hand grips with your palms facing forward. **(b)** Press the weight upward until your arms are extended. Return to the starting position.

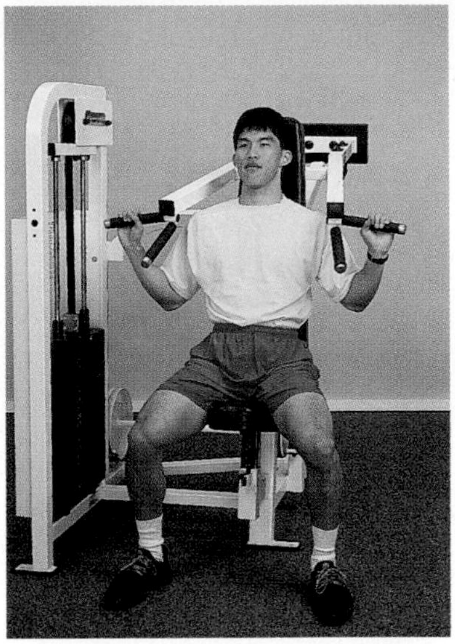

(a)

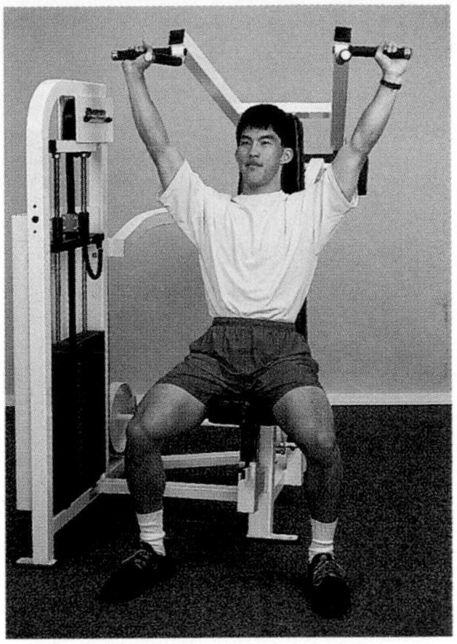

(b)

EXERCISE 3

LAT PULL

Muscles developed: Latissimus dorsi, biceps

Instructions: Begin in a seated or kneeling position, depending on the type of lat machine and the manufacturer's instructions. **(a)** Grasp the bar of the machine with arms fully extended. **(b)** Slowly pull the weight down until it reaches the top of your chest. Slowly return to the starting position.

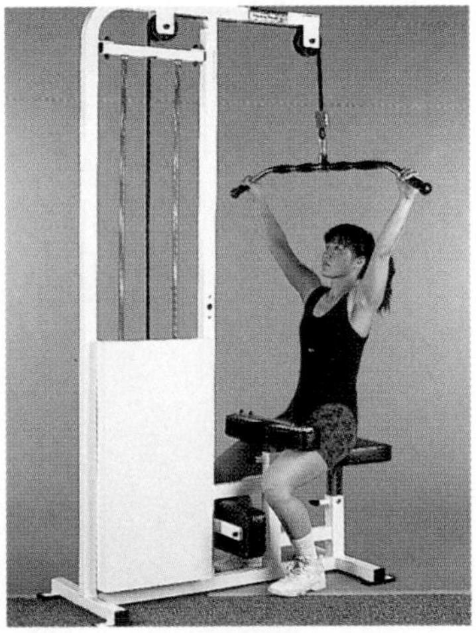

(a)

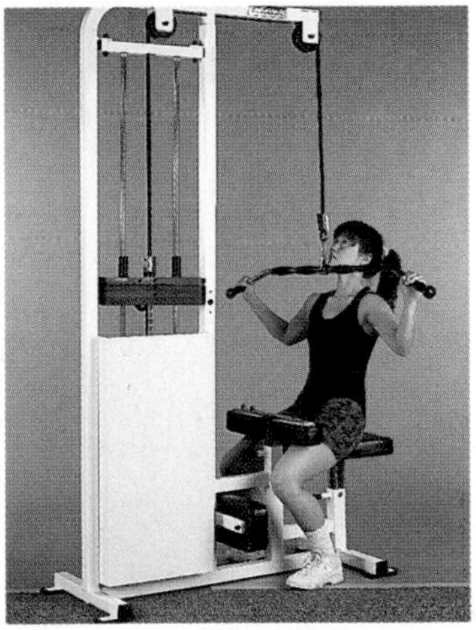

(b)

EXERCISE 4

PULLOVER

Muscles developed: Latissimus dorsi, pectoralis major and minor, triceps, abdominals

Instructions: Adjust the seat so your shoulders are aligned with the cams. Push down on the foot pads with your feet to bring the bar forward until you can place your elbows on the pads. Rest your hands lightly on the bar. If possible, place your feet flat on the floor. **(a)** To get into the starting position, let your arms go backward as far as possible. **(b)** Pull your elbows forward until the bar almost touches your abdomen. Return to the starting position.

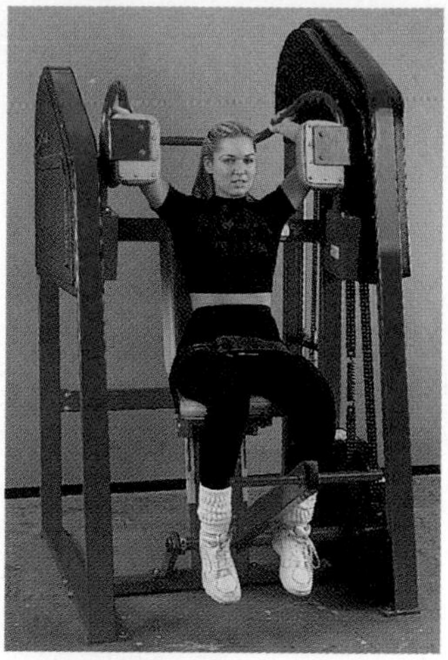

(a)

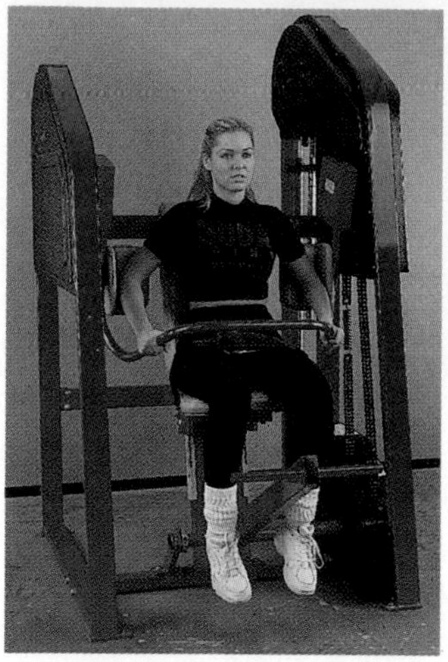

(b)

EXERCISE 5

LATERAL RAISE

Muscles developed: Deltoids, trapezius

Instructions: **(a)** Adjust the seat so the pads rest just above your elbows when your upper arms are at your sides, your elbows are bent, and your forearms are parallel to the floor. Lightly grasp the handles. **(b)** Push outward and up with your arms until the pads are shoulder height. Lead with your elbows rather than trying to lift the bars with your hands. Return to the starting position.

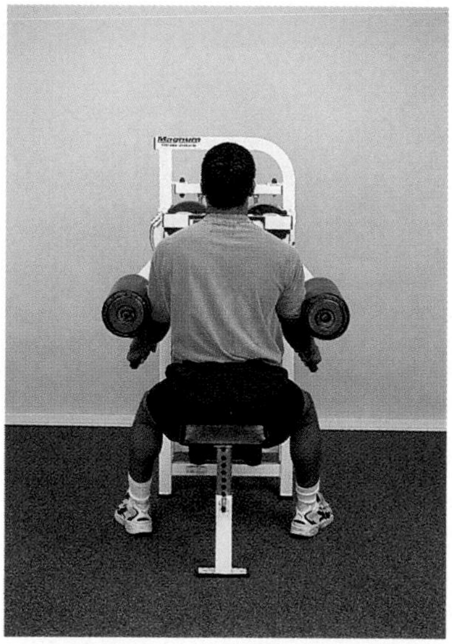

(a)

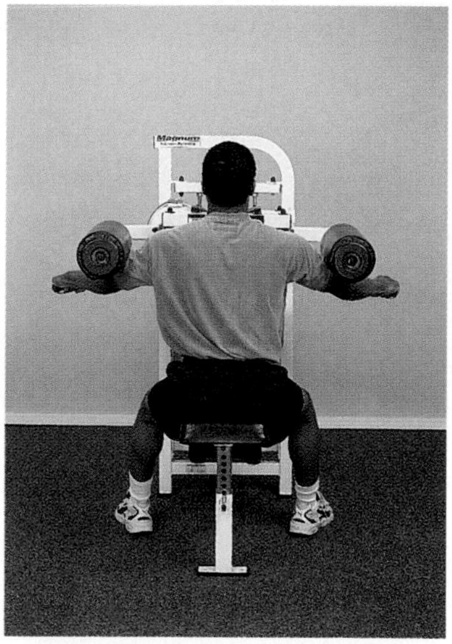

(b)

EXERCISE 6

BICEPS CURL

Muscles developed: Biceps, brachialis

Instructions: **(a)** Adjust the seat so that your back is straight and your arms rest comfortably against the top and side pads. Place your arms on the support cushions and grasp the hand grips with your palms facing up.
(b) Keeping your upper body still, flex (bend) your elbows until the hand grips almost reach your collarbone. Return to the starting position.

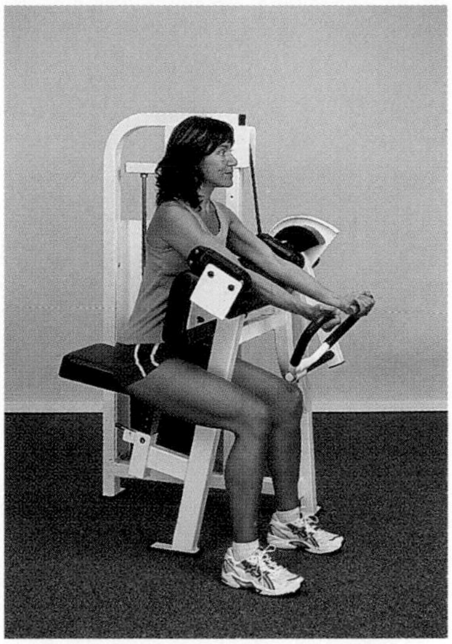

(a)

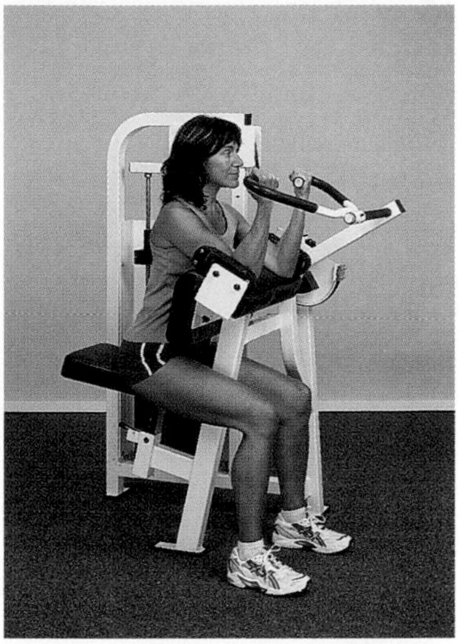

(b)

EXERCISE 7

TRICEPS EXTENSION

Muscles developed: Triceps

Instructions: **(a)** Adjust the seat so that your back is straight and your arms rest comfortably against the top and side pads. Place your arms on the support cushions and grasp the hand grips with palms facing inward.
(b) Keeping your upper body still, extend your elbows as much as possible. Return to the starting position.

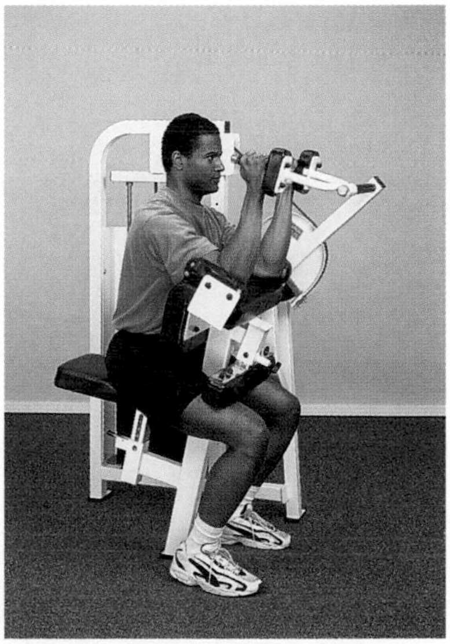

(a)

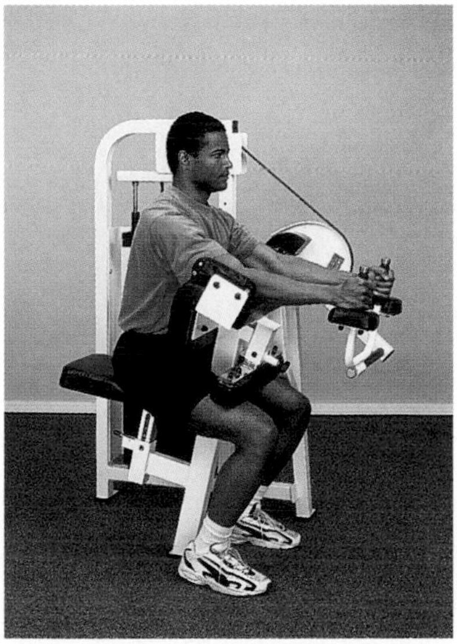

(b)

EXERCISE 8

LEG PRESS

Muscles developed: Gluteus maximus, quadriceps, hamstrings

Instructions: **(a)** Adjust the seat so your knees are bent at a 90-degree angle. **(b)** Sit with your hands on the side handles, your feet on the pedals, and your legs fully extended. **(c)** From this position, bend your right leg 90 degrees and then forcefully extend it. Repeat with your left leg. Alternate between right and left legs.

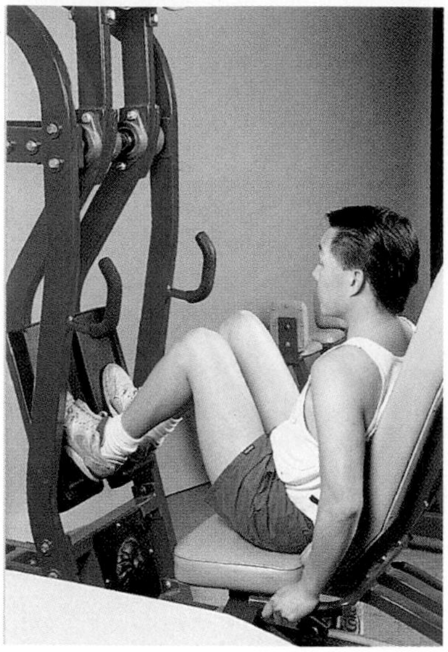
(a)

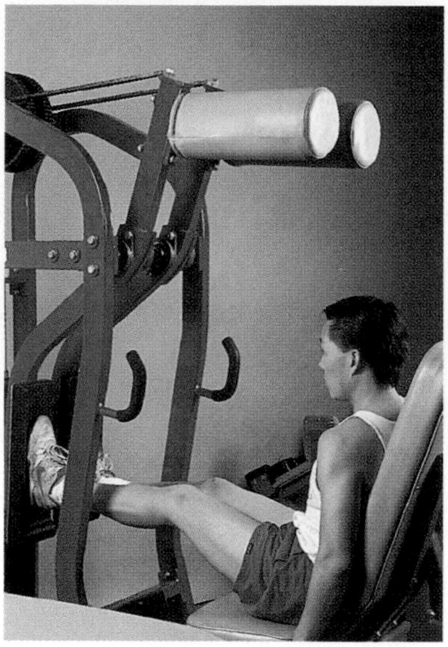
(b)

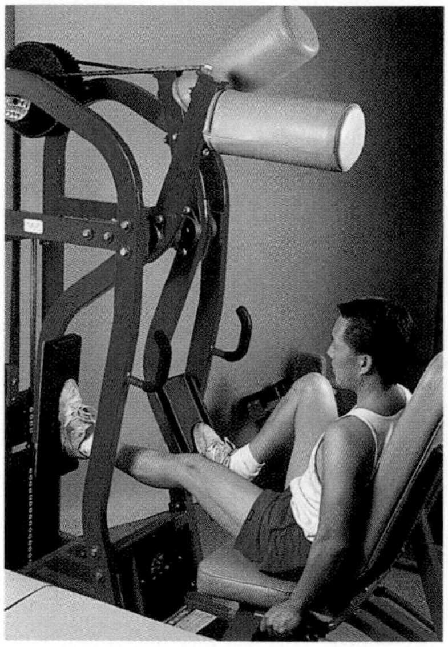
(c)

EXERCISE 9

LEG EXTENSION (Knee Extension)

Muscles developed: Quadriceps

Instructions: **(a)** Adjust the seat so that the pads rest comfortably on top of your lower shins. Loosely grasp the handles. **(b)** Extend your knees until they are almost straight. Return to the starting position.

Knee extensions cause kneecap pain in some people. If you have kneecap pain during this exercise, check with an orthopedic specialist before repeating it.

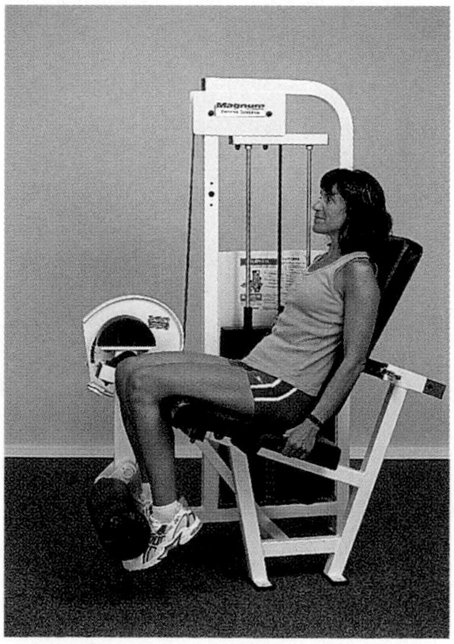
(a)

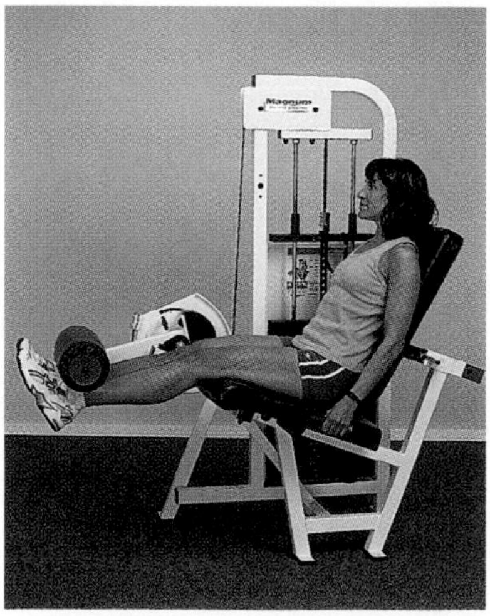
(b)

EXERCISE 10

PRONE LEG CURL (Knee Flexion)

Muscles developed: Hamstrings

Instructions: **(a)** Lie on the front of your body, resting the pads of the machine just below your calf muscles and with your knees just off the edge of the bench. **(b)** Flex your knees until they approach your buttocks. Return to the starting position.

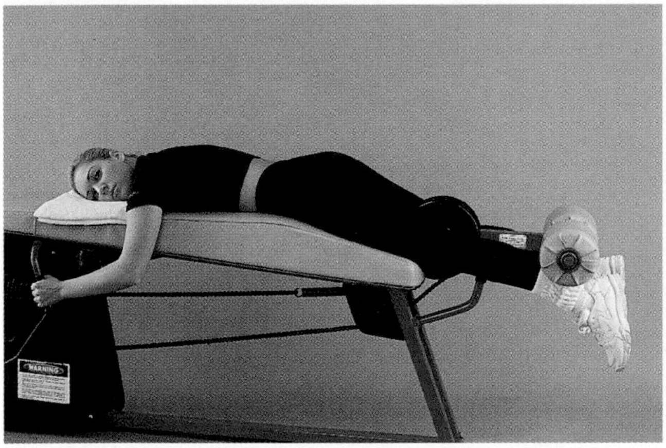

(a)

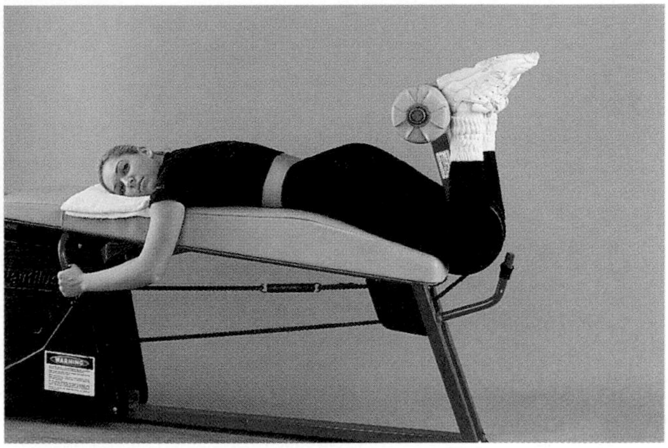

(b)

EXERCISE 11

HEEL RAISE

Muscles developed: Gastrocnemius, soleus

Instructions: **(a)** Stand with your head between the pads and one pad on each shoulder. The balls of your feet should be on the platform. Lightly grasp the handles. **(b)** Press down with your toes while lifting your heels. Return to the starting position. Changing the direction your feet are pointing (straight ahead, inward, and outward) will work different portions of your calf muscles.

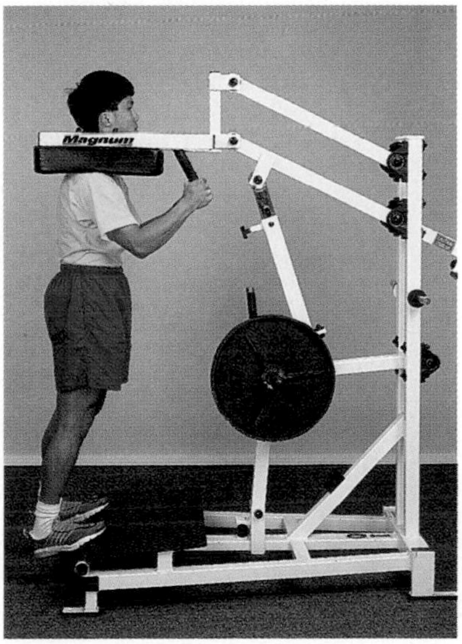

(a)

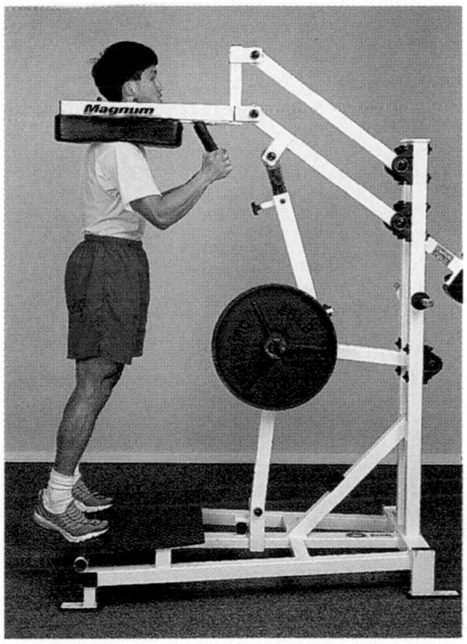

(b)

EXERCISE 12

ABDOMINAL CURL

Muscles developed: Rectus abdominis, internal and external obliques, hip flexors (rectus femoris and iliopsoas muscle group) as stabilizers

Instructions: **(a)** Adjust the seat so the machine rotates at the level of your navel, the pad rests on your upper chest, and your feet can rest comfortably on the floor. **(b)** Move your trunk forward as far as possible. Return to the starting position.

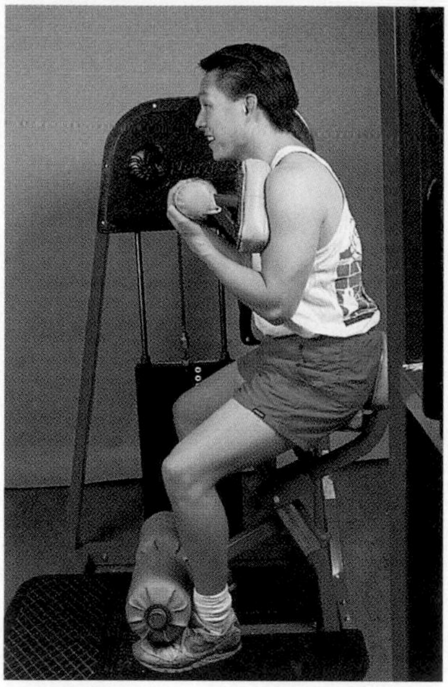

(a)

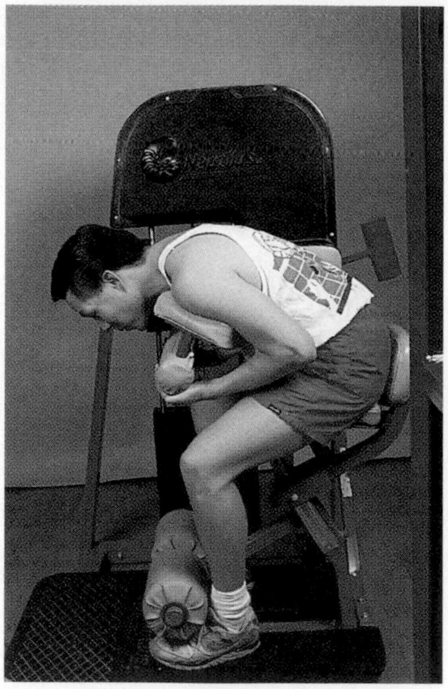

(b)

EXERCISE 13

LOW-BACK MACHINE
(Back Extensions)

Muscles developed: Erector spinae, quadratus lumborum

Instructions: **(a)** Sit on the seat with your upper legs under the thigh-support pads, your back on the back roller pad, and your feet on the platform.
(b) Extend backward until your back is straight. Return to the starting position. Try to keep your spine rigid

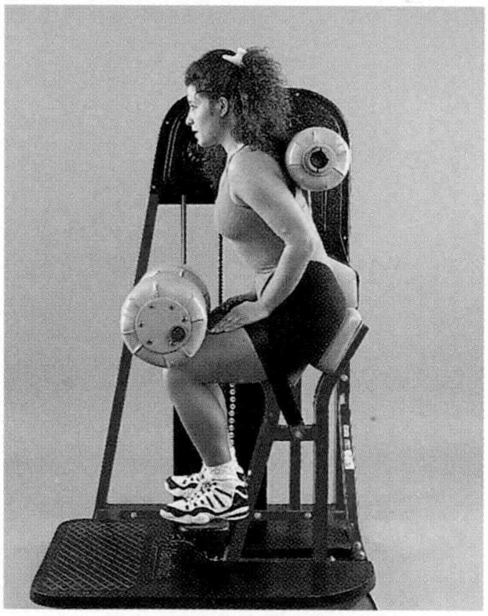

(a)

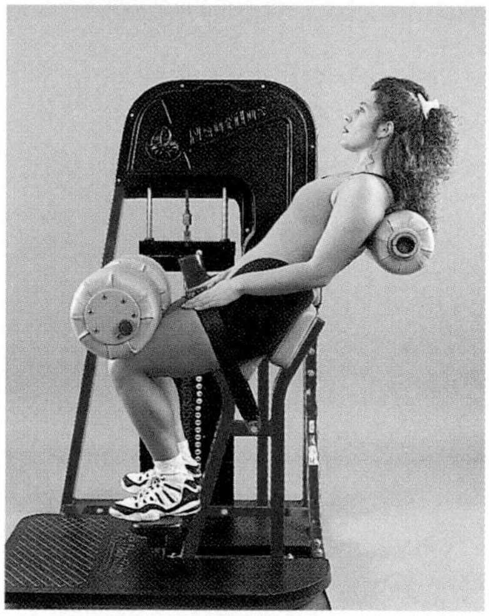

(b)

Tips for Today

Good muscular strength and endurance will enhance your quality of life—both now and in the future. You don't need a complicated or heavy training program to improve strength: Just one set of 8–10 exercises, done 2–3 days per week, is enough for general fitness.

Right now you can

- Think of three things you've done in the past 24 hours that would have been easier or more enjoyable if you increased your level of muscular strength and endurance. Examples might be carrying your books, climbing stairs, or playing recreational sports. Begin to visualize improvements in your quality of life that could come from increased muscular strength and endurance.
- Make a list of five benefits of muscular strength and endurance that are particularly meaningful to you. Put the list on your mirror and use it as a motivational tool for beginning and maintaining your fitness program.
- Do a set of static (isometric) exercises. If you're sitting, try tightening your abdominal muscles as you press your lower back into the seat or work your arms by placing the palms of your hands on top of your thighs and pressing down. Hold the contraction for 6 seconds and do 5–10 repetitions; don't hold your breath.
- Make an appointment with a trainer at your campus or neighborhood fitness facility. A trainer can help you put together an appropriate weight training program and introduce you to the equipment at the facility.
- Invest in an inexpensive set of free weights.

SUMMARY

- Improvements in muscular strength and endurance lead to enhanced physical performance, protection against injury, improved body composition, better self-image, improved muscle and bone health with aging, and reduced risk of chronic disease.
- Muscular strength can be assessed by determining the amount of weight that can be lifted in one repetition of an exercise; muscular endurance can be assessed by determining the number of repetitions of a particular exercise that can be performed.
- Hypertrophy, or increased muscle fiber size, occurs when weight training causes the number of myofibrils to increase; total muscle size thereby increases. Strength also increases through muscle learning.
- Static (isometric) exercises (contraction without movement) are most useful when a person is recovering from an injury or surgery or needs to overcome weak points in a range of motion.
- Dynamic (isotonic) exercises involve contraction that results in movement. The two most common types are constant resistance (free weights) and variable resistance (many weight machines).
- Free weights and weight machines are basically equally effective in producing fitness, although machines tend to be safer.
- Lifting heavy weights for only a few repetitions helps develop strength. Lifting lighter weights for more repetitions helps develop muscular endurance.
- A weight training program for general fitness includes at least 1 set of 8–12 repetitions (enough to cause fatigue) of 8–10 exercises, along with warm-up and cool-down periods; the program should be carried out 2–3 times a week.
- Safety guidelines for weight training include using proper technique, using spotters and collars when necessary, using common sense and remaining alert, and taking care of injuries.
- Supplements or drugs that are promoted as instant or quick "cures" usually don't work and are either dangerous or expensive or both.

COMMON QUESTIONS ANSWERED

How long must I weight train before I begin to see changes in my body? You will increase strength very rapidly during the early stages of a weight training program, primarily the result of muscle learning (the increased ability of the nervous system to recruit muscle fibers to exert force). Actual changes in muscle size usually begin after about 6–8 weeks of training.

I am concerned about my body composition. Will I gain weight if I do resistance exercises? Your weight probably will not change significantly as a result of a recreational-type weight training program: 1 set of 8–12 repetitions of 8–10 exercises. You will tend to increase muscle mass and lose body fat, so your weight will stay about the same. You may notice a change in how your clothes fit, however, because muscle is more dense than fat. Men will tend to build larger muscles than women because of the tissue-building effects of testosterone. Increased muscle mass will help you control body fat. Muscle increases your metabolism, which means you burn more calories every day. If you combine resistance exercises with endurance exercises, you will be on your way to developing a healthier body composition. Concentrate on fat loss rather than weight loss.

Do I need more protein in my diet when I train with weights? No. Although there is some evidence that power athletes involved in heavy training have a higher-than-normal protein

(continued)

requirement, there is no reason for most people to consume extra protein. Most Americans take in more protein than they need, so even if there is an increased protein need during heavy training, it is probably supplied by the average diet. (See Chapter 8 for more on dietary needs of athletes.)

What causes muscle soreness the day or two following a weight training workout? The muscle pain you feel a day or two after a heavy weight training workout is caused by injury to the muscle fibers and surrounding connective tissue. Contrary to popular belief, delayed-onset muscle soreness is not caused by lactic acid buildup. Scientists believe that injury to muscle fibers causes inflammation, which in turn causes the release of chemicals that break down part of the muscle tissue and cause pain. After a bout of intense exercise that causes muscle injury and delayed-onset muscle soreness, the muscles produce protective proteins that prevent soreness during future workouts. If you don't work out regularly, you lose these protective proteins and become susceptible to muscle soreness again.

Will strength training improve my sports performance? Strength developed in the weight room does not automatically increase your power in sports such as skiing, tennis, or cycling. Hitting a forehand in tennis and making a turn on skis are precise skills that require coordination between your nervous system and muscles. In skilled people, movements become reflex—you don't think about them when you do them. Increasing strength can disturb this coordination. Only by simultaneously practicing a sport and improving fitness can you expect to become more powerful in the skill. Practice helps you integrate your new strength with your skills, which makes you more powerful. Consequently, you can hit the ball harder in tennis or make more graceful turns on the ski slopes. (Refer to Chapter 2 for more on the concept of specificity of physical training.)

Will I improve faster if I train every day? No. Your muscles need time to recover between training sessions. Doing resistance exercises every day will cause you to become overtrained, which will increase your chance of injury and impede your progress. If you find that your strength training program has reached a plateau, try one of these strategies:

- Train less frequently. If you are currently training the same muscle groups three or more times per week, you may not be allowing your muscles to fully recover from intense workouts.
- Change exercises. Using different exercises for a particular muscle group may stimulate further strength development.
- Vary the load and number of repetitions. Try increasing or decreasing the loads you are using and changing the number of repetitions accordingly.
- Vary the number of sets. If you have been performing 1 set of each exercise, add sets.
- If you are training alone, find a motivated training partner. A partner can encourage you and assist you with difficult lifts, forcing you to work harder.

If I stop weight training, will my muscles turn to fat? No. Fat and muscle are two different kinds of tissue, and one cannot turn into the other. Muscles that aren't used become smaller (atrophy), and body fat may increase if caloric intake exceeds calories burned. Although the result of inactivity may be smaller muscles and more fat, the change is caused by two separate processes.

Should I wear a weight belt when I lift? Until recently, most experts advised people to wear weight belts. However, several studies have shown that weight belts do not prevent back injuries and may, in fact, increase the risk of injury by encouraging people to lift more weight than they are capable of lifting with good form. Although wearing a belt may allow you to lift more weight in some lifts, you may not get the full benefit of your program because use of a weight belt reduces the effectiveness of the workout on the muscles that help support your spine.

Do abdominal machines advertised on television really work? Studies comparing major types of abdominal exercises have found that all of them develop the abdominal muscles. However, there doesn't appear to be any advantage to using an abdominal machine as compared to performing crunches—and a machine may cost $50 or more.

Can activities such as yoga, tai chi chuan, and Pilates be used to build muscular strength and endurance? Each of these forms of exercise involve carefully controlled body movements and precise body positions, so they can help build muscular strength and endurance—although probably not to the degree of traditional weight training exercises. Yoga involves a series of physical postures that stretch and relax different parts of the body; the emphasis is on breathing, stretching, body awareness, and balance. Tai chi chuan is a martial art consisting of a series of slow, fluid, elegant movements that promote relaxation and concentration as well as the development of body awareness, balance, and muscular strength. Pilates involves the use of specially designed resistance training devices. It focuses on working the core muscles in the back, abdomen, and buttocks; the emphasis is on concentration, control, movement flow, and breathing. To obtain the greatest benefit from these techniques, it's best to begin by finding a qualified instructor. See Chapter 10 for more on the use of yoga and tai chi for stress management.

FOR FURTHER EXPLORATION

Fit and Well Online Learning Center (www.mhhe.com/fahey5e)

Use the learning objectives, study guide questions, and glossary flashcards to review key terms and concepts and prepare for exams. You can extend your knowledge of muscular strength and endurance and gain experience in using the Internet as a resource by completing the activities and checking out the Web links for the topics in Chapter 4 marked with the World Wide Web icon. For this chapter, Internet activities explore the benefits of muscular strength and endurance, different exercises that build strength, and strategies for evaluating supplements; there are Web links for the Critical Consumer box on dietary supplements and the chapter as a whole.

Daily Fitness and Nutrition Journal

Complete the muscular strength and endurance portion of the program plan by setting goals and selecting exercises. Fill in the information for the specific exercises you will perform, including which muscles they develop, how much resistance you plan to start with, and the number of reps and sets you plan to perform.

Health*Quest*

If you haven't already done so, complete the How Fit Are You? section of the Wellness Activities in the fitness module of Health*Quest*. This section provides an overview of your muscular strength and endurance status based on your current level of strength and endurance and your strength training habits.

Books

Bahrke, M., and C. Yesalis. 2002. *Performance-Enhancing Substances in Sport Exercise*. Champaign, Ill.: Human Kinetics. *Provides up-to-date coverage of the issues surrounding supplements as well as the current state of research on major types of supplements and their effects on atheletic performance.*

Delavier, F. 2001. *Strength Training Anatomy*. Champaign, Ill.: Human Kinetics. *Includes exercises for all major muscle groups as well as full anatomical pictures of the muscular system.*

Fahey, T. D. 2000. *Basic Weight Training for Men and Women*, 4th ed. Mountain View, Calif.: Mayfield. *A practical guide to developing training programs, using free weights, tailored to individual needs.*

Graves, J. E., and B. A. Franklin. 2001. *Resistance Training for Health and Rehabilitation*. Champaign, Ill.: Human Kinetics. *Provides detailed information on resistance training for a variety of goals.*

Nelson, M. 2000. *Strong Women Stay Young*. Rev ed New York: Bantam Books. *A program of strengthening exercises geared toward first-time exercisers, written by a Tufts University professor.*

Organizations and Web Sites

American College of Sports Medicine Position Stand: Progression Models in Resistance Training for Healthy Adults. Provides an in-depth look at strategies for setting up a strength training program and making progress based on individual program goals; look for the February 2002 Position Stand.
http://www.acsm-msse.org

Biomechanics World Wide. A resource site with links to many other sites relating to biomechanics; topics include muscle mechanics and sports techniques.
http://www.per.ualberta.ca/biomechanics

Exercise: A Guide from the National Institute on Aging. Provides practical advice on fitness for seniors; includes animated instructions for specific weight training exercises.
http://www.nia.nih.gov/exercisebook

Georgia State University: Strength Training. Provides information about the benefits of strength training and how to develop a safe and effective program; also includes illustrations of a variety of exercises.
http://www.gsu.edu/~wwwfit/strength.html

Human Anatomy On-line. Provides text, illustrations, and animation about the muscular system, nerve-muscle connections, muscular contraction, and other topics.
http://www.innerbody.com/htm/body.html

University of California, San Diego/Muscle Physiology Home Page. Provides an introduction to muscle physiology, including information about types of muscle fibers and energy cycles.
http://muscle.ucsd.edu

University of Michigan/Muscles in Action. Interactive descriptions of muscle movements.
http://www.med.umich.edu/lrc/Hypermuscle/Hyper.html

See also the listings in Chapter 2.

SELECTED BIBLIOGRAPHY

American College of Sports Medicine. 2002. Position Stand: Progression models in resistance training for healthy adults. *Medicine and Science in Sports and Exercise* 34(2): 364-380.

American College of Sports Medicine. 2001. *ACSM's Resource Manual for Guidelines for Exercise Testing and Prescription*, 4th ed. Philadelphia: Lippincott Williams & Wilkins.

American College of Sports Medicine. 2001. Overtraining with resistance exercise. *Current Comment*, January.

American College of Sports Medicine. 2001. Rest during resistance exercise. *Current Comment*, May.

American College of Sports Medicine. 2000. *ACSM's Guidelines for Exercise Testing and Prescription*, 6th ed. Baltimore, Md.: Lippincott Williams & Wilkins.

American College of Sports Medicine. 1998. Position stand: The recommended quantity and quality of exercise for developing and maintaining cardiorespiratory and muscular fitness, and flexibility in healthy adults. *Medicine and Science in Sports and Exercise* 30(6):975–991.

Benzi, G., and A. Ceci. 2001. Creatine as nutritional supplementation and medicinal product. *Journal of Sports Medicine and Physical Fitness* 41(1): 1–10.

Bhasin, S., L. Woodhouse, and T. W. Storer. 2001. Proof of the effect of testosterone on skeletal muscle. *Journal of Endocrinology* 170(1): 27–38.

Brooks, G. A., et al. 2000. *Exercise Physiology: Human Bioenergetics and Its Applications*, 3d ed. Mountain View, Calif.: Mayfield.

Folland, J. P., et al. 2001. Acute muscle damage as a stimulus for training-induced gains in strength. *Medicine and Science in Sports and Exercise* 33(7): 1200–1205.

Galloway, M. T., R. Kadoko, and P. Jokl. 2002. Effect of aging on male and female master athletes' performance in strength versus endurance activities. *American Journal of Orthopedics* 31(2): 93–98.

Green, G. A., D. H. Catlin, and B. Starcevic. 2001. Analysis of over-the-counter dietary supplements. *Clinical Journal of Sports Medicine* 11(4): 254–259.

Hass, C. J., et al. 2000. Single versus multiple sets in long-term recreational weightlifters. *Medicine and Science in Sports and Exercise* 32(1): 235–242.

Ives, J. C., and J. Sosnoff. 2000. Beyond the mind-body exercise hype. *Physician and Sportsmedicine* 28(3).

Izquierdo, M., et al. 2002. Effects of creatine supplementation on muscle power, endurance, and sprint performance. *Medicine and Science in Sports and Exercise* 34(2): 332–343.

Izquierdo, M., et al. 2001. Effects of strength training on muscle power and serum hormones in middle-aged and older men. *Journal of Applied Physiology* 90(4): 1497–1507.

King, D. S., et al. 1999. Effect of oral androstenedione on serum testosterone and adaptations to resistance training in young men: A randomized controlled trial. *Journal of the American Medical Association* 281(21): 2020–2028.

McCarthy, J. P., M. A. Pozniak, and J. C. Agre. 2002. Neuromuscular adaptations to concurrent strength and endurance training. *Medicine and Science in Sports and Exercise* 34(3): 511–519.

Mujika, I., and S. Padilla. 2001. Muscular characteristics of detraining in humans. *Medicine and Science in Sports and Exercise* 33(8): 1297–1303.

Pollock, M. L., et al. 2000. AHA Science Advisory: Resistance exercise in individuals with and without cardiovascular disease. *Circulation* 101: 828–833.

Ryan, A. S., et al. 2000. Changes in plasma leptin and insulin action with resistive training in postmenopausal women. *International Journal of Obesity and Related Metabolic Disorders* 24(1): 27–32.

Shephard, R. J. 2000. Exercise and training in women, part 1: Influence of gender on exercise and training responses. *Canadian Journal of Applied Physiology* 25(1):19–34.

Sports-supplement dangers. 2001. *Consumer Reports*, June.

Trappe, S. D. Williamson, and M. Godard. 2002. Maintenance of whole muscle strength and size following resistance training in older men. *Journals of Gerontology: Biological Sciences and Medical Sciences* 74(4): B138–B143.

Trockel, M. T., M. D. Barnes, and D. L. Eggert. 2000. Health-related variables and academic performance among college students: Implications for sleep and other behaviors. *Journal of American College Health* 49(3): 125–131.

van Aggel-Leijssen, D. P., et al. 2001. Short-term effects of weight loss with or without low-intensity exercise training on fat metabolism in obese men. *American Journal of Clinical Nutrition* 73(3): 523–531.

Williams, P. A., and T. F. Cash. 2001. Effects of a circuit weight training program on the body images of college students. *International Journal of Eating Disorders* 30(1): 75–82.

Strength Ratings for the Maximum Leg Press Test

Men	Very Poor	Poor	Fair	Good	Excellent	Superior
	Pounds Lifted/Body Weight (lb)					
Age: Under 20	Below 1.70	1.70–1.89	1.90–2.03	2.04–2.27	2.28–2.81	Above 2.81
20–29	Below 1.63	1.63–1.82	1.83–1.96	1.97–2.12	2.13–2.39	Above 2.39
30–39	Below 1.52	1.52–1.64	1.65–1.76	1.77–1.92	1.93–2.19	Above 2.19
40–49	Below 1.44	1.44–1.56	1.57–1.67	1.68–1.81	1.82–2.01	Above 2.01
50–59	Below 1.32	1.32–1.45	1.46–1.57	1.58–1.70	1.71–1.89	Above 1.89
60 and over	Below 1.25	1.25–1.37	1.38–1.48	1.49–1.61	1.62–1.79	Above 1.79
Women						
Age: Under 20	Below 1.22	1.22–1.37	1.38–1.58	1.59–1.70	1.71–1.87	Above 1.87
20–29	Below 1.22	1.22–1.36	1.37–1.49	1.50–1.67	1.68–1.97	Above 1.97
30–39	Below 1.09	1.09–1.20	1.21–1.32	1.33–1.46	1.47–1.67	Above 1.67
40–49	Below 1.02	1.02–1.12	1.13–1.22	1.23–1.36	1.37–1.56	Above 1.56
50–59	Below 0.88	0.88–0.98	0.99–1.09	1.10–1.24	1.25–1.42	Above 1.42
60 and over	Below 0.85	0.85–0.92	0.93–1.03	1.04–1.17	1.18–1.42	Above 1.42

SOURCE: Based on norms from the Cooper Institute for Aerobics Research, Dallas, Texas; from *The Physical Specialist Manual*, Revised 2000. Used with permission.

Hand Grip Strength Test

Equipment

Grip strength dynamometer

Preparation

If necessary, adjust the hand grip size on the dynamometer into a position that is comfortable for you; then lock the grip in place. The second joint of your fingers should fit snugly under the handle of the dynamometer.

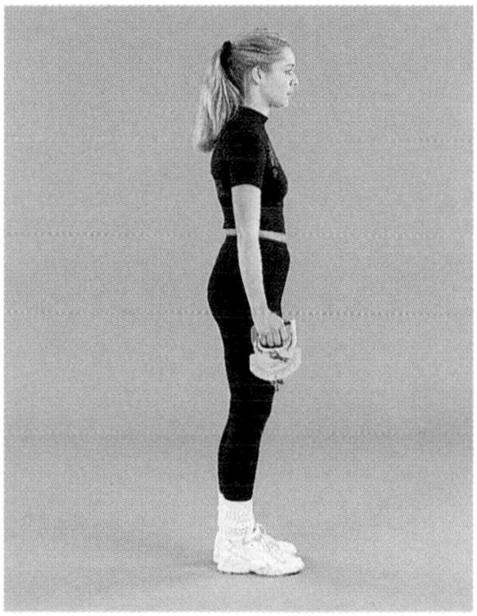

Hand grip strength test.

Instructions

1. Stand with the hand to be tested first at your side, away from your body. The dynamometer should be in line with your forearm and held at the level of your thigh. Squeeze the dynamometer as hard as possible without moving your arm; exhale as you squeeze. During the test, don't let the dynamometer touch your body or any other object.
2. Perform two trials with each hand. Rest for about a minute between trials. Record the scores for each hand to the nearest kilogram.

   Right hand: Trial 1: __________ kg Trial 2: __________ kg

   Left hand: Trial 1: __________ kg Trial 2: __________ kg

(Scores on the dynamometer should be given in kilograms. If the dynamometer you are using gives scores in pounds, convert pounds to kilograms by dividing your score by 2.2.)

Rating Your Hand Grip Strength

Right hand best trial ______ kg Left hand best trial ______ kg

Total score (sum of the best trial for each hand) ______ kg

Refer to the table for a rating of your grip strength. Record the rating below and in the chart at the end of this lab.

Rating for hand grip strength: __________

LABORATORY ACTIVITIES

Grip Strength (kg)*

Men	*Needs Improvement*	*Fair*	*Good*	*Very Good*	*Excellent*
Age: 15–19	Below 84	84–94	95–102	103–112	Above 112
20–29	Below 97	97–105	106–112	113–123	Above 123
30–39	Below 97	97–104	105–112	113–122	Above 122
40–49	Below 94	94–101	102–109	110–118	Above 118
50–59	Below 87	87–95	96–101	102–109	Above 109
60–69	Below 79	79–85	86–92	93–101	Above 101
Women					
Age: 15–19	Below 54	54–58	59–63	64–70	Above 70
20–29	Below 55	55–60	61–64	65–70	Above 70
30–39	Below 56	56–60	61–65	66–72	Above 72
40–49	Below 55	55–58	59–64	65–72	Above 72
50–59	Below 51	51–54	55–58	59–64	Above 64
60–69	Below 48	48–50	51–53	54–59	Above 59

*Combined right and left hand grip strength.

SOURCE: *The Canadian Physical Activity, Fitness and Lifestyle Appraisal: CSEP's Plan for Healthy Active Living*, 2d ed. 1998. Reprinted by permission from the Canadian Society for Exercise Physiology.

Summary of Results

Maximum bench press test: Weight pressed: ___________ lb Rating: ___________

Maximum leg press test: Weight pressed: ___________ lb Rating: ___________

Hand grip strength test: Total score: ___________ kg Rating: ___________

Remember that muscular strength is specific: Your ratings may vary considerably for different parts of your body.

Using Your Results

How did you score? Are you at all surprised by your rating for muscular strength? Are you satisfied with your current rating?

If you're not satisfied, set a realistic goal for improvement: ___________________________

Are you satisfied with your current level of muscular strength as evidenced in your daily life—for example, your ability to lift objects, climb stairs, and engage in sports and recreational activities?

If you're not satisfied, set some realistic goals for improvement:

What should you do next? Enter the results of this lab in the Preprogram Assessment column in Appendix D. If you've set goals for improvement, begin planning your strength training program by completing the plan in Lab 4.3. After several weeks of your program, complete this lab again and enter the results in the Postprogram Assessment column of Appendix D. How do the results compare?

Ratings for the Push-Up and Modified Push-Up Tests

Men	Number of Push-Ups					
	Very Poor	*Poor*	*Fair*	*Good*	*Excellent*	*Superior*
Age: 18–29	Below 22	22–28	29–36	37–46	47–61	Above 61
30–39	Below 17	17–23	24–29	30–38	39–51	Above 51
40–49	Below 11	11–17	18–23	24–29	30–39	Above 39
50–59	Below 9	9–12	13–18	19–24	25–38	Above 38
60 and over	Below 6	6–9	10–17	18–22	23–27	Above 27
Women	**Number of Modified Push-Ups**					
	Very Poor	*Poor*	*Fair*	*Good*	*Excellent*	*Superior*
Age: 18–29	Below 17	17–22	23–29	30–35	36–44	Above 44
30–39	Below 11	11–18	19–23	24–30	31–38	Above 38
40–49	Below 6	6–12	13–17	18–23	24–32	Above 32
50–59	Below 6	6–11	12–16	17–20	21–27	Above 27
60 and over	Below 2	2–4	5–11	12–14	15–19	Above 19

SOURCE: Based on norms from the Cooper Institute for Aerobics Research, Dallas, Texas; from *The Physical Fitness Specialist Manual*, Revised 2002. Used with permission.

YMCA Bench Press Test

The bench press test is preferred by some researchers as a test of upper body muscular endurance because push-up scores are affected by body composition as well as muscular endurance.

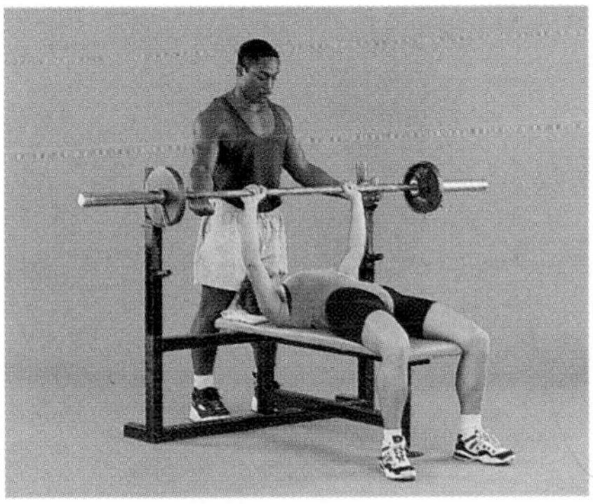

Equipment

1. Flat bench (with or without racks)
2. Barbell
3. Assorted weight plates; collars to hold them in place
4. Metronome
5. One or two spotters

Preparation

1. Try a few bench presses with a small amount of weight so you can practice your technique, warm up your muscles, and coordinate your movements with those of your spotter(s). Once you've warmed up, place the appropriate amount of weight on the barbell for the test. Men should lift 80 lb (36.4 kg); women should lift 35 lb (15.9 kg).
2. Set the metronome at a rate of 60 beats per minute.

Instructions

1. Lie on the bench with your feet firmly on the floor. Grasp the bar at shoulder width with your palms away from you. If you have one spotter, she or he should stand directly behind the bench; if you have two spotters, they should stand to the side, one at each end of the barbell. Lower the bar to your chest in preparation for the lift. Push the barbell until your arms are fully extended. Exhale as you lift. Keep your feet firmly on the floor, don't arch your back, and push the weight evenly with your right and left arms. Don't bounce the weight on your chest. Return the weight to your chest in a controlled manner.
2. Start the metronome and perform bench presses at a steady, continuous rate of 30 per minute. Lift the bar on one beat and lower it on the next. Your spotter counts the number of bench presses you perform.
3. Perform as many bench presses as you can do with good form at the correct rhythm. If at any time during the test you can no longer maintain proper form and keep up with the rhythm set by the metronome, stop the test and record the number of bench presses you performed up to that point.

Number of bench presses: ____________

Rating Your Muscular Endurance

Your score is the number of completed bench presses. Refer to the appropriate portion of the table below for a rating of your upper body endurance. Record your rating below and in the chart at the end of this lab.

Rating: ___________

Ratings for the YMCA Bench Press Test

	Number of Bench Presses						
Men	*Very Poor*	*Poor*	*Below Average*	*Average*	*Above Average*	*Good*	*Excellent*
Age: 18–25	Below 13	13–19	20–23	24–28	29–33	34–43	Above 43
26–35	Below 12	12–16	17–20	21–25	26–29	30–40	Above 40
36–45	Below 9	9–13	14–17	18–21	22–25	26–35	Above 35
46–55	Below 5	5–8	9–11	12–15	16–20	21–27	Above 27
56–65	Below 2	2–4	5–8	9–11	12–16	17–23	Above 23
Over 65	Below 2	2–3	4–6	7–9	10–11	12–19	Above 19
Women							
Age: 18–25	Below 9	9–15	16–19	20–24	25–29	30–41	Above 41
26–35	Below 9	9–13	14–17	18–23	24–28	29–39	Above 39
36–45	Below 6	6–11	12–15	16–20	21–25	26–32	Above 32
46–55	Below 2	2–6	7–9	10–13	14–19	20–28	Above 28
56–65	Below 2	2–4	5–7	8–11	12–16	17–23	Above 23
Over 65	Below 1	1–2	3–4	5–7	8–11	12–17	Above 17

SOURCE: Adapted from norms in *YMCA Fitness Testing and Assessment Manual*. Fourth Edition, 2000. Reprinted and adapted with permission of the YMCA of the USA, 101 N. Wacker Drive, Chicago, IL 60606.

Summary of Results

Curl-up test: Number of curl-ups: ___________ Rating: ___________

Push-up test: Number of push-ups: ___________ Rating: ___________

YMCA bench press test: Number of bench presses: ___________ Rating: ___________

Remember that muscular endurance is specific: Your ratings may vary considerably for different parts of your body.

Using Your Results

How did you score? Are you at all surprised by your ratings for muscular endurance? Are you satisfied with your current ratings?

If you're not satisfied, set realistic goals for improvement: ___________________________

Are you satisfied with your current level of muscular endurance as evidenced in your daily life—for example, your ability to carry groceries or your books, hike, and do yardwork?

If you're not satisfied, set some realistic goals for improvement:

What should you do next? Enter the results of this lab in the Preprogram Assessment column in Appendix D. If you've set goals for improvement, begin planning your weight training program by completing the plan in Lab 4.3. After several weeks of your program, complete this lab again and enter the results in the Postprogram Assessment column of Appendix D. How do the results compare?

Name ______________________ Section ______________ Date ______________

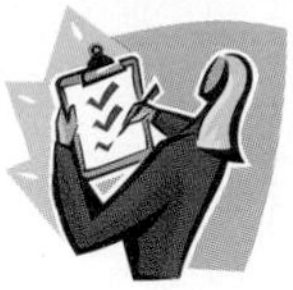

LAB 4.3 *Designing and Monitoring a Strength Training Program*

Ww

1. *Set goals.* List goals for your strength training program. Your goals can be specific or general, short or long term. In the first section, include specific, measurable goals that you can use to track the progress of your fitness program. These goals might be things like raising your upper body muscular strength rating from fair to good or being able to complete 10 repetitions of a lat pull with 125 pounds of resistance. In the second section, include long-term and more qualitative goals, such as improving self-confidence and reducing your risk for back pain.

   Specific Goals: Current Status ______________________ Final Goal ______________________

   ______________________ ______________________

   ______________________ ______________________

   Other goals:

   ____

   ____

2. *Choose exercises.* Based on your goals, choose 8–10 exercises to perform during each weight training session. If your goal is general training for wellness, use one of the sample programs in Figure 4.3 (p.88) and on pp. 98–109. List your exercises and the muscles they develop in the program plan below.
3. *Choose starting weights.* Experiment with different amounts of weight until you settle on a good starting weight, one that you can lift easily for 10–12 repetitions. As you progress in your program, you can add more weight. Fill in the starting weight for each exercise on the program plan.
4. *Choose a starting number of sets and repetitions.* Include at least 1 set of 8–12 repetitions of each exercise. (As you add weight, you may have to decrease the number of repetitions slightly until your muscles adapt to the heavier load.) If your program is focusing on strength alone, your sets can contain fewer repetitions using a heavier load. If you are over approximately 50–60 years of age, your sets should contain more repetitions (10–15) using a lighter load. Fill in the starting number of sets and repetitions of each exercise on the program plan.
5. *Choose the number of training sessions per week.* Work out at least 2 days per week. Indicate the days you will train on your program plan; be sure to include days of rest to allow your body to recover.
6. *Monitor your progress.* Use the workout card on the next page to monitor your progress and keep track of exercises, weights, sets, and repetitions. (A more extensive series of logs is included in the Daily Fitness and Nutrition Journal.)

Program Plan for Weight Training

Exercise	Muscle(s) Developed	Weight (lb)	Repetitions	Sets	Frequency (check ✓)						
					M	T	W	Th	F	Sa	Su

WORKOUT CARD FOR ____________________

Exercise/Date										
	Wt									
	Sets									
	Reps									
	Wt									
	Sets									
	Reps									
	Wt									
	Sets									
	Reps									
	Wt									
	Sets									
	Reps									
	Wt									
	Sets									
	Reps									
	Wt									
	Sets									
	Reps									
	Wt									
	Sets									
	Reps									
	Wt									
	Sets									
	Reps									
	Wt									
	Sets									
	Reps									
	Wt									
	Sets									
	Reps									
	Wt									
	Sets									
	Reps									
	Wt									
	Sets									
	Reps									

Flexibility and Low-Back Health

5

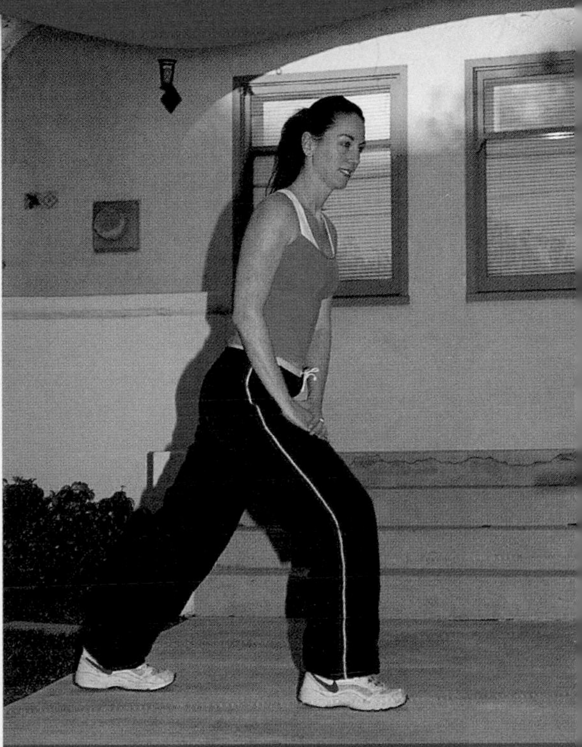

LOOKING AHEAD

After reading this chapter, you should be able to

- Describe the potential benefits of flexibility and stretching exercises
- List the factors that affect the flexibility in a joint
- Explain the different types of stretching exercises and how they affect muscles
- Describe the intensity, duration, and frequency of stretching exercises that will develop the most flexibility with the lowest risk of injury
- List safe stretching exercises for major joints
- Describe how low-back pain can be prevented and managed

TEST YOUR KNOWLEDGE

1. Stretching exercises should be performed
   a. at the start of a warm-up.
   b. following the active part of a warm-up.
   c. after endurance exercise or strength training.
2. If you injure your back, it's usually best to rest in bed for several days. True or false?
3. To gain flexibility, you should stretch until you feel pain. True or false?

TEST YOUR KNOWLEDGE ANSWERS

1. B and/or C. It's best to do stretching exercises when your muscles are warm, after either the active part of a warm-up (5–10 minutes of an activity such as walking or easy jogging) or an endurance or strength training workout.

2. FALSE. Prolonged bed rest may actually worsen back pain. Limit bed rest to a day or less, treat pain and inflammation with cold and then heat, and begin moderate physical activity as soon as possible.

3. FALSE. Stretch to the point of slight tension or mild discomfort, not pain. If you are very sore or sore for more than 24 hours following a stretching workout, you have stretched too intensely.

Fit and Well Online Learning Center

www.mhhe.com/fahey5e

Visit the *Fit and Well* Online Learning Center for study aids, additional information about flexibility and low-back health, links, Internet activities that explore the development of flexibility, and much more.

Flexibility—the ability of a joint to move through its full **range of motion**—is extremely important for general fitness and wellness. The smooth and easy performance of everyday and recreational activities is impossible if flexibility is poor. Flexibility is a highly adaptable physical fitness component. It increases in response to a regular program of stretching exercises and decreases with inactivity. Flexibility is also specific: Good flexibility in one joint doesn't necessarily mean good flexibility in another. Flexibility can be increased through stretching exercises for all major joints.

There are two basic types of flexibility: static and dynamic. Static flexibility refers to the ability to assume and maintain an extended position at one end or point in a joint's range of motion; it is what most people mean by the term *flexibility*. Dynamic flexibility, unlike static flexibility, involves movement; it is the ability to move a joint through its range of motion with little resistance. For example, static shoulder flexibility would determine how far you could extend your arm across the front of your body or out to the side. Dynamic shoulder flexibility would affect your ability to pitch a softball, swing a golf club, or swim the crawl stroke. When gymnasts perform a split on the balance beam, they must have good static flexibility in their legs and hips; to perform a split leap, they must have good dynamic flexibility.

Static flexibility depends on many factors, including the structure of a joint and the tightness of muscles, tendons, and ligaments that are attached to it. Dynamic flexibility depends on static flexibility, but it also involves such factors as strength, coordination, and resistance to movement. Dynamic flexibility can be important for both daily activities and sports. However, because static flexibility is easier to measure and better researched, most assessment tests and stretching programs—including those presented in this chapter—target static flexibility.

This chapter describes the factors that affect flexibility and the benefits of maintaining good flexibility. It provides guidelines for assessing your current level of flexibility and putting together a successful stretching program. It also examines the common problem of low-back pain.

Terms

Ww

range of motion The full motion possible in a joint.

delayed-onset muscle soreness Soreness that occurs 1–2 days after exercising, probably caused by tissue damage and inflammation that leads to further tissue damage.

joint capsules Semielastic structures, composed primarily of connective tissue, that surround major joints.

soft tissues Tissues of the human body that include skin, fat, linings of internal organs and blood vessels, connective tissues, tendons, ligaments, muscles, and nerves.

collagen White fibers that provide structure and support in connective tissue.

elastin Yellow fibers that make connective tissue flexible.

titin A filament in muscle that helps align proteins that cause muscle contraction, titin has elastic properties and also plays a role in flexibility.

BENEFITS OF FLEXIBILITY AND STRETCHING EXERCISES

Good flexibility provides benefits for the entire musculoskeletal system; it may also prevent injuries and soreness and improve performance in all physical activities.

Joint Health

Good flexibility is essential to good joint health. When the muscles and other tissues that support a joint are tight, the joint is subject to abnormal stresses that can cause joint deterioration. For example, tight thigh muscles cause excessive pressure on the kneecap, leading to pain in the knee joint. Tight shoulder muscles can compress sensitive soft tissues in the shoulder, leading to pain and disability in the joint. Poor joint flexibility can also cause abnormalities in joint lubrication, leading to deterioration of the sensitive cartilage cells lining the joint; pain and further joint injury can result.

Improved flexibility can greatly improve your quality of life, particularly as you get older. Aging decreases the natural elasticity of muscles, tendons, and joints, resulting in stiffness. The problem is compounded if you have arthritis. Flexibility exercises improve the elasticity in your tissues, making it easier to move your body. When you're flexible, everything from tying your shoes to reaching for a jar on an upper shelf becomes easier.

Prevention of Low-Back Pain and Injuries

Low-back pain can be related to poor spinal alignment, which puts pressure on the nerves leading out from the spinal column. Strength and flexibility in the back, pelvis, and thighs may help prevent this type of back pain. Unfortunately, research studies have not yet clearly defined the relationship between back pain and lack of flexibility. Few studies have found that trunk flexibility improves back health or reduces the risk of injury; in some people, greater spinal mobility may actually increase the risk of low-back problems. However, good hip and knee flexibility has been found to protect the spine from excessive motion during the tasks of daily living.

Poor flexibility does increase one's risk for injury. A general stretching program has been shown to be effective in reducing the frequency of injuries as well as their severity. When injuries do occur, flexibility exercises can be used in treatment: They reduce symptoms and help restore normal range of motion in affected joints.

Overstretching—stretching muscles to extreme ranges of motion—may actually decrease the stability of a joint. Although some activities, such as gymnastics and ballet, require extreme joint movements, such flexibility is not recommended for the average person. In fact, extreme flexibility may increase the risk of injury in activities such as skiing, basketball, and volleyball. Again, as with other types of exercise, moderation is the key to safe training.

Additional Potential Benefits

- *Temporary reduction of postexercise muscle soreness.* **Delayed-onset muscle soreness,** occurring 1–2 days after exercise, is thought to be caused by damage to the muscle fibers and supporting connective tissue. Some studies have shown that stretching after exercise decreases the degree of muscle soreness—but this improvement appears to be temporary. Postexercise stretching does not appear to relieve muscle soreness for an extended period of time.
- *Relief of aches and pains.* Flexibility exercises help relieve pain that develops from stress or prolonged sitting. Studying or working in one place for a long time can make your muscles tense. Stretching helps relieve tension, so you can go back to work refreshed and effective.
- *Improved body position and strength for sports (and life).* Good flexibility lets a person assume more efficient body positions and exert force through a greater range of motion. For example, swimmers with more flexible shoulders have stronger strokes because they can pull their arms through the water in the optimal position. Flexible joints and muscles let you move more fluidly. Some studies also suggest that flexibility training enhances strength development.
- *Maintenance of good posture.* Good flexibility also contributes to body symmetry and good posture. Bad posture can gradually change your body structures. Sitting in a slumped position, for example, can lead to tightness in the muscles in the front of your chest and overstretching and looseness in the upper spine, causing a rounding of the upper back. This condition, called kyphosis, is common in older people. It may be prevented by stretching regularly.
- *Relaxation.* Flexibility exercises are a great way to relax. Studies have shown that doing flexibility exercises reduces mental tension, slows your breathing rate, and reduces blood pressure.

Flexibility and Lifetime Wellness

Part of wellness is being able to move without pain or hindrance. Flexibility exercises are an important part of this process. Sedentary people often effectively lose their mobility at an early age. Even relatively young people are often handicapped by back, shoulder, knee, and ankle pain. As they age, the pain can become debilitating, leading to injuries and a lower quality of life. Good flexibility helps keep your joints and muscles moving without pain so that you can do all the things you enjoy.

WHAT DETERMINES FLEXIBILITY?

The flexibility of a joint is affected by its structure, by muscle elasticity and length, and by nervous system activity. Some factors—joint structure, for example—can't be changed. Other factors, such as the length of resting muscle fibers, can be changed through exercise; these factors should be the focus of a program to develop flexibility.

Joint Structure

The amount of flexibility in a joint is determined in part by the nature and structure of the joint. Hinge joints such as those in your fingers and knees allow only limited forward and backward movement; they lock when fully extended. Ball-and-socket joints like the hip enable movement in many different directions and have a greater range of motion. Major joints are surrounded by **joint capsules,** semielastic structures that give joints strength and stability but limit movement. Heredity also plays a part in joint structure and flexibility; for example, although everyone has a broad range of motion in the ball-and-socket hip joint, not everyone can do a split.

Muscle Elasticity and Length

Soft tissues, including skin, muscles, tendons, and ligaments, also limit the flexibility of a joint. Muscle tissue is the key to developing flexibility because it can be lengthened if it is regularly stretched. As described in Chapter 4, muscles contain proteins that create movement by causing muscles to contract. These contractile proteins can also stretch, and they are involved in the development of flexibility. However, the most important component of muscle tissue related to flexibility is the connective tissue that surrounds and envelops every part of muscle tissue, from individual muscle fibers to entire muscles. Connective tissue provides structure, elasticity, and bulk and makes up about 30% of muscle mass. Two principal types of connective tissue are **collagen,** white fibers that provide structure and support, and **elastin,** yellow fibers that are elastic and flexible. Muscles contain both collagen and elastin, closely intertwined, so muscle tissue exhibits the properties of both types of fibers. A recently discovered structural protein in muscles called **titin** also has elastic properties and contributes to flexibility.

When a muscle is stretched, the wavelike elastin fibers straighten; when the stretch is relieved, they rapidly snap back to their resting position. If gently and regularly stretched, connective tissues will lengthen and flexibility will improve. Without regular stretching, the process reverses: These tissues shorten, resulting in decreased flexibility. Regular stretching also contributes to flexibility by lengthening muscle fibers through the addition of contractile units called sarcomeres.

The stretch characteristics of connective tissue in muscle are important considerations for a stretching program. The amount of stretch a muscle will tolerate is limited, and as the limits of its flexibility are reached, connective tissue becomes more brittle and may rupture if overstretched (Figure 5.1). A safe and effective program stretches muscles enough to slightly elongate the tissues but not so much that they are damaged. Research has shown that flexibility is improved best by stretching when muscles are warm (following exercise or the application of heat) and the stretch is applied gradually and conservatively. Sudden, high-stress stretching is less effective and can lead to muscle damage.

Nervous System Activity

Muscles contain **stretch receptors** that control their length. If a muscle is stretched suddenly, stretch receptors send signals to the spinal cord, which then sends a signal back to the same muscle, causing it to contract. These reflexes occur frequently in active muscles. They help the body know what the muscles are doing and allow for fine control of muscle length.

Small movements that only slightly stimulate these receptors cause small reflex actions. Rapid, powerful, and sudden movements that strongly stimulate the receptors cause large, powerful reflex muscle contractions. Stretches that involve rapid, bouncy movements are considered dangerous because they may stimulate a reflex muscle contraction during a stretch. A muscle that contracts at the same time it's being stretched can be easily injured, so slow, gradual stretches are always safest.

Strong muscle contractions produce a reflex of the opposite type—one that causes muscles to relax and keeps them from contracting too hard. This inverse stretch reflex has recently been introduced as an aid to improving flexibility: Contracting a muscle prior to stretching it causes it to relax, allowing it to stretch farther. The contraction-stretch technique for developing flexibility is called **proprioceptive neuromuscular facilitation (PNF).** More research needs to be done, however, to determine precisely the degree to which PNF techniques cause muscle relaxation and help develop flexibility.

Doing each stretching exercise several times in a row can "reset" the sensitivity of muscle stretch receptors. Stretching a muscle, relaxing, and then stretching it again cause the stretch receptors to become slightly less sensitive, thereby enabling the muscle to stretch farther. It is not known if stretch receptor sensitivity continues to change following prolonged flexibility training, but it's likely that neural changes do occur to help increase flexibility.

ASSESSING FLEXIBILITY

Because flexibility is specific to each joint, there are no tests of general flexibility. The most commonly used flexibility test is the sit-and-reach test, which rates the flexibility of the muscles in the lower back and hamstrings. To assess your flexibility and identify inflexible joints, complete Lab 5.1.

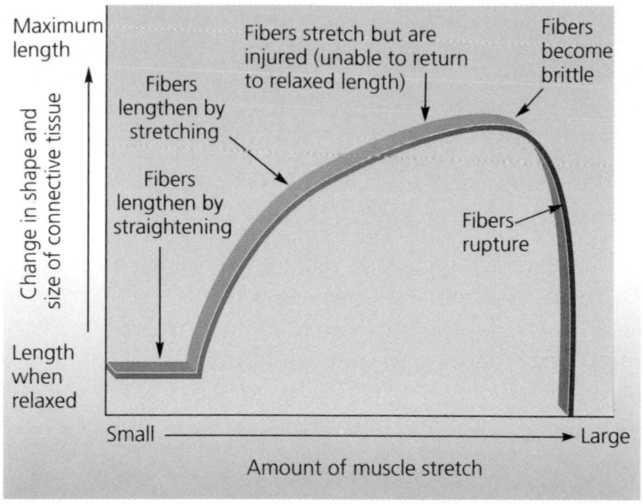

Figure 5.1 The effect of stretch on connective tissue.

CREATING A SUCCESSFUL PROGRAM TO DEVELOP FLEXIBILITY

A successful program for developing flexibility contains safe exercises executed with the most effective techniques.

Types of Stretching Techniques

Stretching techniques vary from simply stretching the muscles during the course of normal activities to sophisticated methods based on patterns of muscle reflexes. Improper stretching techniques can do more harm than good, so it's important to understand the different types of stretching exercises and how they affect the muscles. Three common techniques are static stretches, ballistic stretches, and PNF.

Static Stretching In **static stretching,** each muscle is gradually stretched, and the stretch is held for 10–30 seconds. (Holding the stretch longer than 30 seconds will not further improve flexibility, whereas stretching for less than 10 seconds will provide little benefit.) A slow stretch prompts less reaction from stretch receptors, and the muscles can safely stretch farther than usual. Static stretching is the type most often recommended by fitness experts because it's safe and effective. The key to this technique is to stretch the muscles and joints to the point where a pull is felt, but not to the point of pain.

Ballistic Stretching In **ballistic stretching,** the muscles are stretched suddenly in a bouncing movement. For example, touching the toes repeatedly in rapid succession is a ballistic stretch for the hamstrings. The problem with this technique is that the heightened activity of stretch receptors caused by the rapid stretches can continue for some time, possibly causing injuries during any physical activities that follow. For this reason, ballistic stretching is usually not recommended.

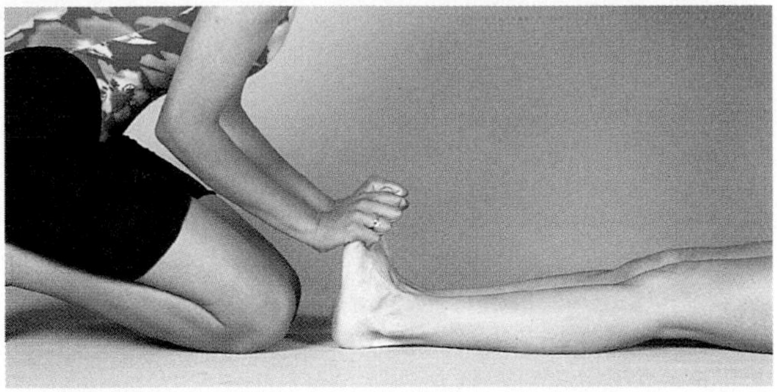
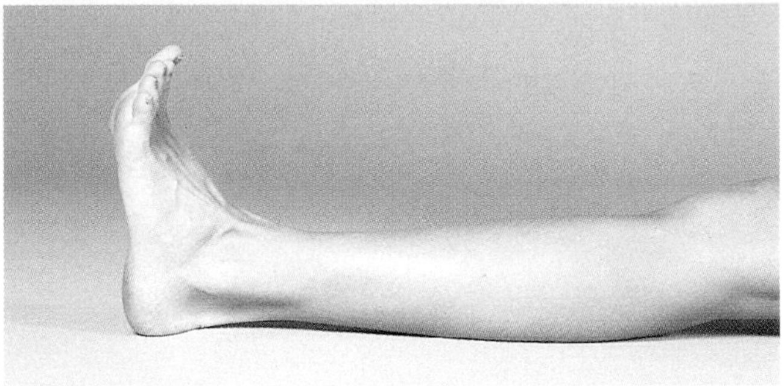

In passive stretching (left), an outside force—such as pressure exerted by another person—helps move the joint and stretch the muscles. In active stretching (right), the force to move the joint and stretch the muscles is provided by a contraction of the opposing muscles.

Proprioceptive Neuromuscular Facilitation (PNF) PNF techniques use reflexes initiated by both muscle and joint receptors to cause greater training effects. The most popular PNF stretching technique is the contract-relax stretching method, in which a muscle is contracted before it is stretched. For example, in a seated stretch of calf muscles, the first step in PNF is to contract the calf muscles. The individual or a partner can provide resistance for an isometric contraction. Following a brief period of relaxation, the next step is to stretch the calf muscles by pulling the tops of the feet toward the body. A duration of 6 seconds for the contraction and 10–30 seconds for the stretch is recommended.

Another example of a PNF stretch is the contract-relax-contract pattern. In this technique, begin by contracting the muscle to be stretched and then relaxing it. Next, contract the opposing muscle (the antagonist). Finally, stretch the first muscle. For example, using this technique to stretch the hamstrings (the muscles in the back of the thigh) would require the following steps: contract the hamstrings, relax the hamstrings, contract the quadriceps (the muscles in the front of the thigh), stretch the hamstrings.

PNF appears to allow more effective stretching, but it tends to cause more muscle stiffness and soreness than static stretching. It also usually requires a partner and takes more time.

Passive and Active Stretching

Stretches can be done either passively or actively.

Passive Stretching In **passive stretching,** an outside force or resistance provided by yourself, a partner, gravity, or a weight helps your joints move through their range of motion. For example, a seated stretch of the hamstring and back muscles can be done by reaching the hands toward the feet until a "pull" is felt in those muscles. You can achieve a greater range of motion (a more intense stretch) using passive stretching. However, because the stretch is not controlled by the muscles themselves, there is a greater risk of injury. Communication between partners in passive stretching is very important so joints aren't forced outside their normal functional range of motion.

Active Stretching In **active stretching,** a muscle is stretched by a contraction of the opposing muscle (the muscle on the opposite side of the limb). For example, an active seated stretch of the calf muscles occurs when a person actively contracts the muscles on the top of the shin. The contraction of this opposing muscle produces a reflex that relaxes the muscles to be stretched. The muscle can be stretched farther with a low risk of injury.

The only disadvantage of active stretching is that a person may not be able to produce enough stress (enough stretch) to increase flexibility using only the contraction of opposing muscle groups. The safest and most convenient technique is active static stretching, with an occasional passive assist. For example, you might stretch your calves both by contracting the muscles on the top of your shin and by pulling your feet toward you. This way you combine the advantages of active stretching—safety and the relaxation reflex—with those of passive stretching—greater range of motion.

Terms

Ww

stretch receptors Sense organs in skeletal muscles that initiate a nerve signal to the spinal cord in response to a stretch; a contraction follows.

proprioceptive neuromuscular facilitation (PNF) A technique for stretching and strengthening muscles; PNF relies on neuromuscular reflexes to stimulate training effects.

static stretching A technique in which a muscle is slowly and gently stretched and then held in the stretched position.

ballistic stretching A technique in which muscles are stretched by the force generated as a body part is repeatedly bounced, swung, or jerked.

passive stretching A technique in which muscles are stretched by force applied by an outside source.

active stretching A technique in which muscles are stretched by the contraction of the opposing muscles.

- Do stretching exercises statically. Stretch to the point of mild discomfort, hold the position for 10–30 seconds, rest for 30–60 seconds, and repeat, trying to stretch a bit farther.
- Do not stretch to the point of pain. Any soreness after a stretching workout should be mild and last no more than 24 hours. If you are sore for a longer period, you stretched too intensely.
- Relax and breathe easily as you stretch. Inhale through the nose and exhale through pursed lips during the stretch. Try to relax the muscles being stretched.
- Perform all exercises on both sides of your body.
- Increase intensity and duration gradually over time. Improved flexibility takes many months to develop.
- Stretch when your muscles are warm. Do gentle warm-up exercises such as easy jogging or calisthenics before doing a pre-exercise stretching routine.
- There are large individual differences in joint flexibility. Don't feel you have to compete with others during stretching workouts.

Intensity and Duration

For each exercise, slowly apply stretch to your muscles to the point of slight tension or mild discomfort. Hold the stretch for 10–30 seconds. As you hold the stretch, the feeling of slight tension should slowly subside; at that point, try to stretch a bit farther. Throughout the stretch, try to relax and breathe easily. Rest for about 30–60 seconds between each stretch, and do at least 4 repetitions of each stretch. A complete flexibility workout usually takes about 20–30 minutes (Figure 5.2).

Frequency

The ACSM recommends that stretching exercises be performed a minimum of 2–3 days a week. Many people do flexibility training more often—3–5 days a week—for even greater benefits. It's best to stretch when your muscles are warm, so try incorporating stretching into your cool-down after cardiorespiratory endurance exercise or weight training. Stretching can also be a part of your warm-up, but it's important to increase the temperature of your muscles first by doing the active part of the warm-up (for example, walking or slow jogging) for 5–10 minutes. Stretching before exercise without warming up does not prevent injury and may even cause injury.

Refer to the box "Safe Stretching" for additional tips on creating a safe and successful stretching program, and complete Lab 5.2 when you're ready to start your own program.

Making Progress

As with any type of physical training, you will make progress and improve your flexibility if you stick with your program. Follow the guidelines outlined in this chapter and train at least 2–3 days per week. The best way to judge your progress is to note your body position while stretching. For example, note how far you can lean forward during a modified hurdler stretch. If you wish, you can repeat the assessment tests that appear in Lab 5.1 periodically; be sure to take the test at the same time of day each time. You will likely notice some improvement in flexibility after only 2–3 weeks of a stretching program; however, attaining significant improvements will take at least 2 months. By then, you can expect flexibility increases of about 10–20% in many joints.

Exercises to Improve Flexibility

There are hundreds of exercises that can improve flexibility. Your program should include exercises that work all the major joints of the body by stretching their associated muscles. The exercises illustrated here are simple to do and pose a minimum risk of injury. Use these exercises, or substitute your favorite stretches, to create a well-rounded program for developing flexibility. Be sure to perform each stretch using the proper technique. Hold each position for 10–30 seconds and perform at least 4 repetitions of each exercise.

Warm-up 5–10 minutes or following an endurance or strength training workout

Stretching exercises for major joints

Sample program

Exercise	*Areas stretched*
Head turns and tilts	Neck
Towel stretch	Triceps, shoulders, chest
Across-the-body stretch	Shoulders, upper back
Upper back stretch	Upper back
Lateral stretch	Trunk muscles
Step stretch	Hip, front of thigh
Side lunge	Inner thigh, hip, calf
Sole stretch	Inner thigh, hip
Trunk rotation	Trunk, outer thigh, hip, lower back
Alternate leg stretcher	Back of thigh, hip, knee, ankle, buttocks
Modified hurdler stretch	Back of thigh, lower back
Lower-leg stretch	Calf, soleus, Achilles tendon

Type of activity: Stretching exercises that focus on major joints

Frequency: 2–3 days per week or more

Intensity: Stretch to the point of mild discomfort, not pain

Duration: All stretches should be held for 10–30 seconds and performed at least 4 times

Figure 5.2 A flexibility workout.

FLEXIBILITY EXERCISES

EXERCISE 1

HEAD TURNS AND TILTS

Areas stretched: Neck

Instructions

Head turns: Turn your head to the right and hold the stretch. Repeat to the left.

Head tilts: Tilt your head to the left and hold the stretch. Repeat to the right.

Variation: Place your right palm on your right cheek; try to turn your head to the right as you resist with your hand. Repeat on the left side.

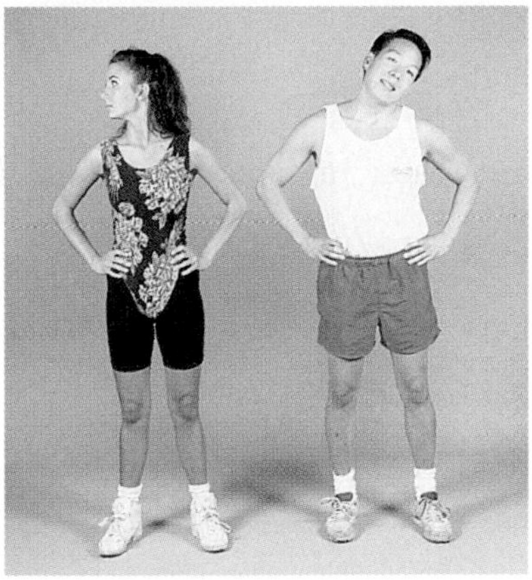

EXERCISE 2

TOWEL STRETCH

Areas stretched: Triceps, shoulders, chest

Instructions: Roll up a towel and grasp it with both hands, palms down. With your arms straight, slowly lift it back over your head as far as possible. The closer together your hands are, the greater the stretch.

Variation: Repeat the stretch with your arms down and the towel behind your back. Grasp the towel with your palms forward and thumbs pointing out. Gently raise your arms behind your back.

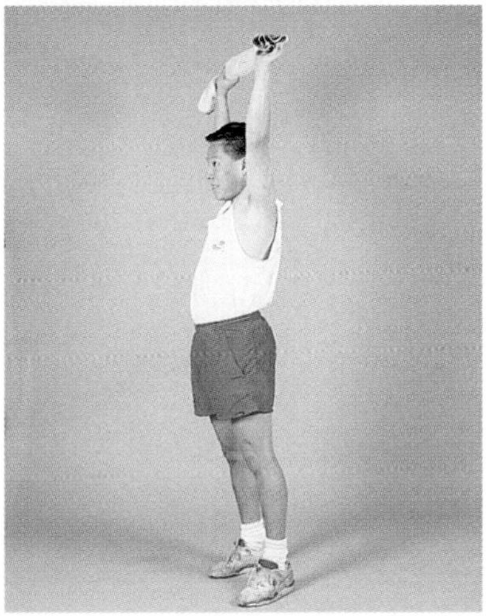

EXERCISE 3

ACROSS-THE-BODY STRETCH

Areas stretched: Shoulders, upper back

Instructions: Keeping your back straight, cross your left arm in front of your body and grasp it with your right hand. Stretch your arm, shoulders, and back by gently pulling your arm as close to your body as possible. Repeat the stretch with your right arm.

Variation: Bend your right arm over and behind your head. Grasp your right hand with your left, and gently pull your arm until you feel the stretch. Repeat for your left arm.

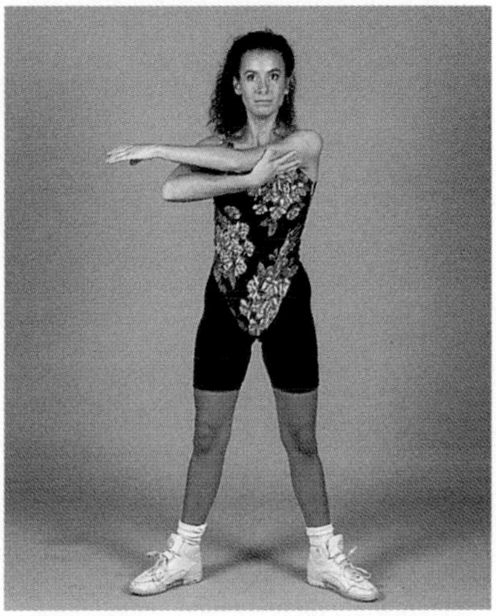

EXERCISE 4

UPPER-BACK STRETCH

Areas stretched: Upper back

Instructions: Stand with your feet shoulder-width apart, knees slightly bent, and pelvis tucked under. Clasp your hands in front of your body and press your palms forward.

Variation: In the same position, wrap your arms around your body as if you were giving yourself a hug.

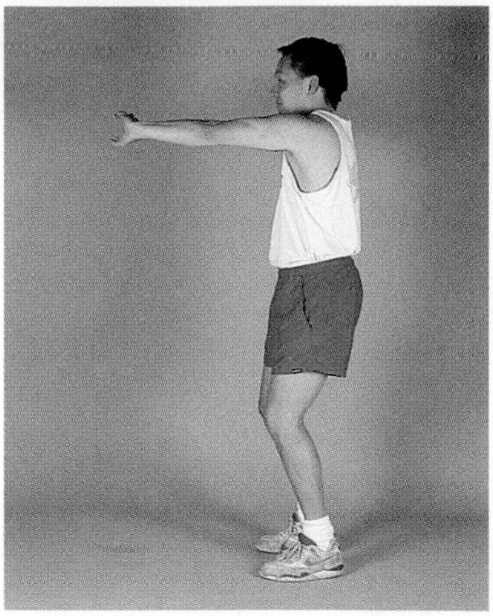

EXERCISE 5

LATERAL STRETCH

Areas stretched: Trunk muscles

Instructions: Stand with your feet shoulder-width apart, knees slightly bent, and pelvis tucked under. Raise one arm over your head and bend sideways from the waist. Support your trunk by placing the hand or forearm of your other arm on your thigh or hip for support. Be sure you bend directly sideways and don't move your body below the waist. Repeat on the other side.

Variation: Perform the same exercise in a seated position.

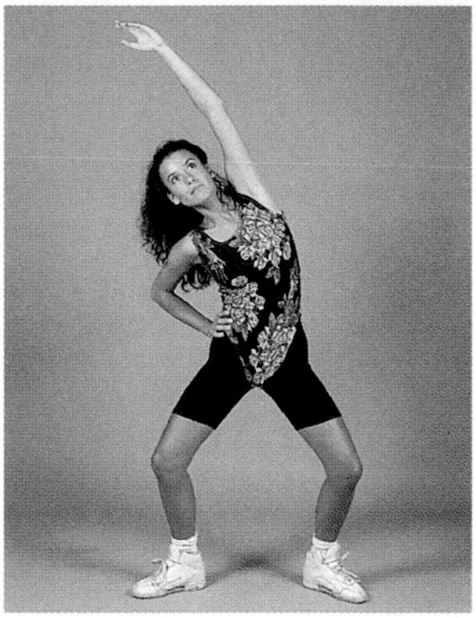

EXERCISE 6

STEP STRETCH

Areas stretched: Hip, front of thigh (quadriceps)

Instructions: Step forward and flex your forward knee, keeping your knee directly above your ankle. Stretch your other leg back so that it is parallel to the floor. Press your hips forward and down to stretch. Your arms can be at your sides, on top of your knee, or on the ground for balance. Repeat on the other side.

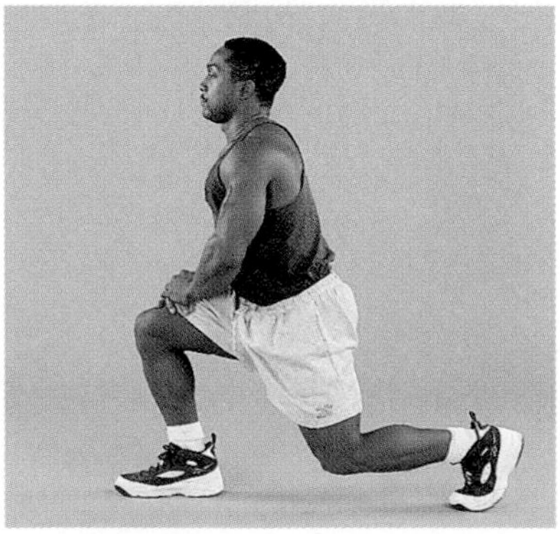

EXERCISE 7

SIDE LUNGE

Areas stretched: Inner thigh, hip, calf

Instructions: Stand in a wide straddle with your legs turned out from your hip joints and your hands on your thighs. Lunge to one side by bending one knee and keeping the other leg straight. Keep your knee directly over your ankle; do not bend it more than 90 degrees. Repeat on the other side.

Variation: In the same position, lift the heel of the bent knee to provide additional stretch. The exercise may also be performed with your hands on the floor for balance.

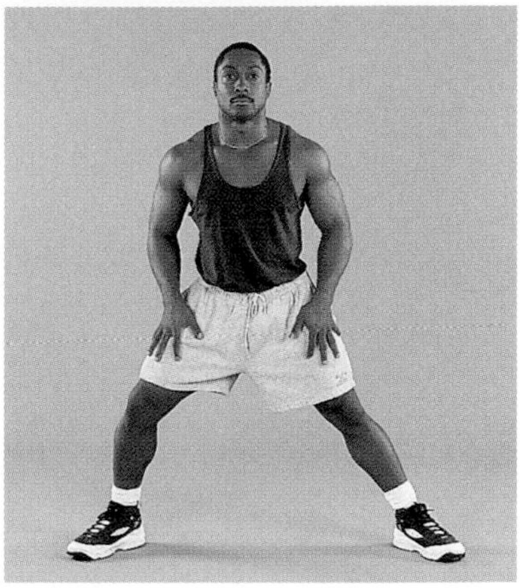

EXERCISE 8

SOLE STRETCH

Areas stretched: Inner thigh, hip

Instructions: Sit with the soles of your feet together. Push your knees toward the floor using your hands or forearms.

Variation: When you first begin to push your knees toward the floor, use your legs to resist the movement. Then relax and press your knees down as far as they will go.

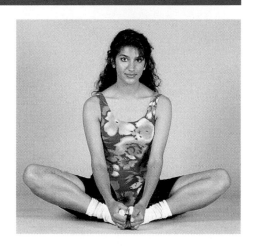

EXERCISE 9

TRUNK ROTATION

Areas stretched: Trunk, outer thigh and hip, lower back

Instructions: Sit with your right leg straight, left leg bent and crossed over the right knee, and left hand on the floor next to your left hip. Turn your trunk as far as possible to the left by pushing against your left leg with your right forearm or elbow. Keep your left foot on the floor. Repeat on the other side.

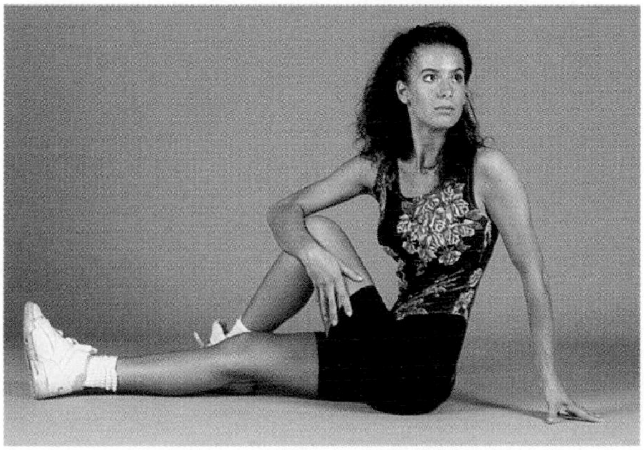

EXERCISE 10

ALTERNATE LEG STRETCHER

Areas stretched: Back of the thigh (hamstring), hip, knee, ankle, buttocks

Instructions: Lie flat on your back with both legs straight.**(a)** Grasp your left leg behind the thigh, and pull in to your chest. **(b)** Hold this position, and then extend your left leg toward the ceiling. **(c)** Hold this position, and then bring your left knee back to your chest and pull your toes toward your shin with your left hand. Stretch the back of the leg by attempting to straighten your knee. Repeat for the other leg.

Variation: Perform the stretch on both legs at the same time.

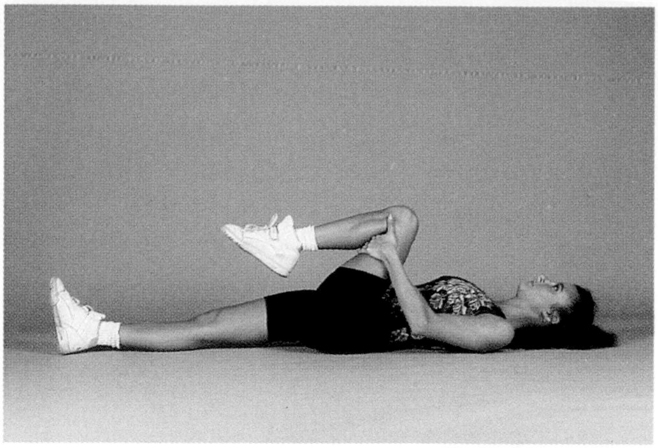

(a)

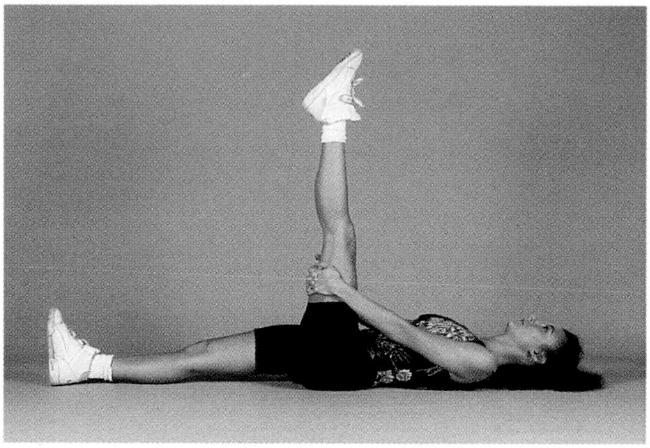

(b)

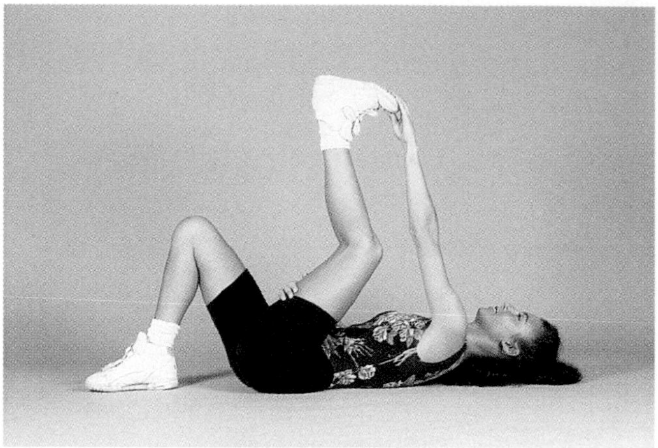

(c)

EXERCISE 11

MODIFIED HURDLER STRETCH
(Seated Single-Toe Touch)

Areas stretched: Back of the thigh (hamstring), lower back

Instructions: Sit with your right leg straight and your left leg tucked close to your body. Reach toward your right foot as far as possible. Repeat for the other leg.

Variation: As you stretch forward, alternately flex and point the foot of your extended leg.

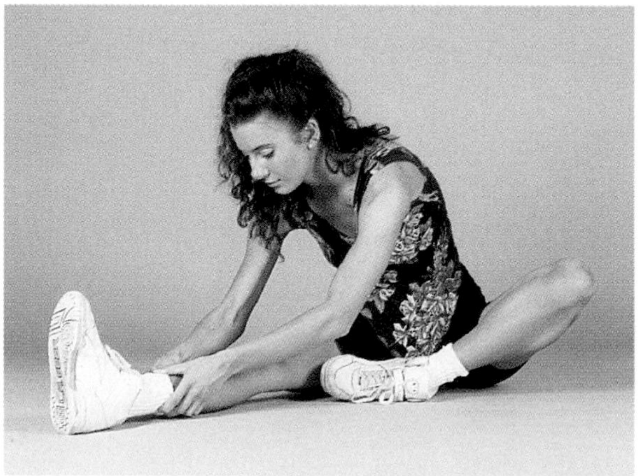

EXERCISE 12

LOWER-LEG STRETCH

Areas stretched: Back of the lower leg (calf, soleus, Achilles tendon)

Instructions: Stand with one foot about 1–2 feet in front of the other, with both feet pointing forward. **(a)** Keeping your back leg straight, lunge forward by bending your front knee and pushing your rear heel backward. Hold. **(b)** Then pull your back foot in slightly, and bend your back knee. Shift your weight to your back leg. Hold. Repeat on the other side.

Variation: Place your hands on a wall and extend one foot back, pressing your heel down to stretch; or stand with the balls of your feet on a step or bench and allow your heels to drop below the level of your toes.

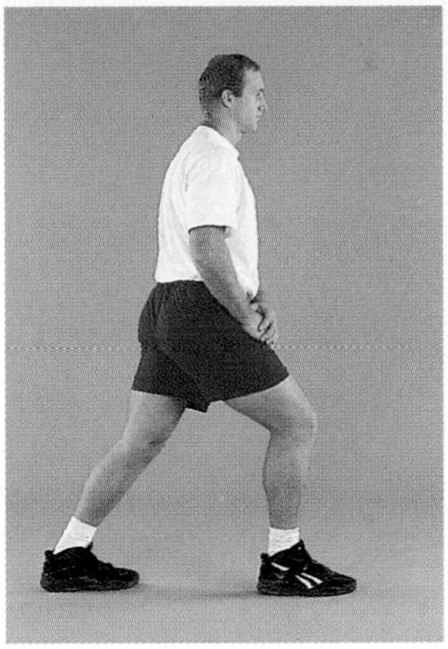

(a)

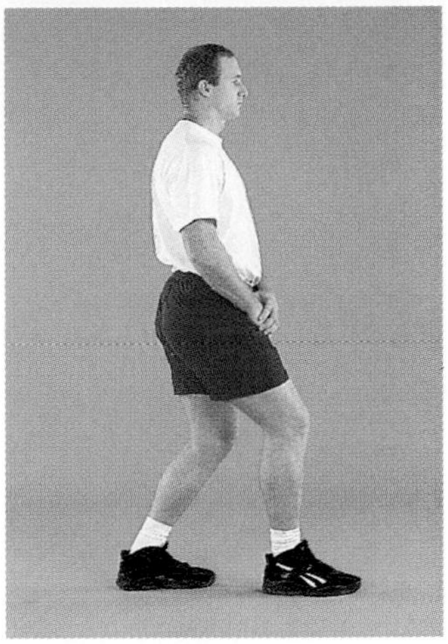

(b)

PREVENTING AND MANAGING LOW-BACK PAIN

More than 85% of Americans experience back pain at some time in their lives. Low-back pain is the second most common ailment in the United States—headache tops the list—and the second most common reason for absences from work. Low-back pain is estimated to cost as much as $50 billion a year in lost productivity, medical and legal fees, and disability insurance and compensation.

Back pain can result from sudden traumatic injuries, but it is more often the long-term result of weak and inflexible muscles, poor posture, or poor body mechanics during activities like lifting and carrying. Any abnormal strain on the back can result in pain. Most cases of low back pain clear up within a few weeks or months, but some people have recurrences or suffer from chronic pain.

Function and Structure of the Spine

The spinal column performs many important functions in the body.

- It provides structural support for the body, especially the thorax (upper-body cavity).
- It surrounds and protects the spinal cord.
- It supports much of the body's weight and transmits it to the lower body.
- It serves as an attachment site for a large number of muscles, tendons, and ligaments.
- It allows movement of the neck and back in all directions.

The spinal column is made up of bones called **vertebrae** (Figure 5.3, p. 134). The spine consists of 7 cervical vertebrae in the neck, 12 thoracic vertebrae in the upper back, and 5 lumbar vertebrae in the lower back. The 9 vertebrae at the base of the spine are fused into two sections and form the sacrum and the coccyx (tailbone). The spine has four curves: the cervical, thoracic, lumbar, and sacral curves. These curves help bring the body weight supported by the spine in line with the axis of the body.

Although the structure of vertebrae depends on their location on the spine, the different types of vertebrae do share common characteristics. Each consists of a body, an arch, and several bony processes (Figure 5.4, p. 134). The vertebral body is cylindrical, with flattened surfaces where **intervertebral disks** are attached. The vertebral body is designed to carry the stress of body weight and physical activity. The vertebral arch surrounds and protects the spinal cord. The bony processes serve as joints for adjacent vertebrae and attachment sites for muscles and ligaments. **Nerve roots** from the spinal cord pass through notches in the vertebral arch.

Intervertebral disks, which absorb and disperse the stresses placed on the spine, separate vertebrae from each other. Disks are made up of a gel- and water-filled nucleus surrounded by a series of fibrous rings. The liquid nucleus can change shape when it is compressed, allowing the disk to absorb shock. The intervertebral disks also help maintain the spaces between vertebrae where the spinal nerve roots are located.

Terms

vertebrae Bony segments composing the spinal column that provide structural support for the body and protect the spinal cord.

intervertebral disk A touch, elastic disk located between adjoining vertebrae consisting of a gel- and water-filled nucleus surrounded by fibrous rings; it serves as a shock absorber for the spinal column.

nerve root Base of one of the 31 pairs of spinal nerves that branch off the spinal cord through spaces between vertebrae.

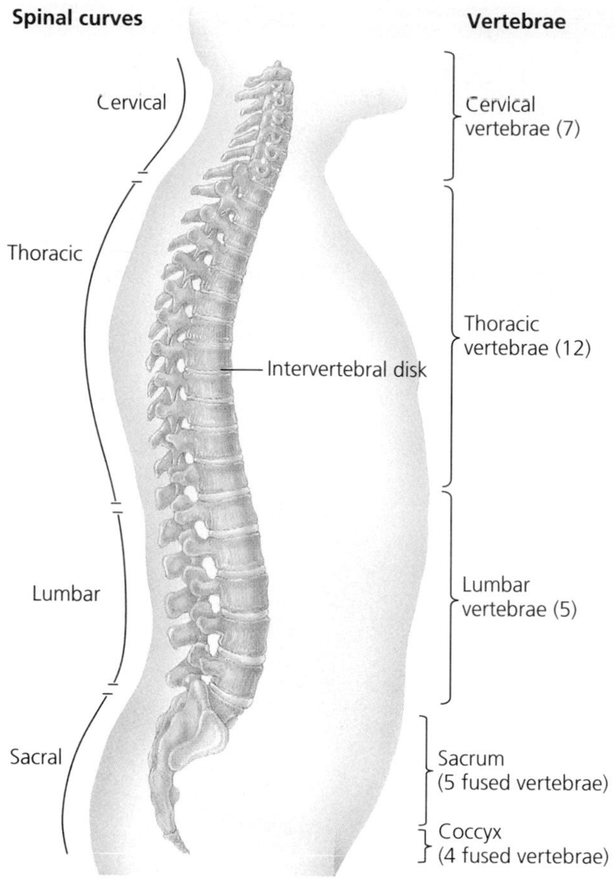

Figure 5.3 The spinal column. The spine is made up of five separate regions and has four distinct curves. An intervertebral disk is located between vertebrae.

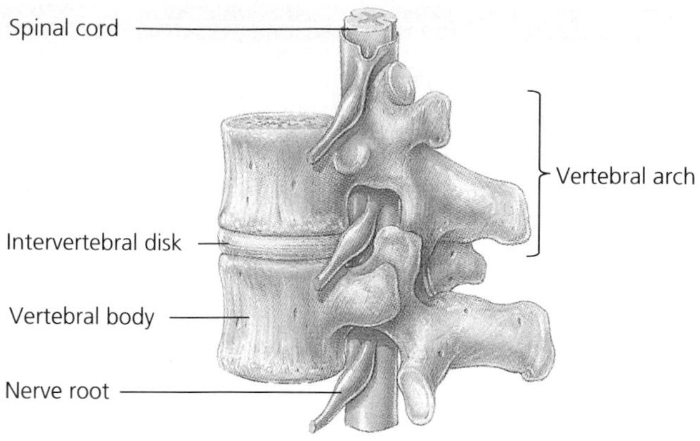

Figure 5.4 Vertebrae and an intervertebral disk.

Causes of Back Pain

Back pain can occur at any point along your spine; the lumbar area, because it bears the majority of your weight, is the most common site. Any movement that causes excessive stress on the spinal column can cause injury and pain. The spine is well equipped to bear body weight and the force or stress of body movements along its long axis. However, it is less capable of bearing loads at an angle to its long axis. You do not have to carry a heavy load or participate in a vigorous contact sport to injure your back. Picking a pencil up from the floor using poor body mechanics—reaching too far out in front of you or bending over with your knees straight, for example—can also result in back pain.

Risk factors associated with low-back pain include age greater than 34 years, degenerative diseases such as arthritis or osteoporosis, a family or personal history of back pain or trauma, a sedentary lifestyle, low job satisfaction, and low socioeconomic status. Smoking increases risk because smoking appears to increase degenerative changes in the spine. Excess body weight also increases strain on the back, and psychological stress or depression can cause muscle tension and back pain. Occupations and activities associated with low-back pain are those involving physically hard work, such as frequent lifting, twisting, bending, standing up, or straining in forced positions; those requiring high concentration demands (such as computer programming); and those involving vibrations affecting the entire body (such as truck driving).

Underlying causes of back pain include poor muscle endurance and strength in the muscles of the abdomen, back, hips, and legs; excess body weight; poor posture or body position when standing, sitting, or sleeping; and poor body mechanics when performing actions like lifting and carrying, or sports movements. Abnormal spinal loading resulting from any of these causes can have short-term or long-term direct and indirect effects on the spine. Strained muscles, tendons, or ligaments can cause pain and can, over time, lead to injuries to vertebrae or the intervertebral disks.

Stress can cause disks to break down and lose some of their ability to absorb shock. A damaged disk may bulge out between vertebrae and put pressure on a nerve root, a condition commonly referred to as a slipped disk. Painful pressure on nerves can also occur if damage to a disk narrows the space between two vertebrae. With age, you lose fluid from the disks, making them more likely to bulge and put pressure on nerve roots. Depending on the amount of pressure on a nerve, symptoms may include numbness in the back, hip, leg, or foot; radiating pain; loss of muscle function; depressed reflexes; and muscle spasm. If the pressure is severe enough, loss of function can be permanent.

Preventing Low-Back Pain

Incorrect posture when standing, sitting, lying, and lifting is responsible for many back injuries. In general, think about moving your spine as a unit, with the force directed through its long axis. Strategies for maintaining good posture during daily activities are presented in the box "Good Posture and Low-Back Health," p. 136. Follow the same guidelines for posture and movement when you engage in sports or recreational activities. Maintain control over your body movements and warm up thoroughly before you exercise. Take special care when lifting weights as part of a resistance training program (see Chapter 4).

The role of exercise in preventing and treating back pain is still being investigated. However, many experts do recommend exercise, especially for people who have already experienced an episode of low-back pain. Regular exercise aimed at increasing muscle endurance and strength in the back and abdomen is often recommended to prevent back pain, as is lifestyle physical activity such as walking. Movement helps lubricate your spinal disks and increases muscle fitness in your trunk and legs. Other lifestyle recommendations for preventing back pain include:

- Lose weight, stop smoking; and reduce emotional stress.
- Avoid sitting, standing, or working in the same position for too long.
- Use a supportive seat and a firm mattress.
- Warm up thoroughly before engaging in vigorous exercise or sports.
- Progress gradually when attempting to improve strength or fitness.

Managing Acute Back Pain

Sudden back pain usually involves tissue injury. Symptoms may include pain, muscles spasms, stiffness, and inflammation. Many cases of acute back pain go away by themselves within a few days or weeks. You may be able to reduce pain and inflammation by applying cold and then heat. Begin with a cold treatment: Apply ice several times a day; once inflammation and spasms subside, you can apply heat using a heating pad or a warm bath. (See Chapter 3 for more on injury treatment and the use of ice.) If the pain is bothersome, an over-the-counter nonsteroidal anti-inflammatory medication such as ibuprofen or naproxen may be helpful; stronger pain medications and muscle relaxants are available by prescription.

Bed rest immediately following the onset of back pain may make you feel better, but it should be of very short duration. Prolonged bed rest—5 days or more—was once thought to be an effective treatment for back pain, but most physicians now advise against it because it may weaken muscles and actually worsen pain. Limit bed rest to one day and begin moderate physical activity as soon as possible. Exercise can increase muscular endurance and flexibility and protect your disks from loss of fluid. Three of the back exercises discussed later in the chapter may be particularly helpful following an episode of acute back pain: curl-ups, side bridges, and back extensions.

See your physician if acute back pain doesn't resolve within a short time. Other warning signals of a more severe problem that requires a professional evaluation include the following: severe pain, numbness, pain that radiates down one or both legs, problems with bladder or bowel control, fever, or rapid weight loss.

Managing Chronic Back Pain

Low-back pain is considered chronic if it persists for more than 3 months. Symptoms vary—some people experience stabbing or shooting pain, others a steady ache accompanied by stiffness. Sometimes pain is localized; in other cases, it radiates to another part of the body. Psychological symptoms may also occur. Underlying causes of chronic back pain include injuries, infection, muscle or ligament strains, and disk herniations.

Because symptoms and causes are so varied, different people benefit from different treatment strategies, and researchers have found that many treatments have only limited benefits. Potential treatments may include over-the-counter or prescription medications; exercise; physical therapy, massage, or chiropractic care; acupuncture; percutaneous electrical nerve stimulation (PENS), in which acupuncture-like needles are used to deliver an electrical current; education and advice about posture, exercise, and body mechanics; and surgery.

Psychological therapy may also be beneficial in some cases. Reducing emotional stress that causes muscle tension can provide direct benefits, and other therapies can help people deal better with chronic pain and its effects on their daily lives. Support groups and expressive writing are strategies that have been found beneficial for people with chronic pain and other conditions (see the box "Expressive Writing and Chronic Conditions," p. 137).

Exercises for the Prevention and Management of Low-Back Pain

The tests in Lab 5.3 can help you assess low-back muscular endurance and posture. The exercises that follow are designed to help you maintain a healthy back by stretching and strengthening the major muscle groups that affect the back—the abdominal muscles, the muscles along your spine and sides, and the muscles of your hips and thighs. If you have back problems, check with your physician before beginning any exercise program. Perform the exercises slowly and progress very gradually. Stop and consult your physician if any exercise causes back pain. General guidelines for back exercise programs include the following:

- Do low-back exercises at least 3 days per week; many experts recommend that back exercises be done daily.
- Emphasize muscular endurance rather than muscular strength—endurance may be more protective. Many back injuries are caused by problems with motor control: If you attempt complex trunk movements (such as picking up a book from the floor) when your muscles are tired, you are more likely to strain muscles and/or put pressure on nerves, thereby causing pain.
- Don't do spine exercises involving a full range of motion early in the morning because your disks have a high fluid content early in the day and injuries may occur as a result.
- Engage in regular endurance exercise such as cycling or walking in addition to performing exercises that specifically build muscular endurance and flexibility.
- Be patient and stick with your program. Increased back fitness and pain relief may require as long as 3 months of regular exercise.

TAKE CHARGE Good Posture and Low-Back Health

Changes in everyday posture and behavior can help prevent and alleviate low-back pain.

- *Lying down.* When resting or sleeping, lie on your side with your knees and hips bent. If you lie on your back place a pillow under your knees. Don't lie on your stomach. If your mattress isn't firm, place a plywood board under it.

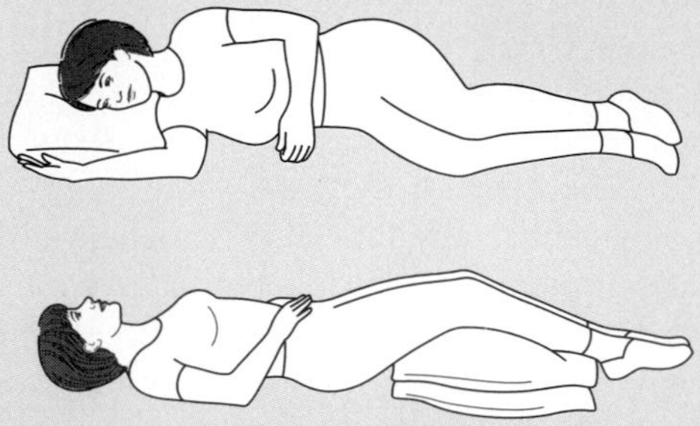

- *Sitting.* Sit with your lower back slightly rounded, knees bent, and feet flat on the floor. Alternate crossing your legs, or use a footrest to keep your knees higher than your hips. If this position is uncomfortable or if your back flattens when you sit, try using a lumbar roll pillow behind your lower back.

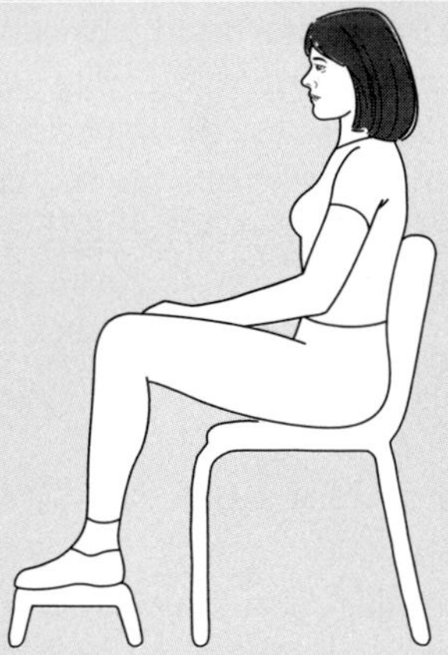

- *Lifting.* If you need to lower yourself to grasp an object, bend at the knees and hips rather than at the waist. Your feet should be about shoulder-width apart. Lift gradually, keeping your arms straight, by standing up or by pushing with your leg muscles. Keep the object close to your body. Don't twist, if you have to turn with the object, change the position of your feet.

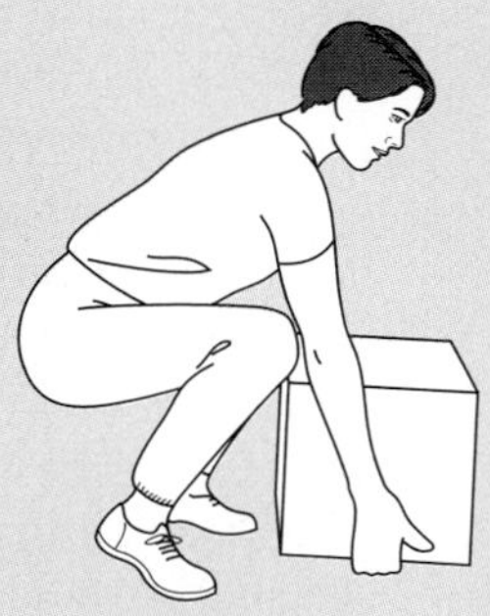

- *Standing.* When you are standing, a straight line should run from the top of your ear through the center of your shoulder, the center of your hip, the back of your kneecap, and the front of your ankle bone. Support your weight mainly on your heels, with one or both knees slightly bent. Try to keep your lower back flat by placing one foot on a stool. Don't let your pelvis tip forward or your back arch. Shift your weight back and forth from foot to foot. Avoid prolonged standing. (To check your posture, stand in a normal way with your back to a wall. Your upper back and buttocks should touch the wall; your heels may be a few inches away. Slide one hand into the space between your lower back and the wall. It should slide in easily but should almost touch both your back and the wall. Adjust your posture as needed, and try to hold this position as you walk away from the wall.)

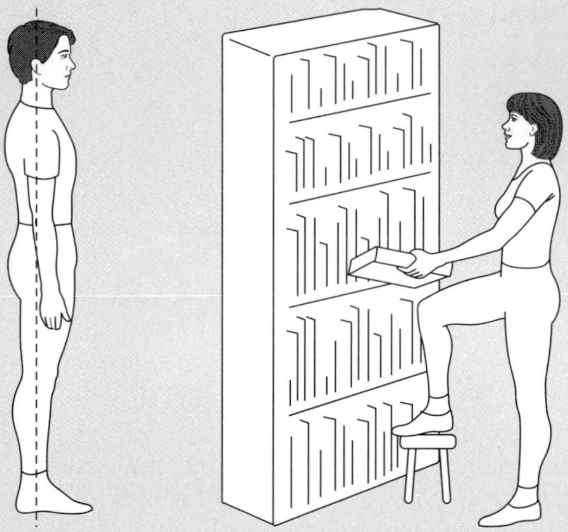

- *Walking.* Walk with your toes pointed straight ahead. Keep your back flat, head up and centered over your body, and chin in. Swing your arms freely. Don't wear high-heeled shoes.

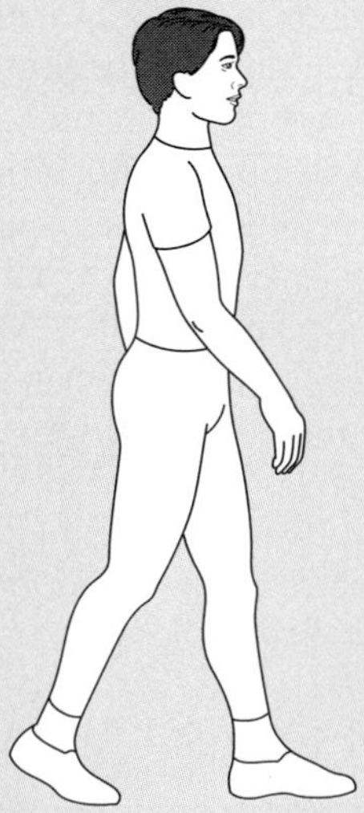

The act of writing down feelings and thoughts about stressful life events has been shown to help people with chronic conditions improve their health. In one recent study, people with asthma or rheumatoid arthritis were asked to write down their feelings about the most stressful event in their lives; they wrote for 20 minutes a day over a three-day period. In follow-up exams four months later, nearly half of the patients who engaged in expressive writing experienced positive changes in their condition such as reduced joint pain. Only about a quarter of the control group, who wrote about their daily plans, experienced a positive change in health.

Investigators remain unsure why writing about one's feelings has beneficial effects. It is possible that expressing feelings about a traumatic event helps people work through the event and put it behind them. The resulting sense of release and control may reduce stress levels and have positive physical effects. Alternatively, expressive writing may change the way people think about previous stressful events in their lives and help them cope with new stressors. Whatever the cause, it's clear that expressive writing can be a safe, inexpensive, and effective supplement to standard treatment of certain chronic conditions.

What about the effects of expressive writing on otherwise healthy individuals? Other studies have, in fact, found such a benefit: People who wrote about traumatic experiences reported fewer symptoms, fewer days off work, fewer visits to the doctor, improved mood, and a more positive outlook.

If you'd like to try expressive writing to help you deal with a traumatic event, set aside a special time—15 minutes a day for four consecutive days, for example, or one day a week for four weeks. Write in a place where you won't be interrupted or distracted. Explore your very deepest thoughts and feelings and why you feel the way you do. Don't worry about grammar or coherence or about what someone else might think about what you're writing; you are writing just for yourself. You may find the writing exercise to be distressing in the short term—sadness and depression are common when dealing with feelings about a stressful event—but most people report relief and contentment soon after writing for several days.

SOURCES: Smyth, J. M., et al. 1999. Effects of writing about stressful experiences on symptom reduction in patients with asthma or rheumatoid arthritis: A randomized trial. *Journal of the American Medical Association* 281(14): 1304–1309. Spiegel, D. 1999. Healing words: Emotional expression and disease outcome. *Journal of the American Medical Association* 281(14): 1328–1329. Pennebaker, J. 1997. *Opening Up: The Healthy Power of Expressing Emotions.* New York: Guilford Press.

LOW-BACK EXERCISES

EXERCISE 1

CAT STRETCH

Target: Improved flexibility, relaxation, and reduced stiffness in the spine

Instructions: Begin on all fours with your knees below your hips and your hands below your shoulders. Slowly and deliberately move through a cycle of extension and flexion of your spine. Begin by slowly pushing your back up and dropping your head slightly until your spine is extended (rounded). Then slowly lower your back and lift your chin slightly until your spine is flexed (relaxed and slightly arched). *Do not press at the ends of the range of motion.* Stop if you feel pain. Do 10 slow, continuous cycles of the movement.

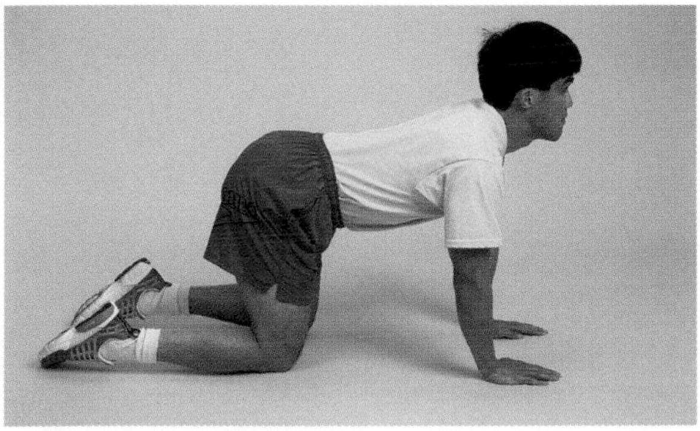

(a)

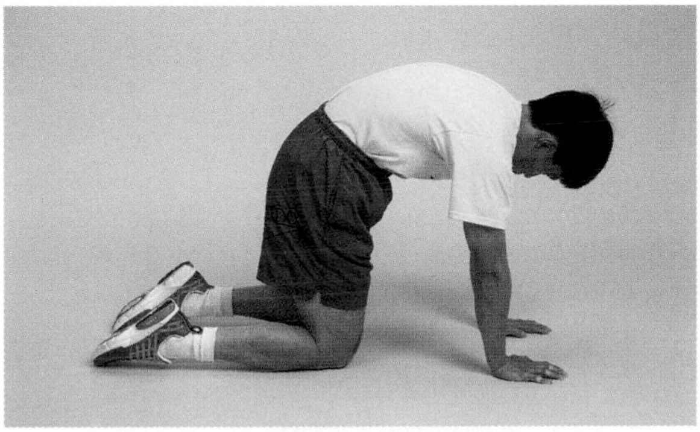

(b)

EXERCISE 2

STEP STRETCH (see Exercise 6 in the flexibility program, p. 130)

Target: Improved flexibility, strength, and endurance in the muscles of the hip and the front of the thigh

Instructions: Hold each stretch for 10–30 seconds and do at least 4 repetitions on each side.

EXERCISE 3

ALTERNATE LEG STRETCHER (see Exercise 10 in the flexibility program, p. 132)

Target: Improved flexibility in the back of the thigh, hip, knee, and buttocks

Instructions: Hold each stretch for 10–30 seconds and do at least 4 repetitions on each side.

EXERCISE 4

DOUBLE KNEE-TO-CHEST

Target: Improved flexibility in the lower back and hips

Instructions: Lie on your back with both knees bent and feet flat on the floor. **(a)** With one hand on the back of each thigh, slowly pull both knees to your chest; hold the stretch. **(b)** Then straighten your knees so that both legs are extended toward the ceiling. Return to the starting position by drawing your legs back to your chest and then placing your feet on the floor. Hold each stretch for 10–30 seconds and do at least 4 repetitions.

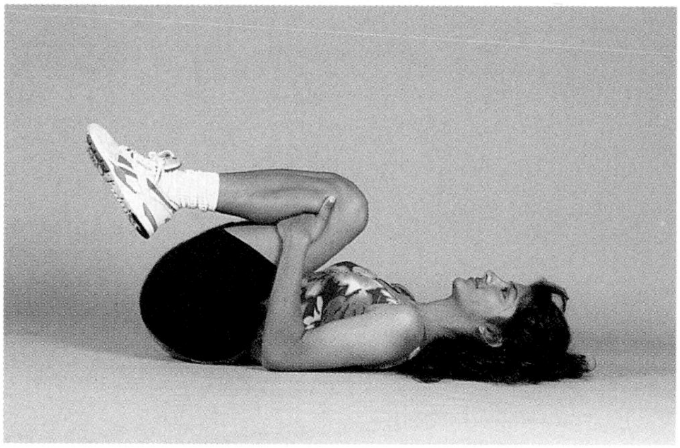

(a)

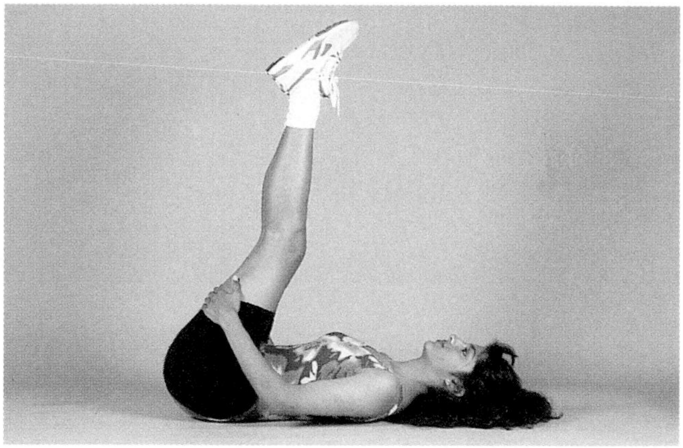

(b)

EXERCISE 5

TRUNK TWIST

Target: Improved flexibility in the lower back and sides

Instructions: Lie on your side with top knee bent, lower leg straight, lower arm extended out in front of you on the floor, and upper arm at your side. Push down with your upper knee while you twist your trunk backward. Try to get your shoulders and upper body flat on the floor, turning your head as well. Return to the starting position, and then repeat on the other side. Hold the stretch for 10–30 seconds and do at least 4 repetitions on each side.

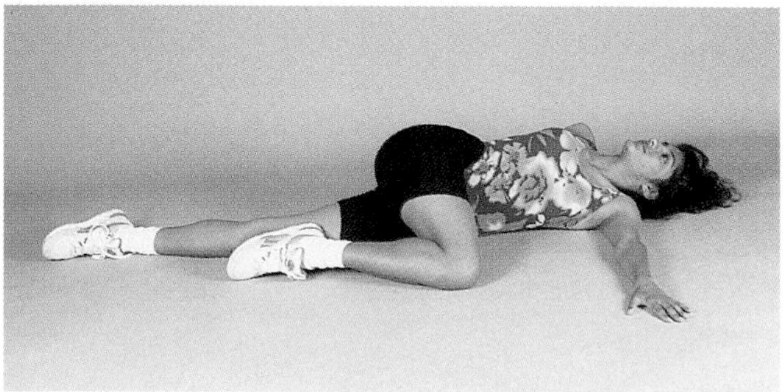

EXERCISE 6

CURL-UP

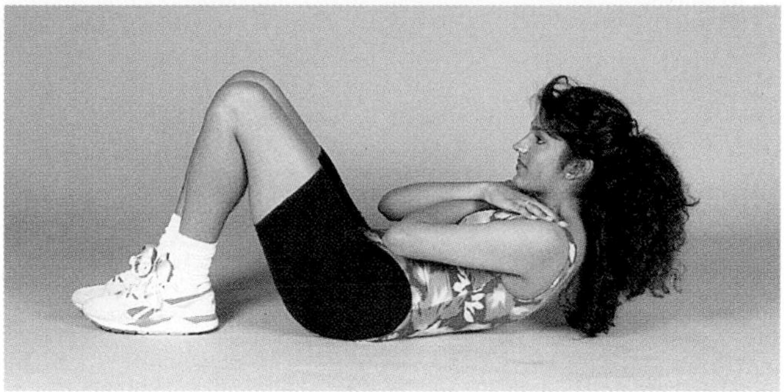

Target: Improved strength and endurance in the abdomen

Instructions: Lie on your back with one or two knees bent and arms crossed on your chest or hands under your lower back. Tilt your pelvis under, flattening your back. Tuck your chin in and slowly curl up, one vertebra at a time, as you lift your head first and then your shoulders. Stop when you can see your knees and hold for 5–10 seconds before returning to the starting position. Do 10 or more repetitions.

Variation: Add a twist to develop other abdominal muscles. When you have curled up so that your shoulder blades are off the floor, twist your upper body so that one shoulder is higher than the other; reach past your knee with your upper arm. Hold and then return to the starting position. Repeat on the opposite side. Curl-ups can also be done using an exercise ball (see p. 142).

EXERCISE 7

ISOMETRIC SIDE BRIDGE

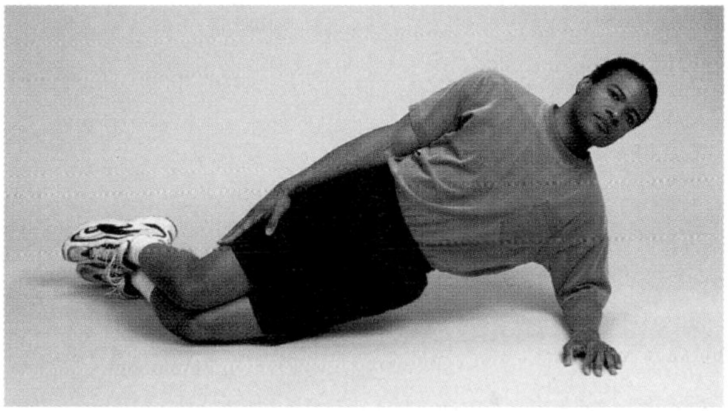

Target: Increased strength and endurance in the muscles along the sides of the abdomen

Instructions: Lie on the ground on your side with your knees bent and your top arm lying alongside your body. Lift your hips so that your weight is supported by your forearm and knee. Hold this position for 10 seconds, breathing normally. Repeat on the other side. Work up to a 60-second hold; perform one or more repetitions on each side.

Variation: You can make the exercise more difficult by keeping your legs straight and supporting yourself with your feet and forearm (see Lab 5.3) or with your feet and hand (with elbow straight).

EXERCISE 8

SPINE EXTENSIONS (see Exercise 9 in the free weights program in Chapter 4, p. 101)

Target: Increased strength and endurance in the back, buttocks, and back of the thighs

Instructions: Hold each position for 10–30 seconds. Begin with one repetition on each side and work up to several repetitions.

Variation: If you have experienced back pain in the past or if this exercise is very difficult for you, do the exercise with both hands on the ground rather than with one arm lifted.

EXERCISE 9

WALL SQUAT (Phantom Chair)

Target: Increased strength and endurance in the lower back, thighs, and abdomen

Instructions: Lean against a wall and bend your knees as though you are sitting in a chair. Support your weight with your legs. Begin by holding the position for 5–10 seconds. Build up to 1 minute or more. Perform one or more repetitions.

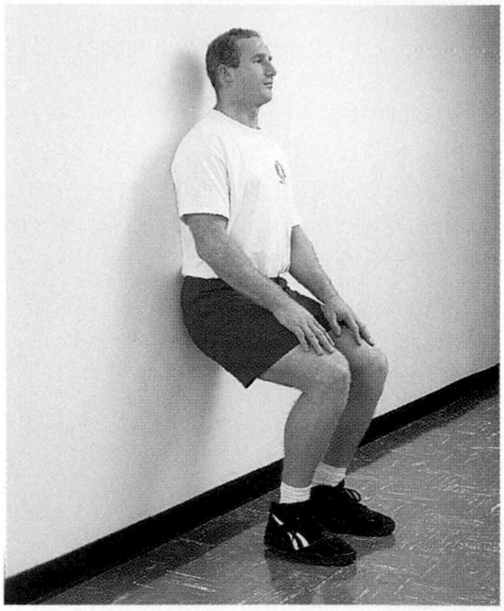

EXERCISE 10

PELVIC TILT

Target: Increased strength and endurance in the abdomen and buttocks

Instructions: Lie on your back with knees bent and arms extended to the side. Tilt your pelvis under and try to flatten your lower back against the floor. Tighten your buttock and abdominal muscles while you hold this position for 5–10 seconds. Don't hold your breath. Work up to 10 repetitions of the exercise. Pelvic tilts can also be done standing or leaning against a wall. (Note: Although this is a popular exercise with many therapists, some experts question the safety of pelvic tilts. Stop if you feel pain in your back at any time during the exercise.)

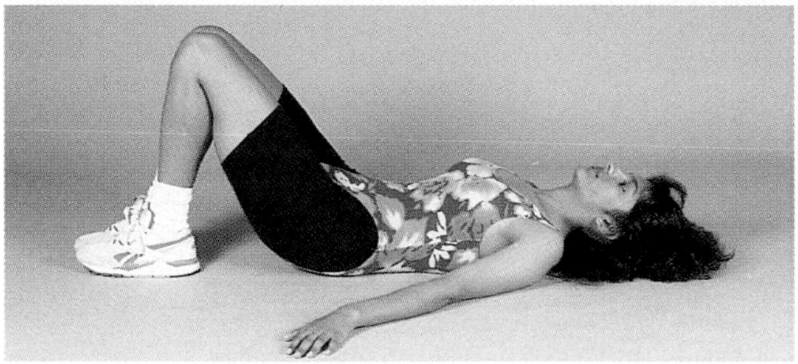

EXERCISE 11

BACK BRIDGE

Target: Increased strength and endurance in the hips and buttocks

Instructions: Lie on your back with knees bent and arms extended to the side. Tuck your pelvis under, and then lift your tailbone, buttocks, and lower back from the floor. Hold this position for 5–10 seconds with your weight resting on your feet, arms, and shoulders, and then return to the starting position. Work up to 10 repetitions of the exercise. (Note: Although this is a popular exercise with many therapists, some experts question the safety of back bridges. Stop if you feel pain in your back at any time during the exercise.)

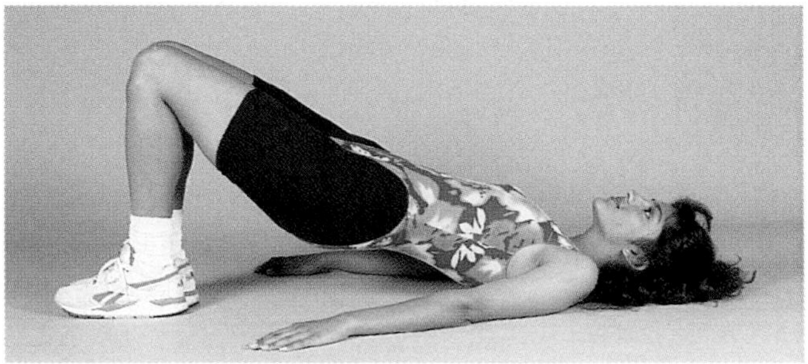

Tips for Today

Good flexibility and proper posture improve the health of your joints and muscles and may prevent injuries and low-back pain, contributing to long-term quality of life. Stretching exercises are also a great way to relax and relieve aches and pains. To improve and maintain your flexibility, perform stretches that work the major joints at least twice a week.

Right now you can

- Make a list of five benefits of flexibility that are particularly meaningful to you. Put the list on your mirror and use it as a motivational tool for beginning and maintaining your fitness program.
- Stand up and stretch—do either the upper-back stretch or the across-the-body stretch shown in the chapter.
- Practice the recommended sitting and standing postures suggested in the chapter (see p. 136). If needed, adjust your chair or find something to use as a footrest.
- If you frequently work at a computer, check the position in which you typically sit and make any needed adjustments to improve your posture. Your back should be flat or slightly rounded, feet flat on the floor (or a footrest), and knees at or slightly above hip level. When your hands are on the keyboard, your shoulders should be relaxed, your forearms and hands should be in a straight line, and the top of the monitor screen should be at or slightly below eye level. Your eyes should be about 18–30 inches from the screen.

SUMMARY

- Flexibility, the ability of joints to move through their full range of motion, is highly adaptable and specific to each joint.
- The benefits of flexibility include preventing abnormal stresses that lead to joint deterioration and possibly reducing the risk of injuries and low-back pain.
- Range of motion can be limited by joint structure, muscle inelasticity, and stretch receptor activity.
- Developing flexibility depends on stretching the elastic tissues within muscles regularly and gently until they lengthen. Overstretching can make connective tissue brittle and lead to rupture.
- Signals sent between stretch receptors and the spinal cord can enhance flexibility because contracting a muscle stimulates a relaxation response, thereby allowing a longer muscle stretch, and because stretch receptors become less sensitive after repeated stretches, initiating fewer contractions.
- Static stretching is done slowly and held to the point of mild tension; ballistic stretching consists of bouncing stretches and can lead to injury. Proprioceptive neuromuscular facilitation uses muscle receptors in contracting and relaxing a muscle.
- Passive stretching, using an outside force in moving muscles and joints, achieves a greater range of motion (and has a higher injury risk) than active stretching, which uses opposing muscles to initiate a stretch.
- Stretches should be held for 10–30 seconds; perform at least 4 repetitions. Flexibility training should be done 2 or more days a week, preferably following activity, when muscles are warm.
- The spinal column consists of vertebrae separated by intervertebral disks. It provides structure and support for the body and protects the spinal cord.
- Acute back pain can be treated as a soft tissue injury, with cold treatment followed by application of heat (once swelling subsides); prolonged bed rest is not recommended. A variety of treatments have been suggested for chronic back pain, including regular exercise, physical therapy, acupuncture, education, and psychological therapy.
- In addition to good posture, proper body mechanics, and regular physical activity, a program for preventing low-back pain includes exercises that stretch and strengthen major muscle groups that affect the lower back.

COMMON QUESTIONS ANSWERED

Are there any stretching exercises I shouldn't do? Yes. Avoid exercises that put excessive pressure on your joints, particularly your spine and knees. Previous injuries and poor flexibility may make certain exercises dangerous for some people. Exercises that may cause problems are described in the box "Stretches to Avoid."

Is stretching the same as warming up? People often confuse stretching and pre-exercise warm-up. Although they are complementary, they are two distinct activities. A warm-up involves light exercise that increases body temperature so your metabolism works better when you're exercising at high intensity. Stretching increases the movement capability of your joints, so you can move more easily with less risk of injury. Stretching may also induce cellular changes that protect muscles from injury.

Whenever you stretch, first spend 5–10 minutes engaged in some form of low-intensity exercise, such as walking, jogging, or low-intensity calisthenics. When your muscles are warmed, begin your stretching routine. Warmed muscles stretch better than cold ones and are less prone to injury.

(continued)

COMMON QUESTIONS ANSWERED (continued)

How much flexibility do I need? This question is not always easy to answer. If you're involved in a sport such as gymnastics, figure skating, or ballet, you are often required to reach extreme joint motions to achieve success. However, nonathletes do not need to reach these extreme joint positions. In fact, too much flexibility may, in some cases, increase your risk of injury. As with other types of fitness, moderation is the key. You should regularly stretch your major joints and muscle groups but not aspire to reach extreme flexibility.

Can I stretch too far? Yes. As muscle tissue is progressively stretched, it reaches a point where it becomes damaged and may rupture. The greatest danger occurs during passive stretching when a partner is doing the stretching for you. It is critical that your stretching partner not force your joint outside its normal functional range of motion.

Can physical training limit flexibility? Weight training, jogging, or any physical activity will decrease flexibility if the exercises are not performed through a full range of motion. When done properly, weight training increases flexibility. However, because of the limited range of motion used during the running stride, jogging tends to compromise flexibility. It is very important for runners to practice flexibility exercises for the hamstrings and quadriceps regularly.

Does stretching affect muscular strength? Several recent studies have found that stretching decreases strength and power for about 5 minutes following the stretch. This is one reason why some experts suggest that people not stretch as part of their exercise warm-up. However, the effects of stretching on muscle strength and athletic performance are still being investigated. Regardless of when you choose to stretch, it is still important to warm up before any workout by engaging in 5–10 minutes of light exercise such as walking or slow jogging.

Can a workout with an exercise ball be useful in preventing and managing low-back pain? The exercise or stability ball is an extra-large inflatable ball. It was originally developed for use in physical therapy but has recently become a popular piece of exercise equipment for use in the home or gym. The exercise ball is particularly effective for working the so-called stability muscles in the abdomen, chest, and back—muscles that are important for preventing back problems. The ball's instability forces an exerciser to use the stability muscles to balance the body. Moves such as crunches have been found to be more effective when they are performed with an exercise ball. Beginners should use caution (and choose a larger-sized ball) until they feel comfortable with the movements.

FOR FURTHER EXPLORATION

Fit and Well Online Learning Center (www.mhhe.com/fahey5e)

Use the learning objectives, study guide questions, and glossary flashcards to review key terms and concepts and prepare for exams. You can extend your knowledge of flexibility and low-back health and gain experience in using the Internet as a resource by completing the activities and checking out the Web links for the topics in Chapter 5 marked with the World Wide Web icon. For this chapter, Internet activities explore the types of stretching techniques, different exercises that build flexibility, and techniques for preventing and managing back pain; there is also a helpful set of Web links.

Daily Fitness and Nutrition Journal

Complete the flexibility portion of the program plan by setting goals and selecting exercises. Fill in the information for the specific exercises you will perform, including which joints they work.

Health*Quest*

If you haven't already done so, complete the How Fit Are You? section of the Wellness Activities in the fitness module of Health*Quest*. This section provides an overview of your flexibility status based on your current level of flexibility and your stretching habits.

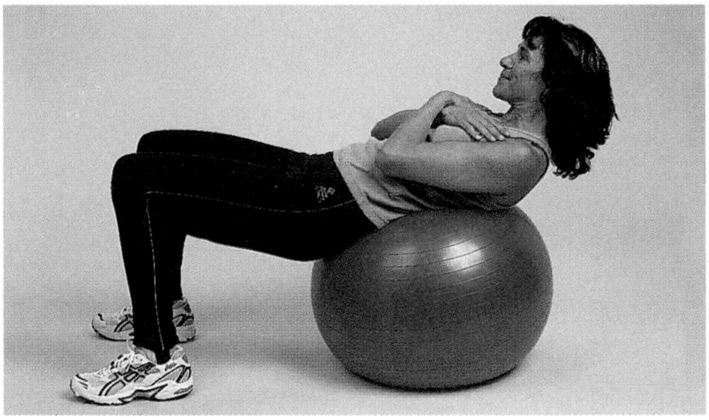

Using an exercise ball for curl-ups works the muscles in the chest, back, buttocks, and legs in addition to those in the abdomen.

Books

Alter, M. J. 1996. *Science of Flexibility,* 2d ed. Champaign, Ill.: Human Kinetics. *An extremely well-researched book that discusses the scientific basis of stretching exercises and flexibility.*

Anderson, B., and J. Anderson. 2000. *Stretching,* 20th anniv. ed. Bolinas, Calif.: Shelter Publications. *A best-selling exercise book, updated with more than 200 stretches for 60 sports and activities.*

Andes, K. 2000. *Fitness Stretching.* Pittsburgh, Pa.: Three Rivers Press. *Takes you through every muscle group with fully illustrated, step-by-step instructions for more than 100 yoga- and sport-inspired stretches.*

Gallagher-Mundy, C. 2001. *Stretching for Health and Fitness.* Alexandria, Va.: Time Life. *A brief guide to safe and effective stretching exercises.*

Hochschuler, S., and B. Reznik. 2002. Treat Your Back without Surgery. 2nd ed. Alameda, Calif.: Hunter House. Provides information about exercises and other nonsurgical techniques for treating back problems.

The safe alternatives listed here are described and illustrated on pages 129–133 as part of the complete program of safe flexibility exercises presented in this chapter.

Standing Toe Touch

Problem: Puts excessive strain on the spine.

Alternatives: Alternate leg stretcher (Exercise 10), modified hurdler stretch (Exercise 11), and lower leg stretch (Exercise 12)

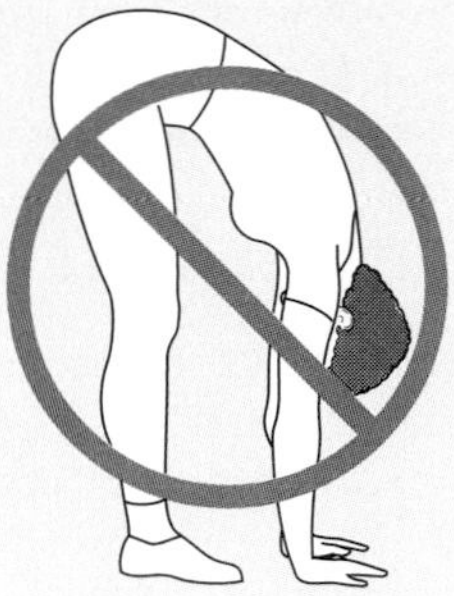

Standing Hamstring Stretch

Problem: Puts excessive strain on the knee and lower back

Alternatives: Alternate leg stretcher (Exercise 10) and modified hurdler stretch (Exercise 11)

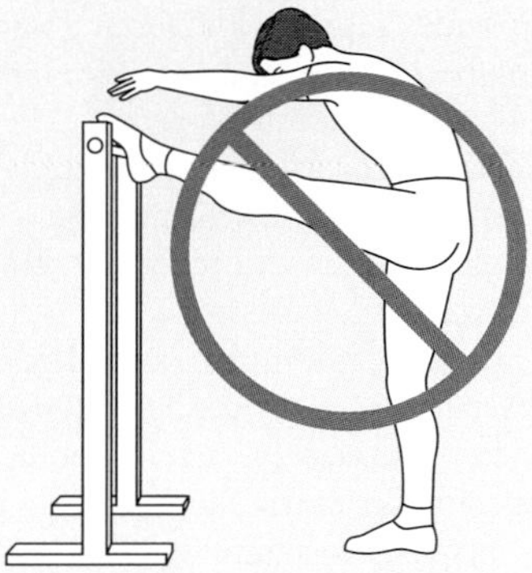

Standing Ankle-to-Buttocks Quadriceps Stretch

Problem: Puts excessive strain on the ligaments of the knee.

Alternative: Step stretch (Exercise 6)

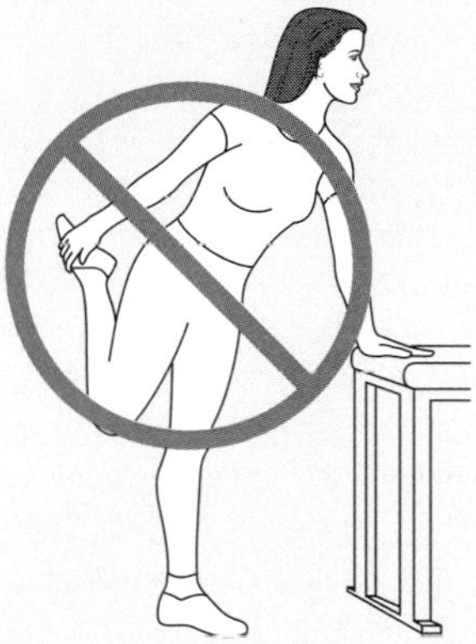

Yoga Plow

Problem: Puts excessive strain on the neck, shoulders and back

Alternatives: Head turns and tilts (Exercise 1), across-the-body stretch (Exercise 3), and upper-back stretch (Exercise 4)

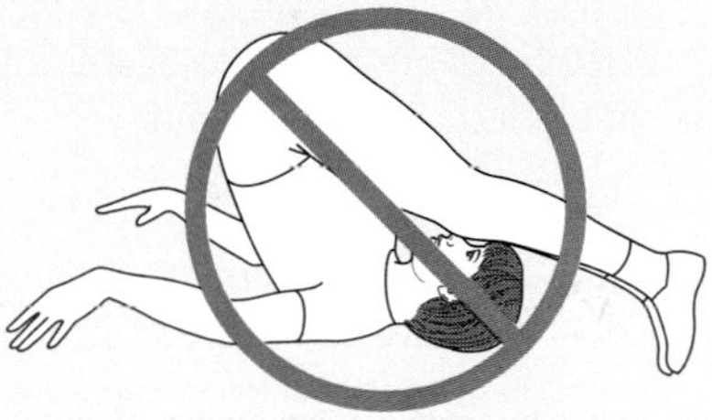

Full Squat

Problem: Puts excessive strain on the ankles, knees, and spine

Alternatives: Alternate leg stretcher (Exercise 10) and lower leg stretch (Exercise 12)

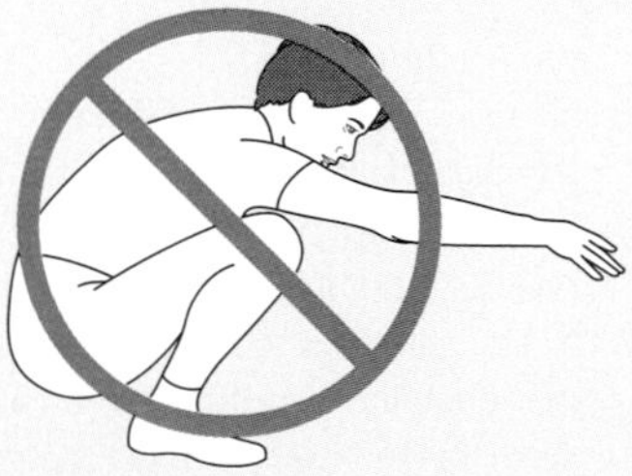

Prone Arch

Problem: Puts excessive strain on the spine, knees, and shoulders

Alternatives: Towel stretch (Exercise 2) and step stretch (Exercise 6)

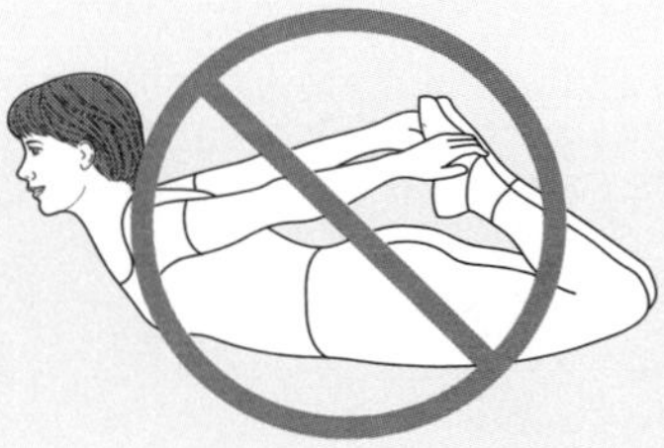

Hurdler Stretch

Problem: Turning out the bent leg can put excessive strain on the ligaments of the knee

Alternatives: Modified hurdler stretch (Exercise 11)

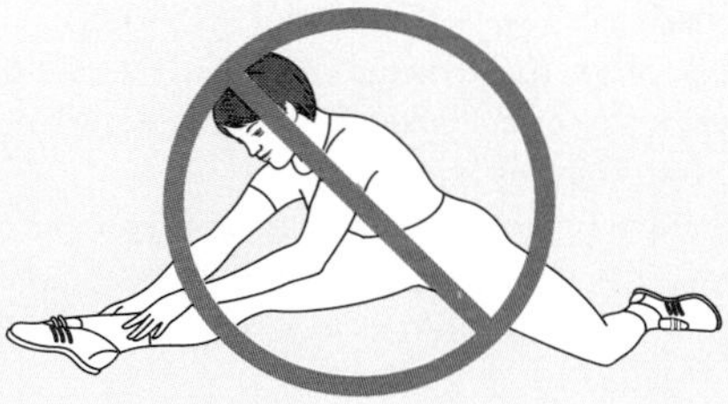

Jemmet, M. 2001. *Spinal Stabilization: The New Science of Back Pain.* Halifax, Nova Scotia: RMJ Fitness and Rehabilitation Consultants. *Provides information on anatomy, biomechanics, common back problems, and helpful exercises.*

WW Organizations and Web Sites

American Academy of Orthopaedic Surgeons: Public Information. Provides information about a variety of joint problems, including back, neck, and shoulder pain.
http://orthoinfo.aaos.org

CUErgo: Cornell University Ergonomics Web Site. Provides information about how to arrange a computer workstation to prevent back pain and repetitive strain injuries as well as other topics related to ergonomics.
http://ergo.human.cornell.edu

Exercise: A Guide from the National Institute on Aging. Practical advice on fitness for seniors; includes animated instructions for specific flexibility exercises.
http://www.n.a.nih.gov/exercisebook

Georgia State University: Flexibility. Provides information about the benefits of stretching and how to develop a safe and effective program; includes illustrations of stretches.
http://www.gsu.edu/~wwwfit/flexibility.html

MedlinePlus Back Pain Tutorial. An interactive, illustrated tutorial of the causes and prevention of back pain.
http://www.nlm.nih.gov/medlineplus/tutorials/backpain.html>

NIH Back Pain Fact Sheet. Basic information on the prevention and treatment of back pain.
http://www.ninds.nih.gov/health_and_medical/disorders/backpain_doc.htm

Southern California Orthopedic Institute. Provides information about a variety of orthopedic problems, including back injuries; also has illustrations of spinal anatomy.
http://www.scoi.com

Stretching and Flexibility. Provides information about the physiology of stretching and different types of stretching exercises.
http://www.ifafitness.com/stretch/index.html

See also the listings for Chapters 2 and 4.

SELECTED BIBLIOGRAPHY

Abenheim, L., et al. 2000. The role of activity in the therapeutic management of back pain. *Spine* 25 (4 Suppl.): 1S–33S.

American College of Sports Medicine. 2001. *ACSM's Resource Manual for Guidelines for Exercise Testing and Prescription,* 4th ed. Philadelphia: Lippincott Williams & Wilkins.

Back pain: Does anything work? 2000. *Consumer Reports on Health,* May.

Canham-Chervak, M., B. H. Jones, and J. J. Knapik. 2000. Does stretching before exercise prevent lower-limb injury? *Clinical Journal of Sport Medicine* 10(3): 216.

Fatouros, I. G., et al. 2002. The effects of strength training, cardiovascular training, and their combination on flexibility of inactive older adults. *International Journal of Sports Medicine* 23(20): 112–119.

Ghoname, E. A., et al., 1999. Percutaneous electrical nerve stimulation for low back pain. *Journal of the American Medical Association* 281:818–823.

Hodges, P., and G. Jull. 2000. Does strengthening the abdominal muscles prevent low back pain? *Journal of Rheumatology* 27(9): 2286–2288.

Knudson, D. V. 2000. Current issues in flexibility fitness. *President's Council on Physical Fitness and Sports: Research Digest* 3(1).

Lieber, R. L., and J. Friden. 2000. Mechanisms of muscle injury after eccentric contraction. *Journal of Science and Medicine in Sport* 2(3): 253–265.

Luebbers, P. 2002. Enhancing your flexibility. *ACSM Fit Society Page,* Spring, pp. 5, 8.

McGill, S. M. 2001. Low back stability: From formal description to issues for performance and rehabilitation. *Exercise and Sport Science Review* 29(1): 26–31.

McGill, S. M. 1998. Low back exercises: Evidence for improving exercise regimens. *Physical Therapy* 78(7): 754–765.

Moffett, J. K., et al. 1999. Randomised controlled trial of exercise for low back pain: Clinical outcomes, costs, and preferences. *British Medical Journal* 319:279–283.

Mundell, E. J. 2002. *Reuters Health: Pre-Workout Stretch Does Protect Muscle* (http://www.nlm.nih.gov/medlineplus/news/fullstory_7301.html; retrieved May 1, 2002).

National Institutes of Health. 2001. *Chronic Pain—Hope Through Research* (http://www.ninds.nih.gov/health_and_medical/pubs/chronic_pain_htr.htm; retrieved October 31, 2001).

Nieman, D. C. 2003. *Exercise Testing and Prescription: A Health-Related Approach,* 5th ed. New York: McGraw-Hill.

Parente, D. 2000. Influence of aerobic and stretching exercise on anxiety and sensation-seeking mood state. *Perceptual and Motor Skills* 90(1): 347–348.

Patel, A. T., and A. A. Ogle. 2000. Diagnosis and management of acute low back pain. *American Family Physician* 61(6): 1779–1786, 1789–1790.

Power, C., et al. 2001. Predictors of low back pain onset in a prospective British study. *American Journal of Public Health* 91(10): 1671–1678.

Schrier, I. 2000. Stretching before exercise: An evidence based approach. *British Journal of Sports Medicine* 34(5): 324–325.

Takala, E. P., and E. Viikari-Juntura. 2000. Do functional tests predict low back pain? *Spine* 25(16): 2126–2132.

Underwood, M. R. 2000. Exercise and the prevention of back pain disability. *British Journal of Sports Medicine* 34(1): 5.

Wilk, K. E., K. Meister, and J. R. Andrews. 2002. Current concepts in the rehabilitation of the overhead throwing athlete. *American Journal of Sports Medicine* 30(1): 136–151.

Willy, R. W., et al. 2001. Effect of cessation and resumption of static hamstring muscle stretching on joint range of motion. *Journal of Orthopaedic and Sports Physical Therapy* 31(3): 138–144.

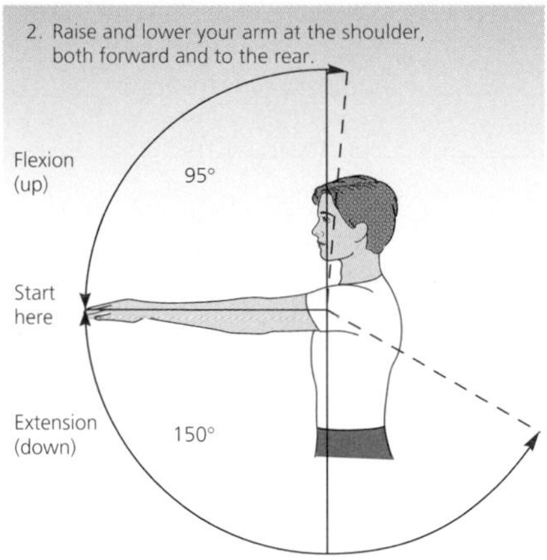

A. Comparison Method (✓)

Flexion: Average or above ______ Needs improvement ______

Extension: Average or above ______ Needs improvement ______

B. Measurement Method

Flexion: ______ ° Rating: ____________

Extension: ______ ° Rating: ____________

Ratings

	Flexion	*Extension*
Below average	<92°	<145°
Average	92°–95°	145°–150°
Above average	96°–99°	151°–156°
Excellent	>99°	>156°

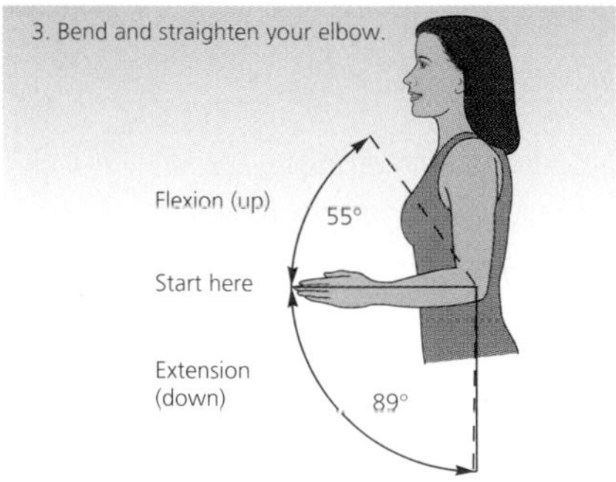

A. Comparison Method (✓)

Flexion: Average or above ______ Needs improvement ______

Extension: Average or above ______ Needs improvement ______

B. Measurement Method

Flexion: ______ ° Rating: ____________

Extension: ______ ° Rating: ____________

Ratings

	Flexion	*Extension*
Below average	<51°	<88°
Average	51°–55°	88°–89°
Above average	56°–60°	90°–91°
Excellent	>60°	>91°

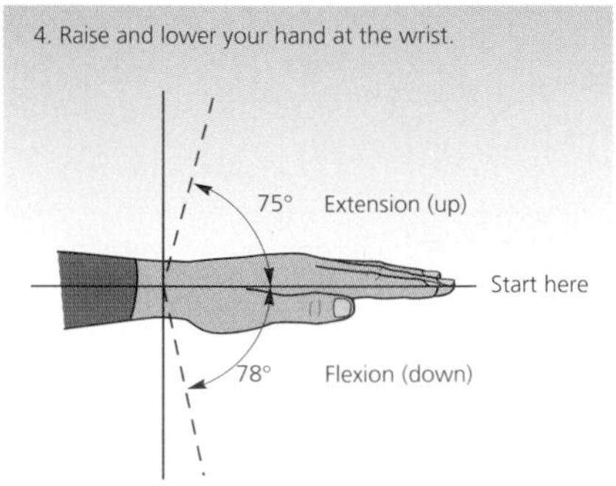

A. Comparison Method (✓)

Extension: Average or above ______ Needs improvement ______

Flexion: Average or above ______ Needs improvement ______

B. Measurement Method

Extension: ______ ° Rating: ____________

Flexion: ______ ° Rating: ____________

Ratings

	Extension	*Flexion*
Below average	<70°	<73°
Average	70°–75°	73°–78°
Above average	76°–81°	79°–84°
Excellent	>81°	>84°

5. Bend directly sideways at your waist. (To prevent injury, keep your knees slightly bent, and support your trunk by placing your hand or forearm on your thigh.)

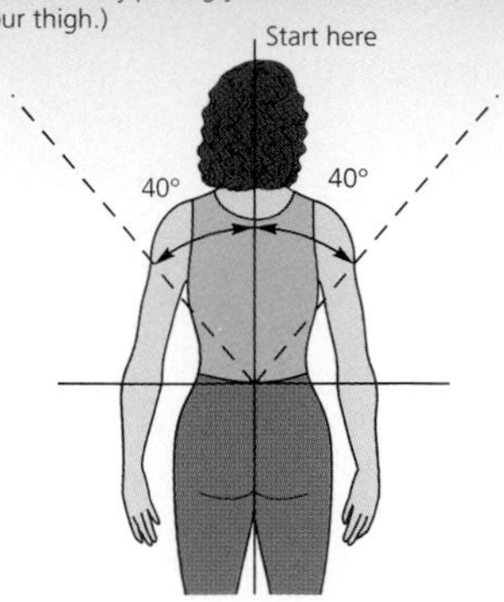

A. Comparison Method (✓)

Right lateral flexion: Average or above ______ Needs improvement ______

Left lateral flexion: Average or above ______ Needs improvement ______

B. Measurement Method:

Right lateral flexion: ______ ° Rating: ____________

Left lateral flexion: ______ ° Rating: ____________

Ratings

	Right or Left Lateral Flexion
Below average	<36°
Average	36°–40°
Above average	41°–45°
Excellent	>45

6. Raise leg to the side at the hip.

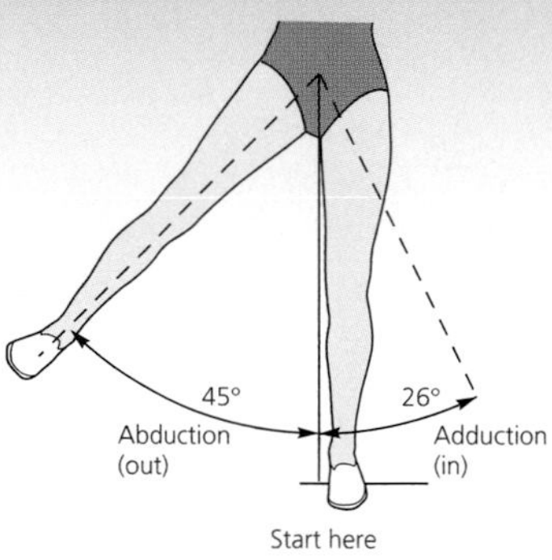

A. Comparison Method (✓)

Abduction: Average or above ______ Needs improvement ______

Adduction: Average or above ______ Needs improvement ______

B. Measurement Method

Abduction: ______ ° Rating: ____________

Adduction: ______ ° Rating: ____________

Ratings

	Abduction	*Adduction*
Below average	<40°	<23°
Average	40°–45°	23°–26°
Above average	46°–51°	27°–30°
Excellent	>51°	>30°

7. Raise and lower your leg forward at the hip.

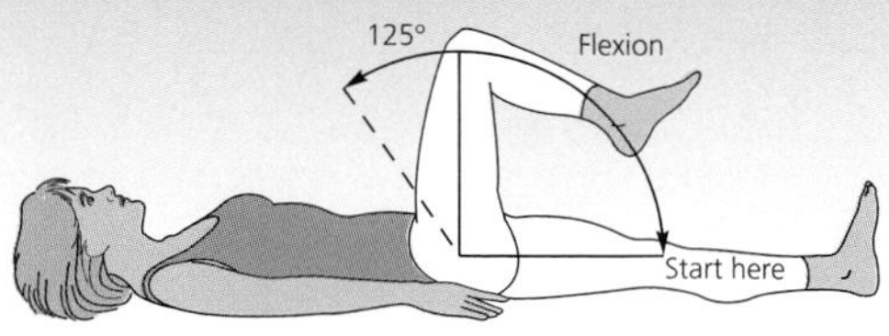

A. Comparison Method (✓)

Average or above ______ Needs improvement ______

B. Measurement Method

Flexion: ______ ° Rating: ____________

Ratings

	Flexion
Below average	<121°
Average	121°–125°
Above average	126°–130°
Excellent	>130°

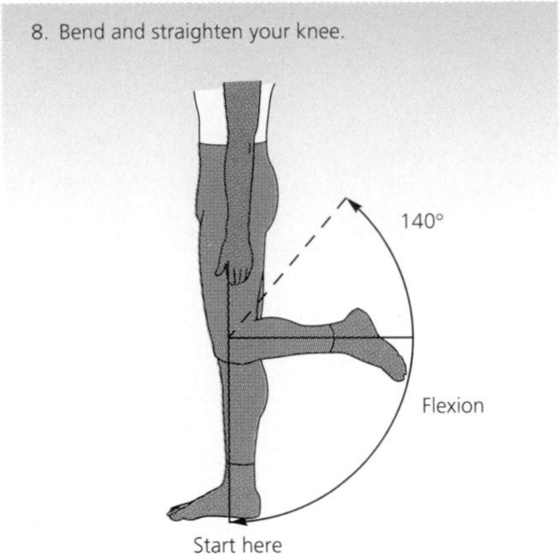

A. Comparison Method (✓)

Average or above ______ Needs improvement ______

B. Measurement Method

Flexion: ______ ° Rating: ____________

	Ratings
	Flexion
Below average	<136°
Average	136°–140°
Above average	141°–145°
Excellent	>145°

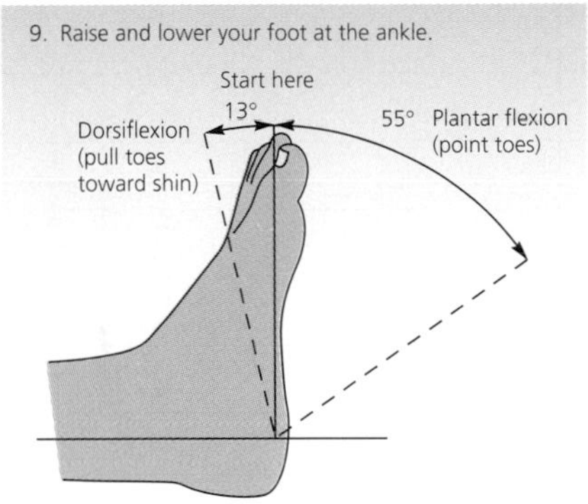

A. Comparison Method (✓)

Dorsiflexion: Average or above ______ Needs improvement ______

Plantar flexion: Average or above ______ Needs improvement ______

B. Measurement Method

Dorsiflexion: ______ ° Rating: ____________

Plantar flexion: ______ ° Rating: ____________

	Ratings	
	Dorsiflexion	*Plantar flexion*
Below average	<9°	<50°
Average	9°–13°	50°–55°
Above average	14° 17°	56°–60°
Excellent	>17°	>60°

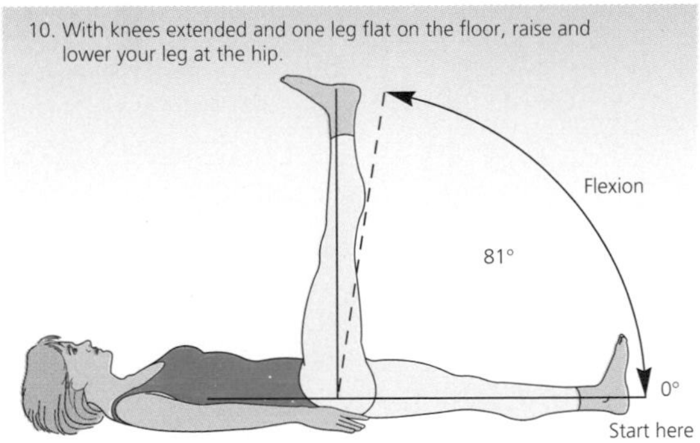

10. With knees extended and one leg flat on the floor, raise and lower your leg at the hip.
Flexion
81°
0°
Start here

A. Comparison Method (✓)

Average or above ______ Needs improvement ______

B. Measurement Method

Flexion: ______ ° Rating: ____________

	Ratings
	Flexion
Below average	<79°
Average	79°–81°
Above average	82°–84°
Excellent	>84°

LABORATORY ACTIVITIES

Rating Your Flexibility

Sit-and-Reach Test: Score: ____________ in. Rating: ____________

Range of Motion Assessment

Joint		*Average ROM*	*Comparison Method (✓)* *Average or above*	*Needs improvement*	*Measurement Method* *Current range of motion (°)*	*Rating*
Shoulder (side-to-side)	Abduction	95°				
	Adduction	127°				
Shoulder (front-to-back)	Flexion	95°				
	Extension	150°				
Elbow (up-and-down)	Flexion	55°				
	Extension	89°				
Wrist (up-and-down)	Extension	75°				
	Flexion	78°				
Low back (side-to-side)	Right flexion	40°				
	Left flexion	40°				
Hip (side-to-side)	Abduction	45°				
	Adduction	26°				
Hip (bent knee)	Flexion	125°				
Knee	Flexion	140°				
Ankle	Dorsiflexion	13°				
	Plantar flexion	55°				
Hip (straight knee)	Flexion	81°				

Using Your Results

How did you score? Are you at all surprised by your ratings for flexibility? Are you satisfied with your current ratings?

If you're not satisfied, set a realistic goal for improvement: ______________________________

Are you satisfied with your current level of flexibility as expressed in your daily life—for example, your ability to maintain good posture and move easily and without pain?

If you're not satisfied, set some realistic goals for improvement:

What should you do next? Enter the results of this lab in the Preprogram Assessment column in Appendix D. If you've set goals for improvement, begin planning your flexibility program by completing the plan in Lab 5.2. After several weeks of your program, complete this lab again and enter the results in the Postprogram Assessment column of Appendix D. How do the results compare?

Name ______________________ Section ____________ Date ______________

LAB 5.2 *Creating a Personalized Program for Developing Flexibility*

Goals: List goals for your flexibility program. In the first section, include specific, measurable goals that you can use to track the progress of your fitness program. These goals might be things like raising your sit-and-reach score from fair to good or your bent-leg hip flexion rating from below average to average. In the second section, include long-term and more qualitative goals, such as reducing your risk for back pain.

Specific Goals: Current Status	Final Goal
______________________	______________________
______________________	______________________
______________________	______________________

Other goals: ____

____

Exercises: The exercises in the program plan below are from the general stretching program presented in Chapter 5. You can add or delete exercises depending on your needs, goals, and preferences. For any exercises you add, fill in the areas of the body affected.

Frequency: A minimum frequency of 2–3 days per week is recommended. You may want to do your stretching exercises the same days you plan to do cardiorespiratory endurance exercise or weight training, because muscles stretch better following exercise, when they are warm.

Intensity: All stretches should be done to the point of mild discomfort, not pain.

Duration: All stretches should be held for 10–30 seconds. (PNF techniques should include a 6-second contraction followed by a 10–30-second assisted stretch.) All stretches should be performed at least 4 times.

Program Plan for Flexibility

Exercise	Areas Stretched	Frequency (check ✔)						
		M	T	W	Th	F	Sa	Su
Head turns and tilts	Neck							
Towel stretch	Triceps, shoulders, chest							
Across-the-body stretch	Shoulders, upper back							
Upper-back stretch	Upper back							
Lateral stretch	Trunk muscles							
Step stretch	Hip, front of thigh							
Side lunge	Inner thigh, hip, calf							
Sole stretch	Inner thigh, hip							
Trunk rotation	Trunk, outer thigh and hip, lower back							
Alternate leg stretcher	Back of the thigh, hip, knee, ankle, buttocks							
Modified hurdler stretch	Back of the thigh, lower back							
Lower-leg stretch	Back of the lower leg							

You can monitor your program using a chart like the one on the next page.

Flexibility Program Chart

Fill in the dates you perform each stretch, the number of seconds you hold each stretch (should be 10–30), and the number of repetitions of each (should be at least 4). For an easy check on the duration of your stretches, count "one thousand one, one thousand two," and so on. You will probably find that over time you'll be able to hold each stretch longer (in addition to being able to stretch farther).

Exercise/Date																				
	Duration																			
	Reps																			
	Duration																			
	Reps																			
	Duration																			
	Reps																			
	Duration																			
	Reps																			
	Duration																			
	Reps																			
	Duration																			
	Reps																			
	Duration																			
	Reps																			
	Duration																			
	Reps																			
	Duration																			
	Reps																			
	Duration																			
	Reps																			
	Duration																			
	Reps																			
	Duration																			
	Reps																			
	Duration																			
	Reps																			
	Duration																			
	Reps																			
	Duration																			
	Reps																			
	Duration																			
	Reps																			
	Duration																			
	Reps																			
	Duration																			
	Reps																			

Body Composition

6

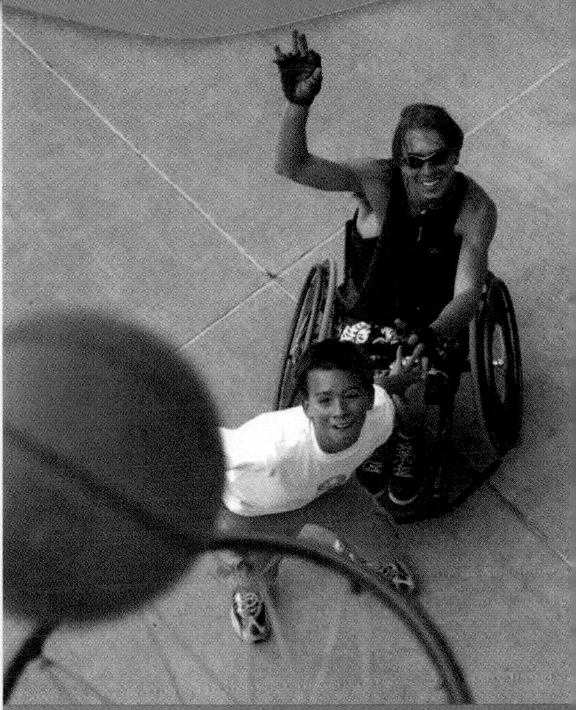

LOOKING AHEAD

After reading this chapter, you should be able to

- Define fat-free mass, essential fat, and nonessential fat and describe their functions in the body
- Explain how body composition affects wellness
- Describe how body composition and body fat distribution are measured and assessed
- Explain how to determine recommended body weight and body fat distribution

TEST YOUR KNOWLEDGE

1. Exercise helps reduce the risks associated with overweight and obesity even if it doesn't result in improvements in body composition.
   True or false?
2. Which of the following is the most significant risk factor for the most common type of diabetes (Type 2 diabetes)?
   a. smoking
   b. low-fiber diet
   c. overweight or obesity
   d. inactivity
3. In women, excessive exercise and low energy (calorie) intake can cause which of the following?
   a. unhealthy reduction in body fat levels
   b. amenorrhea (absent menstruation)
   c. bone density loss and osteoporosis
   d. muscle wasting and fatigue

TEST YOUR KNOWLEDGE ANSWERS

1. TRUE. Regular physical activity provides protection against the health risks of overweight and obesity. People who are fit and obese live longer, healthier lives than normal weight people who are sedentary.

2. C. All four are risk factors for diabetes, but overweight/obesity is the most significant. It's estimated that 90% of cases of Type 2 diabetes could be prevented if people adopted healthy lifestyle behaviors.

3. ALL FOUR. Very low levels of body fat, and the behaviors used to achieve them, have serious health consequences for both men and women.

Fit and Well Online Learning Center

www.mhhe.com/fahey5e

Visit the *Fit and Well* Online Learning Center for study aids, additional information about body composition, links, Internet activities that explore how body composition can influence wellness, and much more.

Body composition, the body's relative amount of fat and fat-free mass, is an important component of fitness for wellness. People whose body composition is optimal tend to be healthier, to move more efficiently, and to feel better about themselves. To reach wellness, you must determine what body composition is right for you and then work to achieve and maintain it.

Although people pay lip service to the idea of exercising for health, a more immediate goal for many is to look fit and healthy. Unfortunately, many people don't succeed in their efforts to obtain a fit and healthy body because they set unrealistic goals and emphasize short-term weight loss rather than the permanent changes in lifestyle that lead to fat loss and a healthy body composition. Successful management of body composition requires the long-term, consistent coordination of many aspects of a wellness program. However, even in the absence of changes in body composition, an active lifestyle can improve wellness (see the box "Can You Be Fit and Fat?"). This chapter focuses on defining and measuring body composition.The aspects of lifestyle that affect body composition are discussed in detail in other chapters: physical activity and exercise in Chapters 2–5 and 7, sound nutritional habits in Chapter 8, specific strategies for weight management in Chapter 9, and healthy techniques for managing stress in Chapter 10.

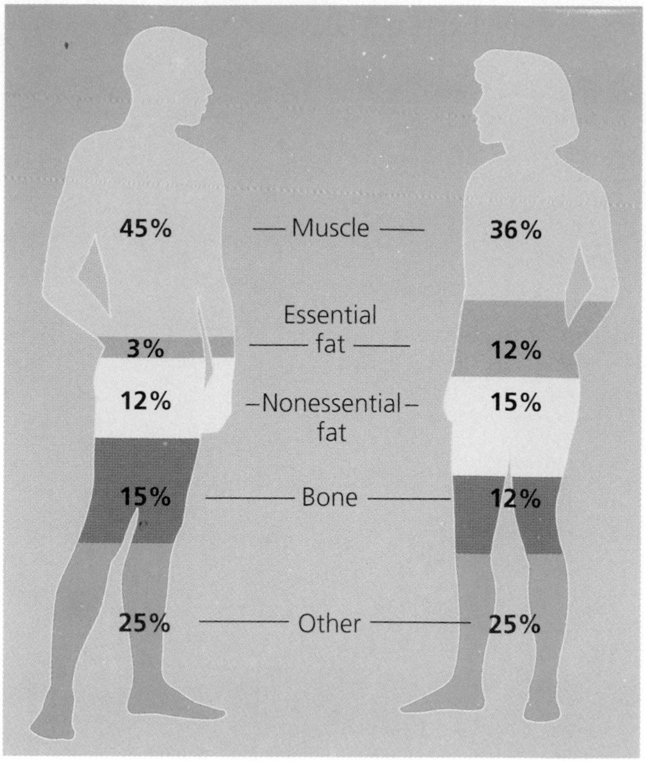

Figure 6.1 Body composition of a typical man and woman, 20–24 years old. SOURCE: Adapted from Brooks, G. A., et al. 2000. *Exercise Physiology: Human Bioenergetics and Its Applications,* 3d ed. Mountain View, Calif.: Mayfield.

WHAT IS BODY COMPOSITION, AND WHY IS IT IMPORTANT?

The human body can be divided into fat-free mass and body fat. Fat-free mass is composed of all the body's nonfat tissues: bone, water, muscle, connective tissue, organ tissues, and teeth. Body fat includes both essential and nonessential body fats (Figure 6.1). **Essential fat** includes lipids incorporated into the nerves, brain, heart, lungs, liver, and mammary glands. These fat deposits, crucial for normal body functioning, make up approximately 3–5% of total body weight in men and 8–12% in women. (The larger percentage in women is due to fat deposits in the breasts, uterus, and other sites specific to females.) **Nonessential (storage) fat** exists primarily within fat cells, or **adipose tissue,** often located just below the skin and around major organs. The amount of storage fat varies from individual to individual based on many factors, including gender, age, heredity, metabolism, diet, and activity level. Excess storage fat is usually the result of consuming more energy (as food) than is expended (in metabolism and physical activity).

How much body fat is too much? In the past, many people relied on height-weight tables based on insurance company mortality statistics to answer this question. Unfortunately, these tables can be highly inaccurate for some people; at best, they provide only an indirect measure of fatness. Because, as explained in Chapter 4, muscle tissue is denser and heavier than fat, a fit person can easily weigh more and an unfit person weigh less than recommended weights on a height-weight table.

The most important consideration when a person is looking at body composition is the proportion of the body's total weight that is fat—the **percent body fat.** For example, two women may both be 5 feet, 5 inches tall and weigh 130 pounds. But one women, a runner, may have only 18% of her body weight as fat, whereas the second, sedentary woman could have 38% body fat. Although neither woman is overweight by most standards, the second woman is overfat. Too much body fat (not total weight) has a negative effect on health and well-being.

Terms

Ww

essential fat The fat in the body necessary for normal body functioning.

nonessential (storage) fat Extra fat or fat reserves stored in the body.

adipose tissue Connective tissue in which fat is stored.

percent body fat The percentage of total body weight that is composed of fat.

overweight Characterized by a body weight above a recommended range for good health; ranges are set through large-scale population surveys.

obese Severely overweight, characterized by an excessive accumulation of body fat; overfat. Obesity may also be defined in terms of some measure of total body weight.

IN FOCUS Can You Be Fit and Fat?

> If a larger percentage of the population became physically active, the public health burden associated with obesity would be greatly reduced. This conclusion should not be interpreted to dismiss the health risks associated with obesity, but rather to emphasize the moderating influence of physical activity and physical fitness on these risks.

This quote from a recent article in the *President's Council on Physical Fitness and Sports Research Digest*—based on years of scientific studies—indicates that for adults, it may be possible to be both fit and fat.

Obesity is linked to many serious diseases and physical problems, including cardiovascular disease, diabetes, certain cancers, gallbladder disease, arthritis, and premature death. Regular physical activity can help prevent obesity, but activity is also extremely important for health even if it results in no changes in body composition. Exercise blocks many of the destructive health effects of obesity even in individuals who remain overweight. It improves blood pressure, blood fat and blood glucose levels, and body fat distribution; it lowers the risk of diabetes, heart disease, and early death. Researchers have found that active obese people have fewer health problems and live longer than normal weight people who are inactive.

Is physical activity or physical fitness more important for fighting the adverse health effects of obesity? The results of large number of published studies suggest that physical activity and fitness are both important—the more fit and active you are, the lower your risk of dying prematurely or having health problems. Of the two, however, daily physical activity appears to be more important for health than physical fitness. So, while reducing body fat and building fitness are important for wellness, many health benefits can be obtained by simply being more physically active each day.

SOURCES: Blair, S. N., Y. Cheng, and J. S. Holder. 2001. Is physical activity or physical fitness more important in defining health benefits? *Medicine and Science in Sports and Exercise* 33(Suppl): S379–S399. Welk, G. J., and S. N. Blair. 2000. Physical activity protects against the health risks of obesity. *President's Council on Physical Fitness and Sports Research Digest* 3(12). Blair, S. N., and S. Brodney. 1999. Effects of physical inactivity and obesity on morbidity and mortality: Current evidence and research issues. *Medicine and Science in Sports and Exercise* 31(Suppl): S646–S662.

Some of the most commonly used methods to assess and classify body composition are described later in the chapter. Although less accurate than standards based on body fat, some methods are based on total body weight because it is easier to measure. **Overweight** is usually defined as total body weight above the recommended range for good health (as determined by large-scale population surveys). **Obesity** is defined as a more serious degree of overweight; the cutoff point for obesity may be set in terms of percent body fat, as in Figure 6.2 (p. 158), or in terms of some measure of total body weight.

By any measure, Americans are getting fatter. The prevalence of obesity has increased from about 12% two decades ago to about 20% today, and more than 50% of American adults are now overweight. Possible explanations for this increase include more time spent in sedentary work and leisure activities, fewer short trips on foot and more by automobile, fewer daily gym classes for students, more meals eaten outside the home, greater consumption of fast food, increased portion sizes, and increased consumption of soft drinks and convenience foods. Fewer than half of Americans meet the minimum recommendation of 30 minutes per day of moderate physical activity, and the Centers for Disease Control and Prevention has estimated that caloric intake has increased by 100–300 calories a day during the past decade. (For more on the causes of obesity, see Chapter 9.)

Though not as prevalent a problem, having too little body fat is also dangerous (see Figure 6.2). Too much or too little body fat can have negative effects on health, performance, and self-image.

WW Health

Obese people have an overall mortality rate almost twice that of nonobese people, and even mild to moderate overweight is associated with a substantial increase in the risk of premature death. Obesity is associated with unhealthy blood fat levels, impaired heart function, and death from cardiovascular disease. It is estimated that if all Americans had a healthy body composition, the incidence of coronary heart disease would drop by more than 24%. Other health problems associated with obesity include hypertension, many kinds of cancer, impaired immune function, gallbladder and kidney diseases, skin problems, sleep and breathing disorders, impotence, pregnancy complications, impaired immune function, back pain, arthritis, and other bone and joint disorders. Of particular note is the strong association between excess body fat and diabetes mellitus: Obese people are more than three times as likely as nonobese people to develop diabetes, and the incidence of diabetes among Americans has increased dramatically as the rate of obesity has climbed (see the box "Diabetes," p. 159).

The distribution of fat is also an important indicator of future health. Studies suggest that people who tend to gain weight in the abdominal area ("apples") have a risk of coronary heart disease, high blood pressure, diabetes, and stroke twice as high as that of people who tend to gain weight in the hip area ("pears"). The reason for this increased risk is not entirely clear, but it appears that fat in the abdomen is more easily mobilized and sent into the bloodstream, increasing disease-related blood fat levels.

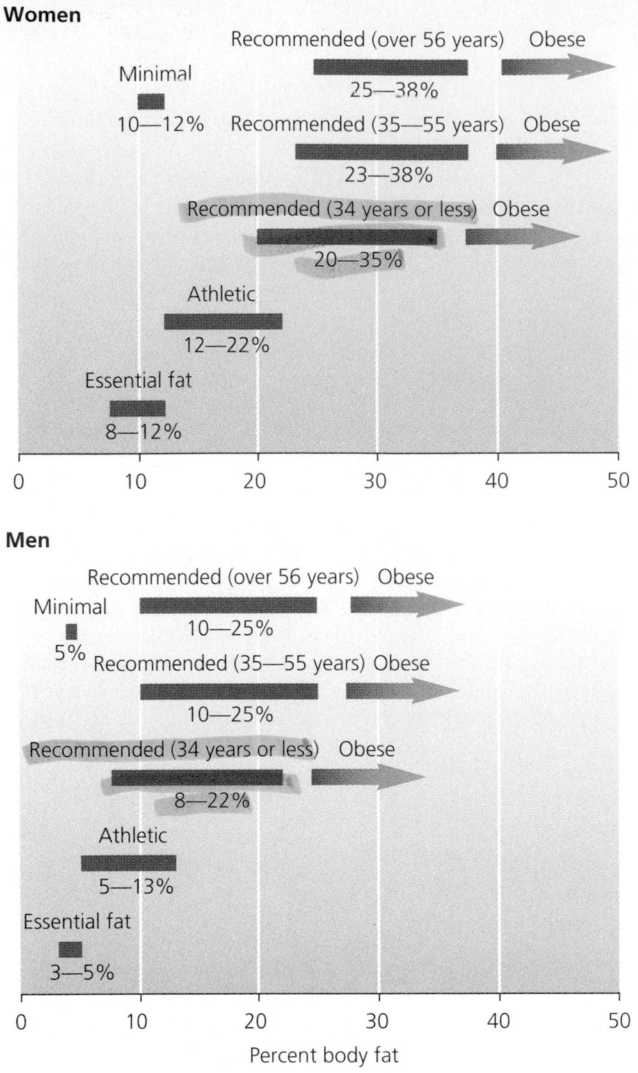

Figure 6.2 Percent body fat standards for men and women.
SOURCE: American College of Sports Medicine. 2001. *ACSM's Resource Manual for Guidelines for Exercise Testing and Prescription*, 4th ed. Philadelphia: Lippincott Williams & Wilkins. Reprinted by permission of Lippincott Williams & Wilkins

In general, men tend to gain weight in the abdominal area and women in the hip area, but women who exhibit the male pattern of fat distribution face the increased health risks associated with it. Researchers have also found ethnic differences in the relative significance of increased abdominal fat, but more studies are needed to clarify the relationships among fat distribution, ethnicity, and disease.

Is it possible to be too lean? Health experts have generally viewed too little body fat—less than 10–12% for women and 5% for men—as a threat to health and well-being. Extreme leanness has been linked with reproductive, circulatory, and immune system disorders. Extremely lean people may experience muscle wasting and fatigue; they are also more likely to suffer from a dangerous eating disorder. For women, an extremely low percentage of body fat is associated with **amenorrhea** and loss of bone mass (see the box "The Female Athlete Triad," p. 160). Additional research is needed to determine all the effects of extremely low body fat levels on health. (See Chapter 9 for more on eating disorders.)

Terms **Ww**

amenorrhea Absent or infrequent menstruation, sometimes related to low levels of body fat and excessive quantity or intensity of exercise.

Performance of Physical Activities

Too much body fat makes all types of physical activity more difficult because just moving the body through everyday activities means working harder and using more energy. In general, overfat people are less fit than others and don't have the muscular strength, endurance, and flexibility that make normal activity easy. Because exercise is more difficult, they do less of it, depriving themselves of an effective way to improve body composition.

Self-Image

The "fashionable" body image has changed dramatically during the past 50 years, varying from slightly plump to an almost unhealthy thinness. Today a fit and healthy-looking body, developed through a healthy lifestyle, is the goal for most people (see the box "Exercise, Body Image and Self-Esteem," p. 161). The key to this "look" is a balance of proper nutrition and exercise—in short, a lifestyle that emphasizes wellness.

Goals for body composition should be realistic, however; a person's ability to change body composition through diet and exercise depends not only on a wellness program, but also on heredity. The "ideal" body presented in the media—from dolls and action figures to fashion models—is an unrealistic goal for the vast majority of Americans. Unrealistic expectations about body composition can have a negative impact on self-image and can lead to the development of eating disorders. (For more information on body image and eating disorders, see Chapter 9.)

For most people, body fat percentage falls somewhere between ideal and a level that is significantly unhealthy. If they consistently maintain a wellness lifestyle that includes a healthy diet and regular exercise, the right body composition will naturally develop.

Wellness for Life

A healthy body composition is vital for wellness throughout life. Strong scientific evidence suggests that controlling your weight will increase your life span; reduce the risk of heart disease, cancer, diabetes, insulin resistance, and back pain; increase your energy level; and improve your self-esteem.

ASSESSING BODY COMPOSITION

The morning weighing ritual on the bathroom scale can't reveal whether a fluctuation in weight is due to a change

Diabetes mellitus is a disease that causes a disruption of normal metabolism. The pancreas, a long, thin organ located behind the stomach, normally secretes the hormone insulin, which stimulates cells to take up glucose to produce energy. In a person with diabetes, this process is disrupted, causing a buildup of glucose in the bloodstream. Over the long term, diabetes is associated with kidney failure; nerve damage; circulation problems; retinal damage and blindness; and increased rates of heart attack, stroke, and hypertension. The rate of diabetes has increased steadily over the past 40 years, jumping a dramatic 33% in the 1990s; it is currently the sixth leading cause of death in the United States.

Types of Diabetes

Approximately 18 million Americans—nearly 7% of the population—have one of two major forms of diabetes. About 5–10% of people with diabetes have the more serious form, known as Type 1 diabetes. In this type of diabetes, the pancreas produces little or no insulin, so daily doses of insulin are required. (Without insulin, a person with Type 1 can lapse into a coma.) Type 1 diabetes usually strikes before age 30.

The remaining 90% of Americans with diabetes have Type 2 diabetes. This condition can develop slowly, and about half of affected individuals are unaware of their condition. In Type 2 diabetes, the pancreas doesn't produce enough insulin, cells are resistant to insulin, or both. This condition is usually diagnosed in people over age 40, but the recent rise in rates of obesity has led to a significant increase in the number of children and young adults with Type 2 diabetes. About one-third of people with Type 2 diabetes must inject insulin; others may take medications that increase insulin production or stimulate cells to take up glucose.

A third type of diabetes occurs in about 2–5% of women during pregnancy. So-called gestational diabetes usually disappears after pregnancy but more than half of women who experience it eventually develop Type 2 diabetes.

The major factors involved in the development of diabetes are age, obesity, physical inactivity, a family history of diabetes, and lifestyle. Excess body fat reduces cell sensitivity to insulin, and it is a major risk factor for Type 2 diabetes. Ethnic background also plays a role. African Americans and people of Hispanic background are 55% more likely than non-Hispanic whites to develop Type 2 diabetes; more than 20% of Hispanics over age 65 have diabetes. Native Americans also have a higher-than-average incidence of diabetes.

Treatment

There is no cure for diabetes, but it can be successfully managed by keeping blood sugar levels within safe limits through diet, exercise, and, if necessary, medication. Blood sugar levels can be monitored using a home test, and close control of glucose levels can significantly reduce the rate of serious complications. Nearly 90% of people with Type 2 diabetes are overweight when diagnosed, and an important step in treatment is to lose weight. Even a small amount of exercise and weight loss can be beneficial. People with diabetes should obtain carbohydrate from whole grains, fruits, vegetables, and low-fat dairy products; carbohydrate and monounsaturated fat together should provide 60–70% of total daily calories. Regular exercise and a healthy diet are often sufficient to control Type 2 diabetes.

Prevention

Exercise can help prevent the development of Type 2 diabetes, a benefit especially important in individuals with one or more risk factors for the disease. Exercise burns excess sugar and makes cells more sensitive to insulin. Exercise also helps keep body fat at healthy levels. Researchers found that people with high blood sugar who exercised for 30 minutes a day and ate a low-fat diet decreased their risk of getting diabetes by more than 58%. Improving lifestyle was much more effective than taking a drug that is commonly used to fight the disease.

Eating a moderate diet to help control body fat is perhaps the most important dietary recommendation for the prevention of diabetes. However, there is some evidence that the composition of the diet may also be important. Studies have linked diets low in fiber and high in sugar, refined carbohydrates, red meat, and high-fat dairy products to increased risk of diabetes; diets rich in whole grains, produce, legumes, fish, and poultry may be protective. Specific foods linked to higher diabetes risk include regular (nondiet) cola beverages, white bread, white rice, french fries, processed meats (bacon, sausage, hot dogs), and sugary desserts. (See Chapter 8 for more information on different types of carbohydrates.)

Warning Signs and Testing

A wellness lifestyle that includes a healthy diet and regular exercise is the best strategy for preventing diabetes. If you do develop diabetes, the best way to avoid complications is to recognize the symptoms and get early diagnosis and treatment. Be alert for the following warning signs:

- Frequent urination
- Extreme hunger or thirst
- Unexplained weight loss
- Extreme fatigue
- Blurred vision
- Frequent infections
- Cuts and bruises that are slow to heal
- Tingling or numbness in the hands and feet
- Generalized itching, with no rash

Type 2 diabetes is often asymptomatic in the early stages, and major health organizations now recommend routine screening for people over age 45 and anyone younger who is at high risk, including anyone who is obese. (The Web site for the American Diabetes Association, listed in the For Further Exploration section at the end of the chapter, includes an interactive diabetes risk assessment). Screening involves a blood test to check glucose levels after either a period of fasting or the administration of a set dose of glucose. If you are concerned about your risk for diabetes, talk with your physician about being tested.

DIMENSIONS OF DIVERSITY The Female Athlete Triad

While obesity is at epidemic levels in the United States, many girls and women strive for unrealistic thinness in response to pressure from peers and a society obsessed with appearance. This quest for thinness has led to an increasingly common, underreported condition called the **female athlete triad.**

The triad consists of three interrelated disorders: abnormal eating patterns (and excessive exercising), followed by lack of menstrual periods (amenorrhea), followed by decreased bone density (premature osteoporosis). Left untreated, the triad can lead to decreased physical performance, increased incidence of bone fractures, disturbances of heart rhythm and metabolism, and even death.

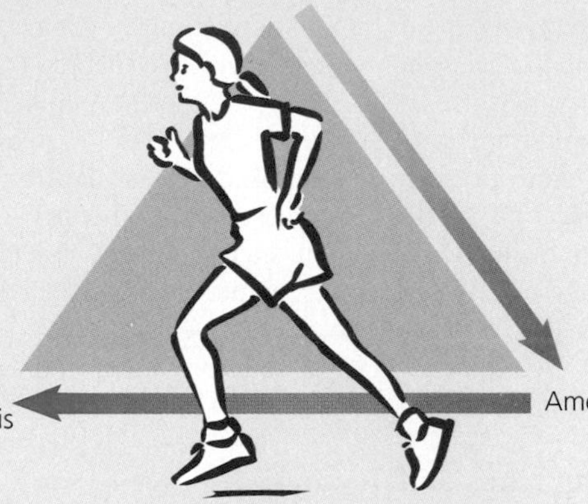

Abnormal eating patterns and excessive exercising
Premature osteoporosis
Amenorrhea

Abnormal eating is the event from which the other two components of the triad flow. Abnormal eating ranges from moderately restricting food intake, to binge eating and purging (bulimia), to severely restricting food intake (anorexia nervosa). Whether serious or relatively mild, eating disorders prevent women from consuming enough calories to meet their bodies' needs.

Disordered eating, combined with intense exercise and emotional stress, can suppress the hormones that control the menstrual cycle. If the menstrual cycle stops for three consecutive months, the condition is called amenorrhea. Prolonged amenorrhea can lead to osteoporosis; bone density may erode to the point that a woman in her 20s will have the bone density of a woman in her 60s. Women with osteoporosis have fragile, easily fractured bones. Some researchers have found that even a few missed menstrual periods can decrease bone density.

All physically active women and girls have the potential to develop one or more components of the female athlete triad; for example, it is estimated that 5–20% of women who exercise regularly and vigorously may develop amenorrhea. But the triad is most prevalent among athletes who participate in certain sports: those in which appearance is highly important, those that emphasize a prepubertal body shape, those that require contour-revealing clothing for competition, those that require endurance, and those that use weight categories for participation. Such sports include gymnastics, figure skating, swimming, distance running, cycling, cross-country skiing, track, volleyball, rowing, horse racing, and cheerleading.

The female athlete triad can be life-threatening, and health professionals are taking it seriously. Typical signs of the eating disorders that trigger the condition are extreme weight loss, dry skin, loss of hair, brittle fingernails, cold hands and feet, low blood pressure and heart rate, swelling around the ankles and hands, and weakening of the bones. Female athletes who have repeated stress fractures may be suffering from the condition. Early intervention is the key to stopping this series of interrelated conditions. Unfortunately, once the condition has progressed, long-term consequences, especially bone loss, are unavoidable. Teenagers may need only to learn about good eating habits; college-age women with a long-standing problem may require intense psychological counseling.

SOURCES: Otis, C. 1998. Too slim, amenorrheic, fracture-prone: The female athlete triad. *ACSM's Health and Fitness Journal* 2(1): 20–25. Smith, A. 1996. The female athlete triad: Causes, diagnosis, and treatment. *Physician and Sportsmedicine* 24(7). Art: Adapted from Yeager, K. K., et al. 1993. The female athlete triad: Disordered eating, amenorrhea, osteoporosis. *Medicine and Science in Sports and Exercise* 25:775–777. Reprinted by permission of Lippincott, Williams & Wilkins.

in muscle, body water, or fat and can't differentiate between overweight and overfat. A 260-pound football player may be overweight according to population height-weight standards yet actually have much less body fat than average. Likewise, a 40-year-old woman may weigh the same as she did 20 years earlier yet have a considerably different body composition.

There are a number of simple, inexpensive ways to estimate body composition that are superior to the bathroom scale. These methods include body mass index and skinfold measurements.

Ww Body Mass Index

Body mass index (BMI) is a rough measure of body composition that is useful for classifying the health risks of body weight if you don't have access to sophisticated equipment. Though more accurate than height-weight tables, body mass index is also based on the concept that a person's weight should be proportional to height. The measurement is fairly accurate for people who do not

Terms Ww

female athlete triad A condition consisting of three interrelated disorders: abnormal eating patterns (and excessive exercising) followed by lack of menstrual periods (amenorrhea) and decreased bone density (premature osteoporosis).

body mass index (BMI) A measure of relative body weight correlating highly with more direct measures of body fat, calculated by dividing total body weight (in kilograms) by the square of body height (in meters).

If you gaze into the mirror and wish you could change the way your body looks, consider getting some exercise—not to reshape your contours but to firm up your body image and enhance your self-esteem. In a recent study, 82 adults completed a 12-week aerobic exercise program (using cycle ergometry) and had 12 months of follow-up. Compared with the control group, the participants improved their fitness and also benefited psychologically in tests of mood, anxiety, and self-concept. These same physical and psychological benefits were still significant at the 1-year follow-up.

One reason for the findings may be that people who exercise regularly often gain a sense of mastery and competence that enhances their self-esteem and body image. In addition, exercise contributes to a more toned look, which many adults prefer. Research suggests that physically active people are more comfortable with their bodies and their image than sedentary people are. In one workplace study, 60 employees were asked to complete a 36-session stretching program whose main purpose was to prevent muscle strains at work. At the end of the program, besides the significant increase by all participants in measurements of flexibility, their perceptions of their bodies improved and so did their overall sense of self-worth.

Similar results were obtained in a Norwegian study, in which 219 middle-aged people at risk for heart disease were randomly assigned to one of four groups: diet, diet plus exercise, exercise, and no intervention. The greater the participation of individuals in the exercise component of the program, the higher were their scores in perceived competence/self-esteem and coping.

SOURCES: DiLorenzo, T. M., et al. 1999. Long-term effects of aerobic exercise on psychological outcomes. *Preventive Medicine* 28(1): 75–85. Sorensen, M., et al. 1999. The effect of exercise and diet on mental health and quality of life in middle-aged individuals with elevated risk factors for cardiovascular disease. *Journal of Sports Science* 17(5): 369–377. Moore, T. M. 1998. A workplace stretching program. *AAOHN Journal* 46(12): 563–568.

have an unusual amount of muscle mass (such as some athletes) and who are not very short. BMI is calculated by dividing your body weight (expressed in kilograms) by the square of your height (expressed in meters). For example, a person who weighs 130 pounds (59 kilograms) and is 5 feet, 3 inches tall (1.6 meters) would have a BMI of 59 kg ÷ $(1.6\text{ m})^2$, or 23 kg/m^2. (Refer to Lab 6.1 for instructions on how to calculate your BMI.) At high values of BMI, the risk of arthritis, diabetes, hypertension, endometrial cancer, and other disorders increases substantially. The increased risk of diabetes at even fairly low values of BMI, especially among women, is of particular concern (Figure 6.3).

Under new federal guidelines from the National Institutes of Health (NIH), a person is classified as overweight if he or she has a BMI of 25 or above and obese if he or she has a BMI of 30 or above (Table 6.1, p. 162). Nearly 55% of American adults have a BMI of 25 or above.

In classifying the health risks associated with overweight and obesity, the NIH guidelines consider body fat distribution and other disease risk factors in addition to BMI. As described earlier, excess fat in the abdomen is of greater concern than excess fat in other areas. Methods of assessing body fat distribution are discussed later in the chapter; the NIH guidelines use measurement of waist circumference (see Table 6.1). At a given level of overweight, people with a large waist circumference and/or additional disease risk factors are at greater risk for health problems. For example, a man with a BMI of 27, a waist circumference of more than 40 inches, and high blood pressure is at greater risk for health problems than another man who has a BMI of 27 but has a smaller waist circumference and no other risk factors.

Thus, optimal BMI for good health depends on many factors; if your BMI is 25 or above, consult a physician for help in determining a healthy BMI for you. (Weight loss

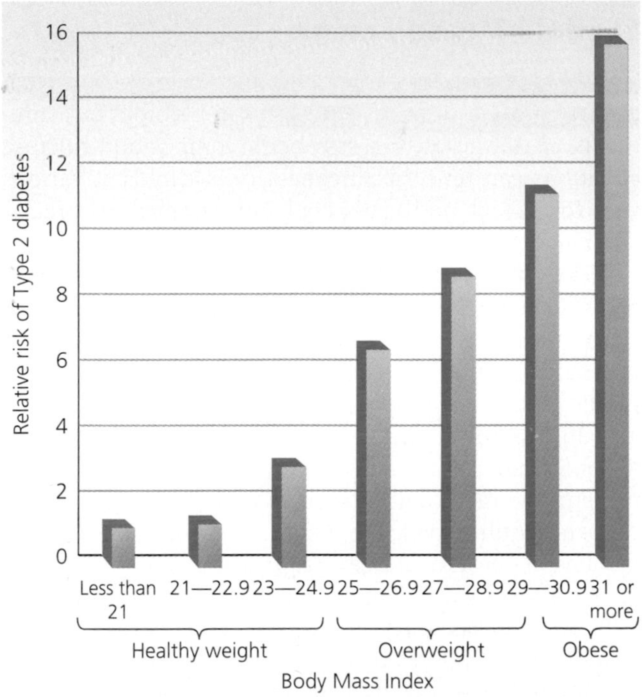

Figure 6.3 Body mass index (BMI) and risk of Type 2 diabetes in women. The risk of diabetes goes up even for women at the high end of the healthy BMI range, but it is extremely high in overweight and obese women. SOURCE: Hankinson, S. E., et al. 2001. *Healthy Women, Healthy Lives: A Guide to Preventing Disease from the Landmark Nurses' Health Study.* New York: Simon & Schuster.

Table 6.1 *Body Mass Index (BMI) Classification and Disease Risk*

Classification	BMI (kg/m²)	Obesity Class	DISEASE RISK RELATIVE TO NORMAL WEIGHT AND WAIST CIRCUMFERENCE[a]: Men ≤ 40 in. (102 cm) Women ≤ 35 in. (88 cm)	> 40 in. (102 cm) > 35 in. (88 cm)
Underweight[b]	<18.5		—	—
Normal[c]	18.5–24.9		—	—
Overweight	25.0–29.9		Increased	High
Obesity	30.0–34.9	I	High	Very high
	35.0–39.9	II	Very high	Very high
Extreme obesity	≥ 40.0	III	Extremely high	Extremely high

[a]Disease risk for Type 2 diabetes, hypertension, and cardiovascular disease. The waist circumference cutoff points for increased risk are 40 inches (102 cm) for men and 35 inches (88 cm) for women.

[b]Research suggests that a low BMI can be healthy in some cases, as long as it is not the result of smoking, an eating disorder, or an underlying disease process.

[c]Increased waist circumference can also be a marker for increased risk, even in persons of normal weight.

SOURCE: Adapted from National Heart, Lung, and Blood Institute. 1998. *Clinical Guidelines on the Identification, Evaluation, and Treatment of Overweight and Obesity in Adults: The Evidence Report.* Bethesda, Md.: National Institutes of Health.

recommendations based on the NIH guidelines are discussed further in Chapter 9.) Despite its widespread use, BMI does have limitations. Although it is good for large population studies, it is less useful for measuring changes in body composition in individuals.

Skinfold Measurements

Skinfold measurement is a simple, inexpensive, and practical way to assess body composition. Skinfold measurements can be used to assess body composition because equations can link the thickness of skinfolds at various sites to percent body fat calculations from more precise laboratory techniques.

Skinfolds are measured with a device called a **caliper**, which consists of a pair of spring-loaded, calibrated jaws. High-quality calipers are made of metal and have parallel jaw surfaces and constant spring tension. Inexpensive plastic calipers are also available; to ensure accuracy, plastic calipers should be spring-loaded and have metal jaws. Refer to Lab 6.1 for the procedure for taking skinfold measurements. Taking accurate measurements with calipers requires patience, experience, and considerable practice. It's best to take several measurements at each site (or have several different people take each measurement) to help ensure accuracy. Be sure to take the measurements in the exact location called for in the procedure. Because the amount of water in your body changes during the day, skinfold measurements taken in the morning and evening often differ. If you repeat the measurements in the future to track changes in your body composition, measure skinfolds at approximately the same time of day.

Terms

caliper A pressure-sensitive measuring instrument with two jaws that can be adjusted to determine thickness.

Ww

Other Methods of Measuring Body Composition

Most of the many other methods for determining body composition are very sophisticated and require expensive equipment. For example, the DXA (dual energy X-ray absorptiometry) technique lets scientists measure body fat by splitting an X-ray beam into two levels. The TOBEC (total body electrical conductivity) technique lets scientists estimate lean body mass by passing a body through a magnetic field. Less expensive methods are available in many health clubs and sports medicine clinics, including underwater weighing, the Bod Pod, and bioelectrical impedance analysis.

Underwater Weighing Hydrostatic (underwater) weighing is considered one of the most accurate indirect ways to measure body composition. It is the standard used for other techniques, including skinfold measurements. For this method, an individual is submerged and weighed under water. The percentages of fat and fat-free weight are calculated from body density. Muscle has a higher density and fat a lower density than water (1.1 grams per cubic centimeter for fat-free mass, 0.91 gram per cubic centimeter for fat, and 1 gram per cubic centimeter for water). Therefore, fat people tend to float and weigh less under water, and lean people tend to sink and weigh more under water. Most university exercise physiology departments or sports medicine laboratories have an

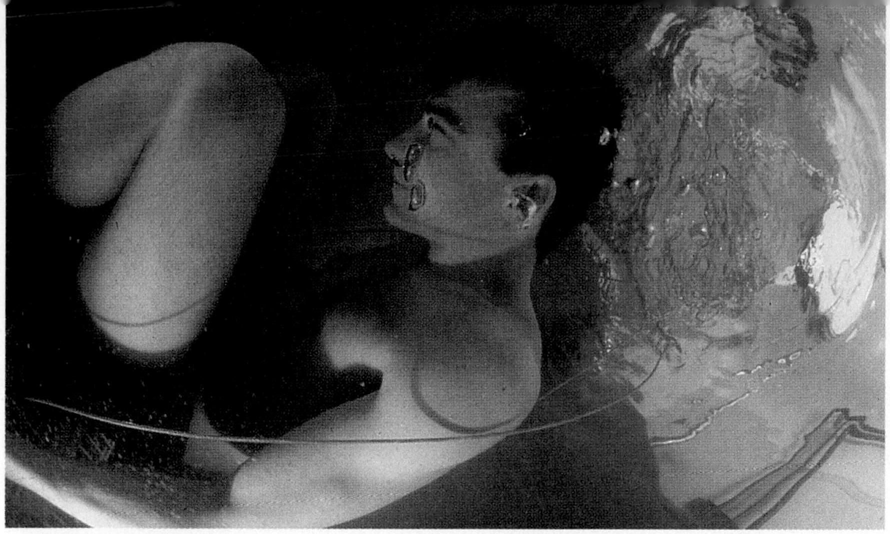

This man is having his body composition assessed in an underwater weighing tank. Muscle has a higher density than water, so people with more lean body mass weigh more under water.

underwater weighing facility. If you want an accurate assessment of your body composition, find a place that does underwater weighing.

The Bod Pod The Bod Pod, a small chamber containing computerized sensors, measures body composition by air displacement rather than water displacement. It determines the percentage of fat by calculating how much air is displaced by the person sitting inside the chamber. Many people prefer this short, 5-minute test over underwater weighing because it takes the place of the difficult "dunking" process and is just as accurate.

Bioelectrical Impedance Analysis (BIA) The BIA technique works by sending a small electrical current through the body and measuring the body's resistance to it. Fat-free tissues, where most body water is located, are good conductors of electrical current, whereas fat is not. Thus, the amount of resistance to electrical current is related to the amount of fat-free tissue in the body (the lower the resistance, the greater the fat-free mass) and can be used to estimate percent body fat. Bioelectrical impedance analysis is fairly accurate for most people (about the same as skinfold measurements). To avoid error, it is important to follow the manufacturer's instructions carefully and to avoid overhydration or underhydration (more or less body water than normal). Because measurement varies with the type of BIA analyzer, use the same instrument to compare measurements over time.

Assessing Body Fat Distribution

Researchers have studied many different methods for determining the risk associated with body fat distribution. Two of the simplest to perform are waist circumference measurement and waist-to-hip ratio calculation. In the first method, you measure your waist circumference; in the second, you divide your waist circumference by your hip circumference. Waist circumference has been found to be a better indicator of abdominal fat than waist-to-hip ratio. More research is needed to determine the precise degree of risk associated with specific values for these two assessments of body fat distribution. However, a total waist measurement of more than 40 inches (102 cm) for men and 35 inches (88 cm) for women and a waist-to-hip ratio above 0.94 for young men and 0.82 for young women are associated with a significantly increased risk of disease. Follow the instructions in Lab 6.1 to measure and rate your body fat distribution.

SETTING BODY COMPOSITION GOALS

If assessment tests indicate that fat loss would be beneficial for your health, your first step is to establish a goal. You can use the ratings in Figure 6.2 or Table 6.1 to choose a target value for percent body fat or BMI (depending on which assessment you completed).

Make sure your goal is realistic and will ensure good health. Genetics limits your capacity to change your body composition, and few people can expect to develop the body of a fashion model or competitive bodybuilder. However, you can improve your body composition through a program of regular exercise and a healthy diet. If your body composition is in or close to the recommended range, you may want to set a lifestyle goal rather than a specific percent body fat or BMI goal. For example, you might set a goal of increasing your daily physical activity from 20 to 60 minutes or beginning a program of weight training, and then let any improvements in body composition occur as a secondary result of your primary target (physical activity).

If you are significantly overfat or if you have known risk factors for disease (such as high blood pressure or high cholesterol), consult your physician to determine a body composition goal for your individual risk profile. For people who are obese, small losses of body weight (5–15%) over a 6–12 month period can result in significant health improvements. And as described earlier, a lifestyle that includes regular exercise may be more important for health than trying to reach any "ideal" weight.

Once you've established a body composition goal, you can then set a target range for body weight. Although body weight is not an accurate method of assessing body composition, it's a useful method for tracking progress in a program to change body composition. If you're losing a small or moderate amount of weight and exercising, you're probably losing fat while building muscle mass. Lab 6.2 will help you determine a range for recommended body weight.

Using percent body fat or BMI will generate a fairly accurate target body weight for most people. However, it's best not to stick rigidly to a recommended body weight calculated from any formula; individual genetic, cultural, and lifestyle factors are also important. Decide whether the body weight that the formulas generate for you is realistic, meets all your goals, is healthy, *and* is reasonable for you to maintain.

MAKING CHANGES IN BODY COMPOSITION

Chapter 9 includes specific strategies for losing or gaining weight and improving body composition. In general, lifestyle should be your focus—regular physical activity, endurance exercise, strength training, and a moderate energy intake. Making significant cuts in food intake in order to lose weight and body fat is a difficult strategy to maintain; focusing on increased physical activity is a better approach for many people. In studies of people who have lost weight and maintained the loss, physical activity was the key to long-term success.

You can track your progress toward your target body composition by checking your body weight periodically. However, it is best not to focus too much on body weight, especially if your goal is modest. Look instead at other factors, such as how much energy you have and how your clothes fit.

To get a more accurate idea of your progress, you should directly reassess your body composition occasionally during your program: Body composition changes as weight changes. Losing a lot of weight usually includes losing some muscle mass no matter how hard a person exercises, partly because carrying less weight requires the muscular system to bear a smaller burden. (Conversely, a large gain in weight without exercise still causes some gain in muscle mass because muscles are working harder to carry the extra weight.)

Tips for Today

Your current body composition is the result of many factors, including gender, heredity, and your activity and eating habits. A healthy body composition reduces your risk of premature death and many diseases, and it improves the quality of your life. Adopting a wellness lifestyle can lead naturally to a body composition that is healthy and appropriate for you.

Right now you can

- Find out what types of body composition assessment techniques are available at facilities on your campus or in your community.
- Do 15 minutes of physical activity—walk, jog, bike, swim, or climb stairs.
- Drink a glass of water instead of a regular (nondiet) soda, and include a high-fiber food such as whole-grain bread or cereal, popcorn, apples, berries, or beans in your next snack or meal. (These types of dietary changes are associated with reduced risk for diabetes.)
- Think about your image of the ideal body type for your sex. Consider where your idea comes from, whether you use this image to judge your own body shape and body composition, and whether it is a realistic goal for you. Write down five positive things about your body.

SUMMARY

- The human body is composed of fat-free mass (which includes bone, muscle, organ tissues, and connective tissues) and body fat (essential and nonessential).
- Having too much body fat has negative health consequences, especially in terms of cardiovascular disease and diabetes. Distribution of fat is also a significant factor in health.
- A fit and healthy-looking body, with the right body composition for a particular person, develops from habits of proper nutrition and exercise.
- Measuring body weight is not an accurate way to assess body composition because it does not differentiate between muscle weight and fat weight.
- Two measurements of body composition are body mass index (formulated through weight and height measurements) and percent body fat (formulated through skinfold measurements). Other techniques for determining percent body fat are hydrostatic weighing, the Bod Pod, and bioelectrical impedance analysis.
- Body fat distribution can be assessed through the total waist measurement or the waist-to-hip ratio.
- Recommended body composition and weight can be determined by choosing a target BMI or target body fat percentage. Keep heredity in mind when setting a goal, and focus on positive changes in lifestyle.

COMMON QUESTIONS ANSWERED

How accurate are body composition tests? Scientists use three different types of procedures for determining body composition: direct, indirect, and doubly indirect methods. The direct measure of body composition involves an autopsy—the dissection and chemical analysis of the body. This method has obvious limitations and can only be done once. Indirect techniques such as underwater weighing attempt to predict the results of autopsy. These methods are fairly accurate but still have an error of about ±3%, meaning that if a person is actually 17% fat, the test result may be between 14% and 20%. Doubly indirect methods such as skinfold measurement predict the results of indirect tests, often underwater weighing, and have higher error rates (about ±6%). Use results of these tests with caution, and don't focus too much on precise values. If you plan to track changes in body composition over time, be sure to use the same method each time to perform the assessment.

Is spot reducing effective? No. Spot reducing refers to attempts to lose body fat in specific parts of the body by doing exercises for those parts. For example, a person might try to spot reduce in the legs by doing leg lifts. Spot-reducing exercises contribute to fat loss only to the extent that they burn calories. The only way you can reduce fat in any specific area is to create an overall negative energy balance: Take in less energy (food) than you use up through exercise and metabolism.

How does exercise affect body composition? Cardiorespiratory endurance exercise burns calories, thereby helping create a negative energy balance. Weight training does not use many calories and therefore is of little use in creating a negative energy balance. However, weight training increases muscle mass, which maintains a high metabolic rate (the body's energy level) and helps improve body composition. To minimize body fat and increase muscle mass, thereby improving body composition, combine cardiorespiratory endurance exercise and weight training (Figure 6.4).

How do I develop a toned, healthy-looking body? The development of a healthy-looking body requires regular exercise, proper diet, and other good health habits. However, it helps to have heredity on your side. Some people put on or take off fat more easily than others just as some people are taller than others. Be realistic in your goals, and be satisfied with the improvements in body composition you can make by observing the principles of a wellness lifestyle.

Are people who have a desirable body composition physically fit? Having a healthy body composition is not necessarily associated with overall fitness. For example, many bodybuilders have very little body fat but have poor cardiorespiratory capacity and flexibility. To be fit, you must rate high on all the components of fitness.

What is liposuction, and will it help me lose body fat? Suction lipectomy, popularly known as liposuction, has become the most popular type of elective surgery in the United States. The procedure involves removing limited amounts of fat from specific areas. Typically, no more than 2.5 kg (5.5 lb) of adipose tissue is removed at a time. The procedure is usually successful if the amount of excess fat is limited and skin elasticity is good. The procedure is most effective if integrated into a program of dietary restriction and exercise. Side effects include infection, dimpling, and wavy skin contours. Liposuction has a death rate of 1 in 5000 patients, primarily from pulmonary thromboembolism (a blood clot in the lungs) or fat embolism (circulatory blockage caused by a dislodged piece of fat). Other serious complications include shock, bleeding, and impaired blood flow to vital organs.

What is cellulite, and how do I get rid of it? Cellulite is the name commonly given to ripply, wavy fat deposits that collect just under the skin. However, these rippling fat deposits are really the same as fat deposited anywhere else in the body. The only way to control them is to create a negative energy balance—burn up more calories than are taken in. There are no creams or lotions that will rub away surface (subcutaneous) fat deposits, and spot reducing is also ineffective. The solution is sensible eating habits and exercise.

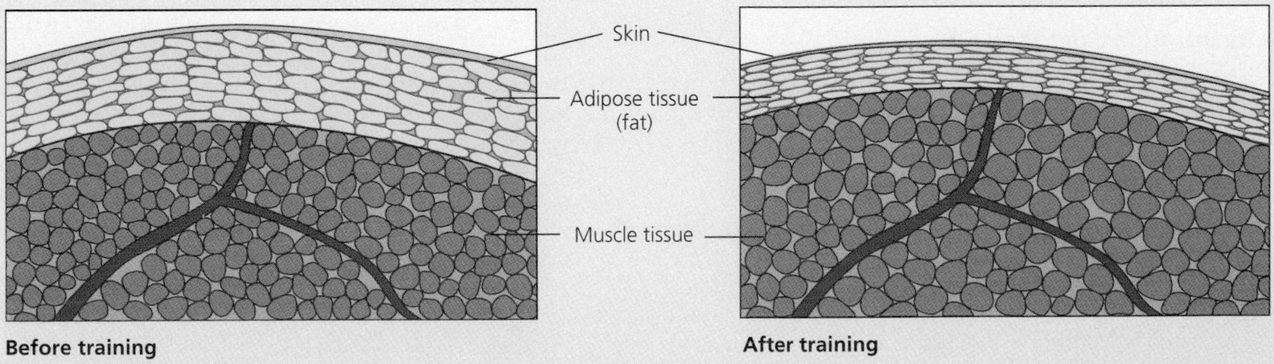

Figure 6.4 Effects of exercise on body composition. Endurance exercise and strength training reduce body fat and increase muscle mass.

FOR FURTHER EXPLORATION

Fit and Well Online Learning Center (www.mhhe.com/fahey5e)

Use the learning objectives, study guide questions, and glossary flashcards to review key terms and concepts and prepare for exams. You can extend your knowledge of body composition and gain experience in using the Internet as a resource by completing the activities and checking out the Web links for the topics in Chapter 6 marked with the World Wide Web icon. For this chapter, Internet activities explore the health risks of too much or too little body fat, body mass index, and diabetes; there are also Web links for major chapter topics.

Daily Fitness and Nutrition Journal

Fill in the body composition portion of the fitness program plan. If you plan to make changes in your body composition, you may also want to begin reviewing the steps in the weight management section of the journal.

Health*Quest*

As a shortcut, use the body mass index calculator included on the Health*Quest* CD-ROM (look in the Wellness Activities for the Fitness module or the Nutrition and Weight Control module).

Books

American Diabetes Association. 2000. *American Diabetes Association Complete Guide to Diabetes,* 2d ed. Alexandria, Va.: American Diabetes Association. *Explains the causes, symptoms, diagnosis, treatment, and self-care of diabetes.*

Bray, G. A., and C. A. Bray. 2002. *An Atlas of Obesity and Weight Control.* London: CRC Press. Provides detailed information about assessment, classification, and treatment of obesity.

Gaesser, G. A. 1999. *Big Fat Lies: The Truth About Your Weight and Your Health.* New York: Ballantine Books. *Emphasizes the importance of diet and exercise in maintaining metabolic health.*

Heyward, V. H., and L. M. Stolarczyk. 1996. *Applied Body Composition Assessment.* Champaign, Ill.: Human Kinetics. *Describes different methods of measuring and assessing body composition.*

Otis, C. L., and R. Goldingay. 2000. *The Athletic Woman's Survival Guide.* Champaign, Ill.: Human Kinetics. *Information on the female athlete triad and suggestions for changing attitudes toward weight, self-esteem, and body image.*

Organizations and Web Sites

American Diabetes Association. Provides information, a free newsletter, and referrals to local support groups; the Web site includes an online diabetes risk assessment.

800-342-2383

http://www.diabetes.org

National Heart, Lung, and Blood Institute. Provides information on the latest federal obesity standards and a BMI calculator.

http://www.nhlbi.nih.gov/guidelines/obesity/ob_home.htm

National Institute of Diabetes and Digestive and Kidney Diseases Health Information/Nutrition and Obesity. Provides information about adult obesity: how it is defined and assessed, the risk factors associated with it, and its causes.

877-946-4627

http://www.niddk.nih.gov/health/nutrit/nutrit.htm

Shape Up America. A site devoted to promoting healthy weight management; calculates and rates BMI and looks at why BMI is an important measure of health.

http://shapeup.org

See also the listings for Chapters 2, 8, and 9.

SELECTED BIBLIOGRAPHY

American College of Sports Medicine. 2001. *ACSM's Resource Manual for Guidelines for Exercise Testing and Prescription,* 4th ed. Philadelphia: Lippincott Williams & Wilkins.

American Diabetes Association. 2002. Evidence-based nutrition principles and recommendations for the treatment and prevention of diabetes and related complications. *Diabetes Care* 25: 148–198.

Ellis, K. J. 2000. Selected body composition methods can be used in field studies. *Journal of Nutrition* 131(5): 1589S–1595S.

Forbes, G. B. 2001. On the matter of ethnic differences in body composition. *American Journal of Clinical Nutrition* 74(4): 555.

Frankenfield, D. C., et al. 2001. Limits of body mass index to detect obesity and predict body composition. *Nutrition* 17(1): 26–30.

Guagnano, M. T., et al. 2001. Large waist circumference and risk of hypertension. *International Journal of Obesity Related Metabolic Disorders* 25(9): 1360–1364.

Hoffman, C. J., and L. A. Hildebrandt. 2001. Use of the air displacement plethysmograph to monitor body composition: A beneficial tool for dietitians. *Journal of the American Dietetic Association* 101(9): 986, 988.

Knowler, W. C., et al. 2002. Reduction in the incidence of type 2 diabetes with lifestyle intervention or metformin. *New England Journal of Medicine* 346(6): 393–403.

Kromhout, D., et al. 2001. Physical activity and dietary fiber determine population body fat levels: The Seven Countries Study. *International Journal of Obesity Related Metabolic Disorders* 25(3): 301–306.

Lewis, C. 2002. Diabetes: A growing public health concern. *FDA Consumer,* January/February.

Lukashi, H. C. 2001. Body composition distribution with age-growth charts for adults? *Nutrition* 17(7–8): 675.

Megnien, J. L., et al. 1999. Predictive value of waist-to-hip ratio on cardiovascular risk events. *International Journal of Obesity and Related Metabolic Disorders* 23:90–97.

Mokdad, A. H., et al. 2001. The continuing epidemics of obesity and diabetes in the United States. *Journal of the American Medical Association* 286(10): 1195–2000.

National Heart, Lung, and Blood Institute. 1998. *Clinical Guidelines on the Identification, Evaluation, and Treatment of Overweight and Obesity in Adults: The Evidence Report.* Bethesda, Md.: National Institutes of Health.

Overweight, obesity threaten U.S. health gains. 2002. *FDA Consumer,* March/April.

Rubinstein, S., and B. Caballero. 2000. Is Miss America an undernourished role model? *Journal of the American Medical Association* 283(12): 1569.

Schmidt, H., and M. Rauchhaus. 2001. Ideal weight, body composition and lipid levels: An unresolved dilemma? *Journal of the American College of Cardiology* 37(7): 2010–2011.

Tuomilehto, J., et al. 2001. Prevention of type 2 diabetes mellitus by changes in lifestyle among subjects with impaired glucose tolerance. *New England Journal of Medicine* 344(18): 1343–1350.

Van Dam, R. M., et al. 2002. Dietary patterns and risk for type 2 diabetes mellitus in U.S. men. *Annals of Internal Medicine* 136(3): 201–209.

Percent Body Fat Estimate for Men: Sum of Chest, Abdomen, and Thigh Skinfolds

Sum of Skinfolds (mm)	*Age*								
	Under 22	*23–27*	*28–32*	*33–37*	*38–42*	*43–47*	*48–52*	*53–57*	*Over 57*
8–10	1.3	1.8	2.3	2.9	3.4	3.9	4.5	5.0	5.5
11–13	2.2	2.8	3.3	3.9	4.4	4.9	5.5	6.0	6.5
14–16	3.2	3.8	4.3	4.8	5.4	5.9	6.4	7.0	7.5
17–19	4.2	4.7	5.3	5.8	6.3	6.9	7.4	8.0	8.5
20–22	5.1	5.7	6.2	6.8	7.3	7.9	8.4	8.9	9.5
23–25	6.1	6.6	7.2	7.7	8.3	8.8	9.4	9.9	10.5
26–28	7.0	7.6	8.1	8.7	9.2	9.8	10.3	10.9	11.4
29–31	8.0	8.5	9.1	9.6	10.2	10.7	11.3	11.8	12.4
32–34	8.9	9.4	10.0	10.5	11.1	11.6	12.2	12.8	13.3
35–37	9.8	10.4	10.9	11.5	12.0	12.6	13.1	13.7	14.3
38–40	10.7	11.3	11.8	12.4	12.9	13.5	14.1	14.6	15.2
41–43	11.6	12.2	12.7	13.3	13.8	14.4	15.0	15.5	16.1
44–46	12.5	13.1	13.6	14.2	14.7	15.3	15.9	16.4	17.0
47–49	13.4	13.9	14.5	15.1	15.6	16.2	16.8	17.3	17.9
50–52	14.3	14.8	15.4	15.9	16.5	17.1	17.6	18.2	18.8
53–55	15.1	15.7	16.2	16.8	17.4	17.9	18.5	19.1	19.7
56–58	16.0	16.5	17.1	17.7	18.2	18.8	19.4	20.0	20.5
59–61	16.9	17.4	17.9	18.5	19.1	19.7	20.2	20.8	21.4
62–64	17.6	18.2	18.8	19.4	19.9	20.5	21.1	21.7	22.2
65–67	18.5	19.0	19.6	20.2	20.8	21.3	21.9	22.5	23.1
68–70	19.3	19.9	20.4	21.0	21.6	22.2	22.7	23.3	23.9
71–73	20.1	20.7	21.2	21.8	22.4	23.0	23.6	24.1	24.7
74–76	20.9	21.5	22.0	22.6	23.2	23.8	24.4	25.0	25.5
77–79	21.7	22.2	22.8	23.4	24.0	24.6	25.2	25.8	26.3
80–82	22.4	23.0	23.6	24.2	24.8	25.4	25.9	26.5	27.1
83–85	23.2	23.8	24.4	25.0	25.5	26.1	26.7	27.3	27.9
86–88	24.0	24.5	25.1	25.7	26.3	26.9	27.5	28.1	28.7
89–91	24.7	25.3	25.9	26.5	27.1	27.6	28.2	28.8	29.4
92–94	25.4	26.0	26.6	27.2	27.8	28.4	29.0	29.6	30.2
95–97	26.1	26.7	27.3	27.9	28.5	29.1	29.7	30.3	30.9
98–100	26.9	27.4	28.0	28.6	29.2	29.8	30.4	31.0	31.6
101–103	27.5	28.1	28.7	29.3	29.9	30.5	31.1	31.7	32.3
104–106	28.2	28.8	29.4	30.0	30.6	31.2	31.8	32.4	33.0
107–109	28.9	29.5	30.1	30.7	31.3	31.9	32.5	33.1	33.7
110–112	29.6	30.2	30.8	31.4	32.0	32.6	33.2	33.8	34.4
113–115	30.2	30.8	31.4	32.0	32.6	33.2	33.8	34.5	35.1
116–118	30.9	31.5	32.1	32.7	33.3	33.9	34.5	35.1	35.7
119–121	31.5	32.1	32.7	33.3	33.9	34.5	35.1	35.7	36.4
122–124	32.1	32.7	33.3	33.9	34.5	35.1	35.8	36.4	37.0
125–127	32.7	33.3	33.9	34.5	35.1	35.8	36.4	37.0	37.6

SOURCE: Jackson, A. S., and M. L. Pollock. 1985. Practical assessment of body composition. *Physician and Sportsmedicine* 13(5): 76–90. Reproduced by permission of The McGraw-Hill Companies.

Percent Body Fat Estimate for Women: Sum of Triceps, Suprailium, and Thigh Skinfolds

Sum of Skinfolds (mm)	Age								
	Under 22	23–27	28–32	33–37	38–42	43–47	48–52	53–57	Over 57
23–25	9.7	9.9	10.2	10.4	10.7	10.9	11.2	11.4	11.7
26–28	11.0	11.2	11.5	11.7	12.0	12.3	12.5	12.7	13.0
29–31	12.3	12.5	12.8	13.0	13.3	13.5	13.8	14.0	14.3
32–34	13.6	13.8	14.0	14.3	14.5	14.8	15.0	15.3	15.5
35–37	14.8	15.0	15.3	15.5	15.8	16.0	16.3	16.5	16.8
38–40	16.0	16.3	16.5	16.7	17.0	17.2	17.5	17.7	18.0
41–43	17.2	17.4	17.7	17.9	18.2	18.4	18.7	18.9	19.2
44–46	18.3	18.6	18.8	19.1	19.3	19.6	19.8	20.1	20.3
47–49	19.5	19.7	20.0	20.2	20.5	20.7	21.0	21.2	21.5
50–52	20.6	20.8	21.1	21.3	21.6	21.8	22.1	22.3	22.6
53–55	21.7	21.9	22.1	22.4	22.6	22.9	23.1	23.4	23.6
56–58	22.7	23.0	23.2	23.4	23.7	23.9	24.2	24.4	24.7
59–61	23.7	24.0	24.2	24.5	24.7	25.0	25.2	25.5	25.7
62–64	24.7	25.0	25.2	25.5	25.7	26.0	26.7	26.4	26.7
65–67	25.7	25.9	26.2	26.4	26.7	26.9	27.2	27.4	27.7
68–70	26.6	26.9	27.1	27.4	27.6	27.9	28.1	28.4	28.6
71–73	27.5	27.8	28.0	28.3	28.5	28.8	29.0	29.3	29.5
74–76	28.4	28.7	28.9	29.2	29.4	29.7	29.9	30.2	30.4
77–79	29.3	29.5	29.8	30.0	30.3	30.5	30.8	31.0	31.3
80–82	30.1	30.4	30.6	30.9	31.1	31.4	31.6	31.9	32.1
83–85	30.9	31.2	31.4	31.7	31.9	32.2	32.4	32.7	32.9
86–88	31.7	32.0	32.2	32.5	32.7	32.9	33.2	33.4	33.7
89–91	32.5	32.7	33.0	33.2	33.5	33.7	33.9	34.2	34.4
92–94	33.2	33.4	33.7	33.9	34.2	34.4	34.7	34.9	35.2
95–97	33.9	34.1	34.4	34.6	34.9	35.1	35.4	35.6	35.9
98–100	34.6	34.8	35.1	35.3	35.5	35.8	36.0	36.3	36.5
101–103	35.3	35.4	35.7	35.9	36.2	36.4	36.7	36.9	37.2
104–106	35.8	36.1	36.3	36.6	36.8	37.1	37.3	37.5	37.8
107–109	36.4	36.7	36.9	37.1	37.4	37.6	37.9	38.1	38.4
110–112	37.0	37.2	37.5	37.7	38.0	38.2	38.5	38.7	38.9
113–115	37.5	37.8	38.0	38.2	38.5	38.7	39.0	39.2	39.5
116–118	38.0	38.3	38.5	38.8	39.0	39.3	39.5	39.7	40.0
119–121	38.5	38.7	39.0	39.2	39.5	39.7	40.0	40.2	40.5
122–124	39.0	39.2	39.4	39.7	39.9	40.2	40.4	40.7	40.9
125–127	39.4	39.6	39.9	40.1	40.4	40.6	40.9	41.1	41.4
128–130	39.8	40.0	40.3	40.5	40.8	41.0	41.3	41.5	41.8

SOURCE: Jackson, A. S., and M. L. Pollock. 1985. Practical assessment of body composition. *Physician and Sportsmedicine* 13(5): 76–90. Reproduced by permission of McGraw-Hill, Inc.

Rating Your Body Composition

Refer to the figure to rate your percent body fat. Record it below and in the chart at the end of this lab.

Rating: ___________

Body Composition Ratings

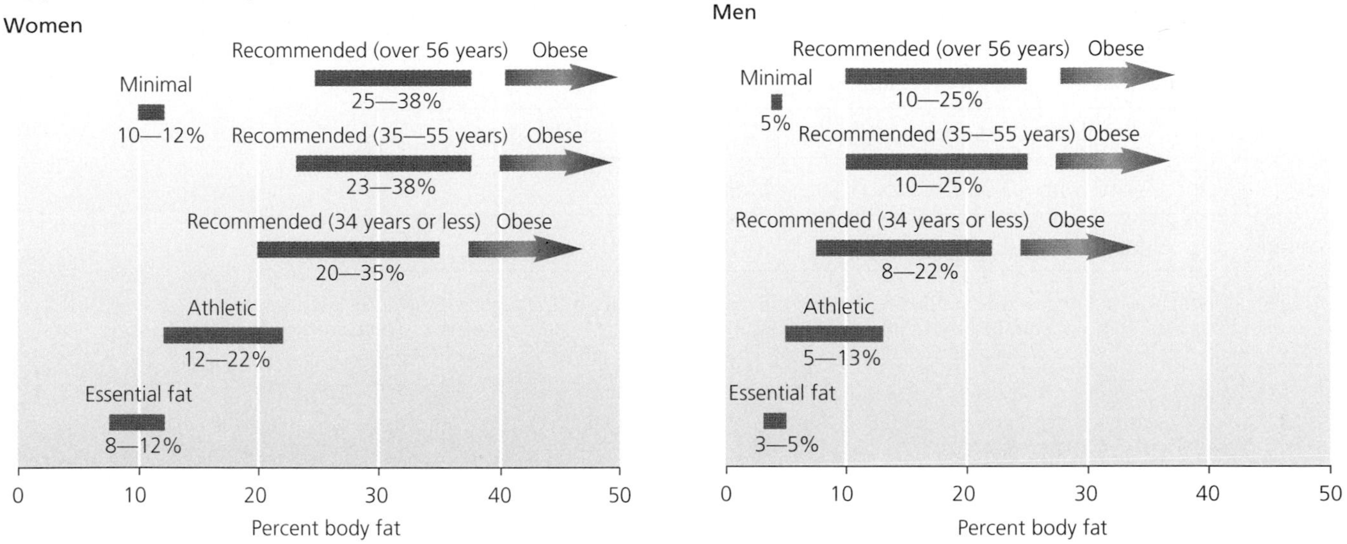

SOURCE: American College of Sports Medicine. 2001. *ACSM's Resource Manual for Guidelines for Exercise Testing and Prescription,* 4th ed. Philadelphia: Lippincott Williams & Wilkins. Reprinted by permission of Lippincott Williams & Wilkins.

Other Methods of Assessing Percent Body Fat

If you use a different method, record the name of the method and the result below and in the chart at the end of this lab. Find your body composition rating on the chart above.

Method used: ___________ Percent body fat: ___________ % Rating (from chart above): ___________

Waist Circumference and Waist-to-Hip Ratio

Equipment

1. Tape measure
2. Partner to take measurements

Preparation

Wear clothes that will not add significantly to your measurements.

Instructions

Stand with your feet together and your arms at your sides. Raise your arms only high enough to allow for taking the measurements. Your partner should make sure the tape is horizontal around the entire circumference and pulled snugly against your skin. The tape shouldn't be pulled so tight that it causes indentations in your skin. Record measurements to the nearest millimeter or one-sixteenth of an inch.

Waist. Measure at the smallest waist circumference. If you don't have a natural waist, measure at the level of your navel. Waist measurement: ___________

Hip. Measure at the largest hip circumference. Hip measurement: ___________

Waist-to-Hip Ratio: You can use any unit of measurement (for example, inches or centimeters), as long as you're consistent. Waist-to-hip ratio equals waist measurement divided by hip measurement.

Waist-to-hip ratio: ___________ (waist measurement) ÷ ___________ (hip measurement) = ___________

Determining Your Risk

The table below indicates values for waist circumference and waist-to-hip ratio above which the risk of health problems increases significantly. If your measurement or ratio is above either cutoff point, put a check on the appropriate line below and in the chart on the final page of this lab.

Waist circumference: ___________ (✔ high risk) Waist-to-hip ratio: ___________ (✔ high risk)

Body Fat Distribution

Cutoff Points for High Risk

	Waist Circumference	*Waist-to-Hip Ratio*
Men	more than 40 in. (102 cm)	more than 0.94
Women	more than 35 in. (88 cm)	more than 0.82

SOURCES: National Heart, Lung, and Blood Institute. 1998. *Clinical Guidelines on the Identification, Evaluation, and Treatment of Overweight and Obesity in Adults: The Evidence Report.* Bethesda, Md.: National Institutes of Health. American College of Sports Medicine. 2001. *ACSM's Resource Manual for Guidelines for Exercise Testing and Prescription,* 4th ed. Philadelphia: Lippincott Williams & Wilkins.

Rating Your Body Composition

Assessment	*Value*	*Classification*
BMI	___________ kg/m^2	___________
Skinfold measurements or alternative method of determining percent body fat Specify method: ___________	___________ % body fat	___________
Waist circumference Waist-to-hip ratio	___________ in. or cm ___________ (ratio)	______ (✔ high risk) ______ (✔ high risk)

Using Your Results

How did you score? Are you at all surprised by your ratings for body composition and body fat distribution? Are your current ratings in the range for good health? Are you satisfied with your current body composition? Why or why not?

If you're not satisfied, set a realistic goal for improvement: ___________

What should you do next? Enter the results of this lab in the Preprogram Assessment column in Appendix D. If you've determined that you need to improve your body composition, set a specific goal by completing Lab 6.2, and then plan your program using the labs in Chapters 8 and 9 and the weight management section of the Daily Fitness and Nutrition Journal. After several weeks or months of an exercise and/or dietary change program, complete this lab again and enter the results in the Postprogram Assessment column of Appendix D. How do the results compare?

Putting Together a Complete Fitness Program

7

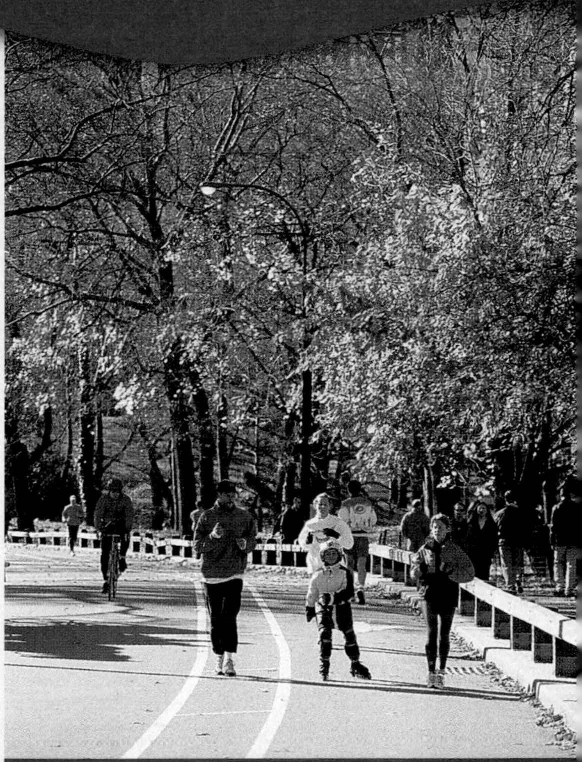

LOOKING AHEAD

After reading this chapter, you should be able to

- Explain the steps for putting together a successful personal fitness program
- Describe strategies that can help you maintain a fitness program over the long term
- Tailor a fitness program to accommodate special health concerns and different life stages

TEST YOUR KNOWLEDGE

1. In surveys, how many Americans report that they've engaged in no physical activity in the past month?
   a. 7%
   b. 17%
   c. 27%
2. Falling asleep in a boring class doesn't necessarily mean a person needs more sleep. True or false?
3. Exercise is not recommended for people with asthma or diabetes. True or false?

TEST YOUR KNOWLEDGE ANSWERS

1. C. More than a quarter of Americans are completely sedentary, putting them at risk for early death and a wide variety of diseases and disabling conditions.

2. FALSE. A fully rested person may become bored during an uninteresting or monotonous event but will not fall asleep. Daytime sleepiness is a sign of inadequate sleep, which negatively affects health and athletic performance.

3. FALSE. Although special precautions may be needed, people with many types of chronic conditions can exercise safely and obtain significant health benefits. Regular exercise reduces the risks of acute asthma attacks and improves insulin sensitivity.

WW *Fit and Well* Online Learning Center

www.mhhe.com/fahey5e

Visit the *Fit and Well* Online Learning Center for study aids, additional information about putting together a complete fitness program, links, Internet activities that explore fitness, consumer resources, and much more.

Understanding the physiological basis and wellness benefits of health-related physical fitness, as explained in Chapters 1–6, is the first step toward creating a well-rounded exercise program. The next challenge is to combine activities into a program that develops all the fitness components and maintains motivation.

This chapter presents a step-by-step procedure for creating and maintaining a well-rounded program. Following the chapter, you'll find sample programs based on popular activities. The structure these programs provide can be helpful if you're beginning an exercise program for the first time.

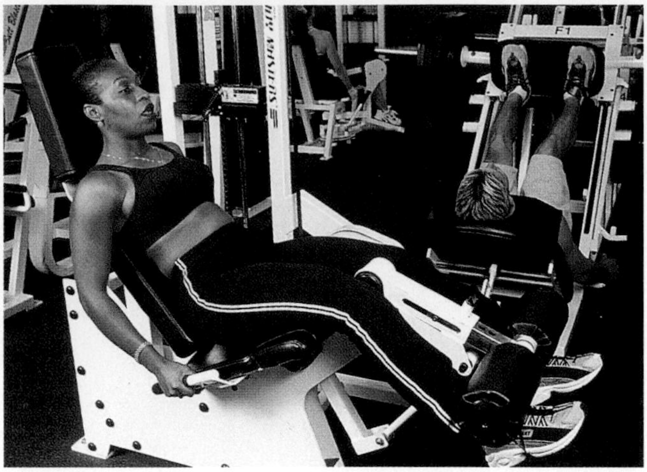

Weight training does little to develop cardiorespiratory endurance but is excellent for developing muscular strength and endurance. An overall fitness program includes exercises to develop all the components of physical fitness.

DEVELOPING A PERSONAL FITNESS PLAN

If you're ready to create a complete fitness program based around the activities you enjoy most, begin by preparing the program plan and contract in Lab 7.1. By carefully developing your plan and signing a contract, you'll increase your chances of success. The step-by-step procedure outlined here (adapted from *Your Guide to Getting Fit,* by Ivan Kusinitz and Morton Fine) will guide you through the steps of Lab 7.1 to the creation of an exercise program that's right for you. Refer to Figure 7.1 for a sample personal fitness program plan and contract.

If you'd like additional help in setting up your program, choose one of the sample programs at the end of this chapter (pp. 190–198). Sample programs are provided for walking/jogging/running, cycling, swimming, and inline skating; they include detailed instructions for starting a program and developing and maintaining fitness.

1. Set Goals

Setting goals to reach through exercise is a crucial first step. Ask yourself, "What do I want from my fitness program?" Develop different types of goals—general and specific, long term and short term. General or long-term goals might include things like lowering your risk for chronic disease, improving posture, having more energy, and improving the fit of your clothes. It's a good idea to also develop some specific, short-term goals based on measurable factors. Specific goals might be raising $\dot{V}O_{2max}$ by 10%, reducing the time it takes you to jog 2 miles from 22 minutes to 19 minutes, increasing the number of push-ups you can do from 15 to 25, and lowering BMI from 26 to 24.5. Having specific goals will allow you to track your progress and enjoy the measurable changes brought about by your fitness program.

Physical fitness assessment tests are essential to determining your goals. They help you decide which types of exercise you should emphasize, and they help you understand the relative difficulty of attaining specific goals. If you have health problems, such as high blood pressure, heart disease, obesity, or serious joint or muscle disabilities, see your physician before taking assessment tests. Measure your progress by taking these tests about every 3 months.

You'll find it easier to stick with your program if you choose goals that are both important to you and realistic. Remember that heredity, your current fitness level, and other individual factors influence the amount of improvement and the ultimate level of fitness you can expect to obtain through physical training. Fitness improves most quickly during the first 6 months of an exercise program. After that, gains come more slowly and usually require a higher-intensity program. So don't expect to improve indefinitely. Improve your fitness to a reasonable target level, and then train consistently to maintain it. Sometimes you may lose fitness—due to illness, injury, missed workouts, or a vacation—so you must begin again at a lower level. Developing fitness is a dynamic process that involves gains and losses. Even if you lose ground occasionally, stay with your program, and you'll be able to achieve your goals.

Think carefully about your reasons for exercising, and then fill in the goals portion of your plan in Lab 7.1.

2. Select Activities

If you have already chosen activities and created separate program plans for different fitness components in Chapters 3, 4, and 5, you can put those plans together into a single program. It's usually best to include exercises to develop each of the health-related components of fitness.

- Cardiorespiratory endurance is developed by activities such as walking, cycling, and aerobic dance that involve continuous rhythmic movements of large-muscle groups like those in the legs (see Chapter 3).
- Muscular strength and endurance are developed by training against resistance (see Chapter 4).

A. I Tracie Kaufman (name) am contracting with myself to follow a physical fitness program to work toward the following goals:

Specific or short-term goals

1. Improving cardiorespiratory fitness by raising my $\dot{V}O_{2max}$ from 34 to 37 ml/kg/min
2. Improving upper body muscular strength and endurance rating from fair to good
3. Improving body composition (from 28% to 25% body fat)
4. Improving my tennis game (hitting 20 playable shots in a row against the ball machine)

General or long-term goals

1. Developing a more positive attitude about myself
2. Improving the fit of my clothes
3. Building and maintaining bone mass to reduce my risk of osteoporosis
4. Increasing my life expectancy and reducing my risk for diabetes and heart disease

B. My program plan is as follows:

Activities	Components (Check ✓) CRE	MS	ME	F	BC	Intensity*	Duration	Frequency (Check ✓) M	Tu	W	Th	F	Sa	Su
Swimming	✓	✓	✓	✓	✓	140-170 bpm	35min	✓		✓		✓		
Tennis	✓	✓	✓	✓	✓	RPE = 13–16	90min						✓	
Weight training		✓	✓	✓	✓	see Lab 4.3	30min		✓		✓		✓	
Stretching				✓		—	25min	✓		✓		✓	✓	

*List your target heart rate range or an RPE value if appropriate.

C. My program will begin on Sept. 21. My program includes the following schedule of mini-goals. For each step in my program, I will give myself the reward listed.

Mini-goal	Date	Reward
Completing 2 full weeks of program (mini-goal 1)	Oct 5	movie with friends
$\dot{V}O_{2max}$ of 35 ml/kg/min (mini-goal 2)	Nov 2	new CD
Completing 10 full weeks of program (mini-goal 3)	Nov 30	new sweater
Percent body fat of 27% (mini-goal 4)	Dec 22	weekend away
$\dot{V}O_{2max}$ of 36 ml/kg/min (mini-goal 5)	Jan 18	new CD

D. My program will include the addition of physical activity to my daily routine (such as climbing stairs or walking to class):

1. Walking to and from campus job
2. Taking the stairs to dorm room instead of elevator
3. Bicycling to the library instead of driving
4. Doing one active chore a day
5.

E. I will use the following tools to monitor my program and my progress toward my goals: I'll use a chart that lists the number of laps and minutes I swim and the charts for strength and flexibility from Labs 4.3 & 5.2.

I sign this contract as an indication of my personal commitment to reach my goal.

Tracie Kaufman (your signature) Sept 10 (date)

I have recruited a helper who will witness my contract and swim with me three days per week

(list any way your helper will participate in your program)

Russell Walker (witness's signature) Sept 10 (date)

Figure 7.1 A sample personal fitness program plan and contract.

Table 7.1 A Summary of Sports and Fitness Activities

This table classifies sports and activities as high (H), moderate (M), or low (L) in terms of their ability to develop each of the five components of physical fitness: cardiorespiratory endurance (CRE), muscular strength (MS), muscular endurance (ME), flexibility (F), and body composition (BC). The skill level needed to obtain fitness benefits is noted: Low (L) means little or no skill is required to obtain fitness benefits; moderate (M) means average skill is needed to obtain fitness benefits; and high (H) means much skill is required to obtain fitness benefits. The fitness prerequisite, or conditioning needs of a beginner, is also noted: Low (L) means not fitness prerequisite is required, moderate (M) means some preconditioning is required, and high (H) means substantial fitness is required. The last two columns list the calorie cost of each activity when performed moderately and vigorously. To determine how many calories you burn, multiply the value in the appropriate column by your body weight and then by the number of minutes you exercise. Work up to using 300 or more calories per workout.

	COMPONENTS							APPROXIMATE CALORIE COST (CAL/LB/MIN)	
Sports and Activities	CRE	MS*	ME*	F*	BC	Skill Level	Fitness Prerequisite	Moderate	Vigorous
Aerobic dance	H	M	H	H	H	L	L	.046	.062
Backpacking	H	M	H	M	H	L	M	.032	.078
Badminton, skilled, singles	H	M	M	M	H	M	M	—	.071
Ballet (floor combinations)	M	M	H	H	M	M	L	—	.058
Ballroom dancing	M	L	M	L	M	M	L	.034	.049
Baseball (pitcher and catcher)	M	M	H	M	M	H	M	.039	—
Basketball, half court	H	M	H	M	H	M	M	.045	.071
Bicycling	H	M	H	M	H	M	L	.049	.071
Bowling	L	L	L	L	L	L	L	—	—
Calisthenic circuit training	H	M	H	M	H	L	L	—	.060
Canoeing and kayaking (flat water)	M	M	H	M	M	M	M	.045	—
Cheerleading	M	M	M	M	M	M	L	.033	.049
Fencing	M	M	H	H	M	M	L	.032	.078
Field hockey	H	M	H	M	H	M	M	.052	.078
Folk and square dancing	M	L	M	L	M	L	L	.039	.049
Football, touch	M	M	M	M	M	M	M	.049	.078
Frisbee, ultimate	H	M	H	M	H	M	M	.049	.078
Golf (riding cart)	L	L	L	M	L	L	L	—	—
Handball, skilled, singles	H	M	H	M	H	M	M	—	.078
Hiking	H	M	H	L	H	L	M	.051	.073
Hockey, ice and roller	H	M	H	M	H	M	M	.052	.078
Horseback riding	M	M	M	L	M	M	M	.052	.065
Interval circuit training	H	H	H	M	H	L	L	—	.062
Jogging and running	H	M	H	L	H	L	L	.060	.104

*Ratings are for the muscle groups involved.

- Flexibility is developed by stretching the major muscle groups (see Chapter 5).
- Healthy body composition can be developed by combining a sensible diet and a program of regular exercise, including cardiorespiratory endurance exercise to burn calories and resistance training to build muscle mass (see Chapter 6).

Table 7.1 rates many popular activities for their ability to develop each of the health-related components of fitness. Check the ratings of the activities you're considering to make sure the program you put together will develop all fitness components and help you achieve your goals. One strategy is to select one activity for each component of fitness—bicycling, weight training, and stretching, for example. Another strategy applies the principle of **cross-training,** using several different activities to develop a particular fitness component—aerobics classes, swimming, and volleyball for cardiorespiratory endurance, for example. Cross-training is discussed in the next section.

If you select activities that support your commitment rather than activities that turn exercise into a chore, the right program will be its own incentive for continuing. Consider the following factors in making your choices.

- *Fun and interest.* Your fitness program is much more likely to be successful if you choose activities that you enjoy doing. Start by considering any activities you cur-

Table 7.1	A Summary of Sports and Fitness Activities (continued)								
	COMPONENTS							APPROXIMATE CALORIE COST (CAL/LB/MIN)	
Sports and Activities	CRE	MS*	ME*	F*	BC	Skill Level	Fitness Prerequisite	Moderate	Vigorous
Judo	M	H	H	M	M	M	L	.049	.090
Karate	H	M	H	H	H	L	M	.049	.090
Lacrosse	H	M	H	M	H	H	M	.052	.078
Modern dance (moving combinations)	M	M	H	H	M	L	L	—	.058
Orienteering	H	M	H	L	H	L	M	.049	.078
Outdoor fitness trails	H	M	H	M	H	L	L	—	.060
Popular dancing	M	L	M	M	M	M	L	—	.049
Racquetball, skilled, singles	H	M	M	M	H	M	M	.049	.078
Rock climbing	M	H	H	H	M	H	M	.033	.033
Rope skipping	H	M	H	L	H	M	M	.071	.095
Rowing	H	H	H	H	H	L	L	.032	.097
Rugby	H	M	H	M	H	M	M	.052	.097
Sailing	L	L	M	L	L	M	L	—	—
Skating, ice, roller, and in-line	M	M	H	M	M	H	M	.049	.095
Skiing, alpine	M	H	H	M	M	H	M	.039	.078
Skiing, cross-country	H	M	H	M	H	M	M	.049	.104
Soccer	H	M	H	M	H	M	M	.052	.097
Squash, skilled, singles	H	M	M	M	H	M	M	.049	.078
Stretching	L	L	L	H	L	L	L	—	—
Surfing (including swimming)	M	M	M	M	M	H	M	—	.078
Swimming	H	M	H	M	H	M	L	.032	.088
Synchronized swimming	M	M	H	H	M	H	M	.032	.052
Table tennis	M	L	M	M	M	M	L	—	.045
Tennis, skilled, singles	H	M	M	M	H	M	M	—	.071
Volleyball	M	L	M	M	M	M	M	—	.065
Walking	H	L	M	L	H	L	L	.029	.048
Water polo	H	M	H	M	H	H	M	—	.078
Water skiing	M	M	H	M	M	H	M	.039	.055
Weight training	L	H	H	H	M	L	L	—	—
Wrestling	H	H	H	H	H	H	H	.065	.094
Yoga	L	L	M	H	L	H	L	—	—

*Ratings are for the muscle groups involved.

SOURCE: Kusinitz, I., and M. Fine 1995. *Your Guide to Getting Fit,* 3d ed. Mountain View, Calif.: Mayfield. Reprinted with permission from The McGraw-Hill Companies.

rently engage in and enjoy. Often you can modify your current activities to fit your fitness program. As you consider new activities, ask yourself, "Is this activity fun?" "Will it hold my interest over time?" For new activities, it is a good idea to undertake a trial period before making a final choice. Table 7.2 on p. 180 shows popular fitness activities of Americans.

• *Your current skill and fitness level.* Although many activities are appropriate for beginners, some sports and activities require participants to have a moderate level of skill to obtain fitness benefits. For example, a beginning tennis player will probably not be able to sustain rallies long enough to develop cardiorespiratory endurance. Refer to the skill level column in Table 7.1 to determine the level of skill needed for full participation in the activities you're considering. If your current skill level doesn't meet the requirement, you may want to begin your program with a different activity. For example, a beginning tennis player may be better off with a walking program while improving his or her tennis game—or practicing with a ball machine to guarantee steady

cross-training Alternating two or more activities to improve a single component of fitness.

Terms

VW

VITAL STATISTICS

Table 7.2 Popular Fitness Activities of Americans

Activity	Number of Participants (millions)
Exercise walking[a]	81.3
Swimming[a]	59.3
Cycling/mountain biking[b]	56.8
Exercising with equipment[a]	43.2
Aerobic exercising[a]	27.2
Weight lifting[a]	24.6
Running/jogging[a]	22.5
In-line skating[b]	21.8
Calisthenics[a]	13.5

[a]Participants are those age 7 and over who participated in the activity more than five times per year.

[b]Participants are those age 7 and over who participated in the activity more than once per year.

SOURCE: National Sporting Goods Association, Mt. Prospect, IL 60056. (http://www.nsga.org/public/articles/details.cfm?id=28; retrieved November 11, 2001). Reprinted by permission of National Sporting Goods Association.

activity. To build skill for a particular activity, consider taking a class or getting some instruction from a coach or fellow participant.

Your current fitness level may also limit the activities that are appropriate for your program. For example, if you have been inactive, a walking program would be more appropriate than a jogging program. Activities in which participants control the intensity of effort—walking, cycling, and swimming, for example—are more appropriate for a beginning fitness program than sports and activities that are primarily "other paced"—soccer, basketball, and tennis, for example. Refer to the fitness prerequisite column of Table 7.1 to determine the minimum level of fitness required for participation in the activities you're considering. However, staying active is the most important thing. If you like to play tennis but don't like to take walks or jog, then play tennis.

- *Time and convenience*. Unless exercise fits easily into your daily schedule, you are unlikely to maintain your program over the long term. As you consider activities, think about whether a special location or facility is required. Can you participate in the activity close to your residence, school, or job? Are the necessary facilities open and available at times convenient to you (see Lab 7.2)? Do you need a partner or a team to play? Can you participate in the activity year-round, or will you need to find an alternative during the summer or winter? Would a home treadmill make you more likely to exercise regularly?
- *Cost*. Some sports and activities require equipment, fees, or some type of membership investment. If you are on a tight budget, limit your choices to activities that are inexpensive or free. Investigate the facilities on your campus, which you may be able to use at little or no cost. Many activities require no equipment beyond an appropriate pair of shoes (see the box "Choosing Exercise Footwear" for more information). Refer back to Chapters 2 and 3 for consumer guidelines for evaluating exercise equipment and facilities.
- *Special health needs*. If you have special exercise needs due to a particular health problem, choose activities that will conform to your needs and enhance your ability to cope. If necessary, consult your physician about how best to tailor an exercise program to your particular needs and goals. Guidelines and safety tips for exercisers with common chronic conditions are provided later in the chapter.

3. Set a Target Intensity, Duration, and Frequency for Each Activity

The next step is to set a target starting intensity, duration, and frequency for each activity you've chosen (see the sample in Figure 7.1). Refer to the calculations and plans you completed in Chapters 3, 4, and 5.

Cardiorespiratory Endurance Exercise For intensity, note your target heart rate zone or RPE value. Your target total duration should be about 20–60 minutes, depending on the intensity of the activity (shorter durations are appropriate for high-intensity activities, longer durations for activities of more moderate intensity). You can exercise in a single session or in multiple sessions of 10 or more minutes. One way to check whether the total duration you've set is appropriate is to use the **Calorie costs** (calories per minute per pound of body weight) given in Table 7.1. Your goal should be to work up to burning about 300 calories per workout; beginners should start with a calorie cost of about 100–150 calories per workout. You can calculate the calorie cost of your activities by multiplying the appropriate factor from Table 7.1 by your body weight and the duration of your workout. For example, walking at a moderate pace burns about 0.029 calorie per minute per pound of body weight. A person weighing 150 pounds could begin her exercise program by walking for 30 minutes, burning about 130 calories. Once her fitness improves, she might choose to start cycling for her cardiorespiratory endurance workouts. Cycling at a moderate pace has a higher calorie cost than walking (0.049 calorie per minute per pound), and if she cycled for 40 minutes, she would burn the target 300 calories during her workout.

Terms

calorie cost The amount of energy used to perform a particular activity, usually expressed in calories per minute per pound of body weight.

Footwear is perhaps the most important item of equipment for almost any activity. Shoes protect and support your feet and improve your traction. When you jump or run, you place as much as six times more force on your feet than when you stand still. Shoes can help cushion against the stress that this additional force places on your lower legs, thereby preventing injuries. Some athletic shoes are also designed to help prevent ankle rollover, another common source of injury.

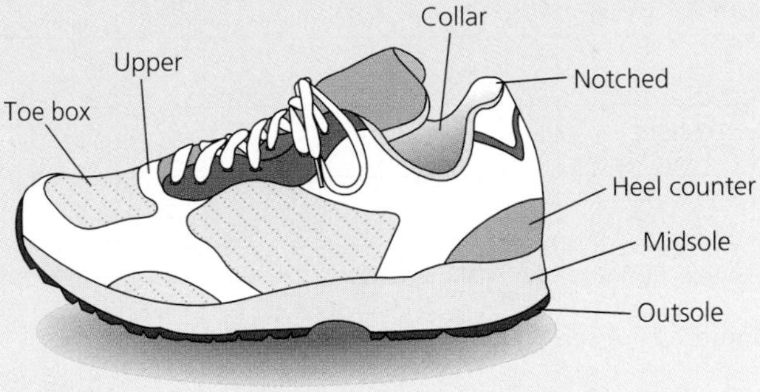

General Guidelines

When choosing athletic shoes, first consider the activity you've chosen for your exercise program. Shoes appropriate for different activities have very different characteristics. For example, running shoes typically have highly cushioned midsoles, rubber outsoles with elevated heels, and a great deal of flexibility in the forefoot. The heels of walking shoes tend to be lower, less padded, and more beveled than those designed for running. For aerobic dance, shoes must be flexible in the forefoot and have straight, nonflared heels to allow for safe and easy lateral movements. Court shoes also provide substantial support for lateral movements; they typically have outsoles made from white rubber that will not damage court surfaces.

Also consider the location and intensity of your workouts. If you plan to walk or run on trails, you should choose shoes with water-resistant, highly durable uppers and more outsole traction. If you work out intensely or have a relatively high body weight, you'll need thick, firm midsoles to avoid bottoming-out the cushioning system of your shoes.

Foot type is another important consideration. If your feet tend to roll inward excessively, you may need shoes with additional stability features on the inner side of the shoe to counter-act this movement. If your feet tend to roll outward excessively, you may need highly flexible and cushioned shoes that promote foot motion. For aerobic dancers with feet that tend to roll inward or outward, mid-cut to high-cut shoes may be more appropriate than low-cut aerobic shoes or cross-trainers (shoes designed to be worn for several different activities). Compared with men, women have narrower feet overall and narrower heels relative to the forefoot. Most women will get a better fit if they choose shoes that are specifically designed for women's feet rather than those that are downsized versions of men's shoes.

Successful Shopping

For successful shoe shopping, keep the following strategies in mind:

- Shop at an athletic shoe or specialty store that has personnel trained to fit athletic shoes and a large selection of styles and sizes.
- Shop late in the day or, ideally, following a workout. Your foot size increases over the course of the day and as a result of exercise.
- Wear socks like those you plan to wear during exercise. If you have an old pair of athletic shoes, bring them with you. The wear pattern on your old shoes can help you select a pair with extra support or cushioning in the places you need it the most.
- Ask for help. Trained salespeople know which shoes are designed for your foot type and your level of activity. They can also help fit your shoes properly.
- Don't insist on buying shoes in what you consider to be your typical shoe size. Sizes vary from shoe to shoe. In addition, foot sizes change over time, and many people have one foot that is larger or wider than the other. Try several sizes in several widths, if necessary. Don't buy shoes that are too small.
- Try on both shoes and wear them around for 10 or more minutes. Try walking on a noncarpeted surface. Approximate the movements of your activity: walk, jog, run, jump, and so on.
- Check the fit and style carefully:

  Is the toe box roomy enough? Your toes will spread out when your foot hits the ground or you push off. There should be at least one thumb's width of space from the longest toe to the end of the toe box.

  Do the shoes have enough cushioning? Do your feet feel supported when you bounce up and down? Try bouncing on your toes and on your heels.

  Do your heels fit snugly into the shoe? Do they stay put when you walk, or do they rise up?

  Are the arches of your feet right on top of the shoes' arch supports?

  Do the shoes feel stable when you twist and turn on the balls of your feet? Try twisting from side to side while standing on one foot.

  Do you feel any pressure points?
- If the shoes are not comfortable in the store, don't buy them. Don't expect athletic shoes to stretch over time in order to fit your feet properly.

Name Tracie Kaufman

Enter duration, distance, or other factor to track your progress.

Activity/Date	M	Tu	W	Th	F	S	S	Weekly Total	M	Tu	W	Th	F	S	S	Weekly Total
1 Swimming	800 yd		725 yd		800 yd			2325 yd	800 yd		800 yd		850 yd			2450 yd
2 Tennis						90 min		90 min						95 min		95 min
3 Weight Training		✓		✓		✓				✓		✓		✓	✓	
4 Stretching	✓		✓		✓	✓			✓			✓	✓	✓	✓	

Figure 7.2 A sample program log.

An appropriate frequency for cardiorespiratory endurance exercise is 3–5 times per week.

Muscular Strength and Endurance Training As described in Chapter 4, a general fitness strength training program includes 1 or more sets of 8–12 repetitions of 8–10 exercises that work all major muscle groups. For intensity, choose a weight that is heavy enough to fatigue your muscles but not so heavy that you cannot complete the full number of repetitions with proper form. A frequency of 2–3 days per week is recommended.

Flexibility Training Stretches should be performed for all major muscle groups. For each exercise, stretch to the point of slight tension or mild discomfort and hold the stretch for 10–30 seconds; do at least 4 repetitions of each exercise. Stretches should be performed at least 2–3 days per week, preferably when muscles are warm.

4. Set Up a System of Mini-Goals and Rewards

To keep your program on track, it is important to set up a system of goals and rewards. Break your specific goals into several steps, and set a target date for each step. For example, if one of the goals of an 18-year-old male student's program is to improve upper-body strength and endurance, he could use the push-up test in Lab 4.2 to set intermediate goals. If he can currently perform 15 push-ups (for a rating of "very poor"), he might set intermediate goals of 17, 20, 25, and 30 push-ups (for a final rating of "fair"). By allowing several weeks between mini-goals and specifying rewards, he'll be able to track his progress and reward himself as he moves toward his final goal. Reaching a series of small goals is more satisfying than working toward a single, more challenging goal that may take months to achieve. Realistic goals, broken into achievable mini-goals, can boost your chances of success. For more on choosing appropriate rewards, refer to pp. 13–14 in Chapter 1 and Activity 4 in the Behavior Change Workbook at the end of the text.

5. Include Lifestyle Physical Activity in Your Program

As described in Chapter 2, daily physical activity is an important part of a fit and well lifestyle. As part of your fitness program plan, specify ways to be more active during your daily routine. You may find it helpful to first use your health journal to track your activities for several days. Review the records in your journal, identify routine opportunities to be more active, and add these to your program plan in Lab 7.1.

6. Develop Tools for Monitoring Your Progress

A record that tracks your daily progress will help remind you of your ongoing commitment to your program and give you a sense of accomplishment. Figure 7.2 shows you how to create a general program log and record the activity type, frequency, and durations. Or if you wish, complete specific activity logs like those in Labs 3.2, 4.3, and 5.2 in addition to, or instead of, a general log. Post your log in a place where you'll see it often as a reminder and as an incentive for improvement. If you have specific, measurable goals, you can also graph your weekly or monthly progress toward your goal (Figure 7.3).

7. Make a Commitment

Your final step in planning your program is to make a commitment by signing a contract. Find a witness for your contract—preferably one who will be actively involved in your program. Keep your contract in a visible spot to remind you of your commitment.

PUTTING YOUR PLAN INTO ACTION

Once you've developed a detailed plan and signed your contract, you are ready to begin your fitness program. Refer to the specific training suggestions provided in Chapters 2–5 for advice on beginning and maintaining your pro-

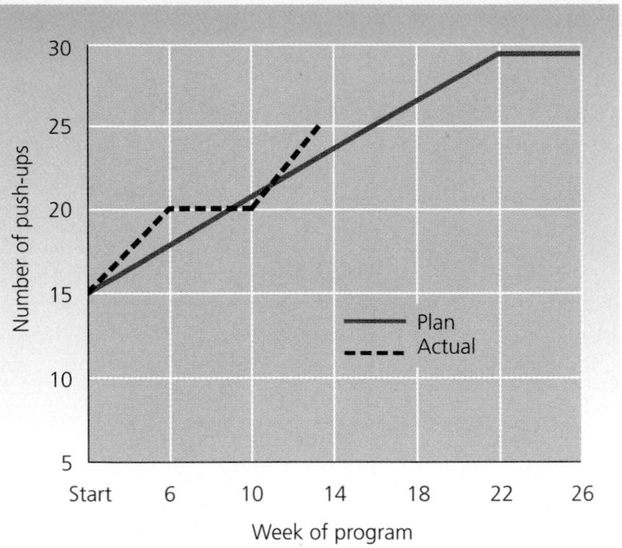

Figure 7.3 A sample program progress chart.

gram. Some key guidelines for putting your plan into action are summarized below.

• *Start slowly and increase fitness gradually*. Overzealous exercising can result in discouraging discomforts and injuries. Your program is meant to last a lifetime. The important first step is to break your established pattern of inactivity. Be patient and realistic. Once your body has adjusted to your starting level of exercise, slowly increase the amount of overload. Small increases are the key—achieving a large number of small improvements will eventually result in substantial gains in fitness. It's usually best to increase duration and frequency before increasing intensity.

• *Find an exercise buddy.* The social side of exercise is an important factor for many regular exercisers. Working out with a friend will make exercise more enjoyable and increase your chances of sticking with your program. Find an exercise partner who shares your goals and general fitness level.

• *Vary your activities.* You can make your program more fun over the long term if you participate in a variety of different activities that you enjoy. You can also add interest by strategies such as varying the routes you take when walking, running, biking, or in-line skating; finding a new tennis or racquetball partner; changing your music for aerobic dance; or switching to a new volleyball or basketball court.

Varying your activities, a strategy known as cross-training, has other benefits. It can help you develop balanced, total body fitness. For example, by alternating running with swimming, you build both upper- and lower-body strength. Cross-training can thus prepare you for a wider range of activities and physical challenges. It can also reduce the risk of injury and overtraining because the same muscles, bones, and joints are not continuously subjected to the stresses of the same activity. Cross-training can be done either by choosing different activities on different days or by alternating activities within a single workout.

• *Cycle the volume and intensity of your workouts.* Olympic athletes use a training technique called periodization of training, meaning that they vary the volume and intensity of their workouts. Sometimes they exercise very intensely; at other times they train lightly or rest. You can use the same technique to improve fitness faster and make your training program more varied and enjoyable. For example, if your program consists of walking, weight training, and stretching, pick one day a week for each activity to train a little harder or longer than you normally do. If you usually walk 2 miles in 16 minutes per mile, increase the pace to 15 minutes per mile once a week. If you lift weights twice a week, train more intensely during one of the workouts by using more resistance or performing multiple sets.

• *Adapt to changing environments and schedules.* Most people are creatures of habit and have trouble adjusting to change. Don't use wet weather or a new job as excuses to give up your exercise program. If you walk in the summer, put on a warm coat and walk in the winter. If you can't go out because of darkness, join a gym and walk on a treadmill. Changes in your job or family situation can also affect your exercise program. Taking a job with a longer commute or having a new baby can rob you of the time you used to spend exercising. Remember that physical activity is important for your energy level, self-esteem, and well-being. You owe it to yourself to include physical activity in your day. Try to exercise before going to work or do some physical activity during your lunch hour—even if it's only a short walk or a few trips up and down the stairs.

• *Expect fluctuations and lapses.* On some days, your progress will be excellent, but on others, you'll barely be able to drag yourself through your scheduled activities. Don't let off-days or lapses discourage you or make you feel guilty. Instead, feel a renewed commitment for your fitness program (see the box "Getting Your Fitness Program Back on Track," p. 184).

MAINTAINING YOUR PROGRAM: FIT FOR LIFE

Exercise should not be something you do just during January and February to satisfy a New Year's resolution—or during a class to satisfy a course requirement. You must make it a permanent part of your life. Choose activities you enjoy and make them part of your daily routine, just like sleeping, eating, brushing your teeth, and going to school and work. Scientists gather more evidence every year that regular exercise is the most important activity you can do to contribute to wellness. It is not a frill or a

TAKE CHARGE Getting Your Fitness Program Back on Track

Lapses are a normal part any behavior change program. The important point is to move on and avoid becoming discouraged. Try again, and keep trying. Know that continued effort will lead to success.

- Don't judge yourself harshly. Focus on the improvements you've already obtained from your program and how good you feel after exercise—both physically and mentally.
- Visualize what it will be like to reach your goals. Keep these pictures in your mind as an incentive to stick with your program.
- Use your exercise journal to identify thoughts and behaviors that are causing noncompliance. Devise strategies to combat these problematic patterns. If needed, make additional changes in your environment or obtain more social support. Call a friend to walk with you. Put your exercise clothes in your car or backpack.
- Make changes in your plan and reward system to help renew your enthusiasm and commitment to your program. Try changing fitness activities or your exercise schedule. Build in more opportunities to reward yourself.
- Plan ahead for difficult situations. Think about what circumstances might make it tough to keep up your fitness routine. Develop strategies to increase your chances of sticking with your program. For example, devise strategies for your program during vacation, travel, bad weather, and so on.
- If you're in a bad mood or just don't feel like exercising, remind yourself that physical activity is probably the one thing you can do that will make you feel better. Even if you can only do half your scheduled workout, you'll boost your energy, improve your mood, and help keep your program on track.

treat—it is a necessity. You will be a healthier, more vital person if you make physical activity a habit. The following strategies can help keep you active for life:

- *Be safe.* Minimize the risk of injury or problems from activity by following safety guidelines, using proper technique and equipment, respecting signals from your body that something may be wrong, and treating any injuries that occur. Warm up, cool down, and drink plenty of fluids before and after exercise.
- *Have several exercise options.* Don't depend on a single location, activity, or person to be active. Cultivate many enjoyable activities that can be done in all seasons and circumstances. Take up a new sport or activity to keep your program fresh and enjoyable. And don't forget to include lifestyle physical activity in your daily routine.
- *Keep an exercise journal.* A journal can help keep your program on track, identify sources of problems, and give you a continuing sense of accomplishment.
- *Reward yourself.* Don't stop rewarding yourself once you reach your fitness goals. Continue to give yourself regular rewards for sticking with your program.
- *Choose other healthy lifestyle behaviors.* Exercise provides huge benefits for your health, but other behaviors are also important. Choose a nutritious diet and avoid harmful habits like smoking and overconsumption of alcohol. Don't skimp on sleep, which has a mutually beneficial relationship with exercise. Physical activity improves sleep, and adequate sleep can improve physical performance (see the box "Sleep").

Terms

interval training A training technique that alternates exercise intervals with rest intervals or intense exercise intervals with low to moderate intervals.

EXERCISE GUIDELINES FOR PEOPLE WITH SPECIAL HEALTH CONCERNS

Regular, appropriate exercise is safe and beneficial for many people with chronic conditions or other special health concerns. For example, people with heart disease or hypertension who exercise may lower their blood pressure and improve their cholesterol levels. For people with diabetes, exercise can improve insulin sensitivity and body composition. For people with asthma, regular exercise may reduce the risk of acute attacks during exertion. For many people with special health concerns, the risks associated with *not* exercising are far greater than those associated with a moderate program of regular exercise.

The fitness recommendations for the general population presented in this text can serve as a general guideline for any exercise program. However, for people with special health concerns, certain precautions and monitoring may be required. Anyone with special health concerns should consult a physician before beginning an exercise program. Guidelines and cautions for some common conditions are described below.

Arthritis

- Begin an exercise program as early as possible in the course of the disease.
- Warm up thoroughly before each exercise session to loosen stiff muscles and lower the risk of injury.
- For cardiorespiratory endurance exercise, avoid high-impact activities that may damage arthritic joints; consider swimming, water walking, or another type of exercise in a warm pool.
- Perform strength training exercises for the whole body; pay special attention to muscles that support

If you could do something simple, safe, and free to dramatically improve your mental, physical, and psychological health, would you do it? The opportunity is yours starting tonight—all you have to do is go to bed earlier! The majority of Americans suffer from chronic sleep deprivation. Most of us get between one-half and two fewer hours of sleep each night than we need in order to be fully alert during the day. One hundred years ago, Americans slept on average one and a half more hours each night than we do now. With the advent of electric lights, sleep times decreased dramatically. Today, we live in a twenty-four-hour nonstop culture, but our bodies still require sleep for about one-third of every day.

Many people view sleep as a luxury or a waste of time. Being able to function without sleep is considered macho. But sleep is absolutely essential for life and health. Humans and other animals who are deprived of sleep for many days will become ill and even die. Less extreme sleep deprivation over a long period of time makes us vulnerable to a wide variety of illnesses including CVD, diabetes, high blood pressure, and psychological disorders such as anxiety and depression. Inadequate sleep also depresses the immune system, making people more likely to become ill with infectious diseases. Inadequate sleep affects learning, memory, and attention span, all critical to academic performance. Athletes who fail to get sufficient sleep cannot perform at their peak because fatigue slows reaction time and lessens endurance. Every aspect of life is easier and more pleasurable when you are well rested.

Sleep deprivation also takes a huge toll on society as a whole. The National Sleep Foundation estimates that sleepy employees cost U.S. businesses $18 billion every year in lost productivity alone. The costs are much higher if you factor in mistakes, accidents, and health problems caused by lack of sleep. Drowsiness is estimated to be a factor in at least one-third of all auto crashes; it impairs driving ability as much as alcohol use. Many of us think that no matter how tired we may be, we can force ourselves to be alert. Researchers have found that people who are sleep deprived may think they are wide awake but often fall asleep at the wheel for brief periods without even realizing it.

College students are particularly vulnerable to sleep deprivation and poor quality of sleep. Most students lead hectic lives as they juggle studies, work, socializing, and family obligations. Students who live in dormitories are often awakened by nighttime noise. Partying, especially if alcohol and other drugs are used, further disrupts sleep. Students who are out partying several nights a week are likely to be significantly sleep deprived, increasing the risk of school failure, car crashes, and illnesses such as frequent colds. To make matters worse, teens and young adults actually need more sleep than older individuals—more than 9 hours of sleep a night—to be well rested.

Financial necessity dictates that many students work part time or even full time. Realistically, there are only so many hours in the day, and many working students find it nearly impossible to get enough sleep to function well in school or at work. What can you do if you are faced with this dilemma? Cut back on work hours if at all possible. Financial aid or a loan from a family member may be what it takes to get your life under control. Taking an extra year to get your degree may be worth it to preserve your health and happiness.

How do you know if you're getting enough sleep? If you need an alarm to get yourself up every morning, rather than awakening naturally at the appropriate time, chances are you are significantly sleep deprived. Another clue is if you fall asleep within just a few minutes of getting into bed, or if you fall asleep during the day when you don't intend to, such as during lectures or while reading or watching TV. Sleep you need but don't get is referred to as "sleep debt." Whenever you get less sleep than your body requires, you add to your sleep debt. Week after week, sleep debt can build, leaving you chronically groggy. If you have a large sleep debt, sleeping in a few extra hours on the weekends won't solve the problem, although it can help a bit. The real solution is to make sleep a priority in your daily life. Remember that the time you spend sleeping will pay for itself in increased productivity. For example, if you go to bed one hour earlier instead of trying to study when you're half awake, you are likely to get the work done in a fraction of the time when you're more alert the next day. Knowing that the quality of your life depends on getting adequate sleep, make sleep a priority part of your wellness lifestyle.

and protect affected joints (for example, build quadriceps, hamstring, and calf strength for the knee). Start with small loads and build intensity gradually.

- Perform flexibility exercises regularly to maintain joint mobility.

Asthma

- Exercise regularly. Acute attacks are more likely if you exercise only occasionally.
- Carry medication during workouts and avoid exercising alone.
- Warm up and cool down slowly to reduce the risk of acute attacks.
- When starting an exercise program, choose self-paced endurance activities, especially those involving **interval training** (short bouts of exercise followed by a rest period). Increase the intensity of cardiorespiratory endurance exercise gradually.
- Cold, dry air can trigger or worsen an attack. Drink water before, during, and after a workout to moisten your airways. In cold weather, cover your mouth with a mask or scarf to warm and humidify the air you breathe. Swimming in a heated pool is an excellent activity choice for people with asthma.
- Avoid outdoor activities during pollen season or when the air is polluted. Avoid exercise in dry or dusty indoor environments.

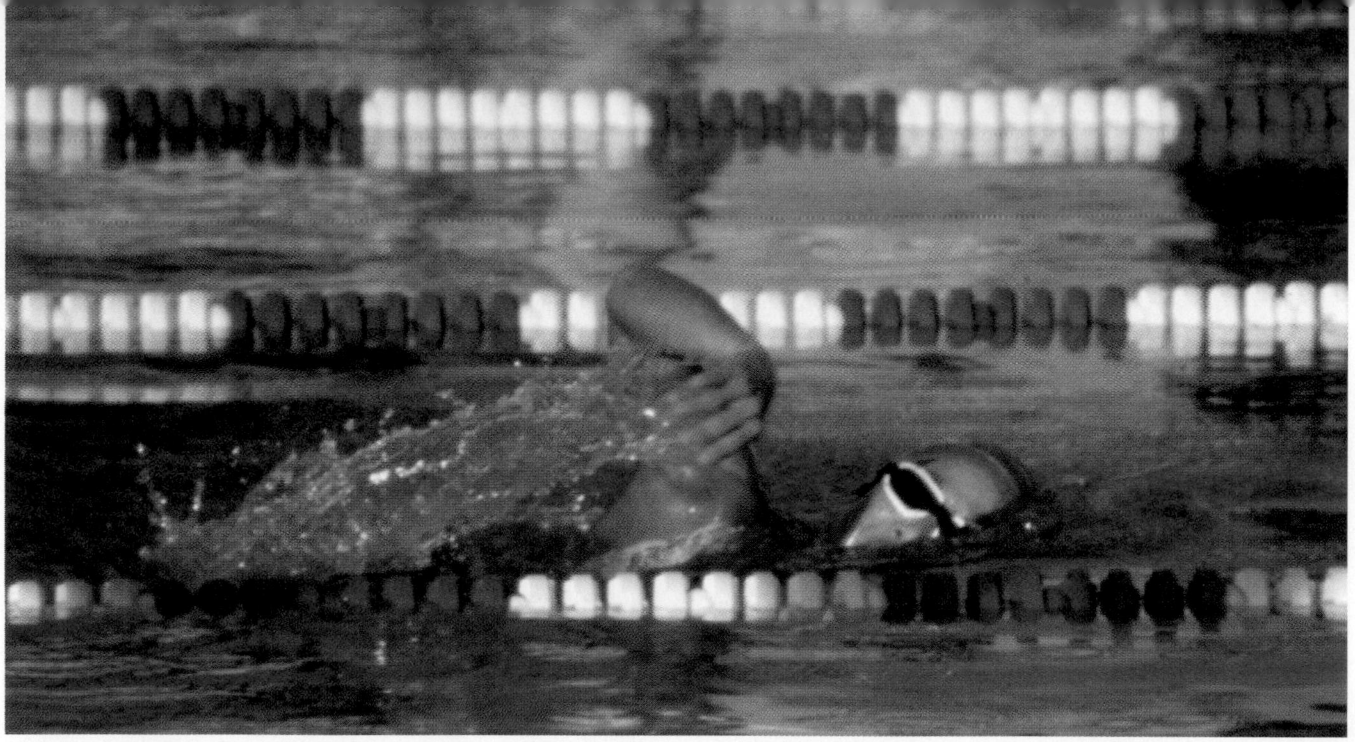

An individual with special health concerns can develop a safe and effective fitness program by choosing activities carefully and making appropriate modifications in the program. Swimming is an excellent activity choice for this man with asthma because breathing warm, moist air reduces the risk of asthma attacks during exercise.

Diabetes

- Don't begin an exercise program unless your diabetes is under control and you have checked about exercise safety with your physician. Because people with diabetes have an increased risk for heart disease, an exercise stress test may be recommended.
- Don't exercise alone. Wear a bracelet identifying yourself as having diabetes.
- If you are taking insulin or another medication, you may need to adjust the timing and amount of each dose. Work with your physician and check your blood sugar levels regularly so you can learn to balance your energy intake and output and your medication dosage.
- To prevent abnormally rapid absorption of injected insulin, inject it over a muscle that won't be exercised and wait at least an hour before exercising.
- Check blood sugar levels before, during, and after exercise and adjust your diet or insulin dosage if needed. Carry high-carbohydrate foods during a workout.
- Don't lift heavy weights. Straining can damage blood vessels.
- If you have poor circulation or numbness in your extremities, check your skin regularly for blisters and abrasions, especially on your feet. Avoid high-impact activities and wear comfortable shoes.
- For maximum benefit and minimum risk, choose low-to-moderate-intensity activities.

Heart Disease and Hypertension

- Check with your physician about exercise safety before increasing your activity level.
- Exercise at a moderate rather than a high intensity. Keep your heart rate below the level at which abnormalities appear on an exercise stress test.
- Warm-up and cool-down sessions should be gradual and last at least 10 minutes.
- Monitor your heart rate during exercise and stop if you experience dizziness or chest pain.
- If your physician has prescribed it, carry nitroglycerin with you during exercise. If you are taking beta-blockers for hypertension, use RPE rather than heart rate to monitor exercise intensity (beta-blockers reduce heart rate). Exercise at an RPE level of "somewhat hard"; your breathing should be unlabored, and you should be able to talk.
- Don't hold your breath when exercising. Doing so can cause sudden, steep increases in blood pressure. Take special care during weight training; don't lift extremely heavy loads.
- Increase exercise intensity, duration, and frequency very gradually.

Obesity

- For maximum benefit and minimum risk, choose low-to-moderate-intensity activities.

- Choose non- or low-weight-bearing activities such as swimming, water exercises, cycling, or walking. Low-impact activities are less likely to lead to joint problems or injuries.
- Stay alert for symptoms of heat-related problems during exercise (see Chapter 3). People who are obese are particularly vulnerable to problems with heat intolerance.
- Ease into an exercise program and increase overload gradually. Increase duration and frequency of exercise before increasing intensity.
- Include strength training in your fitness program to build or maintain muscle mass.
- Try to include as much lifestyle physical activity in your daily routine as possible.

Osteoporosis

- For cardiorespiratory endurance activities, exercise at the maximum intensity that causes no significant discomfort. If possible, choose low-impact weight-bearing activities to help safely maintain bone density (see Chapter 8 for more strategies for building and maintaining bone density).
- To prevent fractures, avoid any activity or movement that stresses the back or carries a risk of falling.
- Include weight training in your exercise program to improve strength and balance and reduce the risk of falls and fractures. Avoid lifting heavy loads.

Exercise guidelines for people with disabilities are discussed in Chapter 2 and for people with low-back pain, in Chapter 5.

EXERCISE GUIDELINES FOR LIFE STAGES

A fitness program may also need to be adjusted to accommodate the requirements of different life stages.

Children and Adolescents

Only about half of all young people age 12–21 in the United States participate regularly in vigorous activity, and 25% report no vigorous activity at all. This lack of physical activity has led to alarming increases in overweight and obesity in children and adolescents. If you have children or are in a position to influence children, keep these guidelines in mind:

- Provide opportunities for children and adolescents to exercise every day. Minimize sedentary activities, such as watching television and playing video games. Children and adolescents should aim for 60 minutes of moderate physical activity most, but preferably all, days.
- During family outings, choose dynamic activities. For example, go for a walk, park away from a mall and then walk to the stores, and take the stairs instead of the escalator.
- For children younger than 12 years, emphasize skill development and fitness rather than excellence in competitive sports. For adolescents, combine participation and training in lifetime sports with traditional, competitive sports.
- Make sure children are developmentally capable of participating in an activity. For example, catching skills are difficult for young children because their nervous system is not developed enough to fully master the skill. When teaching a child to catch a ball, start with a large ball and throw it from a short range. Gradually increase the complexity of the skill once the child has mastered the simpler skill.
- Make sure children get plenty of water when exercising in the heat. Make sure they are dressed properly when doing sports in the cold.

Pregnant Women

Exercise is important during pregnancy, but women should be cautious because some types of exercise can pose increased risk to the mother and the unborn child. The following guidelines are consistent with the recommendations of the American College of Obstetrics and Gynecology.

- See your physician about possible modifications needed for your particular pregnancy.
- Continue mild-to-moderate exercise routines at least three times a week. Avoid exercising vigorously or to exhaustion, especially in the third trimester. Monitor exercise intensity by assessing how you feel rather than by monitoring your heart rate.
- Favor non- or low-weight-bearing exercises such as swimming or cycling over weight-bearing exercises, which can carry increased risk of injury.
- Avoid exercise in a supine position—lying on your back—after the first trimester. Research indicates that this position restricts blood flow to the uterus. Also avoid prolonged periods of motionless standing.
- Avoid exercise that could cause loss of balance, especially in the third trimester, and exercise that might injure the abdomen, stress the joints, or carry a risk of falling (such as contact sports, vigorous racquet sports, skiing, and in-line skating).
- Avoid activities involving extremes in altitude—for example, scuba diving and mountain climbing.
- Especially during the first trimester, drink plenty of fluids and exercise in well-ventilated areas to avoid heat stress.
- After giving birth, resume prepregnancy exercise routines gradually, based on how you feel.

Older Adults

Older people readily adapt to endurance exercise and strength training. Exercise principles are the same as for younger people, but some specific guidelines apply:

- Include the three basic types of exercise—resistance, endurance, and flexibility.
- Drink plenty of water and avoid exercising in excessively hot or cold environments. (Older people sometimes have a decreased ability to regulate body temperature during exercise.) Wear clothes that speed heat loss in warm environments and that prevent heat loss in cold environments.
- Warm up slowly and carefully. Increase intensity and duration of exercise gradually.
- Cool down slowly, continuing very light exercise until the heart rate is below 100.
- To help prevent soft tissue pain, do static stretching after a normal workout.

Sample fitness programs begin on p. 190.

Tips for Today

A complete fitness program includes activities to build and maintain cardiorespiratory endurance, muscular strength and endurance, and flexibility. It takes time, energy, and commitment to begin and maintain a fitness program, but the many benefits are well worth the effort. Begin today, and you'll be on your way to enjoying fitness and wellness for the rest of your life.

Right now you can

- Obtain a journal to track your daily physical activity and exercise routine.
- Put away your remote control devices—every bit of physical activity can benefit your health.
- Put the clothes and equipment for your next workout in a convenient and obvious location.
- Plan to go to bed 15 minutes earlier than usual.
- Make a list of situations such as bad weather that may challenge your ability to stick with your fitness program. Develop a strategy for dealing with each one.

COMMON QUESTIONS ANSWERED

Should I exercise every day? Some daily exercise is beneficial, and health experts recommend that you engage in at least 30 minutes of moderate physical activity over the course of every day. Back experts suggest that you also do back pain prevention exercises daily. However, if you train intensely every day without giving yourself a rest, you will likely get injured or become overtrained. When strength training, for example, rest at least 1 day between workouts before exercising the same muscle group. For cardiorespiratory endurance exercise, rest or exercise lightly the day after an intense or long-duration workout. Balancing the proper amount of rest and exercise will help you feel better and improve your fitness faster.

I'm just starting an exercise program. How much activity should I do at first? Be conservative. Walking is a good way to begin almost any fitness program. At first, walk for approximately 10 minutes, and then increase the distance and pace. After several weeks, you can progress to something more vigorous. Let your body be your guide. If the intensity and duration of a workout seem easy, increase them a little the next time. The key is to be progressive; don't try to achieve physical fitness in one or two workouts. Build your fitness gradually.

What are kickboxing and Tae Bo? Are they effective forms of exercise? Kickboxing and Tae Bo are group fitness workouts that combine martial arts maneuvers, boxing moves, and traditional group exercise activities. Participants in martial arts workouts repetitively execute a variety of punches and kicks, building movement combinations that involve the entire body. Workouts are often choreographed to moderately paced popular music and are continuous. Although more research is needed to clarify the actual training effects, the workouts certainly develop cardiovascular endurance, muscular endurance, and flexibility. Because of the potential for injury, classes should be led either by a certified fitness professional who has had ancillary training in teaching martial arts skills or a martial artist with qualifications as a fitness instructor. Other key safety elements include precise skill modeling and verbal instruction, moderate pacing, and an emphasis on health-related fitness development.

I'm concerned about my safety when I go for a jog or walk. What can I do to make sure that my training sessions are safe and enjoyable? A person exercising alone in the park can be a tempting target for criminals. Don't exercise alone. You are much safer training in a group or with a partner. Another alternative is to take an exercise class. Classes are fun and much safer than exercising by yourself. If you must train alone, try to exercise where there are plenty of people. A good bet is the local high school or college track.

Make sure you're wearing proper safety equipment. If you're riding a bike, wear a helmet. If you're playing racquetball or handball, wear eye protectors. Don't go in-line skating unless you're wearing the proper pads and protective equipment. If you are jogging at night, wear reflective clothing that can be seen easily.

Refer to Appendix A for more on personal safety.

SUMMARY

- Steps for putting together a complete fitness program include (1) setting realistic goals; (2) selecting activities to develop all the health-related components of fitness; (3) setting a target intensity, duration, and frequency for each activity; (4) setting up a system of mini-goals and rewards; (5) making lifestyle physical activity a part of the daily routine; (6) developing tools for monitoring progress; and (7) making a commitment.
- In selecting activities, consider fun and interest, your current skill and fitness levels, time and convenience, cost, and any special health concerns.
- Keys to beginning and maintaining a successful program include starting slowly, increasing intensity and duration gradually, finding a buddy, varying the activities and intensity of the program, and expecting fluctuations and lapses.
- Regular exercise is appropriate and highly beneficial for people with special health concerns or in particular stages of life; program modifications may be necessary to maximize safety.

FOR FURTHER EXPLORATION

Fit and Well Online Learning Center (www.mhhe.com/fahey5e)

Use the learning objectives, study guide questions, and glossary flashcards to review key terms and concepts and prepare for exams. You can extend your knowledge of personal fitness and gain experience in using the Internet as a resource by completing the activities and checking out the Web links for the topics in Chapter 7 marked with the World Wide Web icon. For this chapter, Internet activities explore fitness activities and strategies for creating a complete fitness program; there are also helpful Web links for chapter topics.

Daily Fitness and Nutrition Journal

Complete the program plan and fitness contract, and begin your program. Use the journal to record your activities and track your progress.

Health*Quest*

Use the Fitness Wizard on the Health*Quest* CD-ROM to create a schedule for your complete fitness program; select the Fitness Wizard option from the Fitness Planner portion of the Wellness Activities in the Fitness module. Once in the Fitness Wizard, choose the Physical Fitness Program option to build a program that includes activities to build all the health-related fitness components.

Books, Organizations, and Web Sites

See the listings for Chapters 2–7.

SELECTED BIBLIOGRAPHY

American College of Sports Medicine. 2001. *ACSM's Resource Manual for Guidelines for Exercise Testing and Prescription,* 4th ed. Philadelphia: Lippincott Williams & Wilkins.

American College of Sports Medicine. 2000. *ACSM's Guidelines for Exercise Testing and Prescription,* 6th ed. Baltimore, Md.: Lippincott Williams & Wilkins.

American College of Sports Medicine. 1998. ACSM position stand: Exercise and physical activity for older adults. *Medicine and Science in Sports and Exercise* 30(6): 992–1008.

American College of Sports Medicine. 1998. ACSM position stand: The recommended quantity and quality of exercise for developing and maintaining cardiorespiratory and muscular fitness, and flexibility in healthy adults. *Medicine and Science in Sports and Exercise* 30(6): 975–991.

American College of Sports Medicine and American Diabetes Association. 1997. Joint position statement: Diabetes mellitus and exercise. *Medicine and Science in Sports and Exercise* 29(12): I–VI.

Carroll, J. F., C. K. Kyser. 2002. Exercise training in obesity lowers blood pressure independent of weight change. *Medicine and Science in Sports and Exercise* 34(4): 596–601.

Chodzko-Zajko, W. J. 2001. Dispelling exercise myths promotes healthy aging. *ACSM Fit Society Page,* Fall.

Clapp, J. F., et al. 2002. Continuing regular exercise during pregnancy: effect of exercise volume on fetoplacental growth. *American Journal of Obstetrics and Gynecology* 186(1): 142–147.

Cooper, C. B. 2001. Exercise in chronic pulmonary disease: Aerobic exercise prescription. *Medicine and Science in Sports and Exercise* 33(7 Suppl): S671–S679.

Eriksson J. G. 1999. Exercise and the treatment of Type 2 diabetes mellitus: An update. *Sports Medicine* 27(6): 381–391.

Foster, C. K., et al. 2001. Physical activity and exercise training prescription for patients. *Cardiology Clinic* 19(3): 447–457.

Friedman, E. H. 2000. Exercise and don't smoke. *Journal of Pediatrics* 136(4): 564.

Galloway, M. T., and P. Jokl. 2000. Aging successfully: The importance of physical activity in maintaining health and function. *Journal of the American Academy of Orthopaedic Surgeons* 8(1): 37–44.

International Inline Skating Association. Health benefits: Burn, baby, burn (http://www.iisa.org/numbers/health.htm; retrieved December 4, 1999).

Karani, R., M. A. McLaughlin, and C. K. Cassel. 2001. Exercise in the healthy older adult. *American Journal of Geriatric Cardiology* 10(5): 269–273.

Mazzeo, R. S., and H. Tanaka. 2001. Exercise prescription for the elderly: Current recommendations. *Sports Medicine* 31(11): 809–818.

Moore, P. J., et al. 2002. Socioeconomic status and health: The role of sleep. *Psychosomatic Medicine* 64(2): 337–344.

National Sleep Foundation. 2002. *2002 Sleep in America Poll* (http://www.sleepfoundation.org/2002poll.html; retrieved May 14, 2002).

Olson, M. D., and H. N. Williford. 1999. Martial arts exercise. *ACSM's Health and Fitness Journal* 3(6): 6–14.

Reid, C. M., T. Maher, and G. L. Jennings. 2000. Substituting lifestyle management for pharmacological control of blood pressure. *Blood Pressure* 9(50): 267–274.

Satta, A. 2000. Exercise training in asthma. *Journal of Sports Medicine and Physical Fitness* 40(4): 277–283.

Walters, P. H. 2000. Sleep facts. *ACSM's Health and Fitness Journal* 4(6): 17–19, 28.

Workouts for special disorders. 2000. *Consumer Reports on Health,* January, 9.

SAMPLE PROGRAMS FOR POPULAR ACTIVITIES

Sample programs based on four different types of cardiorespiratory activities—walking/jogging/running, bicycling, swimming, and in-line skating—are presented below. Each sample program includes regular cardiorespiratory endurance exercise, resistance training, and stretching. To choose a sample program, first compare your fitness goals with the benefits of the different types of endurance exercise featured in the sample programs (see Table 7.1). Identify the programs that meet your fitness needs. Next, read through the descriptions of the programs you're considering, and decide which will work best for you based on your present routine, the potential for enjoyment, and adaptability to your lifestyle. If you choose one of these programs, complete the personal fitness program plan in Lab 7.1, just as if you had created a program from scratch.

No program will produce enormous changes in your fitness level in the first few weeks. Give your program a good chance. Follow the specifics of the program for 3–4 weeks. Then if the exercise program doesn't seem suitable, make adjustments to adapt it to your particular needs. But retain the basic elements of the program that make it effective for developing fitness.

General Guidelines

The following guidelines can help make the activity programs more effective for you.

- *Intensity.* To work effectively for cardiorespiratory endurance training or to improve body composition, you must raise your heart rate into its target zone. Monitor your pulse or use rates of perceived exertion to monitor your intensity.

  If you've been sedentary, begin very slowly. Give your muscles a chance to adjust to their increased workload. It's probably best to keep your heart rate below target until your body has had time to adjust to new demands. At first you may not need to work very hard to keep your heart rate in its target zone, but as your cardiorespiratory endurance improves, you will probably need to increase intensity.
- *Duration and frequency.* To experience training effects, you should exercise for 20–60 minutes at least three times a week.
- *Interval training.* Some of the sample programs involve continuous activity. Others rely on interval training, which calls for alternating a relief interval with exercise (walking after jogging, for example, or coasting after biking uphill). Interval training is an effective way to achieve progressive overload: When your heart rate gets too high, slow down to lower your pulse rate until you're at the low end of your target zone. Interval training can also prolong the total time you spend in exercise and delay the onset of fatigue.
- *Warm-up and cool-down.* Begin each exercise session with a 10-minute warm-up. Begin your activity at a slow pace and work up gradually to your target heart rate. Always slow down gradually at the end of your exercise session to bring your system back to its normal state. It's a good idea to do stretching exercises to increase your flexibility after cardiorespiratory exercise or strength training because your muscles will be warm and ready to stretch.
- *Record keeping.* After each exercise session, record your daily distance or time on a progress chart.

WALKING/JOGGING/RUNNING SAMPLE PROGRAM

Walking, jogging, and running are the most popular forms of training for people who want to improve cardiorespiratory endurance; they also improve body composition and muscular endurance of the legs. It's not always easy to distinguish among these three endurance activities. For clarity and consistency, we'll consider walking to be any on-foot exercise of less than 5 miles per hour, jogging any pace between 5 and 7.5 miles per hour, and running any pace faster than that. Table 1 divides walking, jogging, and running into nine categories, with rates of speed (in both miles per hour and minutes per mile) and calorie costs for each. The faster your pace or the longer you exercise, the more calories you burn. The greater the number of calories burned, the higher the potential training effects of these activities. Tables 2 and 3 on p. 192 contain sample walking/jogging programs by time and distance.

Equipment and Technique

These activities require no special skills, expensive equipment, or unusual facilities. Comfortable clothing, well-fitted walking or running shoes, and a stopwatch or ordinary watch with a second hand are all you need.

Developing Cardiorespiratory Endurance

The four variations of the basic walking/jogging/running sample program that follow are designed to help you regulate the intensity, duration, and frequency of your program. Use the following guidelines to choose the variation that is right for you.

- *Variation 1: Walking (Starting).* Choose this program if you have medical restrictions, are recovering from illness or surgery, tire easily after short walks, are obese, or have a sedentary lifestyle, and if you want to prepare for the advanced walking program to improve cardiorespiratory endurance, body composition, and muscular endurance.
- *Variation 2: Advanced Walking.* Choose this program if you already can walk comfortably for 30 minutes and if you want to develop and maintain cardiorespiratory fitness, a lean body, and muscular endurance.
- *Variation 3: Preparing for a Jogging Program.* Choose this program if you already can walk comfortably for 30 minutes and if you want to prepare for the jogging/running program to improve cardiorespiratory endurance, body composition, and muscular endurance.
- *Variation 4: Jogging/Running.* Choose this program if you already can jog comfortably without muscular discomfort, if you already can jog for 15 minutes without stopping or 30 minutes with brief walking intervals within your target heart rate range, and if you want to develop and maintain a high level of cardiorespiratory fitness, a lean body, and muscular endurance.

SAMPLE PROGRAM TABLE 1 *Caloric Costs for Walking/Jogging/Running*

This table gives the calorie costs of walking, jogging, and running for slow, moderate, and fast paces. Calculations for calorie costs are approximate and assume a level terrain. A hilly terrain would result in higher calorie costs. To get an estimate of the number of calories you burn, multiply your weight by the calories per minute per pound for the speed at which you're doing the activity (listed in the right-hand column), and then multiply that by the number of minutes you exercise.

Activity	SPEED: Miles per Hour	SPEED: Minutes: Seconds per Mile	Calories per Minute per Pound
Walking			
Slow	2.0	30:00	.020
	2.5	24:00	.023
Moderate	3.0	20:00	.026
	3.5	17:08	.029
Fast	4.0	15:00	.037
	4.5	13:20	.048
Jogging			
Slow	5.0	12:00	.060
	5.5	11:00	.074
Moderate	6.0	10:00	.081
	6.5	9:00	.088
Fast	7.0	8:35	.092
	7.5	8:00	.099
Running			
Slow	8.5	7:00	.111
Moderate	9.0	6:40	.116
Fast	10.0	6:00	.129
	11.0	5:30	.141

SOURCE: Kusinitz, I., and M. Fine. 1995. *Your Guide to Getting Fit*, 3d ed. Mountain View, Calif.: Mayfield. Reprinted with permission from The McGraw-Hill Companies.

Variation 1: Walking (Starting)

Intensity, duration, and frequency: Walk at first for 15 minutes at a pace that keeps your heart rate below your target zone. Gradually increase to 30-minute sessions. The distance you travel will probably be 1–2 miles. At the beginning, walk every other day. You can gradually increase to daily walking if you want to burn more calories (helpful if you want to change body composition).

Calorie cost: Work up to using 90–135 calories in each session (see Table 1). To increase calorie costs to the target level, walk for a longer time or for a longer distance rather than sharply increasing speed.

At the beginning: Start at whatever level is most comfortable. Maintain a normal, easy pace, and stop to rest as often as you need to. Never prolong a walk past the point of comfort. When walking with a friend (a good motivation), let a comfortable conversation be your guide to pace.

As you progress: Once your muscles have become adjusted to the exercise program, increase the duration of your sessions—but by no more than 10% each week. Increase your intensity only enough to keep your heart rate just below your target. When you're able to walk 1.5 miles in 30 minutes, using 90–135 calories per session, you should consider moving on to Variation 2 or 3. Don't be discouraged by lack of immediate progress and don't try to speed things up by overdoing. Remember that pace and heart rate can vary with the terrain, the weather, and other factors.

Variation 2: Advanced Walking

Intensity, duration, and frequency: Start at a pace at the lower end of your target heart rate zone and begin soon afterward to increase your pace. This might boost your heart rate into the upper levels of your target zone, which is fine for brief periods. But don't overdo the intervals of fast walking. Slow down after a short time to drop your pulse rate. Vary your pattern to allow for intervals of slow, medium, and fast walking. Walk at first for 30 minutes and gradually increase your walking time until eventually you reach 60 minutes, all the while maintaining your target heart rate. The distance you walk will probably be 2–4 miles. Walk at least every other day.

Calorie cost: Work up to using about 200–350 calories in each session (see Table 1).

At the beginning: Begin by walking somewhat faster than you did in Variation 1. Check your pulse to make sure you keep your heart rate within your target zone. Slow down when necessary to lower your heart rate when going up hills or when extending the duration of your walks.

As you progress: As your heart rate adjusts to the increased workload, gradually increase your pace and your total walking time. Gradually lengthen the periods of fast walking and shorten the relief intervals of slow walking, always maintaining target heart rate. Eventually, you will reach the fitness level you would like to maintain. And to maintain that level of fitness, continue to burn the same amount of calories in each session.

Vary your program by changing the pace and distance walked, or by walking routes with different terrains and views. Gauge your progress toward whatever calorie goal you've set by using Table 1.

Variation 3: Preparing for a Jogging Program

Intensity, duration, and frequency: Start by walking at a moderate pace (3–4 miles per hour or 15–20 minutes per mile). Staying within your target heart rate zone, begin to add brief intervals of slow jogging (5–6 miles per hour or 10–12 minutes per mile). Keep the walking intervals constant at 60 seconds or at 110 yards, but gradually increase the jogging intervals until eventually you jog 4 minutes for each minute of walking. You'll probably cover between 1.5 and 2.5 miles. Each exercise session should last 15–30 minutes. Exercise every other day. If your goals include changing body composition and you want to exercise more frequently, walk on days you're not jogging.

Calorie cost: Work up to using 200–350 calories in each session (see Table 1).

At the beginning: Start slowly. Until your muscles adjust to jogging, you may need to exercise at less than your target heart

SAMPLE PROGRAM TABLE 2 *Walking/Jogging Progression by Time*

This table is based on a walking interval of 3.75 miles per hour, measured in seconds, and a jogging interval of 5.5 miles per hour, measured in minutes:seconds. The combination of the two intervals equals a single set. In the Number of Sets column, the higher figure represents the maximum number of sets to be completed.

	Walk Interval (sec)	Jog Interval (min:sec)	Number of Sets	Total Distance (mi)	Total Time (min:sec)
Stage 1	:60	:30	10–15	1.0–1.7	15:00–22:30
Stage 2	:60	:60	8–13	1.2–2.0	16:00–26:00
Stage 3	:60	2:00	5–19	1.3–2.3	15:00–27:00
Stage 4	:60	3:00	5–7	1.6–2.4	16:00–28:00
Stage 5	:60	4:00	3–6	1.5–2.7	15:00–30:00

SOURCE: Kusinitz, I., and M. Fine. 1995. *Your Guide to Getting Fit,* 3d ed. Mountain View, Calif.: Mayfield. Reprinted with permission from The MacGraw-Hill Companies.

SAMPLE PROGRAM TABLE 3 *Walking/Jogging Progression by Distance*

This table is based on a walking interval of 3.75 miles per hour, measured in yards, and a jogging interval of 5.5 miles per hour, also measured in yards. The combination of the two intervals equals a single set. (One lap around a typical track is 440 yards.)

	Walk Interval (yd)	Jog Interval (yd)	Number of Sets	Total Distance (mi)	Total Time (min:sec)
Stage 1	110	55	11–21	1.0–2.0	15:00–28:12
Stage 2	110	110	16	2.0	26:56
Stage 3	110	220	11	2.0	26:02
Stage 4	110	330	8	2.0	24:24
Stage 5	110	440	7	2.2	26:05
Stage 6	110	440	8	2.5	29:49

SOURCE: Kusinitz, I., and M. Fine. 1995. *Your Guide to Getting Fit,* 3d ed. Mountain View, Calif.: Mayfield. Reprinted with permission from The McGraw-Hill Companies.

rate. At the outset, expect to do two to four times as much walking as jogging, even more if you're relatively inexperienced. Be guided by how comfortable you feel—and by your heart rate—in setting the pace for your progress. Follow the guidelines presented in Chapter 3 for exercising in hot or cold weather. Drink enough liquids to stay adequately hydrated, particularly in hot weather. In addition, use the proper running technique, described below.

- Run with your back straight and your head up. Look straight ahead, not at your feet. Shift your pelvis forward and tuck your buttocks in.
- Hold your arms slightly away from your body. Your elbows should be bent so that your forearms are parallel to the ground. You may cup your hands, but do not clench your fists. Allow your arms to swing loosely and rhythmically with each stride.
- Your heel should hit the ground first in each stride. Then roll forward onto the ball of your foot and push off for the next stride. If you find this difficult, you can try a more flat-footed style, but don't land on the balls of your feet.
- Keep your steps short by allowing your foot to strike the ground in line with your knee. Keep your knees bent at all times.
- Breathe deeply through your mouth. Try to use your abdominal muscles rather than just your chest muscles to take deep breaths.
- Stay relaxed.

As you progress: Adjust your ratio of walking to jogging to keep within your target heart rate zone as much as possible. When you have progressed to the point where most of your 30-minute session is spent jogging, consider moving on to Variation 4. To find a walking/jogging progression that suits you, refer to Tables 2 and 3 (one uses time, the other distance). Which one you choose will depend, to some extent, on where you work out. If you have access to a track or can use a measured distance with easily visible landmarks to indicate yardage covered, you may find it convenient to use distance as your organizing principle. If you'll be using parks, streets, or woods, time intervals (measured with a watch) would probably work better. The progressions in Tables 2 and 3 are not meant to be rigid; they are guidelines to help you develop your own rate of progress. Let your progress be guided by your heart rate and increase your intensity and duration only to achieve your target zone.

Variation 4: Jogging/Running

Intensity, duration, and frequency: The key is to exercise within your target heart rate zone. Most people who sustain a continuous jog/run program will find that they can stay within their target heart rate zone with a speed of 5.5–7.5 miles per hour (8–11 minutes per mile). Start by jogging steadily for 15 minutes. Gradually increase your jog/run session to a regular 30–60 minutes (or about 2.5–7 miles). Exercise at least every other day. Increasing frequency by doing other activities on alternate days will place less stress on the weight-bearing parts of your lower body than will a daily program of jogging/running.

Calorie cost: Use about 300–750 calories in each session (see Table 1).

At the beginning: The greater number of calories you burn per minute makes this program less time-consuming for altering body composition than the three other variations in the walking/jogging/running program.

As you progress: If you choose this variation, you probably already have a moderate-to-high level of cardiorespiratory fitness. To stay within your target heart rate zone, increase your distance or both pace and distance as needed. Add variety to your workouts by varying your route, intensity, and duration. Alternate short runs with long ones. If you run for 60 minutes one day, try running for 30 minutes the next session. Or try doing sets that alternate hard and easy intervals—even walking, if you feel like it. You can also try a road race now and then, but be careful not to do too much too soon.

Developing Muscular Strength and Endurance

Walking, jogging, and running provide muscular endurance workouts for your lower body; they also develop muscular strength of the lower body to a lesser degree. To develop muscular strength and endurance of the upper body, and to make greater and more rapid gains in lower-body strength, you need to include resistance training in your fitness program. Use the general wellness weight training program from Chapter 4, or tailor one to fit your personal fitness goals. If you'd like to increase your running speed and performance, you might want to focus your program on lower-body exercises. (Don't neglect upper-body strength, however; it is important for overall wellness.) Regardless of the strength training exercises you choose, follow the guidelines for successful training:

- Train 2–3 days per week.
- Perform 1 or more sets of 8–12 repetitions of 8–10 exercises.
- Include exercises that work all the major muscle groups: neck, shoulders, chest, arms, upper and lower back, abdomen, thighs, and calves.

Depending on the amount of time you are able to set aside for exercise, you may find it more convenient to alternate between your cardiorespiratory endurance workouts and your muscular strength and endurance workouts. In other words, walk or jog one day and strength train the next day.

Developing Flexibility

To round out your fitness program, you also need to include exercises that develop flexibility. The best time for a flexibility workout is when your muscles are warm, as they are immediately following cardiorespiratory endurance exercise or strength training. Perform the stretching routine presented in Chapter 5 or one that you have created to meet your own goals and preferences. Be sure to pay special attention to the hamstrings and quadriceps, which are not worked through their complete range of motion during walking or jogging. As you put your program together, remember the basic structure of a successful flexibility program:

- Stretch at least 2–3 days per week, preferably when muscles are warm.
- Stretch all the major muscle groups.
- Stretch to the point of mild discomfort and hold for 10–30 seconds.
- Repeat each stretch at least 4 times.

BICYCLING SAMPLE PROGRAM

Bicycling can also lead to large gains in physical fitness. For many people, cycling is a pleasant and economical alternative to driving and a convenient way to build fitness.

Equipment and Technique

Cycling has its own special array of equipment, including headgear, lighting, safety pennants, and special shoes. The bike is the most expensive item, ranging from about $100 to well over $1000. Avoid making a large investment until you're sure you'll use your bike regularly. While investigating what the marketplace has to offer, rent or borrow a bike. Consider your intended use of the bike. Most cyclists who are interested primarily in fitness are best served by a sturdy 10-speed rather than a mountain bike or sport bike. Stationary cycles are good for rainy days and areas that have harsh winters.

Clothing for bike riding shouldn't be restrictive or binding, nor should it be so loose-fitting or so long that it might get caught in the chain. Clothing worn on the upper body should be comfortable but not so loose that it catches the wind and slows you down. Always wear a helmet to help prevent injury in case of a fall or crash. Wearing glasses or goggles can protect the eyes from dirt, small objects, and irritation from wind.

To avoid saddle soreness and injury, choose a soft or padded saddle and adjust it to a height that allows your legs to almost reach full extension while pedaling. Make certain the saddle doesn't put too much pressure on sensitive areas. Wear a pair of well-padded gloves if your hands tend to become numb while riding or if you begin to develop blisters or calluses. To prevent backache and neck strain, warm up thoroughly and periodically shift the position of your hands on the handlebars and your body in the saddle. Keep your arms relaxed and don't lock your elbows. To protect your knees from strain, pedal with your feet pointed straight ahead or very slightly inward and don't pedal in high gear for long periods.

Bike riding requires a number of precise skills that practice makes automatic. If you've never ridden before, consider taking a course. In fact, many courses are not just for beginners. They'll help you develop skills in braking, shifting, and handling emergencies, as well as teach you ways of caring for and repairing your bike. For safe cycling, follow these rules:

- Always wear a helmet.
- Keep on the correct side of the road. Bicycling against traffic is usually illegal and always dangerous.
- Obey all traffic signs and signals.
- On public roads, ride in single file, except in low-traffic areas (if the law permits). Ride in a straight line; don't swerve or weave in traffic.
- Be alert; anticipate the movements of other traffic and pedestrians. Listen for approaching traffic that is out of your line of vision.
- Slow down at street crossings. Check both ways before crossing.
- Use hand signals—the same as for automobile drivers—if you intend to stop or turn. Use audible signals to warn those in your path.
- Maintain full control. Avoid anything that interferes with your vision. Don't jeopardize your ability to steer by carrying anything (including people) on the handlebars.
- Keep your bicycle in good shape. Brakes, gears, saddle, wheels, and tires should always be in good condition.
- See and be seen. Use a headlight at night and equip your bike with rear reflectors. Use side reflectors on pedals, front and rear. Wear light-colored clothing or use reflective tape at night; wear bright colors or use fluorescent tape by day.
- Be courteous to other road users. Anticipate the worst and practice preventive cycling.
- Use a rear-view mirror.

Developing Cardiorespiratory Endurance

Cycling is an excellent way to develop and maintain cardiorespiratory endurance and a healthy body composition.

Intensity, duration, and frequency: If you've been inactive for a long time, begin your cycling program at a heart rate that is 10–20% below your target zone. Once you feel at home on your bike, try 1 mile at a comfortable speed, and then stop and check your heart rate. Increase your speed gradually until you can cycle at 12–15 miles per hour (4–5 minutes per mile), a speed fast enough to bring most new cyclists' heart rate into their target zone. Allow your pulse rate to be your guide: More highly fit individuals may need to ride faster to achieve their target heart rate. Cycling for at least 20 minutes three times a week will improve your fitness.

Calorie cost: Use Table 4 to determine the number of calories you burn during each outing. You can increase the number of calories burned by cycling faster or for a longer duration (it's usually better to increase distance rather than to add speed).

At the beginning: It may require several outings to get the muscles and joints of your legs and hips adjusted to this new activity. Begin each outing with a 10-minute warm-up that includes stretches for your hamstrings and your back and neck muscles. Until you become a skilled cyclist, select routes with the fewest hazards and avoid heavy automobile traffic.

As you progress: Interval training is also effective with bicycling. Simply increase your speed for periods of 4–8 minutes or for specific distances, such as 1–2 miles. Then coast for 2–3 minutes. Alternate the speed intervals and slow intervals for a total of 20–60 minutes, depending on your level of fitness. Hilly terrain is also a form of interval training.

Developing Muscular Strength and Endurance

Bicycling develops a high level of endurance and a moderate level of strength in the muscles of the lower body. To develop muscular strength and endurance of the upper body—and to make greater and more rapid gains in lower-body strength—you need to include resistance training as part of your fitness program. Use the general wellness weight training program from Chapter 4, or tailor one to fit your personal fitness goals. If one of your goals is to increase your cycling speed and performance, be sure to include exercises for the quadriceps, hamstrings, and buttocks muscles in your strength training program. No matter which exercises you include in your program, follow the general guidelines for successful and safe training:

- Train 2–3 days per week.
- Perform 1 or more sets of 8–12 repetitions of 8–10 exercises.
- Include exercises that work all the major muscle groups: neck, shoulders, chest, arms, upper and lower back, abdomen, things, and calves.

Depending on your schedule, you may find it more convenient to alternate between your cardiorespiratory endurance workouts and your muscular strength and endurance workouts. In other words, cycle one day and strength train the next day.

Developing Flexibility

A complete fitness program also includes exercises that develop flexibility. The best time for a flexibility workout is when your muscles are warm, as they are immediately following a session of cardiorespiratory endurance exercise or strength training. Perform the stretching routine presented in Chapter 5, or develop one that meets your own goals and preferences. Pay special attention to the hamstrings and quadriceps, which are not worked through their complete range of motion during bike riding, and to the muscles in your lower back, shoulders, and neck. As you put your stretching program together, remember these basic guidelines:

- Stretch at least 2–3 days per week, preferably when muscles are warm.
- Stretch all the major muscle groups.
- Stretch to the point of mild discomfort and hold for 10–30 seconds.
- Repeat each stretch at least 4 times.

SAMPLE PROGRAM TABLE 4 *Calorie Costs for Bicycling*

This table gives the approximate calorie costs per pound of body weight for cycling from 5 to 60 minutes for distances of .50 mile up to 15 miles on a level terrain. To use the table, find on the horizontal line the time most closely approximating the number of minutes you cycle. Next, locate on the vertical column the approximate distance in miles you cover. The figure at the intersection represents an estimate of the calories used per minute per pound of body weight. Multiply this figure by your own body weight. Then multiply the product of these two figures by the number of minutes you cycle to get the total number of calories burned. For example, assuming you weight 154 pounds and cycle 6 miles in 40 minutes, you would burn 260 calories: 154 × .042 (calories per pound, from table) = 6.5 × 40 (minutes) = 260 calories burned.

	TIME (MIN)											
Distance (mi)	5	10	15	20	25	30	35	40	45	50	55	60
.50	.032											
1.00	.062	.032										
1.50		.042	.032									
2.00		.062	.039	.032								
3.00			.062	.042	.036	.032						
4.00				.062	.044	.039	.035	.032				
5.00				.097	.062	.045	.041	.037	.035	.032		
6.00					.088	.062	.047	.042	.039	.036	.034	.032
7.00						.081	.062	.049	.043	.040	.038	.036
8.00							.078	.062	.050	.044	.041	.039
9.00								.076	.062	.051	.045	.042
10.00								.097	.074	.062	.051	.045
11.00									.093	.073	.062	.052
12.00										.088	.072	.062
13.00											.084	.071
14.00												.081
15.00												.097

SOURCE: Kusinitz, I., and M. Fine. 1995. *Your Guide to Getting Fit,* 3d ed. Mountain View, Calif.: Mayfield. Reprinted with permission from The McGraw-Hill Companies.

SWIMMING SAMPLE PROGRAM

Swimming is excellent for developing all-around fitness. Because water supports the body weight of the swimmer, swimming places less stress than weight-bearing activities on joints, ligaments, and tendons and tends to cause fewer injuries.

Equipment and Safety Guidelines

Aside from having access to a swimming pool, the only equipment required for a swimming program is a swimsuit and a pair of swimming goggles to protect the eyes from irritation in chlorinated pools. Following these few simple rules can help keep you safe and healthy during your swimming sessions:

- Swim only in a pool with a qualified lifeguard on duty.
- Always walk carefully on wet surfaces.
- Dry your ears well after swimming. If you experience the symptoms of swimmer's ear (itching, discharge, or even a partial hearing loss), consult your physician. If you swim while recovering from swimmer's ear, protect your ears with a few drops of lanolin on a wad of lamb's wool.
- To avoid back pain, try not to arch your back excessively when you swim.
- Be courteous to others in the pool.

If you swim in a setting other than a pool with a lifeguard, remember the following important rules:

- Don't swim beyond your skill and endurance limits.
- Avoid being chilled by water colder than 70°F.
- Never drink alcohol before going swimming.
- Never swim alone.

Developing Cardiorespiratory Endurance

Any one or any combination of common swimming strokes—front crawl stroke, breaststroke, backstroke, butterfly stroke, sidestroke, or elementary backstroke—can help develop and maintain cardiorespiratory fitness. (Swimming may not be as helpful as walking, jogging, or cycling for body fat loss.)

Intensity, duration, and frequency: Because swimming is not a weight-bearing activity and is not done in an upright position, it elicits a lower heart rate per minute. Therefore, you need to adjust your target heart rate zone. To calculate your target heart rate for swimming, use this formula:

Maximum swimming heart rate (MSHR) = 205 − age

Target heart rate zone = 65–90% of MSHR

For example, a 19-year-old would calculate her target heart rate zone for swimming as follows:

MSHR = 205 − 19 = 186 bpm

65% intensity: 0.65 × 186 = 121 bpm

90% intensity: 0.90 × 186 = 167 bpm

SAMPLE PROGRAM TABLE 5 *Calorie Costs for Swimming*

To use this table, find on the top horizontal row the distance in yards that most closely approximates the distance you swim. Next, locate on the appropriate vertical column (below the distance in yards) the time it takes you to swim the distance. Then locate in the first column on the left the approximate number of calories burned per minute per pound for the time and distance. To find the total number of calories burned, multiply your weight by the calories per minute per pound. Then multiply the product of these two numbers by the time it takes you to swim the distance (minutes:seconds). For example, assuming you weigh 130 pounds and swim 500 yards in 20 minutes, you would burn 106 calories: 130 × .041 (calories per pound, from table) = 5.33 × 20 (minutes) = 106 calories burned.

	DISTANCE (YD)					
Calories per Minute per Pound	25	100	150	250	500	750
.033	1:15	5:00	7:30	12:30	25:00	30:30
.041	1:00	4:00	6:00	10:00	20:00	30:00
.049	0:50	3:20	5:00	8:20	18:40	25:00
.057	0:43	2:52	4:18	7:10	17:20	21:30
.065	0:37.5	2:30	3:45	6:15	10:00	
.073	0:33	2:13	3:20	5:30	8:50	
.081	0:30	2:00	3:00	5:00	8:00	
.090	0:27	1:48	2:42	4:30	7:12	
.097	0:25	1:40	2:30	4:10	6:30	

SOURCE: Kusinitz, I., and M. Fine. 1995. *Your Guide to Getting Fit,* 3d ed. Mountain View, Calif. Mayfield. Reprinted with permission from The McGraw-Hill Companies.

Base your duration of swimming on your intensity and target calorie costs. Swim at least three times a week.

Calorie cost: Calories burned while swimming are the result of the pace: how far you swim and how fast (see Table 5). Work up to using at least 300 calories per session.

At the beginning: If you are an inexperienced swimmer, invest the time and money for instruction. You'll make more rapid gains in fitness if you learn correct swimming technique. If you've been sedentary and haven't done any swimming for a long time, begin your program with 2–3 weeks, three times a week, of leisurely swimming at a pace that keeps your heart rate 10–20% below your target zone. Start swimming laps of the width of the pool if you can't swim the length. To keep your heart rate below target, take rest intervals as needed. Swim one lap, then rest 15–90 seconds as needed. Start with 10 minutes of swim/rest intervals and work up to 20 minutes. How long it takes will depend on your swimming skills and muscular fitness.

As you progress: Gradually increase the duration, or the intensity, or both duration and intensity of your swimming to raise your heart rate to a comfortable level within your target zone. Gradually increase your swimming intervals and decrease your rest intervals as you progress. Once you can swim the length of the pool at a pace that keeps your heart rate on target, continue swim/rest intervals for 20 minutes. Your rest intervals should be 30–45 seconds. You may find it helpful to get out of the pool during your rest intervals and walk until you've lowered your heart rate. Next, swim two laps of the pool length per swim interval and continue swim/rest intervals for 30 minutes. For the 30-second rest interval, walk (or rest) until you've lowered your heart rate. Gradually increase the number of laps you swim consecutively and the total duration of your session until you reach your target calorie expenditure and fitness level. But take care not to swim at too fast a pace: It can raise your heart rate too high and limit your ability to sustain your swimming. Alternating strokes can rest your muscles and help prolong your swimming time. A variety of strokes will also let you work more muscle groups.

Developing Muscular Strength and Endurance

The swimming program outlined in this section will result in moderate gains in strength and large gains in endurance in the muscles used during the strokes you've chosen. To develop strength and endurance in all the muscles of the body, you need to include resistance training as part of your fitness program. Use the general wellness weight training program from Chapter 4, or tailor one to fit your personal fitness goals. To improve your swimming performance, include exercises that work key muscles. For example, if you swim primarily front crawl, include exercises to increase strength in your shoulders, arms, and upper back. (Training the muscles you use during swimming can also help prevent injuries.) Regardless of which strength training exercise you include in your program, follow the general guidelines for successful training:

- Train 2–3 days per week.
- Perform 1 or more sets of 8–12 repetitions of 8–10 exercises.
- Include exercises that work all the major muscle groups: neck, shoulders, chest, arms, upper and lower back, abdomen, thighs, and calves.

Depending on the amount of time you have for exercise, you might want to schedule your cardiorespiratory endurance workouts and your muscular strength and endurance workouts on alternate days. In other words, swim one day and strength train the next day.

Developing Flexibility

For a complete fitness program, you also need to include exercises that develop flexibility. The best time for a flexibility workout is when your muscles are warm, as they are immediately following cardiorespiratory endurance exercise or strength training. Perform the stretching routine presented in Chapter 5 or one you have created to meet your own goals and preferences. Be sure to pay special attention to the muscles you use during swimming, particularly the shoulders and back. As you put your program together, remember the basic structure of a successful flexibility program:

- Stretch at least 2–3 days per week, preferably when muscles are warm.
- Stretch all the major muscle groups.
- Stretch to the point of mild discomfort and hold for 10–30 seconds.
- Repeat each stretch at least 4 times.

In-line skating is convenient and inexpensive (after the initial outlay for equipment); it can be done on city streets, on paved bike paths and trails, and in parks. If done intensively enough, skating can provide a cardiorespiratory endurance workout comparable to the workouts provided by jogging and cycling. Studies indicate that skating consumes about as many calories as jogging. An advantage of skating over jogging is that skating is low impact, so it is less harmful to the knees and ankles. An advantage of skating over bicycling is that it works the hamstring muscle in the back of the thigh. Skating develops lower-body strength and endurance, working all the muscles of the leg and hip and strengthening the muscles and connective tissues surrounding the ankles, knees, and hips.

Equipment

To skate safely and enjoyably, you will need a pair of comfortable, sturdy, quality skates and adequate safety equipment. The skate consists of a hard polyurethane shell or outer boot; a padded foam liner; and a frame or chassis that holds the wheels, bearings, spacers, and brake. If you want to try out the sport before making a commitment, rent your skates and equipment from a skate shop. If you are buying, plan to spend about \$110–\$200 for skates that meet the basic needs of most recreational skaters. Shop for the best combination of price, quality, comfort, and service.

Essential safety equipment includes a helmet, elbow pads, knee pads, and wrist guards. (Wrist injuries are the most common in-line skating injury.) You may want to put reflective tape on your skates for those occasions when you don't get home before dark. Carry moleskin or adhesive bandages with you in case you start to develop a blister while skating. (For more on safety, see Appendix A.)

Technique

In-line skating uses many of the skills and techniques of ice skating, roller skating, and skiing, so if you have ever participated in any of those activities, you will probably take to in-line skating fairly readily. Many people begin without instruction, but instruction will allow you to progress more quickly.

To begin, center your weight equally over both skates, bend your knees slightly so your nose, knees, and toes are all in the same line, and look straight ahead. Keep your weight forward over the balls of your feet; don't lean back.

To skate, use a stroke, glide, stroke, glide rhythm (rather than a series of quick, short strokes). Push with one leg while gliding with the other. Shift your body weight back and forth so it is always centered over the gliding skate.

To stop, use your brake, located on the back of the right skate in most skates. With knees bent and arms extended in front of your body, move the right foot forward, shift your weight to your left leg, and lift your right toe until the brake pad touches the ground and stops you. An alternative stop is the T-stop, in which you drag one skate behind the other at a 90-degree angle to the direction of your forward motion.

If you lose your balance and are about to fall, lower your center of gravity by bending at the waist and putting your hands on your knees. If you can't regain your balance, try to fall forward, directing the impact to your wrist guards and knee pads. Try not to fall backward.

Again, instruction can help you learn many moves and techniques that will make the sport safer and more enjoyable.

Developing Cardiorespiratory Endurance

Studies have shown that in-line skaters raise their heart rates and oxygen consumption comparably to joggers, bicyclers, and walkers. Skaters reached 60–75% of $\dot{V}O_{2max}$ by skating continuously (not pushing off and gliding for several seconds) at 10.6–12.5 mph for 20–30 minutes. It may be difficult for recreational skaters to safely skate this fast for this long, however, given the typical constraints of city and suburban streets. Experts suggest skating uphill as much as possible to reach the level of intensity that builds cardiorespiratory endurance. If you can reach and maintain higher speeds in parks or on paved paths, do so, but always skate safely.

Intensity, duration, and frequency: Start your early skating sessions at a pace that keeps your heart rate about 10–20% below your target zone. Skate for 5–10 minutes, and then check your heart rate. Increase your speed gradually until you can skate at about 10 miles per hour (6 minutes per mile). Use your pulse as a guide to speed, aiming for 65% of your target heart rate zone. To achieve cardiorespiratory benefits, you will have to skate at a continuous and relatively intense pace for at least 20 minutes three times a week. The more fit you are, the more intensively you will need to skate to reach your target heart rate.

Calorie cost: Use Table 6 on p. 198 to determine the approximate number of calories you burn during each outing. You can increase the number of calories burned by skating faster, for a longer time, or uphill.

At the beginning: If you are a beginner, practice skating in an empty schoolyard or a parking lot. As you become confident with the basic techniques, you can move on to streets, parks, and paved bike trails. Maintain an easy pace, alternating stroking and gliding.

Begin each outing with a 5- to 10-minute warm-up of walking, jogging, or even slow skating. Once your muscles are warm, you can do some stretches to help loosen and warm up the primary muscles used during skating. These muscles include the quadriceps, hamstrings, buttocks, hips, groin, ankles, calves, and lower back. You can also save the stretches for the end of the workout.

To launch an in-line skating fitness program, aim for slow, long-distance workouts at first. Start by skating for 15 minutes and gradually increase your sessions to 20–30 minutes of continuous skating (about 3.5–5 miles). Try to skate about 20 miles a week, or 5 miles a day (about 30 minutes) 4 days a week.

As you progress: After the first week or two, add about a mile a day, up to 40 miles per week (60 minutes a day). To increase intensity, add some hills, sprints (bursts of short, rapid striding), and interval training (periods of intensive exercise at your target heart rate alternating with timed rest periods when your heart rate drops below your target zone). Try to skate 30–60 minutes a day four or more times a week.

The harder and faster you skate, the more intensive your workout will be and the more your cardiorespiratory endurance and muscular strength will improve. The longer and more often you skate, the more your endurance will increase.

Developing Muscular Strength and Endurance

In-line skating develops the muscles in the entire upper leg, buttocks, and hip; lower back; and upper arms and shoulders when arms are swung vigorously. To make greater gains in

SAMPLE PROGRAM TABLE 6 *Calorie Costs for In-Line Skating*

To estimate the number of calories you burn, first determine your approximate speed (use the Minutes: Seconds per Mile column if necessary), multiply the calories per minute per pound by your weight, and then multiply that figure by the number of minutes you skate. For example assuming you weigh 145 pounds and skate at 10 mph for 30 minutes, you would burn 273 calories: 145 × .063 (calories per pound, from table) = 9.1 × 30 (minutes) = 273 calories burned. Calculations are approximate.

SPEED		
Miles per Hour	Minutes: Seconds per Mile	Calories per Minute per Pound
8	7:30	.041
9	6:40	.053
10	6:00	.063
11	5:25	.072
12	5:00	.084
13	4:35	.095
14	4:20	.105
15	4:00	.115

SOURCES: Adapted from International Inline Skating Association. 1999. *Health Benefits of Inline Skating* (http://www.iisa.org/numbers/health.htm, retrieved April 7, 2000); Wallick, M. E., et al. 1995. Physiological responses to in-line skating compared to treadmill running. *Medicine and Science in Sports and Exercise* 27(2): 242–248.

lower-body strength and to develop the entire upper body, include resistance training in your overall fitness program. Use the general wellness weight training program from Chapter 4, or tailor one to fit your personal fitness goals. No matter which exercises you include in your program, follow the general guidelines for successful and safe training:

- Train 2–3 days per week.
- Perform 1 or more sets of 8–12 repetitions of 8–10 exercises.
- Include exercises that work all the major muscle groups: neck, shoulders, chest, arms, upper and lower back, thighs, and calves.

Depending on your schedule, you may find it more convenient to skate and weight train on alternate days.

Developing Flexibility

The best times for a flexibility workout are when your muscles are warm, so stretch after a short warm-up at the beginning of your skating session, or after your skating session, or after a weight training session. Use the stretching routine presented in Chapter 5, or develop one that meets your own goals and preferences. Pay particular attention to your quadriceps, hamstrings, buttocks, hips, groin, ankles, calves, and lower back. Remember these basic guidelines:

- Stretch at least 2–3 days per week, preferably when muscles are warm.
- Stretch all the major muscle groups.
- Stretch to the point of mild discomfort and hold for 10–30 seconds.
- Repeat each stretch at least 4 times.

Name ______________________ Section ______________ Date ______________

LAB 7.1 *A Personal Fitness Program Plan and Contract*

A. I, ______________________ (name), am contracting with myself to follow a physical fitness program to work toward the following goals:

Specific or short-term goals (include current status for each)

1. ______________________
2. ______________________
3. ______________________
4. ______________________

General or long-term goals

1. ______________________
2. ______________________
3. ______________________
4. ______________________

B. My program plan is as follows:

Activities	Components (Check ✓)					*Intensity**	*Duration*	Frequency (Check ✓)						
	CRE	MS	ME	F	BC			M	Tu	W	Th	F	Sa	Su

*Conduct activities for achieving CRE goals in your target range for heart rate or RPE.

C. My program will begin on __________ (date). My program includes the following schedule of mini-goals. For each step in my program, I will give myself the reward listed.

______________________ (mini-goal 1) __________ (date) __________ (reward)

______________________ (mini-goal 2) __________ (date) __________ (reward)

______________________ (mini-goal 3) __________ (date) __________ (reward)

______________________ (mini-goal 4) __________ (date) __________ (reward)

______________________ (mini-goal 5) __________ (date) __________ (reward)

D. My program will include the addition of physical activity to my daily routine (such as climbing stairs or walking to class):

1. ______________________________

2. ______________________________

3. ______________________________

4. ______________________________

5. ______________________________

E. I will use the following tools to monitor my program and my progress toward my goals:

____
(list any charts, graphs, or journals you plan to use)

____

____

I sign this contract as an indication of my personal commitment to reach my goal.

______________________________ ______________
(your signature) (date)

I have recruited a helper who will witness my contract and ______________________________

____
(list any way your helper will participate in your program)

____

______________________________ ______________
(witness's signature) (date)

Name ______________ Section ______________ Date ______________

LAB 7.2 *Getting to Know Your Fitness Facility*

To help create a successful training program, take time out to learn more about the fitness facility you plan to use.

Basic Information

Name and location of facility: ______________

Hours of operation: ______________

Times available for general use: ______________

Times most convenient for your schedule: ______________

Can you obtain an initial session or consultation with a trainer to help you create a program? ____ yes ____ no

If so, what does the initial planning session involve? ______________

____

Are any of the staff certified? Do any have special training? If yes, list/describe: ______________

____

What types of equipment are available for the development of cardiorespiratory endurance? Briefly list/describe:

____

____

____

Are any group activities or classes available? If so, briefly describe: ______________

____

____

What types of weight training equipment are available for use? ______________

____

Yes	No	
____	____	Is there a fee for using the facility? If so, how much? $ ________
____	____	Is a student ID required for access to the facility?
____	____	Do you need to sign up in advance to use the facility or any of the equipment?
____	____	Is there typically a line or wait to use the equipment during the times you use the facility?
____	____	Is there a separate area with mats for stretching and/or cool-down?
____	____	Do you need to bring your own towel?
____	____	Are lockers available? If so, do you need to bring your own lock? ____ yes ____ no
____	____	Are showers available? If so, do you need to bring your own soap and shampoo? ____yes ____ no
____	____	Is drinking water available? (If not, be sure to bring your own bottle of water.)

Describe any other amenities, such as vending machines or saunas, that are available at the facility.

____

____

Information About Equipment

Fill in the specific equipment and exercise(s) that you can use to develop cardiorespiratory endurance and each of the major muscle groups. For cardiorespiratory endurance, list the type(s) of equipment and a sample starting workout: intensity, duration, frequency, and other pertinent information (such as a setting for resistance or speed). For muscular strength and endurance, list the equipment, exercises, and finally indicate the order in which you'll complete them during a workout session (see p. 86 for suggestions on order of weight training exercises).

Cardiorespiratory Endurance Equipment

Equipment	Sample Starting Workout

Muscular Strength and Endurance Equipment

Order	Muscle Groups	Equipment	Exercises(s)
	Neck		
	Chest		
	Shoulders		
	Upper back		
	Front of arms		
	Back of arms		
	Buttocks		
	Abdomen		
	Lower back		
	Front of thighs		
	Back of thighs		
	Calves		
	Other:		
	Other:		

Nutrition

8

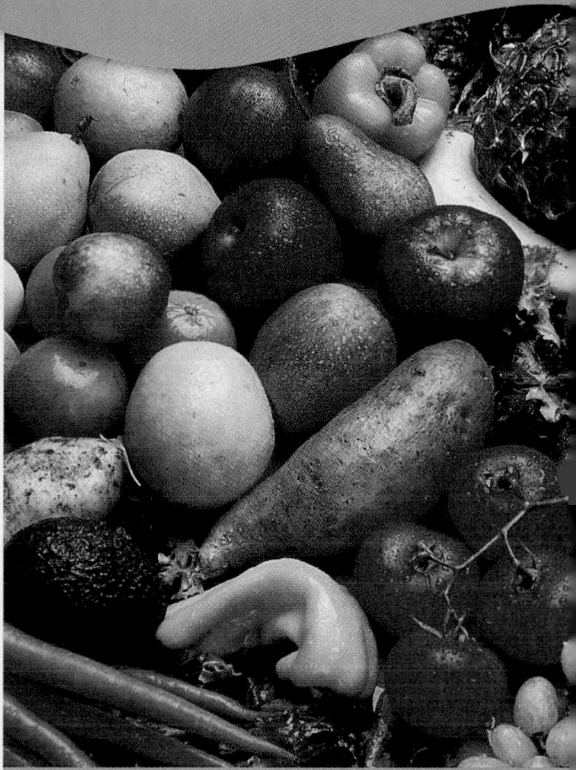

LOOKING AHEAD

After reading this chapter, you should be able to

- List the essential nutrients and describe the functions they perform in the body
- Describe the guidelines that have been developed to help people choose a healthy diet, avoid nutritional deficiencies, and protect themselves from diet-related chronic diseases
- Discuss nutritional guidelines for vegetarians and for special population groups
- Explain how to use food labels and other consumer tools to make informed choices about foods
- Put together a personal nutrition plan based on affordable foods that you enjoy and that will promote wellness, today and in the future

TEST YOUR KNOWLEDGE

1. Three ounces of chicken or meat, the amount considered to be one serving, is approximately the size of which of the following?
   a. a domino
   b. a deck of cards
   c. a small paperback book
2. Candy is the leading source of added sugars in the American diet. True or false?
3. Which of the following is NOT a whole grain?
   a. brown rice
   b. wheat flour
   c. popcorn

TEST YOUR KNOWLEDGE ANSWERS

1. B. Many people underestimate the size of the servings they eat, leading to overconsumption of calories and fat.

2. FALSE. Regular (nondiet) sodas are the leading source, with an average of 54 gallons consumed per person per year. Each 12-ounce soda supplies about 10 teaspoons of sugar, the total recommended daily limit for a 2000-calorie diet.

3. B. Unless labeled "whole wheat," wheat flour is processed to remove the bran and germ and is not a whole grain.

Fit and Well Online Learning Center

www.mhhe.com/fahey5e

Visit the *Fit and Well* Online Learning Center for study aids, additional information about nutrition, links, Internet activities that explore the role of nutrition in wellness, and much more.

In your lifetime, you'll spend about 6 years eating—about 70,000 meals and 60 tons of food. What you eat affects your energy level, well-being, and overall health (see the box "Eating Habits and Total Wellness"). Of particular concern is the connection between lifetime nutritional habits and risk of the major chronic diseases, including heart disease, cancer, stroke, and diabetes. Choosing foods that provide adequate amounts of the nutrients you need while limiting the substances linked to disease should be an important part of your daily life. The food choices you make will significantly influence your health—both now and in the future.

Creating a diet plan to support maximum fitness and protect against disease is a two-part project. First, you have to know which nutrients are necessary and in what amounts. Second, you have to translate those requirements into a diet consisting of foods you like to eat that are both available and affordable. Once you have an idea of what constitutes a healthy diet for you, you may also have to make adjustments in your current diet to bring it into line with your goals.

This chapter provides the basic principles of **nutrition.** It introduces the six classes of essential nutrients, explaining their role in the functioning of the body. It also provides different sets of guidelines that you can use to design a healthy diet plan. Finally, it offers practical tools and advice to help you apply the guidelines to your own life. Diet is an area of your life in which you have almost total control. Using your knowledge and understanding of nutrition to create a healthy diet plan is a significant step toward wellness.

Ww NUTRITIONAL REQUIREMENTS: COMPONENTS OF A HEALTHY DIET

When you think about your diet, you probably do so in terms of the foods you like to eat—a turkey sandwich and a glass of milk, or a steak and a baked potato. What's important for your health, though, are the nutrients contained in those foods. Your body requires proteins, fats, carbohydrates, vitamins, minerals, and water—about 45 **essential nutrients.** The word *essential* in this context means that you must get these substances from food because your body is unable to manufacture them at all, or at least not fast enough to meet your physiological needs. The six classes of nutrients, along with their functions and major sources, are listed in Table 8.1.

Nutrients are released into the body by the process of **digestion,** which breaks them down into compounds that the gastrointestinal tract can absorb and the body can use (Figure 8.1 on p. 206). A diet containing adequate amounts of all essential nutrients is vital because various nutrients provide energy, build and maintain body tissues, and regulate body functions.

The energy in foods is expressed as **kilocalories**. One kilocalorie represents the amount of heat it takes to raise the temperature of 1 liter of water 1°C. A person needs about 2000 kilocalories a day to meet energy needs. In common usage, people usually refer to kilocalories as *calories,* which is a much smaller energy unit: 1 kilocalorie contains 1000 calories. We'll use the familiar word *calorie* in this chapter to stand for the larger energy unit; you'll also find the word *calorie* used on food labels.

Of the six classes of nutrients, three supply energy:

- Fat = 9 calories per gram
- Protein = 4 calories per gram
- Carbohydrate = 4 calories per gram

(Alcohol, although it is not an essential nutrient, also supplies energy, providing 7 calories per gram.) The high caloric content of fat is one reason experts continually advise against high fat consumption; most of us do not need the extra calories to meet energy needs. Calories consumed in excess of energy needs are converted to fat and stored in the body.

But just meeting energy needs is not enough; our bodies need adequate amounts of all the essential nutrients to grow and function properly. Practically all foods contain mixtures of nutrients, although foods are commonly classified according to their predominant nutrients. For example, spaghetti is considered a carbohydrate food although it contains small amounts of other nutrients. Let's take a closer look at the functions and sources of the six classes of nutrients.

Proteins—The Basis of Body Structure

Proteins form important parts of the body's main structural components: muscles and bones. Proteins also form important parts of blood, enzymes, cell membranes, and some hormones. As mentioned above, protein can also provide energy at 4 calories per gram of protein weight.

Amino Acids The building blocks of proteins are called **amino acids.** Twenty common amino acids are found in food; nine of these are essential: histidine, isoleucine, leucine, lysine, methionine, phenylalanine, threonine,

Terms Ww

nutrition The science of food and how the body uses it in health and disease.

essential nutrients Substances the body must get from food because it cannot manufacture them at all or fast enough to meet its needs. These nutrients include proteins, fats, carbohydrates, vitamins, minerals, and water.

digestion The process of breaking down foods in the gastrointestinal tract into compounds the body can absorb.

kilocalorie A measure of energy content in food; 1 kilocalorie represents the amount of heat needed to raise the temperature of 1 liter of water 1°C; commonly referred to as *calorie.*

protein An essential nutrient; a compound made of amino acids that contains carbon, hydrogen, oxygen, and nitrogen.

amino acids The building blocks of proteins.

Healthy eating does more than nourish your body—it enhances your ability to enjoy life to the fullest by improving overall wellness, both physical and mental. A recent study examined a group of adults who followed a healthy eating plan for four years. At the end of this period, the study subjects were more confident with their food choices and more satisfied with their lives in general than their peers who did not make any dietary changes. The reverse is also true—when people overeat they often have feelings of guilt, anger, discouragement, and even self-loathing. Out-of-control eating can erode self-confidence and lead to depression. How we eat is a reflection of how we feel about ourselves. Enjoying food and eating well is a major part of a healthy and happy life.

Can individual foods affect the way we feel? Limited scientific evidence points to some correlation between certain foods and one's mood. Many people, especially women, seem to crave chocolate when they are "blue." Studies show that chocolate, in small quantities, may indeed give you a lift. Sugary foods tend to temporarily raise serotonin levels in the brain, which can improve mood (serotonin is a neurotransmitter associated with a calm, relaxed state). The fat found in chocolate acts to increase endorphins, brain chemicals that reduce pain and increase feelings of well-being. Chocolate also contains caffeine, theobromine, phenylethylamine, and a variety of other less studied chemicals that may have a positive impact on mood.

A commonly held belief about the connection between food and the mind is that eating sugary foods makes people (especially children) hyperactive. Parents often comment on the wild behavior observed at parties and festive events where lots of sweets are consumed. However, several carefully controlled studies showed no correlation between behavior and the consumption of sugary foods. Researchers speculate that high-sugar foods tend to be eaten at birthday parties and other exciting occasions when children tend to be highly stimulated regardless of what they eat.

Some recent research shows that eating certain carbohydrate-rich foods such as a plain baked potato or a bagel with jelly can have a temporary calming effect. Scientists postulate that this occurs because carbohydrates stimulate insulin release, which improves the transport of the amino acid tryptophan (the major building block for serotonin) into the brain. This effect is most pronounced when rapidly digestible carbohydrates are consumed alone, with no fats or protein in the meal. The practical implications of this research are uncertain.

If you are looking for a mental boost, some scientists think that eating a meal consisting primarily of protein-rich foods may be helpful. The theory is that proteins contain the amino acid tyrosine, which is used by the body to manufacture the neurotransmitters dopamine and norepinephrine. Some researchers postulate that eating protein-containing foods could increase the synthesis of these neurotransmitters, which can speed reaction time and increase alertness. Whether this really works, especially in well-nourished individuals who have not been lacking these nutrients to begin with, remains to be seen. In the meantime, it wouldn't hurt, and might even help, to include some protein in the meal you eat prior to your next big exam.

What we know about how food affects mood remains limited. But evidence points to the commonsense conclusion that enjoying reasonable portions of a variety of healthy and tasty foods is a great way to optimize your physical and mental health.

Table 8.1 *The Six Classes of Essential Nutrients*

Nutrient	Function	Major Sources
Proteins (4 calories/gram)	Form important parts of muscles, bone, blood, enzymes, some hormones, and cell membranes; repair tissue; regulate water and acid-base balance; help in growth; supply energy	Meat, fish, poultry, eggs, milk products, legumes, nuts
Carbohydrates (4 calories/gram)	Supply energy to cells in brain, nervous system, and blood; supply energy to muscles during exercise	Grains (breads and cereals), fruits, vegetables, milk
Fats (9 calories/gram)	Supply energy; insulate, support, and cushion organs; provide medium for absorption of fat-soluble vitamins	Animal foods, grains, nuts, seeds, fish, vegetables
Vitamins	Promote (initiate or speed up) specific chemical reactions within cells	Abundant in fruits, vegetables, and grains; also found in meat and dairy products
Minerals	Help regulate body functions; aid in the growth and maintenance of body tissues; act as catalysts for the release of energy	Found in most food groups
Water	Makes up 50–70% of body weight; provides a medium for chemical reactions; transports chemicals; regulates temperature; removes waste products	Fruits, vegetables, and liquids

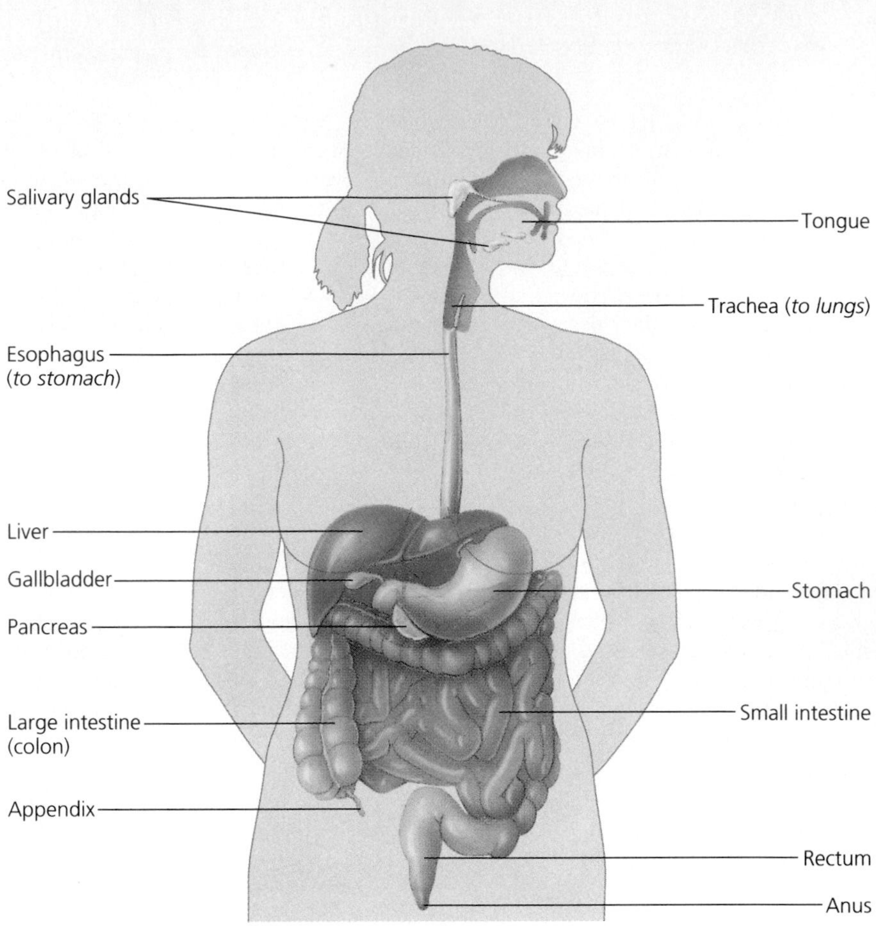

Figure 8.1 The digestive system. Food is partially broken down by being chewed and mixed with saliva in the mouth. As food moves through the digestive tract, it is mixed by muscular contractions and broken down by chemicals. After traveling to the stomach via the esophagus, food is broken down further by stomach acids. Most absorption of nutrients occurs in the small intestine, aided by secretions from the pancreas, gallbladder, and intestinal lining. The large intestine reabsorbs excess water; the remaining solid wastes are collected in the rectum and excreted through the anus.

tryptophan, and valine. The other eleven amino acids can be produced by the body as long as the necessary components are supplied by foods.

Complete and Incomplete Proteins Individual protein sources are considered "complete" if they supply all the essential amino acids in adequate amounts and "incomplete" if they do not. Meat, fish, poultry, eggs, milk, cheese, and soy provide complete proteins. Incomplete proteins, which come from plant sources such as **legumes** and nuts, are good sources of most essential amino acids, but are usually low in one or two.

Combining two vegetable proteins, such as wheat and peanuts in a peanut butter sandwich, allows each vegetable protein to make up for the amino acids missing in the other protein. The combination yields a complete protein. Your concern with amino acids and complete protein in your diet should focus on what you consume throughout the day, rather than at each meal. It was once believed that vegetarians had to "complement" their proteins at each meal in order to receive the benefit of a complete protein. It is now known, however, that proteins consumed throughout the course of the day can complement each other to form a pool of amino acids the body can draw from to produce the necessary proteins. (Healthy vegetarian diets are discussed later in the chapter.)

Recommended Protein Intake The leading sources of protein in the American diet are (1) beef, steaks, and roasts; (2) hamburger and meatloaf; (3) white bread, rolls, and crackers; (4) milk; and (5) pork. About two-thirds of the protein in the American diet comes from animal sources; therefore, the American diet is rich in amino acids. Most Americans consume more protein than they need each day. Protein consumed beyond what the body needs is synthesized into fat for energy storage or burned for energy requirements. Consuming somewhat above our needs is not harmful, but it does contribute fat to the diet because protein-rich foods are often fat-rich as well. A very high protein intake can strain the kidneys and lead to dehydration. The amount of protein you eat should represent about 10–15% of your total daily calories.

Fats—Essential in Small Amounts

Fats, also known as lipids, are the most concentrated source of energy, at 9 calories per gram. The fats stored in your body represent usable energy, help insulate your body, and support and cushion your organs. Fats in the diet help your body absorb fat-soluble vitamins and add important flavor and texture to foods. Fats are the major fuel for the body during periods of rest and light activity. Two fats—linoleic acid and alpha-linolenic acid—are

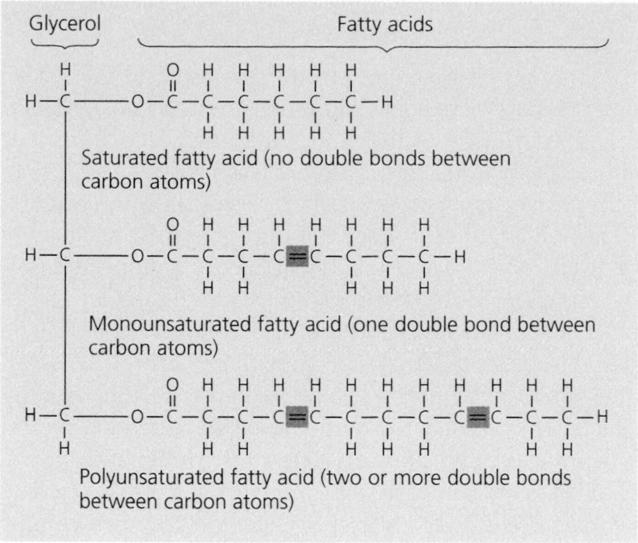

Figure 8.2 Chemical structures of saturated and unsaturated fatty acids. This example of a triglyceride consists of a molecule of glycerol with three fatty acids attached. Fatty acids can differ in the length of their carbon chains and their degree of saturation.

essential to the diet; they are key regulators of such body functions as the maintenance of blood pressure and the progress of a healthy pregnancy.

Types and Sources of Fats Most of the fats in food are in the form of triglycerides, which are composed of a glycerine molecule (an alcohol) plus three fatty acids. A fatty acid is made up of a chain of carbon atoms with oxygen attached at the end and hydrogen atoms attached along the length of the chain. Fatty acids differ in the length of their carbon atom chains and in their degree of saturation (the number of hydrogens attached to the chain). If every available bond from each carbon atom in a fatty acid chain is attached to a hydrogen atom, the fatty acid is said to be **saturated** (Figure 8.2). If not all the available bonds are taken up by hydrogens, the carbon atoms in the chain will form double bonds with each other. Such fatty acids are called unsaturated fats. If there is only one double bond, the fatty acid is called **monounsaturated.** If there are two or more double bonds, the fatty acid is called **polyunsaturated.** The essential fatty acids, linoleic and alpha-linolenic acids, are both polyunsaturated. The different types of fatty acids have different characteristics and different effects on your health.

Food fats are often composed of both saturated and unsaturated fatty acids; the dominant type of fatty acid determines the fat's characteristics. Food fats containing large amounts of saturated fatty acids are usually solid at room temperature; they are generally found naturally in animal products. The leading sources of saturated fat in the American diet are red meats (hamburger, steak, roasts), whole milk, cheese, and hot dogs and lunch meats. Food fats containing large amounts of monounsaturated and polyunsaturated fatty acids are usually from plant sources and are liquid at room temperature. Olive, canola, safflower, and peanut oils contain mostly monounsaturated fatty acids. Corn, soybean, and cottonseed oils contain mostly polyunsaturated fatty acids.

There are notable exceptions to these generalizations. When unsaturated vegetable oils undergo the process of **hydrogenation,** a mixture of saturated and unsaturated fatty acids is produced. Hydrogenation turns many of the double bonds in unsaturated fatty acids into single bonds, increasing the degree of saturation and producing a more solid fat from a liquid oil. Hydrogenation also changes some unsaturated fatty acids into **trans fatty acids,** unsaturated fatty acids with an atypical shape that affects their behavior in the body. Food manufacturers use hydrogenation to increase the stability of an oil so it can be reused for deep frying; to improve the texture of certain foods (to make pastries and pie crusts flakier, for example); and to extend the shelf life of foods made with oil. Hydrogenation is also used to transform liquid vegetable oils into margarine or shortening.

Many baked and fried foods are prepared with hydrogenated vegetable oils, so they can be relatively high in saturated and trans fatty acids. Leading sources of trans fats in the American diet are deep-fried fast foods such as french fries and fried chicken (typically fried in vegetable shortening rather than oil); baked and snack foods such as pot pies, cakes, cookies, pastries, doughnuts, and chips; and stick margarine. In general, the more solid a hydrogenated oil is, the more saturated and trans fats it contains; for example, stick margarines typically contain more saturated and trans fats than do tub or squeeze margarines. Small amounts of trans fatty acids are found naturally in meat and milk.

Hydrogenated vegetable oils are not the only plant fats that contain saturated fats. Palm and coconut oils, although derived from plants, are also highly saturated. Fish oils, derived from an animal source, are rich in polyunsaturated fats.

Terms

Ww

legumes Vegetables such as peas and beans that are high in fiber and are also important sources of protein.

saturated fat A fat with no carbon-carbon double bonds; usually solid at room temperature.

monounsaturated fat A fat with one carbon-carbon double bond; liquid at room temperature.

polyunsaturated fat A fat containing two or more carbon-carbon double bonds; liquid at room temperature.

hydrogenation A process by which hydrogens are added to unsaturated fats, increasing the degree of saturation and turning liquid oils into solid fats. Hydrogenation produces a mixture of saturated fatty acids and standard and trans forms of unsaturated fatty acids.

trans fatty acid A type of unsaturated fatty acid produced during the process of hydrogenation; trans fats have an atypical shape that affects their chemical activity.

Fats and Health Different types of fats have very different effects on health. Many studies have examined the effects of dietary fat intake on blood **cholesterol** levels and the risk of heart disease. Saturated and trans fatty acids raise blood levels of **low-density lipoprotein (LDL)**, or "bad" cholesterol, thereby increasing a person's risk of heart disease. Unsaturated fatty acids, on the other hand, lower LDL. Monounsaturated fatty acids, such as those found in olive and canola oils, may also increase levels of **high-density lipoproteins (HDL)**, or "good" cholesterol, providing even greater benefits for heart health. In large amounts, trans fatty acids may lower HDL. Thus, to reduce the risk of heart disease, it is important to substitute unsaturated fats for saturated and trans fats. (See Chapter 11 for more on cholesterol and a heart-healthy diet.)

Most Americans consume more saturated fat than trans fat (11% versus 2–4% of total daily calories). However, health experts are particularly concerned about trans fats because of their double negative effect on heart health—they both raise LDL and lower HDL—and because there is less public awareness of trans fats. The saturated fat content of prepared foods has been listed on nutrition labels since 1994. The FDA has proposed that information on trans fat content also be listed on food labels, included with the amount of saturated fat. Consumers would thus be able to determine the total amount of unhealthy fats that a food contains. Until trans fat content appears on food labels, consumers can check for the presence of trans fats by examining the ingredient list of a food: If a food contains "partially hydrogenated oil" or "vegetable shortening," it contains trans fat.

For heart health, it's important to limit your consumption of both saturated and trans fats. The best way to reduce saturated fat in your diet is to lower your intake of meat and full-fat dairy products (whole milk, cream, butter, cheese, ice cream). To lower trans fats, decrease your intake of deep-fried foods and baked goods made with hydrogenated vegetable oils; use liquid oils rather than margarine or shortening for cooking; and favor tub or squeeze margarines or those labeled low-trans or trans-free over standard stick margarines. Remember, the softer or more liquid a fat is, the less saturated and trans fat it is likely to contain.

Although saturated and trans fats pose health hazards, other fats are beneficial. Monounsaturated fatty acids, as found in avocados, most nuts, and olive, canola, peanut, and safflower oils, improve cholesterol levels and may help protect against some cancers. **Omega-3 fatty acids,** a form of polyunsaturated fat found primarily in fish, may be even more healthful. Omega-3s are produced when the endmost double bond of a polyunsaturated fat occurs three carbons from the end of the fatty acid chain. (The polyunsaturated fatty acid shown in Figure 8.2 is an omega-3 form.) Omega-3s have a number of heart-healthy effects: They reduce the tendency of blood to clot, inhibit inflammation and abnormal heart rhythms, and reduce blood pressure and risk of heart attack and stroke in some people. Because of these benefits, nutritionists recommend that Americans increase the proportion of omega-3s in their diet by eating fish two or more times a week. Salmon, tuna, trout, mackerel, herring, sardines, and anchovies are all good sources of omega-3s; lesser amounts are found in plant sources, including dark-green leafy vegetables; walnuts; flaxseeds; and canola, walnut, and flaxseed oils.

Another form of polyunsaturated fat, omega-6 fatty acid, is produced if the endmost double bond occurs at the sixth carbon atom. Most of the polyunsaturated fats currently consumed by Americans are omega-6s, primarily from corn oil and soybean oil. Foods rich in omega-6s are important because they contain the essential nutrient linoleic acid. However, some nutritionists recommend that people reduce the proportion of omega-6s they consume in favor of omega-3s. To make this adjustment, use canola oil rather than corn oil in cooking, and check for corn, soybean, or cottonseed oil in products such as mayonnaise, margarine, and salad dressing.

In addition to its effects on heart disease risk, dietary fat can affect health in other ways. Diets high in fatty red meat are associated with an increased risk of certain forms of cancer, especially colon cancer. A high-fat diet can also make weight management more difficult. Because fat is a concentrated source of calories (9 calories per gram versus 4 calories per gram for protein and carbohydrate), a high-fat diet is often a high-calorie diet that can lead to weight gain. In addition, there is some evidence that calories from fat are more easily converted to body fat than calories from protein or carbohydrate.

Although more research is needed on the precise effects of different types and amounts of fat on overall health, a great deal of evidence points to the fact that most people benefit from lowering their overall fat intake to recommended levels and substituting unsaturated fats for saturated and trans fats. The types of fatty acids and their effects on health are summarized in Figure 8.3.

Recommended Fat Intake You need only about 1 tablespoon (15 grams) of vegetable oil per day incorporated

Terms Ww

cholesterol A waxy substance found in the blood and cells and needed for cell membranes, vitamin D, and hormone synthesis.

low-density lipoprotein (LDL) Blood fat that transports cholesterol to organs and tissues; excess amounts result in the accumulation of fatty deposits on artery walls.

high-density lipoprotein (HDL) Blood fat that helps transport cholesterol out of the arteries, thereby protecting against heart disease.

omega-3 fatty acids Polyunsaturated fatty acids commonly found in fish oils that are beneficial to cardiovascular health; the endmost double bond occurs three carbons from the end of the fatty acid chain.

	Type of Fatty Acid	Found In[a]	Possible Effects on Health
Keep Intake Low	SATURATED	Animal fats (especially fatty meats and poultry fat and skin) Butter, cheese, and other high-fat dairy products Palm and coconut oils	Raises total cholesterol and "bad" (LDL) cholesterol levels Increases risk of heart disease May increase risk of colon and prostate cancers
	TRANS	French fries and other deep-fried fast foods Stick margarines, shortening Packaged cookies and crackers Processed snacks and sweets	Raises total cholesterol and "bad" (LDL) cholesterol levels Lowers "good" (HDL) cholesterol levels May increase risk of heart disease and breast cancer
Choose Moderate Amounts	MONOUNSATURATED	Olive, canola, and safflower oils Avocados, olives Peanut butter (without added fat) Many nuts, including almonds, cashews, pecans, pistachios	Lowers total cholesterol and "bad" (LDL) cholesterol levels May reduce blood pressure and lower triglyceride levels (a risk factor for CVD) May reduce risk of heart disease, stroke, and some cancers
	POLYUNSATURATED (two groups)[b]		
	Omega-3 fatty acids	Fatty fish, including salmon, white albacore tuna, mackerel, anchovies, and sardines Lesser amounts in walnut, flaxseed, canola, and soybean oils; tofu; walnuts; flaxseeds; and dark-green, leafy vegetables	Reduces blood clotting and inflammation and inhibits abnormal heart rhythms Lowers triglyceride levels (a risk factor for CVD) May lower blood pressure in some people May reduce risk of fatal heart attack, stroke and some cancers
	Omega-6 fatty acids	Corn, soybean, and cottonseed oils (often used in margarine, mayonnaise, and salad dressing)	Lowers total cholesterol and "bad" (LDL) cholesterol levels May lower "good" (HDL) cholesterol levels May reduce risk of heart disease May slightly increase risk of cancer if omega-6 intake is high and omega-3 intake is low

[a] Food fats contain a combination of types of fatty acids in various proportions; for example, canola oil is composed mainly of monounsaturated fatty acids (62%) but also contains polyunsaturated (32%) and saturated (6%) fatty acids. Food fats are categorized here according to their predominant fatty acid.

[b] The essential fatty acids are polyunsaturated: Linoleic acid is an omega-6 fatty acid and alpha-linolenic acid is an omega-3 fatty acid.

Figure 8.3 Types of fatty acids and their possible effects on health. The health effects of dietary fats are still being investigated. In general, nutritionists recommend that we consume a diet moderate in fat overall and that we substitute unsaturated fats for saturated and trans fats. Monounsaturated fats and omega-3 polyunsaturated fats may be particularly good choices for promoting health. Eating lots of fat of any type can provide excess calories because all types of fats are rich sources of energy (9 calories per gram).

into your diet to supply the essential fats. The average American diet supplies considerably more than this amount; in fact, fats make up about 33% of our total calorie intake. (This is the equivalent of about 75 grams, or 5 tablespoons, of fat per day for someone who consumes 2000 calories.) Although the percentage of calories from fat has declined in the American diet in recent years, the simultaneous increase in total calorie intake means that we're actually consuming more total grams of fat.

The 2000 Dietary Guidelines for Americans recommend that most people limit their total fat intake to 30% or less of total calories, with less than 10% coming from saturated fat. A 2001 report by the National Cholesterol Education Program (NCEP) suggests total fat intake of 25–35%, with less than 7% coming from saturated fat, up to 10% from polyunsaturated fat, and up to 20% from monounsaturated fat. The NCEP diet also recommends that trans fat intake be kept low and that total calorie intake allow for the maintenance of a healthy weight. This slightly higher fat intake (up to 35% of total calories rather than the generally suggested limit of 30%) for people whose weight and calorie intake is under control reflects the recent American Heart Association recommendation that people replace some of the saturated fat in their diets with monounsaturated fat rather than with carbohydrate. This recommendation underscores the growing evidence for the health-conferring benefits of monounsaturated fats.

The number of calories and grams of fat that correspond to the 30% (total fat) and 10% (saturated fat) limits are shown in Table 8.2 for diets consisting of 1600, 2200, and 2800 calories per day. For example, if you consume

Table 8.2 *Recommended Daily Intake for Fat, Protein, and Carbohydrate*

			RECOMMENDED DAILY NUTRIENT INTAKE GOAL OR LIMIT		
			CALORIES AND GRAMS FOR THREE LEVELS OF ENERGY INTAKE		
	Energy/Gram	Percent of Total Calories	1600 Calories	2200 Calories	2800 Calories
Fat	9 calories/gram	30% or less	480 calories = 53 grams	660 calories = 73 grams	840 calories = 93 grams
Saturated fat	*9 calories/gram*	*less than 10%*	*160 calories = 18 grams*	*220 calories = 24 grams*	*280 calories = 31 grams*
Protein	4 calories/gram	15%	240 calories = 60 grams	330 calories = 83 grams	420 calories = 105 grams
Carbohydrate	4 calories/gram	55%	880 calories = 220 grams	1210 calories = 303 grams	1540 calories = 385 grams
Added sugars	*4 calories/gram*		*6 teaspoons = 24 grams*	*12 teaspoons = 48 grams*	*18 teaspoons = 72 grams*

To individualize these goals or limits, multiply the appropriate percentage by total calorie intake and then divide the result by the corresponding calories per gram value. For example, a fat limit of 35% applied to a 2200-calorie diet would be calculated as follows: 0.35 × 2200 = 770 calories total fat ÷ 9 calories per gram = 86 grams total fat. For a saturated fat limit of 7% in a 2200-calorie diet: 0.07 × 2200 = 154 calories saturated fat ÷ 9 calories per gram = 17 grams saturated fat.

about 2200 calories per day, you should limit your total fat intake to 73 grams per day, of which no more than 24 grams should be saturated fat; recommended intakes for protein and carbohydrate are also provided in Table 8.2. To determine how close you are to meeting these intake goals for fat, keep a running total over the course of the day. For prepared foods, food labels list the number of grams of fat, protein, and carbohydrate; the breakdown for many foods and popular fast-food items can be found in Appendixes B and C. Nutrition information is also available in many grocery stores, in published nutrition guides, and online (see For Further Exploration at the end of the chapter). By checking these resources, you can keep track of the total grams of fat, protein, and carbohydrate you eat and assess how close your current diet is to the recommended intake goals.

In reducing fat intake to recommended levels, the emphasis should be on lowering saturated and trans fats (see Figure 8.3). You can still eat high-fat foods, but it makes good sense to limit the size of your portions and to balance your intake with low-fat foods. For example, peanut butter is high in fat, with 8 grams (72 calories) of fat in each 90-calorie tablespoon. Two tablespoons of peanut butter eaten on whole-wheat bread and served with a banana, carrot sticks, and a glass of nonfat milk makes a nutritious lunch—high in protein and carbohydrate, relatively low in total and saturated fat (500 calories, 18 grams of total fat, 4 grams of saturated fat). Four tablespoons of peanut butter on high-fat crackers with potato chips, cookies, and whole milk is a less healthy combination (1000 calories, 62 grams of total fat, 15 grams of saturated fat). So although it's important to evaluate individual food items for their fat content, it is more important to look at them in the context of your overall diet.

Carbohydrates—An Ideal Source of Energy

Carbohydrates are needed in the diet primarily to supply energy to body cells. Some cells, such as those in the brain and other parts of the nervous system and in the blood, use only carbohydrates for fuel. During high-intensity exercise, muscles also get most of their energy from carbohydrates.

Simple and Complex Carbohydrates Carbohydrates are classified into two groups: simple and complex. Simple carbohydrates contain only one or two sugar units in each molecule; they include sucrose (table sugar), fructose (fruit sugar, honey), maltose (malt sugar), and lactose (milk sugar). Providing much of the sweetness in foods, they are found naturally in fruits and milk and are added

Terms Ww

carbohydrate An essential nutrient; sugars, starches, and dietary fiber are all carbohydrates.

glucose A simple sugar that is the body's basic fuel.

glycogen An animal starch stored in the liver and muscles.

whole grain The entire edible portion of a grain such as wheat, rice, or oats, including the germ, endosperm, and bran. During milling or processing, parts of the grain are removed, often leaving just the endosperm.

glycemic index A measure of how the ingestion of a particular food affects blood glucose levels.

Our bodies require adequate amounts of all essential nutrients—water, proteins, carbohydrates, fats, vitamins, and minerals—to grow and function properly. Choosing foods to satisfy these nutritional requirements is an important part of a healthy lifestyle.

to soft drinks, fruit drinks, candy, and sweet desserts. There is no evidence that any type of simple sugar is more nutritious than any other.

Complex carbohydrates consist of chains of many sugar molecules; they include starches and most types of dietary fiber. Starches are found in a variety of plants, especially grains (wheat, rye, rice, oats, barley, millet), legumes, and tubers (potatoes and yams). Most other vegetables contain a mix of starches and simple carbohydrates. Dietary fiber is found in fruits, vegetables, and grains.

During digestion in the mouth and small intestine, your body breaks down starches and double sugars into single sugar molecules, such as **glucose,** for absorption. Once the glucose is in the bloodstream, the pancreas releases insulin, which allows cells to take up glucose and use it for energy. The liver and muscles also take up glucose and store it in the form of a starch called **glycogen.** The muscles use glycogen as fuel during endurance events or long workouts. Carbohydrates consumed in excess of the body's energy needs are changed into fat and stored. Whenever calorie intake exceeds calorie expenditure, fat storage can lead to weight gain. This is true whether the excess calories come from carbohydrates, proteins, fat, or alcohol.

Refined Carbohydrates Versus Whole Grains Complex carbohydrates can be further divided between refined, or processed, carbohydrates and unrefined carbohydrates, or whole grains. Before they are processed, all grains are **whole grains,** consisting of an inner layer of germ, a middle layer called the endosperm, and an outer layer of bran. During processing, the germ and bran are often removed, leaving just the starchy endosperm. The refinement of whole grains transforms whole-wheat flour to white flour, brown rice to white rice, and so on.

Refined carbohydrates usually retain all the calories of their unrefined counterparts, but they tend to be much lower in fiber, vitamins, minerals, and other beneficial compounds. Unrefined carbohydrates tend to take longer to chew and digest than refined ones; they also enter the bloodstream more slowly. This slower digestive pace tends to make people feel full sooner and for a longer period, lessening the chance that they will overeat. Also, a slower rise in blood glucose levels following consumption of complex carbohydrates may help in the management of diabetes. Whole grains are also high in dietary fiber and so have all the benefits of fiber. Consumption of whole grains has been linked to reduced risk for heart disease, diabetes, high blood pressure, stroke, and certain forms of cancer. For all these reasons, whole grains are recommended over those that have been refined. This does not mean that you should never eat refined carbohydrates such as white bread or white rice, simply that whole-wheat bread, brown rice, and other whole grains are healthier choices. See the box "Choosing More Whole-Grain Foods" on p. 212 for tips on increasing your intake of whole grains.

Glycemic Index Insulin and glucose levels rise and fall following a meal or snack containing any type of carbohydrate. Some foods cause a quick and dramatic rise in glucose and insulin levels; others have a slower, more moderate effect. A food that has a strong effect on blood glucose levels is said to have a high **glycemic index.** A meal containing high glycemic index foods may increase appetite in some people; over the long term, diets rich in high glycemic index foods are linked to increased risk of diabetes and heart disease.

Attempting to base food choices on glycemic index is a difficult task, however. Although one can say generally that unrefined complex carbohydrates and high-fiber foods tend to have a low glycemic index, patterns are less clear for other types of foods and do not follow a simple distinction such as that of simple versus complex carbohydrates. For example, some fruits with fairly high levels of simple carbohydrates have only a moderate effect on blood glucose levels, while white rice, potatoes, and white bread, which are rich in complex carbohydrates, have a high glycemic index. Watermelon has a glycemic index more

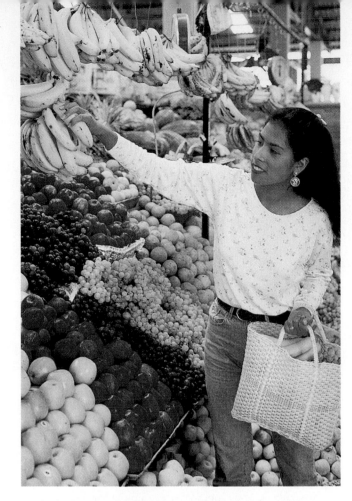

TAKE CHARGE Choosing More Whole-Grain Foods

What Are Whole Grains?

The first step in increasing your intake of whole grains is to correctly identify them. The following are whole grains:

whole wheat	whole-grain corn
whole rye	popcorn
whole oats	brown rice
oatmeal	barley

Other choices include bulgur (cracked wheat), millet, kasha (roasted buckwheat kernels), quinoa, teff, wheat and rye berries, amaranth, graham flour, whole-grain kamut, whole-grain spelt, and whole-grain triticale.

Wheat flour, unbleached flour, enriched flour, and degerminated corn meal are not whole grains. Wheat germ and wheat bran are also not whole grains, but they are the constituents of wheat typically left out when wheat is processed and so are healthier choices than regular wheat flour, which typically contains just the endosperm.

Reading Food Packages to Find Whole Grains

To find packaged foods rich in whole grains, read the list of ingredients and check for special health claims related to whole grains. The *first* item on the list of ingredients should be one of the whole grains listed above. In addition, the FDA allows manufacturers to include special health claims for foods that contain 51% or more whole-grain ingredients. Such products may contain a statement such as the following on their packaging: "Rich in whole grain," "Made with 100% whole grain," or "Diets rich in whole-grain foods may help reduce the risk of heart disease and certain cancers." However, many whole-grain products will not carry such claims.

Incorporating Whole Grains into Your Daily Diet

- *Bread:* Look for sandwich breads, bagels, English muffins, buns, and pita breads with a whole grain listed as the first ingredient. Color and name can be misleading; always check the list of ingredients.
- *Breakfast cereals:* Whole-grain choices include oatmeal, muesli, shredded wheat, and some types of raisin bran, bran flakes, wheat flakes, toasted oats, and granola. Check the ingredient list for whole grains.
- *Rice:* Choose brown rice or rice blends that include brown rice.
- *Pasta:* Look for whole-wheat, whole-grain kamut, or whole-grain spelt pasta.
- *Tortillas:* Choose whole-wheat or whole-corn tortillas.
- *Crackers and snacks:* Some varieties of crackers are made from whole grains, including some flatbreads or crispbreads, woven wheat crackers, and rye crackers. Other whole-grain snack possibilities include popcorn, popcorn cakes, brown rice cakes, whole-corn tortilla chips, and whole-wheat fig cookies. Be sure to check food labels for fat content, as many popular snacks are also high in fat.
- *Mixed-grain dishes:* Combine whole grains with other foods to create healthy mixed dishes such as tabouli; soups made with hulled barley or wheat berries; and pilafs, casseroles, and salads made with brown rice, whole-wheat couscous, kasha, millet, wheat bulgur, and quinoa.

If your grocery store doesn't carry these items, try your local health food store.

than twice that of strawberries, and the glycemic index of a banana changes dramatically as it ripens. Spaghetti has a glycemic index half that of white bread, even when the two items are made from the same ingredients. The acid and fat content of a food also affect glycemic index—the more acidic and higher in fat a food is, the lower its effect on glucose levels.

This complexity is one reason why major health organizations have not issued specific guidelines for glycemic index. For people with particular health concerns, glycemic index may be an important consideration; however, it should not be the sole criterion for food choices. For example, ice cream and chocolate have much lower glycemic index values than brown rice and carrots—but that doesn't make them healthier choices overall. Glycemic index and its effects on appetite and heart health are discussed further in Chapters 9 and 11. For now, remember that most unrefined grains, fruits, vegetables, and legumes are rich in nutrients and have a low-to-moderate glycemic index. Choose a variety of vegetables daily, and avoid heavy consumption of white potatoes.

Recommended Carbohydrate Intake On average, Americans consume over 250 grams of carbohydrate per day, well above the minimum of 50–100 grams of essential carbohydrate required by the body. However, health experts recommend that most Americans increase their consumption of carbohydrates to 55–60% of total daily calories, or about 275–300 grams of carbohydrate for someone consuming 2000 calories per day. A lower consumption of carbohydrate may be appropriate for people who choose to replace saturated fat in their diets with monounsaturated fats rather than carbohydrates; this pattern is associated with reduced risk of heart disease, and the NCEP diet described on p.209 allows for a slightly higher fat intake (up to 35% of total calories as fat, including up to 20% from monounsaturated fat) and a slightly lower carbohydrate intake. Regardless of the total amount of carbohydrate consumed, the focus should be on consuming a variety of foods rich in complex carbohydrates, especially whole grains.

Experts also recommend that Americans alter the proportion of simple and complex carbohydrates in the diet, lowering simple carbohydrate intake from about 25% to 10–15% of total daily calories. To accomplish this change, reduce your intake of foods like soft drinks, candy, sweet desserts, and sweetened fruit drinks, which are high in simple sugars but low in other nutrients. The bulk of the simple carbohydrates in your diet should come from fruits, which are excellent sources of vitamins and minerals, and milk, which is high in protein and calcium.

Athletes in training can especially benefit from high-carbohydrate diets (60–70% of total daily calories), which enhance the amount of carbohydrates stored in their muscles (as glycogen) and therefore provide more carbohydrate fuel for use during endurance events or long workouts. In addition, carbohydrates consumed during prolonged athletic events can help fuel muscles and extend the availability of the glycogen stored in muscles. Caution is in order, however, because overconsumption of carbohydrates can lead to feelings of fatigue and underconsumption of other nutrients. (For more on the special nutritional needs of athletes, see pp. 228–229.)

Dietary Fiber—A Closer Look

Dietary fiber consists of carbohydrate plant substances that are difficult or impossible for humans to digest. Instead, fiber passes through the intestinal tract and provides bulk for feces in the large intestine, which in turn facilitates elimination. In the large intestine, some types of fiber are broken down by bacteria into acids and gases, which explains why consuming too much fiber can lead to intestinal gas.

Types of Dietary Fiber Nutritionists classify dietary fiber as soluble or insoluble. **Soluble fiber** slows the body's absorption of glucose and binds cholesterol-containing compounds in the intestine, lowering blood cholesterol levels and reducing the risk of cardiovascular disease. **Insoluble fiber** binds water, making the feces bulkier and softer so they pass more quickly and easily through the intestines.

Both kinds of fiber contribute to disease prevention. A diet high in soluble fiber can help people manage diabetes and high blood cholesterol levels. A diet high in insoluble fiber can help prevent a variety of health problems, including constipation, hemorrhoids, and **diverticulitis.** Some studies have linked diets high in fiber-rich fruits, vegetables, and grains with a lower risk of some kinds of cancer; however, it is unclear whether fiber or other food components are responsible for this reduction in risk.

Sources of Dietary Fiber All plant foods contain some dietary fiber, but fruits, legumes, oats (especially oat bran), barley, and psyllium (found in some cereals and laxatives) are particularly rich in it. Wheat (especially wheat bran), cereals, grains, and vegetables are all good sources of insoluble fiber. However, the processing of packaged foods can remove fiber, so it's important to depend on fresh fruits and vegetables and foods made from whole grains as sources of dietary fiber.

Recommended Intake of Dietary Fiber Most experts believe the average American would benefit from an increase in daily fiber intake. Currently, most Americans consume about 16 grams of fiber a day, whereas the recommended daily amount is 20–35 grams of fiber—not from supplements, which should be taken only under medical supervision.

To increase the amount of fiber in your diet, try the following:

- Look for breads, crackers, and cereals that list whole grain first in the ingredient list: Whole-wheat flour, whole-grain oats, and whole-grain rice are whole grains; wheat flour is not. Choose a breakfast cereal with 5 or more grams of fiber per serving.
- Eat whole, unpeeled fruits rather than drinking fruit juice. Top cereals, yogurt, and desserts with berries, apple slices, or other fruit.
- Include beans in soups and salads. Combine raw vegetables with pasta, rice, or beans in salads.
- Substitute bean dip for cheese-based or sour cream–based dips or spreads. Use raw vegetables rather than chips for dipping.

Vitamins—Organic Micronutrients

Vitamins are organic (carbon-containing) substances required in very small amounts to regulate various processes within living cells (Table 8.3). Humans need 13 vitamins. Four are fat-soluble (A, D, E, and K), and nine are water-soluble (C and the eight B-complex vitamins: thiamin, riboflavin, niacin, vitamin B-6, folate, vitamin B-12, biotin, and pantothenic acid). Solubility affects how a vitamin is absorbed, transported, and stored in the body. The water-soluble vitamins are absorbed directly into the bloodstream, where they travel freely; excess water-soluble vitamins are detected and removed by the kidneys and excreted in urine. Fat-soluble vitamins require a more complex absorptive process; they are usually carried in the blood by special proteins and are stored in the body in fat tissues rather than excreted.

Terms

Ww

dietary fiber Carbohydrates and other substances in plants that are difficult or impossible for humans to digest.

soluble fiber Fiber that dissolves in water or is broken down by bacteria in the large intestine.

insoluble fiber Fiber that does not dissolve in water and is not broken down by bacteria in the large intestine.

diverticulitis A digestive disorder in which abnormal pouches form in the walls of the intestine and become inflamed.

vitamins Organic substances needed in small amounts to help promote and regulate chemical reactions and processes in the body.

Table 8.3 Facts About Vitamins

Vitamin	Important Dietary Sources	Major Functions	Signs of Prolonged Deficiency	Toxic Effects of Megadoses
Fat-Soluble				
Vitamin A	Liver, milk, butter, cheese, and fortified margarine; carrots, spinach, and other orange and deep-green vegetables and fruits	Maintenance of vision, skin, linings of the nose, mouth, digestive and urinary tracts, immune function	Night blindness; dry, scaling skin; increased susceptibility to infection; loss of appetite; anemia; kidney stones	Liver damage, miscarriage and birth defects, headache, vomiting and diarrhea, vertigo, double vision, bone abnormalities
Vitamin D	Fortified milk and margarine, fish oils, butter, egg yolks (sunlight on skin also produces vitamin D)	Development and maintenance of bones and teeth, promotion of calcium absorption	Rickets (bone deformities) in children; bone softening, loss, and fractures in adults	Kidney damage, calcium deposits in soft tissues, depression, death
Vitamin E	Vegetable oils, whole grains, nuts and seeds, green leafy vegetables, asparagus, peaches	Protection and maintenance of cellular membranes	Red blood cell breakage and anemia, weakness, neurological problems, muscle cramps	Relatively nontoxic, but may cause excess bleeding or formation of blood clots
Vitamin K	Green leafy vegetables; smaller amounts widespread in other foods	Production of proteins essential for blood clotting and bone metabolism	Hemorrhaging	None reported
Water-Soluble				
Biotin	Cereals, yeast, egg yolks, soy flour, liver; widespread in foods	Synthesis of fat, glycogen, and amino acids	Rash, nausea, vomiting, weight loss, depression, fatigue, hair loss	None reported
Folate	Green leafy vegetables, yeast, oranges, whole grains, legumes, liver	Amino acid metabolism, synthesis of RNA and DNA, new cell synthesis	Anemia, weakness, fatigue, irritability, shortness of breath, swollen tongue	Masking of vitamin B-12 deficiency
Niacin	Eggs, poultry, fish, milk, whole grains, nuts, enriched breads and cereals, meats, legumes	Conversion of carbohydrates, fats, and protein into usable forms of energy	Pellagra (symptoms include diarrhea, dermatitis, inflammation of mucous membranes, dementia)	Flushing of the skin, nausea,vomiting, diarrhea, liver dysfunction, glucose intolerance
Pantothenic acid	Animal foods, whole grains, broccoli, potatoes; widespread in foods	Metabolism of fats, carbohydrates, and proteins	Fatigue, numbness and tingling of hands and feet, gastrointestinal disturbances	None reported
Riboflavin	Dairy products, enriched breads and cereals, lean meats, poultry, fish, green vegetables	Energy metabolism; maintenance of skin, mucous membranes, and nervous system structures	Cracks at corners of mouth, sore throat, skin rash, hypersensitivity to light, purple tongue	None reported
Thiamin	Whole-grain and enriched breads and cereals, organ meats, lean pork, nuts, legumes	Conversion of carbohydrates into usable forms of energy, maintenance of appetite and nervous system function	Beriberi (symptoms include muscle wasting, mental confusion, anorexia, enlarged heart, nerve changes)	None reported
Vitamin B-6	Eggs, poultry, fish, whole grains, nuts, soybeans, liver, kidney, pork	Metabolism of amino acids and glycogen	Anemia, convulsions, cracks at corners of mouth, dermatitis, nausea, confusion	Neurological abnormalities and damage
Vitamin B-12	Meat, fish, poultry, fortified cereals	Synthesis of blood cells; other metabolic reactions	Anemia, fatigue, nervous system damage, sore tongue	None reported
Vitamin C	Peppers, cruciferous vegetables, spinach, citrus fruits, strawberries, tomatoes, potatoes, other fruits and vegetables	Maintenance and repair of connective tissue, bones, teeth, and cartilage; promotion of healing; aid in iron absorption	Scurvy, anemia, reduced resistance to infection, loosened teeth, joint pain, poor wound healing, hair loss, poor iron absorption	Urinary stones in some people, acid stomach from ingesting supplements in pill form, nausea, diarrhea, headache, fatigue

SOURCES: Food and Nutrition Board, Institute of Medicine, National Academies. 2001. *Dietary Reference Intakes Tables* (http://www4.nationalacademies.org/IOM/IOMHome.nsf/Pages/Food+and+Nutrition+Board; retrieved November 15, 2001). The complete Dietary Reference Intake reports are available from the National Academy Press (http://www.nap.edu). National Research Council. 1989. *Recommended Dietary Allowances,* 10th ed. Washington, D.C.: National Academy Press. Shils, M. E., et. al., eds. 1998. *Modern Nutrition in Health and Disease,* 9th ed. Baltimore: Williams & Wilkins.

Functions of Vitamins Many vitamins help chemical reactions take place. They provide no energy to the body directly but help unleash the energy stored in carbohydrates, proteins, and fats. Vitamins are critical in the production of red blood cells and the maintenance of the nervous, skeletal, and immune systems. Some vitamins also form substances that act as **antioxidants,** which help preserve healthy cells in the body. Key vitamin antioxidants include vitamin E, vitamin C, and the vitamin A precursor beta-carotene. (The actions of antioxidants are described later in the chapter.)

Sources of Vitamins The human body does not manufacture most of the vitamins it requires and must obtain them from foods. Vitamins are abundant in fruits, vegetables, and grains. In addition, many processed foods, such as flour and breakfast cereals, contain added vitamins. A few vitamins are made in certain parts of the body: The skin makes vitamin D when it is exposed to sunlight, and intestinal bacteria make vitamin K. Nonetheless, you still need to obtain vitamin D and vitamin K from foods.

Vitamin Deficiencies and Excesses If your diet lacks sufficient amounts of a particular vitamin, characteristic symptoms of deficiency develop (see Table 8.3). For example, vitamin A deficiency can cause blindness, and vitamin B-6 deficiency can cause seizures. Vitamin deficiency diseases are most often seen in developing countries; they are relatively rare in the United States because vitamins are readily available from our food supply. However, intakes below recommended levels can have adverse effects on health even if they are not low enough to cause a deficiency disease. For example, low intake of folate increases a woman's chance of giving birth to a baby with a neural tube defect (a congenital malformation of the central nervous system). Low intake of folate and vitamins B-6 and B-12 has been linked to increased heart disease risk. Many Americans consume less-than-recommended amounts of vitamins A, C, B-6, and E.

Extra vitamins in the diet can be harmful, especially when taken as supplements. High doses of vitamin A are toxic and increase the risk of birth defects, for example. Vitamin B-6 can cause irreversible nerve damage when taken in large doses. Megadoses of fat-soluble vitamins are particularly dangerous because the excess will be stored in the body rather than excreted, increasing the risk of toxicity. Even when supplements are not taken in excess, relying on them for an adequate intake of vitamins can be a problem: There are many substances in foods other than vitamins and minerals, and some of these compounds may have important health effects. Later in the chapter we discuss specific recommendations for vitamin intake and when a supplement is advisable. For now, keep in mind that it's best to obtain most of your vitamins from foods rather than supplements.

When preparing foods, remember that vitamins and minerals in vegetables can be easily lost or destroyed during storage or cooking. To retain their value, eat or process vegetables immediately after buying them. If you can't do this, then store them in a cool place, covered to retain moisture—either in the refrigerator (for a few days) or in the freezer (for a longer term). To reduce nutrient losses during food preparation, minimize the amount of water used and the total cooking time. Develop a taste for a crunchier texture in cooked vegetables. Baking, steaming, broiling, and microwaving are all good methods of preparing vegetables.

Minerals—Inorganic Micronutrients

Minerals are inorganic (non-carbon-containing) elements you need in small amounts to help regulate body functions, aid in the growth and maintenance of body tissues, and help release energy (Table 8.4). There are about 17 essential minerals. The major minerals, those that the body needs in amounts exceeding 100 milligrams, include calcium, phosphorus, magnesium, sodium, potassium, and chloride. The essential trace minerals, those that you need in minute amounts, include copper, fluoride, iodide, iron, selenium, and zinc.

Characteristic symptoms develop if an essential mineral is consumed in a quantity too small or too large for good health. The minerals most commonly lacking in the American diet are iron, calcium, zinc, and magnesium. Focus on good food choices for these nutrients (see Table 8.4). Lean meats are rich in iron and zinc; low-fat or fat-free dairy products are excellent choices for calcium. Plant foods such as whole grains and leafy vegetables are good sources of magnesium. Iron-deficiency **anemia** is a problem in some age groups, and researchers fear poor calcium intakes are sowing the seeds for future **osteoporosis,** especially in women. See the box "Eating for Healthy Bones" on p. 217 to learn more.

Water—A Vital Component

Water is the major component in both foods and the human body: You are composed of about 60% water. Your need for other nutrients, in terms of weight, is much less than your need for water. You can live up to 50 days without food but only a few days without water.

Terms

Ww

antioxidant A substance that protects against the breakdown of body constituents by free radicals; actions include binding oxygen, donating electrons to free radicals, and repairing damage to molecules.

minerals Inorganic compounds needed in small amounts for regulation, growth, and maintenance of body tissues and functions.

anemia A deficiency in the oxygen-carrying material in the red blood cells.

osteoporosis A condition in which the bones become thin and brittle and break easily.

Table 8.4 Facts About Selected Minerals

Mineral	Important Dietary Sources	Major Functions	Signs of Prolonged Deficiency	Toxic Effects of Megadoses
Calcium	Milk and milk products, tofu, fortified orange juice and bread, green leafy vegetables, bones in fish	Formation of bones and teeth; control of nerve impulses, muscle contraction, blood clotting	Stunted growth in children, bone mineral loss in adults; urinary stones	Kidney stones, calcium deposits in soft tissues, inhibition of mineral absorption, constipation
Fluoride	Fluoridated water, tea, marine fish eaten with bones	Maintenance of tooth and bone structure	Higher frequency of tooth decay	Increased bone density, mottling of teeth, impaired kidney function
Iodine	Iodized salt, seafood, processed foods	Essential part of thyroid hormones, regulation of body metabolism	Goiter (enlarged thyroid), cretinism (birth defect)	Depression of thyroid activity, hyperthyroidism in susceptible people
Iron	Meat and poultry, fortified grain products, dark-green vegetables, dried fruit	Component of hemoglobin, myoglobin, and enzymes	Iron-deficiency anemia, weakness, impaired immune function, gastrointestinal distress	Nausea, diarrhea, liver and kidney damage, joint pains, sterility, disruption of cardiac function, death
Magnesium	Widespread in foods and water (except soft water); especially found in grains, legumes, nuts, seeds, green vegetables, milk	Transmission of nerve impulses, energy transfer, activation of many enzymes	Neurological disturbances, cardiovascular problems, kidney disorders, nausea, growth failure in children	Nausea, vomiting, diarrhea, central nervous system depression, coma; death in people with impaired kidney function
Phosphorus	Present in nearly all foods, especially milk, cereal, peas, eggs, meat	Bone growth and maintenance, energy transfer in cells	Impaired growth, weakness, kidney disorders, cardiorespiratory and nervous system dysfunction	Drop in blood calcium levels, calcium deposits in soft tissues, bone loss
Potassium	Meats, milk, fruits, vegetables, grains, legumes	Nerve function and body water balance	Muscular weakness, nausea, drowsiness, paralysis, confusion, disruption of cardiac rhythm	Cardiac arrest
Selenium	Seafood, meat, eggs, whole grains	Defense against oxidative stress and regulation of thyroid hormone action	Muscle pain and weakness, heart disorders	Hair and nail brittleness and loss, nausea and vomiting, weakness, irritability
Sodium	Salt, soy sauce, salted foods, tomato juice	Body water balance, acid-base balance, nerve function	Muscle weakness, loss of appetite, nausea, vomiting; deficiency is rarely seen	Edema, hypertension in sensitive people
Zinc	Whole grains, meat, eggs, liver, seafood (especially oysters)	Synthesis of proteins, RNA, and DNA; wound healing; immune response; ability to taste	Growth failure, loss of appetite, impaired taste acuity, skin rash, impaired immune function, poor wound healing	Vomiting, impaired immune function, decline in blood HDL levels, impaired copper absorption

SOURCES: Food and Nutrition Board, Institute of Medicine, National Academies. 2001. *Dietary Reference Intakes Tables* (http://www4.nationalacademies.org/IOM/IOMHome.nsf/Pages/Food+and+Nutrition+Board; retrieved November 15, 2001). The complete Dietary Reference Intake reports are available from the National Academy Press (http://www.nap.edu). Shils, M. E., et al., eds. 1998. *Modern Nutrition in Health and Disease*, 9th ed. Baltimore: Williams & Wilkins.

Water is distributed all over the body, among lean and other tissues and in urine and other body fluids. Water is used in the digestion and absorption of food and is the medium in which most of the chemical reactions take place within the body. Some water-based fluids like blood transport substances around the body; other fluids serve as lubricants or cushions. Water also helps regulate body temperature.

Water is contained in almost all foods, particularly in liquids, fruits, and vegetables. The foods and fluids you consume provide 80–90% of your daily water intake; the remainder is generated through metabolism. You lose

TAKE CHARGE Eating for Healthy Bones

Osteoporosis is a condition in which the bones become dangerously thin and fragile over time. It currently afflicts over 28 million Americans, 80% of them women, and results in over 1.5 million bone fractures each year. Most bone mass is built by age 18. After bone density peaks between the ages of 25 and 35, bone mass is slowly lost over time. To prevent osteoporosis, the best strategy is to build as much bone as possible during your young years and then do everything you can to maintain it as you age. Up to 50% of bone loss is determined by controllable lifestyle factors. Key nutrients include the following:

Calcium Consuming an adequate amount of calcium is important throughout life to build and maintain bone mass. Milk, yogurt, and calcium-fortified orange juice, bread, and cereals are all good sources.

Vitamin D Vitamin D is necessary for bones to absorb calcium, a daily intake of 400–800 IU is recommended by the National Osteoporosis Foundation. Vitamin D can be obtained from foods and is manufactured by the skin when exposed to sunlight. Candidates for vitamin D supplements include people who don't eat many foods rich in vitamin D; those who don't expose their face, arms, and hands to the sun (without sunscreen) for 5–15 minutes a few times each week; and people who live north of an imaginary line roughly between Boston and the Oregon–California border (the sun is weaker in northern latitudes).

Vitamin K Vitamin K promotes the synthesis of proteins that help keep bones strong. Broccoli and leafy-green vegetables are rich in vitamin K.

Other Nutrients Other nutrients that may play an important role in bone health include vitamin C, magnesium, potassium, manganese, zinc, copper, and boron. On the flip side, there are several dietary substances that may have a *negative* effect on bone health, especially if consumed in excess: alcohol, sodium, caffeine, and retinol (a form of vitamin A). Drinking lots of soda, which often replaces milk in the diet and which is high in phosphorus (a mineral that may interfere with calcium absorption), has been shown to increase the risk of bone fracture in teenage girls. For healthy bones, it is important to be moderate in your consumption of alcohol, sodium, caffeine, retinol, and sodas.

Finally, it is important to combine a healthy diet with other wellness behaviors. Weight-bearing aerobic activities, if performed regularly, help build and maintain bone mass throughout life. Strength training improves bone density, muscle mass, strength, and balance, protecting against both bone loss and falls, a major cause of fractures. Drinking alcohol only in moderation, refraining from smoking, and managing depression and stress are also important for maintaining strong bones. For people who do develop osteoporosis, a variety of medications is available to treat the condition.

water each day in urine, feces, and sweat and through evaporation in your lungs. To maintain a balance between water consumed and water lost, you need to take in about 1 milliliter of water for each calorie you burn—about 2 liters, or 8 cups, of fluid per day—more if you live in a hot climate or engage in vigorous exercise. Many Americans fall short of this recommended intake.

Thirst is one of the body's first signs of dehydration that we can actually recognize. However, by the time we are actually thirsty, our cells have been needing fluid for quite some time. A good motto to remember, especially when exercising, is: Drink *before* you're thirsty. If the thirst mechanism is faulty, as it may be during illness or vigorous exercise, hormonal mechanisms can help conserve water by reducing the output of urine. Severe dehydration causes weakness and can lead to death. See p. 228 for more on the fluid needs of athletes and active people.

Other Substances in Food

There are many substances in food that are not essential nutrients but that may influence health.

Antioxidants When the body uses oxygen or breaks down certain fats or proteins as a normal part of metabolism, it gives rise to substances called **free radicals.** Environmental factors such as cigarette smoke, exhaust fumes, radiation, excessive sunlight, certain drugs, and stress can increase free radical production. A free radical is a chemically unstable molecule that is missing an electron; it will react with any molecule it encounters from which it can take an electron. In their search for electrons, free radicals react with fats, proteins, and DNA, damaging cell membranes and mutating genes. Because of this, free radicals have been implicated in aging, cancer, cardiovascular disease, and other degenerative diseases like arthritis.

Antioxidants found in foods can help protect the body by blocking the formation and action of free radicals and repairing the damage they cause. Some antioxidants, such as vitamin C, vitamin E, and selenium, are also essential nutrients; others, such as carotenoids, found in yellow, orange, and dark-green leafy vegetables, are not. Many fruits and vegetables are rich in antioxidants.

Terms

free radical An electron-seeking compound that can react with fats, proteins, and DNA, damaging cell membranes and mutating genes in its search for electrons; produced through chemical reactions in the body and by exposure to environmental factors such as sunlight and tobacco smoke.

Phytochemicals Antioxidants are a particular type of **phytochemical,** a substance found in plant foods that may help prevent chronic disease. Researchers have just begun to identify and study all the different compounds found in foods, and many preliminary findings are promising. For example, certain proteins found in soy foods may help lower cholesterol levels. Sulforaphane, a compound isolated from broccoli and other **cruciferous vegetables,** may render some carcinogenic compounds harmless. Allyl sulfides, a group of chemicals found in garlic and onions, appear to boost the activity of cancer-fighting immune cells. Further research on phytochemicals may extend the role of nutrition to the prevention and treatment of many chronic diseases.

To increase your intake of phytochemicals, it is best to obtain them by eating a variety of fruits and vegetables rather than relying on supplements. Like many vitamins and minerals, isolated phytochemicals may be harmful if taken in high doses. In addition, it is likely that their health benefits are the result of chemical substances working in combination. The role of phytochemicals in disease prevention is discussed further in Chapters 11 and 12.

NUTRITIONAL GUIDELINES: PLANNING YOUR DIET

The second part of putting together a healthy food plan—after you've learned about necessary nutrients—is choosing foods that satisfy nutritional requirements and meet your personal criteria. Various tools have been created by scientific and government groups to help people design healthy diets. The **Dietary Reference Intakes (DRIs)** are standards for nutrient intake designed to prevent nutritional deficiencies and reduce the risk of chronic disease. The **Food Guide Pyramid** translates these nutrient recommendations into a balanced food-group plan that includes all essential nutrients. To provide further guidance, **Dietary Guidelines for Americans** have been established to address the prevention of diet-related chronic diseases. Together, these tools make up a complete set of resources for dietary planning.

Dietary Reference Intakes (DRIs)

How much vitamin C, iron, calcium, and other nutrients do you need to stay healthy? The Food and Nutrition Board of the National Academy of Sciences establishes dietary standards, or recommended intake levels, for Americans of all ages. The current set of standards, called Dietary Reference Intakes (DRIs), is relatively new, having been introduced in 1997. An earlier set of standards, called the **Recommended Dietary Allowances (RDAs),** focused on preventing nutritional deficiency diseases such as anemia; the RDAs were established in 1941 and updated periodically, most recently in 1989. The newer DRIs have a broader focus because recent research has looked not just at the prevention of nutrient deficiencies but also at the role of nutrients in promoting optimal health and preventing chronic diseases such as cancer, osteoporosis, and heart disease.

The DRIs include standards for both recommended intakes and maximum safe intakes. The recommended intake of each nutrient is expressed as either a *Recommended Dietary Allowance (RDA)* or *Adequate Intake (AI)*. An AI is set when there is not enough information available to set an RDA value; regardless of the type of standard used, however, the DRI represents the best available estimate of intake for optimal health. The *Tolerable Upper Intake Level (UL)* sets the maximum daily intake by a healthy person that is unlikely to cause health problems. For example, the RDA for calcium for an 18-year-old female is 1300 mg per day; the UL is 2500 mg per day. Because of lack of data, ULs have not been set for all nutrients. This does not mean that people can tolerate chronic intakes of these vitamins and minerals above recommended levels. Like all chemical agents, nutrients can produce adverse effects if intakes are excessive. There is no established benefit from consuming nutrients at levels above the RDA or AI.

The DRIs are being issued in stages, and, by early 2002, they had been set for most vitamins and minerals. By 2003, the remaining nutrients will have DRI values set, and other substances such as fiber will also be considered by the Food and Nutrition Board. The DRIs established to date can be found in the Nutrition Resources section at the end of the chapter (pp. 242–244); there you can also

Terms

Ww

phytochemical A naturally occurring substance found in plant foods that may help prevent and treat chronic diseases such as heart disease and cancer; *phyto* means plant.

cruciferous vegetables Vegetables of the cabbage family, including cabbage, broccoli, brussels sprouts, kale, and cauliflower; the flower petals of these plants form the shape of a cross, hence the name.

Dietary Reference Intakes (DRIs) An umbrella term for four types of nutrient standards: Adequate Intake (AI), Estimated Average Requirement (EAR), and Recommended Dietary Allowance (RDA) set levels of intake considered adequate to prevent nutrient deficiencies and reduce the risk of chronic disease; Tolerable Upper Intake Level (UL) sets the maximum daily intake that is unlikely to cause health problems.

Food Guide Pyramid A food-group plan that provides practical advice to ensure a balanced intake of the essential nutrients.

Dietary Guidelines for Americans General principles of good nutrition intended to help prevent certain diet-related diseases.

Recommended Dietary Allowances (RDAs) Amounts of certain nutrients considered adequate to prevent deficiencies in most healthy people; will eventually be replaced by the Dietary Reference Intakes (DRIs).

Daily Values A simplified version of the RDAs used on food labels; also included are values for nutrients with no established RDA.

find an abridged version of the 1989 RDAs, which includes recommended intakes for nutrients for which DRIs have not yet been set. (For more on updates and additions to the DRIs, visit the Web site of the Food and Nutrition Board; see For Further Exploration at the end of the chapter.)

Should You Take Supplements? The aim of the DRIs is to guide you in meeting your nutritional needs primarily with food, rather than with vitamin and mineral supplements. This goal is important because recommendations have not yet been set for some essential nutrients. Many supplements contain only nutrients with established recommendations, so using them to meet nutrient needs can leave you deficient in other nutrients. Supplements also lack potentially beneficial phytochemicals that are found only in whole foods. Nutrition scientists generally agree that most Americans can obtain most of the vitamins and minerals they need by consuming a varied, nutritionally balanced diet.

The question of whether to take supplements is a serious one. Some vitamins and minerals are dangerous when ingested in excess, as shown in Tables 8.3 and 8.4. Large doses of particular nutrients can also cause health problems by affecting the absorption of other vitamins and minerals. For all these reasons, you should think carefully about whether to take supplements; consider consulting a physician or registered dietitian.

In setting the DRIs, the Food and Nutrition Board recommended supplements of particular nutrients for the following groups:

- Women who are capable of becoming pregnant should take 400 μg per day of folic acid (the synthetic form of the vitamin folate) from fortified foods and/or supplements in addition to folate from a varied diet. Research indicates that this level of folate intake will reduce the risk of neural tube defects. (This defect occurs early in pregnancy, before most women know they are pregnant; therefore, the recommendation for the folate intake applies to all women of reproductive age rather than only to pregnant women.) Since 1998, enriched breads, flours, corn meals, rice, noodles, and other grain products have been fortified with small amounts of folic acid. Folate is found naturally in leafy green vegetables, legumes, oranges and orange juice, and strawberries.
- People over age 50 should consume foods fortified with vitamin B-12, B-12 supplements, or a combination of the two in order to meet the majority of the DRI of 2.4 mg of B-12 daily. Up to 30% of people over 50 may have problems absorbing protein-bound B-12 in foods. Vitamin B-12 in supplements and fortified foods is more readily absorbed and can help prevent a deficiency.

Because of the oxidative stress caused by smoking, the Food and Nutrition Board also recommends that smokers consume 35 mg *more* vitamin C per day than the DRI intake level set for their age and sex (for adults, recommended daily vitamin C intakes for nonsmokers are 90 mg for men and 75 mg for women). However, supplements are not usually needed because this extra vitamin C can easily be obtained from foods. For example, one cup of orange juice has about 100 mg of vitamin C.

Supplements may also be recommended in other cases. Women with heavy menstrual flows may need extra iron to compensate for the monthly loss. Some vegetarians may need supplemental calcium, iron, zinc, and vitamin B-12, depending on their food choices. Newborns need a single dose of vitamin K, which must be administered under the direction of a physician. People who consume few calories, who have certain diseases, or who take certain medications may need specific vitamin and mineral supplements; such supplement decisions must be made by a physician because some vitamins and minerals counteract the actions of certain medications.

In deciding whether to take a vitamin and mineral supplement, consider whether you already regularly consume a fortified breakfast cereal. Many breakfast cereals contain almost as many nutrients as a vitamin pill! If you do decide to take a supplement, choose a balanced formulation that contains 50–100% of the Daily Value for vitamins and minerals. Avoid supplements containing large doses of particular nutrients. See pp. 230–232 for more on choosing and using supplements.

Daily Values Because the DRIs are far too cumbersome to use as a basis for food labels, the U.S. Food and Drug Administration developed another set of dietary standards, the **Daily Values.** The Daily Values are based on several different sets of guidelines and include standards for fat, cholesterol, carbohydrate, dietary fiber, and selected vitamins and minerals. The Daily Values represent appropriate intake levels for a 2000-calorie diet. The percent Daily Value shown on a food label shows how well that food contributes to your recommended daily intake. Food labels are described in detail later in the chapter.

WW The Food Guide Pyramid

The Food Guide Pyramid is a food-group plan developed by the U.S. Department of Agriculture that gives a recommended number of servings for five different major food groups (Figure 8.4, p. 220). A range of servings is given for each group: The smaller number is for people who consume about 1600 calories a day, such as many sedentary women; the larger number is for those who consume about 2800 calories a day, such as active men. Serving sizes and examples of foods are described below for each group. The fundamental principles of the Food Guide Pyramid are moderation, variety, and balance—a theme echoed throughout this chapter.

It is important to choose a variety of foods within each group because different foods have different combinations of nutrients: for example, within the vegetable

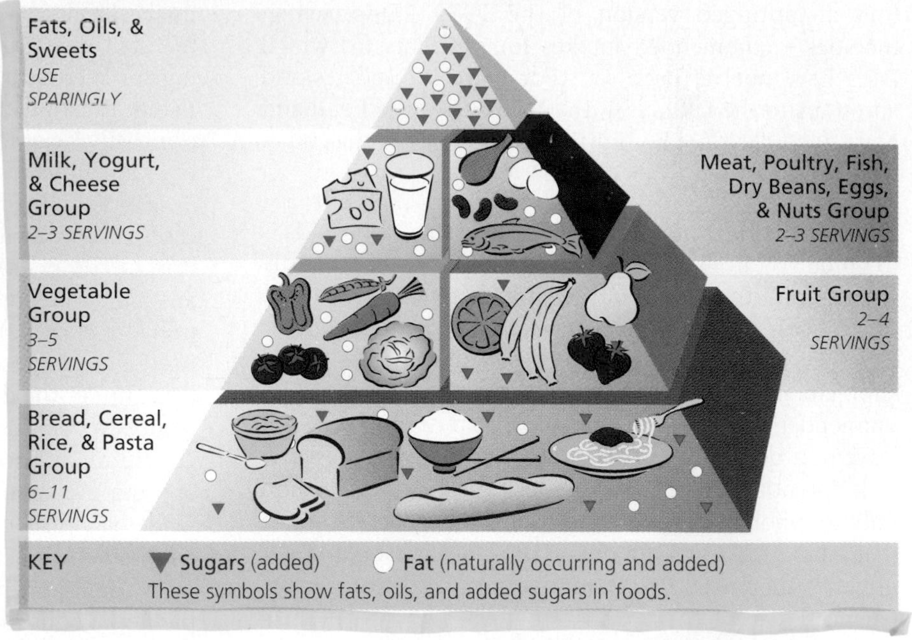

Figure 8.4 The Food Guide Pyramid: A guide to daily food choices. The Pyramid is an outline of what to eat each day—not a rigid prescription, but a general guide that lets you choose a healthful diet that's right for you. It calls for eating a variety of foods to get the nutrients you need and at the same time the right amount of calories to maintain a healthy weight. The Pyramid also focuses on fat because many Americans eat too much fat, especially saturated fat. SOURCE: USDA. Center for Nutrition Policy and Information. 1996. *Food Guide Pyramid.* USDA Home and Garden Bulletin no. 252.

group, potatoes are high in vitamin C, and spinach is a rich source of vitamin A. Foods also vary in their amount of calories and nutrients. People who do not need many calories should focus on nutrient-dense foods within each group (foods that are high in nutrients relative to the number of calories they contain). For example, whole-grain bread is more nutrient-dense than white bread, and 100% orange juice is more nutrient-dense than an orange-flavored drink. Many foods you eat contain servings from more than one food group.

For more on the basic pyramid and alternative pyramids for special populations such as young children and people choosing particular ethnic diets, contact the USDA's Center for Nutrition Policy and Promotion (see For Further Exploration at the end of the chapter).

Bread, Cereals, Rice, and Pasta (6–11 Servings) Foods from this group are usually low in fat and rich in complex carbohydrates, dietary fiber (if grains are unrefined), and many vitamins and minerals, including thiamin, riboflavin, iron, niacin, folate, and zinc. Although 6–11 servings may seem like a large amount of food, many people eat several servings at a time. A single serving is the equivalent of the following:

- 1 slice of bread or half a hamburger bun, English muffin, or bagel
- 1 small roll, biscuit, or muffin
- 1 ounce of ready-to-eat cereal
- ½ cup cooked cereal, rice, or pasta
- 5–6 small or 2–3 large crackers

If you are one of the many people who have trouble identifying an ounce of cereal or half a cup of rice, see the strategies in the box "Judging Serving Sizes." Choose foods that are typically made with little fat or sugars (bread, rice, pasta) over those that are high in fat and sugars (croissants, chips, cookies, doughnuts). For maximum nutrition, choose at least three servings from whole grains, such as whole-wheat bread, high-fiber cereal, whole-wheat pasta, and brown rice.

Vegetables (3–5 Servings) Vegetables are rich in carbohydrates, dietary fiber, vitamin A, vitamin C, folate, magnesium, and other nutrients. They are also naturally low in fat. A serving of vegetables is equivalent to the following:

- 1 cup raw leafy vegetables
- ½ cup raw or cooked vegetables
- ½ cup tomato sauce
- ¾ cup vegetable juice
- ½ cup cooked dry beans

Good choices from this group include dark-green leafy vegetables such as spinach, chard, and collards; deep-orange and red vegetables such as carrots, winter squash, red bell peppers, and tomatoes; broccoli, cauliflower, and other cruciferous vegetables; peas; green beans; potatoes; and corn. Dry beans (legumes) such as pinto, navy, kidney, and black beans can be counted as servings of vegetables *or* as alternatives to meat.

Fruits (2–4 Servings) Like vegetables, fruits are rich in carbohydrates, dietary fiber, and many vitamins, especially vitamin C. They are low in fat and sodium. The serving sizes used in the Pyramid are as follows:

- 1 medium (apple, banana, peach, orange, pear) or 2 small (apricot, plum) whole fruit(s)
- 1 melon wedge
- ½ cup berries, cherries, or grapes

TAKE CHARGE Judging Serving Sizes

Studies have shown that most people underestimate the size of their food portions, in many cases by as much as 50%. If you need to retrain your eye, try using measuring cups and spoons and an inexpensive kitchen scale when you eat at home. With a little practice, you'll learn the difference between 3 and 8 ounces of chicken or meat and what a half-cup of rice really looks like. For quick estimates, use these equivalents:

- 1 teaspoon of margarine = the tip of your thumb
- 1 ounce of cheese = your thumb, four dice stacked together, or an ice cube
- 3 ounces of chicken or meat = a deck of cards or an audiocassette tape
- $\frac{1}{2}$ cup of rice or cooked vegetables = an ice cream scoop or one-third of a soda can
- 2 tablespoons of peanut butter = a Ping-Pong ball or large marshmallow
- 1 cup of pasta = a small fist or a tennis ball
- 1 medium potato = a computer mouse
- 1 2-ounce bagel = a hockey puck or yo-yo
- 1 medium fruit (apple or orange) = a baseball
- $\frac{1}{4}$ cup nuts = a golf ball
- small cookie or cracker = a poker chip

- $\frac{1}{2}$ grapefruit
- $\frac{1}{2}$ cup chopped, cooked, canned, or frozen fruit
- $\frac{3}{4}$ cup fruit juice (100% juice)
- $\frac{1}{4}$ cup dried fruit

Good choices from this group are citrus fruits and juices, melons, pears, apples, bananas, and berries. Choose whole fruits often—they are higher in fiber and often lower in calories than fruit juices. Fruit *juices* typically contain more nutrients than fruit *drinks*. For canned fruits, choose those packed in their own juice rather than in syrup.

Milk, Yogurt, and Cheese (2–3 Servings) Foods from this group are high in protein, carbohydrate, calcium, riboflavin, and vitamin D. To limit the fat in your diet, choose servings of low-fat or nonfat items from this group:

- 1 cup milk or yogurt
- $1\frac{1}{2}$ ounces cheese
- 2 ounces processed cheese

Cottage cheese is lower in calcium than most other cheeses, and 1 cup of cottage cheese counts as only half a serving for this food group. Ice cream is also lower in calcium than many other dairy products ($\frac{1}{2}$ cup is equivalent to $\frac{1}{3}$ serving); in addition, it is high in sugar and fat.

Meat, Poultry, Fish, Dry Beans, Eggs, and Nuts (2–3 Servings) This food group provides protein, niacin, iron, vitamin B-6, zinc, and thiamin; the animal foods in the group also provide vitamin B-12. The Pyramid recommends 2–3 servings each day of foods from this group. The total amount of these servings should be the equivalent of 5–7 ounces of cooked lean meat, poultry, or fish a day. Many people misjudge what makes up a single serving for this food group:

- 2–3 ounces cooked lean meat, poultry, or fish (an average hamburger or a medium chicken breast half is about 3 ounces; 4 slices of bologna, 6 slices of hard salami, or $\frac{1}{2}$ cup of drained canned tuna counts as about 2 ounces)
- The following portions of nonmeat foods are equivalent to 1 ounce of lean meat: $\frac{1}{2}$ cup cooked dry beans (if not counted as a vegetable), 1 egg, 2 tablespoons peanut butter, $\frac{1}{3}$ cup nuts, $\frac{1}{4}$ cup seeds, and $\frac{1}{2}$ cup tofu

One egg at breakfast, a cup of pinto beans at lunch, and a hamburger at dinner would add up to the equivalent of 6 ounces of lean meat for the day. To limit your intake of fat and saturated fat, choose lean cuts of meat and skinless poultry, eat nuts and seeds in moderation, and watch your serving sizes carefully. Choose at least one serving of plant proteins such as black beans, lentils, or tofu every day.

Fats, Oils, and Sweets The tip of the Pyramid includes fats, oils, and sweets—foods such as salad dressings, oils, butter, margarine, gravy, mayonnaise, soft drinks, sugar, candy, jellies and jams, syrups, and sweet desserts. Foods from the Pyramid tip provide calories but few nutrients; they should not replace foods from the other groups. The total amount of fats, oils, and sweets you consume should be determined by your overall energy needs.

The colored triangles and circles in the Pyramid appear in all the other food groups to remind you that food choices in those groups can also be high in fats and added sugars. ("Added sugars" are sugars added in processing, not those found naturally in fruits and milk.) Foods that come from animals (the meat and milk groups) are naturally higher in fats than foods that come from plants, which is why it's important to choose lean meats and low-fat dairy products. Fruits, vegetables, and grains are naturally lower in fat, but they are often prepared in ways that make them higher-fat choices, such as french fries, baked potatoes with sour cream and cheese, fettuccine Alfredo,

Table 8.5 Food Guide Pyramid Recommendations Compared with the Average American Diet

	RECOMMENDED DIETS AT THREE CALORIE LEVELS[a]			AVERAGE AMERICAN DIET	
	1600	2200	2800	Women (1600 calories)	Men (2400 calories)
Grain group (servings)	6	9	11	5.7	7.9
Vegetable group (servings)	3	4	5	2.9	3.9
Fruit group (servings)	2	3	4	1.5	1.5
Dairy group (servings)[b]	2–3	2–3	2–3	1.1	1.5
Meat group (ounces)[c]	5	6	7	4.0	6.7
Total fat (grams)[d]	53	73	93	58.1	90.1
Total added sugars (teaspoons)[d,e]	6	12	18	15.4	22.2

[a]The bottom of the recommended range of servings (1600 calories) is about right for many sedentary women and older adults. The middle range (2200 calories) is about right for most children, teenage girls, active women, and many sedentary men. The top of the range (2800 calories) is about right for teenage boys, many active men, and some very active women.

[b]Women who are pregnant or lactating, teenagers, and young adults to age 24 need 3 servings.

[c]The Pyramid recommends 2–3 servings a day, the equivalent of 5–7 ounces of cooked lean meat, poultry, or fish (see p. 221).

[d]Values for total fat and added sugars include fat and added sugars that are in food choices from the five major food groups as well as fat and added sugars from foods in the Fats, Oils, and Sweets group. The total for added sugars does not include sugars that occur naturally in foods such as fruit and milk. The recommended fat totals are based on a limit of 30% of total calories as fat.

[e]A teaspoon of sugar is equivalent to 4 grams (16 calories).

SOURCES: USDA Agricultural Research Service. 2000. *Pyramid Servings Intakes: CNRG Table Set No 1.* Beltsville, Md.: Community Nutrition Research Group. Shaw, A., et al. 1997. *Using the Food Guide Pyramid: A Resource for Nutrition Educators.* USDA Center for Nutrition Policy and Promotion (http://www.nal.usda.gov/fnic/Fpyr/guide pdf; retrieved April 18, 2000).

and baked goods like cookies and pies. Added sugars are common in the milk group (ice cream, sweetened yogurt), the fruit group (canned fruit in syrup), and the grain group (bakery goods). Reduced-fat versions of prepared foods are often *very* high in added sugars and consequently just as high in calories as their full-fat versions.

The average American diet currently includes more fat and added sugars than recommended. The Pyramid suggests that Americans limit the fat in their diets to 30% of total calories. You can moderate your fat intake by making low-fat choices from each group and minimizing the use of fat in cooking or as toppings such as sour cream and heavy sauces. Added sugars are less of a concern to health than fat, but consumption of large amounts of sugars adds empty calories to the diet and can make weight management more difficult.

Analysis of the average diet of Americans has revealed that the number of servings from the fruit, dairy, and meat groups is below the recommended ranges, and servings from the grain and vegetable groups are near the bottom of the recommended ranges (Table 8.5). Overconsumption of fat and added sugars leaves fewer calories available for healthier food choices from the five major food groups. For example, the average daily diet among American women includes about 9.5 teaspoons (38 grams) of added sugars and 5 grams of fat above recommended limits. The 200 calories in these extra sugars and fats could be better used to increase the number of servings from the food groups for which women typically fall short of Pyramid recommendations.

General strategies for controlling intake of fat and added sugars include choosing lower-fat foods within each food group, eating fewer foods that are high in sugar and fat and low in other nutrients, and limiting the amount of fats and sugars added to foods during cooking or at the table. Consider the nutrient density of your food choices, and favor foods that are rich in nutrients relative to the number of calories they contain.

The Food Guide Pyramid is a general guide to what you should eat every day. By eating a balanced variety of foods from each of the six food groups and including some plant proteins, you can ensure that your daily diet is adequate in all nutrients. A diet using low-fat food choices contains only about 1600 calories but meets all known nutritional needs, except possibly for iron in some women who have heavy menstrual periods. For these women, foods fortified in iron, such as breakfast cereals, can make up the deficit.

Dietary Guidelines for Americans

To provide further guidance for choosing a healthy diet, the U.S. Department of Agriculture (USDA) and the U.S. Department of Health and Human Services (DHHS) have issued Dietary Guidelines for Americans, most recently in

2000. Following these guidelines promotes health and reduces risk for chronic diseases, including heart disease, cancer, diabetes, stroke, osteoporosis, and obesity. Ten guidelines are provided, organized under three messages, the "ABCs for Health":

Aim for fitness.

Build a healthy base.

Choose sensibly.

Here is a brief summary of the guidelines.

Aim for Fitness The two guidelines in this category emphasize that a lifestyle combining sensible eating with regular physical activity promotes long-term health and fitness and enables people to enjoy life and feel their best.

AIM FOR A HEALTHY WEIGHT Evaluate your body weight in terms of body mass index (BMI), a measure of relative body weight that also takes height into account. (See Chapter 6 for instructions on how to determine your BMI.) If your current weight is healthy, aim to avoid weight gain. Do so by eating vegetables, fruits, and whole grains with little added fat or sugar; also focus on selecting sensible portion sizes. If you are overweight, first aim to prevent further weight gain, and then lose weight to improve your health. Plan to lose weight gradually—about 10% of your weight over about 6 months—through a combination of sensible eating, physical activity, and behavior change. Loss of ½ to 2 pounds a week is usually safe. Your health is more likely to improve over the long term if you achieve and maintain a healthy weight than if you lose and regain weight several times. But even if you have regained weight in the past, it's worthwhile to try again.

BE PHYSICALLY ACTIVE EVERY DAY Become active if you are inactive, and maintain or increase physical activity if you are already active. Aim to accumulate at least 30 minutes (adults) or 60 minutes (children) of moderate physical activity on most days, preferably every day. You can do the activity all at once or spread it out over two to three periods during the day. If you already get 30 minutes of physical activity daily, you can gain even more health benefits by increasing the intensity or duration of your activity. Aerobic activities and activities for strength and flexibility are especially beneficial.

Physical activity and nutrition work together for better health. For example, physical activity increases the amount of calories you use, which in turn makes it easier to get the nutrients you need. For those who have intentionally lost weight, being active makes it easier to maintain the weight loss. However, to maintain a healthy weight after weight loss, adults will likely need more than 30 minutes of activity daily.

Build a Healthy Base The four guidelines in this category provide a foundation for healthy eating.

LET THE PYRAMID GUIDE YOUR FOOD CHOICES To ensure that you get all the nutrients and other substances you need, choose the recommended number of daily servings from each of the five major food groups shown in the Food Guide Pyramid (see Figure 8.4). Healthy eating patterns start with plant foods, represented in the three food groups at the base of the Pyramid: grains, vegetables, and fruits. Plan your meals around a variety of foods from these groups, keeping a close eye on serving sizes. Be flexible and adventurous—try new choices in place of some of the less nutritious foods you usually eat. Everyone, especially adolescent girls and women, should take special care to meet their recommended intakes for calcium, iron, and folic acid.

People's food choices are affected by culture, family background, religion, moral beliefs, the cost and availability of food, life experience, food intolerances, and allergies. The Pyramid provides a good guide to healthy eating no matter how the foods are prepared or combined. However, if you avoid all foods from any of the five major groups, be sure to get enough nutrients from other groups. For example, if you eat few dairy products, choose other foods that are good sources of calcium and make sure you get enough vitamin D. If you avoid animal products, be sure you get enough iron, vitamin B-12, calcium, and zinc. Some people may need to consume fortified foods or take a vitamin or mineral supplement to meet a specific nutrient need; however, you should not depend on supplements to meet your usual nutritional needs.

EAT A VARIETY OF GRAINS DAILY, ESPECIALLY WHOLE GRAINS Grains such as wheat, oats, corn, and rice are rich in complex carbohydrates and tend to be low in fat; whole grains provide more fiber and nutrients than refined grains. Make grains the foundation of your diet—eat six or more servings daily. If your calorie needs are low, eat only six servings of a sensible size. Include several servings of whole grains daily, choosing a variety of grains, such as whole wheat, brown rice, oats, and whole corn. Prepare or choose grain products with little added saturated fat and sugar.

EAT A VARIETY OF FRUITS AND VEGETABLES DAILY Different fruits and vegetables are rich in different nutrients, so it's important to choose a variety. For example, carrots, dark-green leafy vegetables, and cantaloupe are excellent sources of carotenoids; citrus fruits, potatoes, and broccoli are rich in vitamin C; spinach, legumes, and orange juice are high in folate; and bananas, winter squash, and dried fruits are good sources of potassium. Fresh fruits and vegetables, especially when eaten with the peel, are also good sources of dietary fiber.

Eat at least two servings of fruit and three servings of vegetables daily. Choose fresh, frozen, dried, or canned forms and a variety of colors and kinds. Favor dark-green leafy vegetables, bright orange fruits and vegetables, and cooked dried peas and beans.

TAKE CHARGE Reducing the Fat in Your Diet

Your overall goal is to limit total fat intake to no more than 30% of total calories. Within that limit, favor unsaturated fats from vegetable oils, nuts, and fish over saturated and trans fats from animal products and foods made with hydrogenated vegetable oils or shortening. Limit saturated fat to less than 10% of total calories.

- Be moderate in your consumption of foods high in fat, including fast food, commercially prepared baked goods and desserts, deep-fried foods, meat, poultry, nuts and seeds, and regular dairy products.
- When you do eat high-fat foods, limit your portion sizes, and balance your intake with foods low in fat.
- Choose lean cuts of meat, and trim any visible fat from meat before and after cooking. Remove skin from poultry before or after cooking.
- Drink fat-free or low-fat milk instead of whole milk, and use lower-fat varieties in puddings, soups, and baked products. Substitute plain low-fat yogurt, blender-whipped low-fat cottage cheese, or buttermilk in recipes that call for sour cream.
- To reduce saturated and trans fat, use vegetable oil instead of butter or margarine. Use tub or squeeze margarine instead of stick margarine. Look for margarines that are free of trans fats.
- Season vegetables, seafood, and meats with herbs and spices rather than with creamy sauces, butter, or margarine.
- Try lemon juice on salad, or use a yogurt-based salad dressing instead of mayonnaise or sour cream dressings.
- Steam, boil, bake, or microwave vegetables, or stir-fry them in a small amount of vegetable oil.
- Roast, bake, or broil meat, poultry, or fish so that fat drains away as the food cooks.
- Use a nonstick pan for cooking so that added fat will be unnecessary; use a vegetable spray for frying.
- Chill broths from meat or poultry until the fat becomes solid. Spoon off the fat before using the broth.
- Substitute egg whites for whole eggs when baking; limit the number of egg yolks when scrambling eggs.
- Choose fruits as desserts most often.
- Eat a low-fat vegetarian main dish at least once a week.

KEEP FOOD SAFE TO EAT Safe foods are those that pose little risk from harmful bacteria, viruses, parasites, or chemical contaminants. It is especially important to be careful with perishable foods such as eggs, meats, poultry, fish, shellfish, milk products, and fresh fruits and vegetables. If food has been left out for too long or refrigerated for too long, it may not be safe to eat even if it looks and smells fine. Refer to the section "Preventing and Treating Foodborne Illness" (p. 233) for specific food safety tips.

Choose Sensibly The four guidelines in this category help you make food choices that promote health and reduce the risk of certain chronic diseases.

CHOOSE A DIET LOW IN SATURATED FAT AND CHOLESTEROL AND MODERATE IN TOTAL FAT A diet low in saturated fat (less than 10% of daily calories) and cholesterol (less than 300 milligrams per day) helps keep blood cholesterol levels low and reduces the risk of cardiovascular disease. Moderate total fat intake (no more than 30% of total calories) also helps with weight control. Refer to the box "Reducing the Fat in Your Diet" for specific strategies for meeting these guidelines.

Cholesterol is found only in animal foods. To limit your cholesterol intake, follow the Pyramid recommendations for consumption of animal foods and pay particular attention to serving sizes. In addition, limit your intake of foods that are particularly high in cholesterol, including egg yolks, dairy fats, and liver and other organ meats. Food labels provide the fat, saturated fat, and cholesterol content of foods.

CHOOSE BEVERAGES AND FOODS TO MODERATE YOUR INTAKE OF SUGARS Sugar doesn't cause hyperactivity, but it does promote tooth decay and it may lower HDL cholesterol levels. In addition, many foods high in sugar are relatively high in calories but low in other nutrients; consuming excess calories from added sugars may contribute to weight gain or lower consumption of more nutritious foods. The Pyramid recommends no more than about 6 teaspoons (24 g) of added sugars a day if you eat 1600 calories, 12 teaspoons (48 g) at 2200 calories, or 18 teaspoons (72 g) at 2800 calories. Most Americans consume much more than this—one can of regular soda, the leading source of added sugars in the American diet, supplies about 10 teaspoons of sugar. On average, Americans consume more than 50 gallons of soda and 25 pounds of candy per year.

Terms Ww

vegan A vegetarian who eats no animal products at all.

lacto-vegetarian A vegetarian who includes milk and cheese products in the diet.

lacto-ovo-vegetarian A vegetarian who eats no meat, poultry, or fish, but does eat eggs and milk products.

partial vegetarian, semivegetarian, or **pesco-vegetarian** A vegetarian who includes eggs, dairy products, and small amounts of poultry and seafood in the diet.

To reduce sugar consumption, cut back on soft drinks, candies, sweet desserts (cakes, cookies, pies), fruit drinks, and other foods high in added sugars. A food is likely high in sugar if one of the following ingredients appears first or second in the list of ingredients or if several are listed: sugar (any type, including beet, brown, raw, and cane), corn syrup or sweetener, fruit juice concentrate, honey, malt syrup, molasses, syrup, cane juice, or dextrose, fructose, glucose, lactose, maltose, mannitol, or sucrose. Try drinking water rather than sweetened drinks and don't let sodas and other sweets crowd out more nutritious foods, such as low-fat milk and fruit.

Choose and Prepare Foods with Less Salt Many people can reduce their chance of developing high blood pressure by consuming less salt. Salt is made up of the minerals sodium and chloride. Although sodium is essential for normal body function, we need only small amounts, the equivalent of less than 1/4 teaspoon of salt daily. It is recommended that you limit sodium intake to no more than 2400 mg per day, the equivalent of about 1 teaspoon of salt.

Salt is found mainly in processed and prepared foods and may also be added during cooking or at the table. To lower your intake of salt, choose fresh or plain frozen meat, poultry, seafood, and vegetables most often; they are lower in salt than more processed forms. Check and compare the sodium content in processed foods, including frozen dinners, cheeses, soups, salad dressings, sauces, and canned mixed dishes. Add less salt during cooking and at the table, and limit your use of high-sodium condiments like soy sauce, ketchup, mustard, pickles, and olives. Use lemon juice, herbs, and spices instead of salt to enhance the flavor of foods.

If You Drink Alcoholic Beverages, Do So in Moderation Alcoholic beverages supply calories but few nutrients; excess alcohol alters judgment and can lead to dependency and other serious health problems (see Chapter 13). Drinking in moderation is defined as no more than one drink a day for women and no more than two drinks a day for men. People who should not drink at all include individuals who cannot restrict their drinking to moderate levels, women who are or may become pregnant, individuals who plan to drive or operate machinery, and individuals taking medications that can interact with alcohol. If you choose to drink alcoholic beverages, do so sensibly, moderately, and with meals; never drink in situations where it may put you or others at risk.

The Vegetarian Alternative

Some people choose a diet with one essential difference from the diets we've already described: Foods of animal origin (meat, poultry, fish, eggs, milk) are eliminated or restricted. Many do so for health reasons; vegetarian diets tend to be lower in saturated fat, cholesterol, and animal protein and higher in complex carbohydrates, dietary fiber, folate, vitamins C and E, carotenoids, and phytochemicals. Some people adopt a vegetarian diet out of concern for the environment, for financial considerations, or for reasons related to ethics or religion.

No matter what your dietary choices or challenges, you need to include water in your daily diet. Drink about 8 cups of fluid a day—more if you live in a hot climate or if you exercise vigorously.

Types of Vegetarian Diets There are various vegetarian styles; the wider the variety of the diet eaten, the easier it is to meet nutritional needs. **Vegans** eat only plant foods. **Lacto-vegetarians** eat plant foods and dairy products. **Lacto-ovo-vegetarians** eat plant foods, dairy products, and eggs. According to recent polls, about 5 million American adults never eat meat, poultry, or fish and fall into one of these three groups. Others can be categorized as **partial vegetarians, semivegetarians,** or **pescovegetarians;** these individuals eat plant foods, dairy products, eggs, and usually a small selection of poultry, fish, and other seafood. Many other people choose vegetarian meals frequently but are not strictly vegetarian. Including

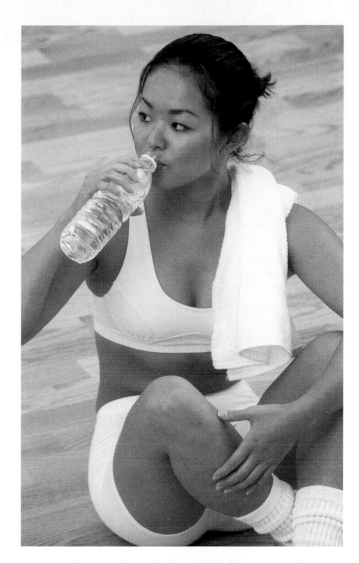

some animal protein (such as dairy products) in a vegetarian diet makes planning easier, but it is not necessary.

A Food Pyramid for Vegetarians The basic USDA pyramid can be adapted for use by vegetarians with only a few key modifications:

- Bread, cereal, rice, and pasta group (6–11 servings per day)
- Vegetable group (3–5 servings per day)
- Fruit group (2–4 servings per day)
- Milk, yogurt, and cheese group (0–3 servings per day); vegans and other vegetarians who do not consume any dairy products must find other rich sources of calcium (see below)
- Dry beans, nuts, seeds, eggs, and meat substitutes group (2–3 servings per day); this group includes such foods as soy milk, legumes, eggs or egg whites, nuts, seeds, tofu (soybean curd), tempeh (a cultured soy product), and peanut butter

A healthy vegetarian diet emphasizes a wide variety of plant foods. Although plant proteins are generally of lower quality than animal proteins, choosing a variety of plant foods will supply all of the essential amino acids. Choosing minimally processed and unrefined foods will maximize nutrient value and provide ample dietary fiber. Daily consumption of a variety of plant foods in amounts that meet total energy needs can provide all needed nutrients, except vitamin B-12 and possibly vitamin D. Strategies for obtaining these and other nutrients of concern include the following:

- *Vitamin B-12* is found naturally only in animal foods; if dairy products and eggs are limited or avoided, B-12 can be obtained from fortified foods such as ready-to-eat cereals, soy beverages, meat substitutes, and special yeast products or from supplements.
- *Vitamin D* can be obtained by spending 5–15 minutes a day out in the sun, by consuming vitamin D-fortified products like ready-to-eat cereals and soy or rice milk, or by taking a supplement.
- *Calcium* is found in legumes, tofu processed with calcium, dark-green leafy vegetables, nuts, tortillas made from lime-processed corn, and fortified orange juice, soy milk, bread, and other foods.
- *Iron* is found in whole grains, fortified bread and breakfast cereals, dried fruits, green leafy vegetables, nuts and seeds, legumes, and soy foods. The iron in plant foods is more difficult for the body to absorb than the iron from animal sources; consuming a good source of vitamin C with most meals is helpful because vitamin C improves iron absorption.
- *Zinc* is found in whole grains, nuts, legumes, and soy foods.

It takes a little planning and common sense to put together a good vegetarian diet. If you are a vegetarian or are considering becoming one, devote some extra time and thought to your diet. It's especially important that you eat as wide a variety of foods as possible to ensure that all your nutritional needs are satisfied. Consulting with a registered dietitian will make your planning even easier. Vegetarian diets for children, teens, and pregnant and lactating women warrant professional guidance.

Dietary Challenges for Special Population Groups

The Food Guide Pyramid and Dietary Guidelines for Americans provide a basis that everyone can use to create a healthy diet. However, some population groups face special dietary challenges.

Women Women tend to be smaller and to weigh less than men, meaning they have lower energy needs and therefore consume fewer calories. Because of this, women have more difficulty getting adequate amounts of all the essential nutrients and need to focus on nutrient-dense foods. Two nutrients of special concern are calcium and iron, minerals for which many women fail to meet the RDAs. Low calcium intake may be linked to the development of osteoporosis in later life. The *Healthy People 2010* report sets a goal of increasing from 40% to 75% the proportion of women age 20–49 who meet the dietary recommendation for calcium. Nonfat and low-fat dairy products and fortified cereal, bread, and orange juice are good choices. Iron is also a concern: Menstruating women have higher iron requirements than other groups, and a lack of iron in the diet can lead to iron-deficiency anemia. Lean red meat, green leafy vegetables, and fortified breakfast cereals are good sources of iron. As discussed earlier, all women capable of becoming pregnant should consume adequate folic acid from fortified foods and/or supplements.

Men Men are seldom thought of as having nutritional deficiencies because they generally have high-calorie diets. However, many men have a diet that does not follow the Food Guide Pyramid but that includes more red meat and fewer fruits, vegetables, and grains than recommended. This dietary pattern is linked to heart disease and some types of cancer. A high intake of calories can lead to weight gain in the long term if a man's activity level decreases as he ages. Men should use the Food Guide Pyramid as a basis for their overall diet and focus on increasing their consumption of fruits, vegetables, and grains to obtain vitamins, minerals, dietary fiber, and phytochemicals.

College Students Foods that are convenient for college students are not always the healthiest choices. It is easy for students who eat in buffet-style dining halls to overeat, and the foods offered are not necessarily high in essential nutrients and low in fat. The same is true of meals at fast-food

TAKE CHARGE Eating Strategies for College Students

General Guidelines

- Eat slowly and enjoy your food. Set aside a separate time to eat. Don't eat while you study.
- Eat a colorful, varied diet. The more colorful your diet is, the more varied and rich in fruits and vegetables it will be. Many Americans eat few fruits and vegetables, despite the fact that these foods are typically inexpensive, delicious, rich in nutrients, and low in fat and calories.
- Eat breakfast. You'll have more energy in the morning and be less likely to grab an unhealthy snack later on.
- Choose healthy snacks—fruits, vegetables, grains, and cereals—as often as you can.
- Drink water more often than soft drinks or other sweetened beverages. Rent a mini-refrigerator for your dorm room and stock up on healthy beverages.
- Pay attention to portion sizes.
- Combine physical activity with healthy eating. You'll look and feel better and have a much lower risk of many chronic diseases. Even a little exercise is better than none.

Eating in the Dining Hall

- Choose a meal plan that includes breakfast—and don't skip it.
- Accept that dining hall food is not going to be as good as home cooking. Find dishes that you like that are nutritious.
- If menus are posted or distributed, decide what you want to eat before getting in line and stick to your choices. Consider what you plan to do and eat for the rest of the day before making your choices.
- Ask for large servings of vegetables and small servings of meat and other high-fat main dishes. Build your meals around grains and vegetables.
- Try whole grains like brown rice, whole-wheat bread, and whole-grain cereals.
- Choose leaner poultry, fish, or bean dishes rather than high-fat meats and fried entrees.
- Ask that gravies and sauces be served on the side; limit your intake.
- Choose broth-based or vegetable soups rather than cream soups.
- At the salad bar, load up on leafy greens, beans, and fresh vegetables. Avoid mayonnaise-coated salads, bacon, croutons, and high-fat dressings. Put dressing on the side; dip your fork into it rather than pouring it over the salad.
- Drink nonfat milk, water, mineral water, or 100% fruit juice rather than heavily sweetened fruit drinks, whole milk, soft drinks, or beer.
- Choose fruit for dessert rather than pastries, cookies, or cakes.
- Do some research about the foods and preparation methods used in your dining hall or cafeteria. Discuss any food and nutrition suggestions you have with your food service manager.

Eating in Fast-Food Restaurants

- Most fast-food chains can provide a brochure with a nutritional breakdown of the foods on the menu. Ask for it. (See also the information in Appendix C.)
- Order small single burgers with no cheese instead of double burgers with many toppings. If possible, ask for them broiled instead of fried.
- Ask for items to be prepared without mayonnaise, tartar sauce, sour cream, or other high-fat sauces. Ketchup, mustard, and fat-free mayonnaise or sour cream are better choices and are available at many fast-food restaurants.
- Choose whole-grain buns or bread for burgers, hot dogs, and sandwiches.
- Choose chicken items made from chicken breast, not processed chicken.
- Order vegetable pizzas.
- If you order french fries or onion rings, get the smallest size and/or share them with a friend.

Eating on the Run

Are you chronically short of time? The following healthy and filling items can be packed for a quick snack or meal: fresh or dried fruit, fruit juices, raw fresh vegetables, plain bagels, bread sticks, whole-wheat fig bars, low-fat cheese sticks or cubes, low-fat crackers or granola bars, nonfat or low-fat yogurt, snack-size cereal boxes, pretzels, rice or corn cakes, plain popcorn, soup (if you have access to a microwave), or water.

restaurants, another convenient source of quick and inexpensive meals for busy students. Although no food is entirely "bad," consuming a wide variety of foods is critical for a healthy diet. See the box "Eating Strategies for College Students" for tips on making healthy eating convenient and affordable.

Older Adults As people age, they tend to become less active, so they require fewer calories to maintain their weight. At the same time, the absorption of nutrients tends to be lower in older adults because of age-related changes in the digestive tract. Thus, they must consume nutrient-dense foods to meet their nutritional requirements. As discussed earlier, foods fortified with vitamin B-12 and/or B-12 supplements are recommended for people over age 50. Because constipation is a common problem, consuming foods high in dietary fiber and obtaining adequate fluids are important goals.

TAKE CHARGE Nutrition for Active People: Focus on Fluids

Jessica, a 25-year-old graduate student, sets out for her daily 3-mile walk. It's first thing in the morning, and she hasn't had anything to eat or drink yet. She starts off at a brisk pace, but about halfway through she feels a bit fatigued. She finishes her walk feeling tired. After a shower and a quick cup of coffee with toast, she drags herself off to work. She feels unenergetic all morning and wonders if she is wearing herself out with her daily walks. Jessica considers giving up the exercise habit, even though she knows it's supposed to be good for her. What would help Jessica enjoy her exercise more and feel less fatigued? Water! Like many Americans, Jessica is chronically mildly dehydrated. She doesn't feel thirsty and has no idea that her fluid intake is not sufficient for optimal performance. Jessica is likely to experience a noticeable increase in energy and enjoyment of her walks if she drinks a glass of fruit juice (for fluid and quick energy) when she first gets up, sips from a water bottle during her walk, and has several cups of water (and a decent breakfast) after she finishes her walk.

Every active person, from the recreational walker to the professional athlete, needs to make a conscious effort to stay well hydrated. Water is perhaps the most crucial and most frequently neglected nutrient among athletes. Mild dehydration is extremely common and even feels "normal" to the many people who suffer from it chronically. Even if you don't feel obviously thirsty or weak, lack of fluid can impair your ability to enjoy physical activity and make peak performance impossible.

Every cell in the body depends on adequate fluid to survive. In particular, the human cooling system relies on water evaporation in the form of sweat to keep the body from overheating. Working muscles produce heat, and the body will rapidly overheat if its cooling systems are not functioning properly due to a lack of fluids. As the environmental temperature rises, the need for fluid also increases. What happens if you are low on fluids? First, optimal muscle performance becomes impossible, and you quickly lose your competitive edge. Fatigue sets in, and your thinking and reaction time may become impaired. When dehydration is very severe, heat stroke, unconsciousness, and even death can occur (see Chapter 3 for more on heat illnesses).

How do you know if you are drinking enough fluids? Thirst alone is not the best guide because you can be significantly dehydrated before you begin to feel thirsty. One-size-fits-all advice such as "drink 8 glasses of water a day" can be inaccurate for some people because fluid needs vary considerably depending on body size, previous conditioning, type of exercise, environmental temperature and humidity, and other factors. One way to tell if you are drinking enough fluid is to take a look at your urine. If it is dark in color and you need to urinate only a few times a day, chances are you are dehydrated. If your urine is pale yellow and clear, and you urinate every few hours throughout the day, you are probably getting enough fluid. Another way to gauge your fluid needs is to weigh yourself before and after exercise. If you lose more than 1–2% of your total body weight, you are dehydrated and should increase your fluid intake before, during, and after exercise.

Prepare yourself for an athletic event—or any strenuous activity—by drinking plenty of fluid the day before. On the day of the event, the American College of Sports Medicine advises consuming 14–22 oz (400–600 ml) of fluid about 2 hours before exercise, and then 6–12 oz (150–350 ml) of fluid every 15–20 minutes during exercise—or as much of this amount that you can tolerate. Afterwards, drink enough to replace lost fluids—16–24 oz for every pound of weight lost. If you don't have a scale to check your weight, drink several glasses of fluid, and when you no longer feel thirsty, have at least 8 oz more. Remember that your body needs plenty of water regardless of the season. Even in the winter, you sweat under your clothing and lose water through your respiratory system as you breathe cool, dry air.

What should you drink? Most of the time water is the best choice, particularly if you are trying to avoid excess calories. Fruit or vegetable juice can also be an excellent option, giving you some quick energy and valuable nutrients along with the liquid. If you are exercising for less than 60–90 minutes, replacing lost fluids with cool water is fine. For longer duration activities, a sports drink can be worthwhile. These contain water, electrolytes, and carbohydrates. The advantage of sports drinks is that they can provide you with some extra energy (in the form of rapidly digestible carbohydrates that help maintain blood glucose levels) and can replace electrolytes that are lost through sweat. Beverages that contain caffeine or alcohol are not good choices for replacing fluids lost during exercise. Caffeine and alcohol are both diuretics that cause you to urinate more, aggravating fluid loss.

Make a habit of drinking plenty of fluid all day, every day, regardless of whether you plan to exercise. Peak athletic performance, as well as the enjoyment of all types of physical activity, depends on staying well hydrated.

Athletes Key dietary concerns for athletes are drinking enough fluids during practice and throughout the day to remain fully hydrated and meeting their increased energy requirements (see the box "Nutrition for Active People: Focus on Fluids" for information on fluid intake). Individuals engaged in vigorous training programs expend more energy (calories) than sedentary and moderately active individuals and may have energy needs ranging from 2000 to more than 6000 calories a day. For athletes, the American Dietetic Association recommends a diet with 60–65% of calories coming from carbohydrate, 10–15% from protein, and no more than 30% from fat.

Endurance athletes involved in competitive events lasting longer than 90 minutes may benefit from increasing carbohydrate intake to 65–70% of total calories; this increase should come in the form of complex, rather than simple, carbohydrates. High carbohydrate intake builds and maintains muscle glycogen stores, resulting in greater endurance and delayed fatigue during competitive events. Some endurance athletes engage in "carbohydrate loading"—a practice that involves increasing carbohydrate intake in the days before a competition. Before exercise, the ACSM recommends that an active adult or athlete consume a meal or snack that is relatively high in carbohydrate, moderate in protein, and low in fat. Soon after exercise, particularly following a strenuous competition or training session, a mixed meal containing carbohydrates, protein, and fat should be consumed to replace muscle glycogen and provide amino acids for building and repairing muscle tissue.

Athletes for whom maintaining low body weight and body fat is important—such as skaters, gymnasts, and wrestlers—should consume adequate calories and nutrients and avoid falling into unhealthy patterns of eating. The combination of low levels of body fat, high physical activity, disordered eating habits, and, in women, amenorrhea is associated with stress fractures and other injuries and with osteoporosis. Eating disorders are discussed in Chapter 9.

There is no evidence that consuming supplements containing vitamins, minerals, protein, or specific amino acids will build muscle or improve sports performance. Strength and muscle are built with exercise, not extra protein, and carbohydrates provide the fuel needed for muscle-building exercise. Strenuous physical activity does increase the need for protein and some vitamins and minerals; however, the increased energy intake of athletes more than compensates for this increased need. (Indeed, the protein intake in the average American diet is already about 50% above the RDA, representing 16% of total calories.) For endurance athletes, the ACSM recommends a protein intake of 1.2–1.4 grams per kilogram of body weight per day, up from the standard RDA of 0.8 gram per kilogram; for athletes engaged in heavy strength training, protein needs may be as high as 1.6–1.7 grams per kilogram of body weight. This level of protein intake is easily obtainable from foods, however. A 160-pound athlete consuming 3500 calories a day needs to obtain only 12% of total calories from protein to achieve the upper end of the protein range for endurance athletes. A balanced high-carbohydrate, moderate-protein, low-fat diet can provide all the nutrients athletes need.

People with Special Health Concerns Many Americans have special health concerns that affect their dietary needs. For example, women who are pregnant or breastfeeding require extra calories, vitamins, and minerals. People with diabetes benefit from a well-balanced diet that is low in simple sugars, high in complex carbohydrates, and relatively rich in monounsaturated fats. And people with high blood pressure need to limit their sodium consumption and control their weight. If you have a health problem or concern that may require a special diet, discuss your situation with a physician or registered dietitian.

NUTRITIONAL PLANNING: MAKING INFORMED CHOICES ABOUT FOOD

Now that you know the nutrients you need and the amounts required for maximum wellness, you are almost ready to create a diet that works for you. Depending on your needs and dietary habits, you may have some specific areas of concern you want to address first, such as interpreting food labels, understanding food additives, or avoiding foodborne illnesses. We turn to these and other topics next.

Food Labels—A Closer Look

Consumers can get help in applying the principles of the Food Guide Pyramid and the Dietary Guidelines for Americans from food labels. Since 1994, all processed foods regulated by either the FDA or the USDA have included standardized nutrition information on their labels. Every food label shows serving sizes and the amount of fat, saturated fat, cholesterol, protein, dietary fiber, and sodium in each serving. To make intelligent choices about food, learn to read and understand food labels (see the box "Using Food Labels," p. 230). Research has shown that people who read food labels eat less fat.

Because most meat, poultry, fish, fruits, and vegetables are not processed, they were not covered by the 1994 law. You can obtain information on the nutrient content of these items from basic nutrition books, registered dietitians, nutrient analysis computer software, the World Wide Web, and the companies that produce or distribute these foods. Also, supermarkets often have large posters or pamphlets listing the nutrient contents of these foods. Lab 8.3 gives you the opportunity to compare foods using the information provided on their labels.

WW Dietary Supplement Labels—New Requirements

Dietary supplements include vitamins, minerals, amino acids, herbs, enzymes, and other compounds. Although dietary supplements are often thought to be safe and "natural," they do contain powerful, bioactive chemicals that have the potential for harm. About one-quarter of all pharmaceutical drugs are derived from botanical sources, and even essential vitamins and minerals can have toxic effects if consumed in excess.

In the United States, supplements are not legally considered drugs and are not regulated the way drugs are. Before they are approved by the FDA and put on the market, drugs undergo clinical studies to determine safety, effectiveness, side effects and risks; possible interactions with other substances; and appropriate dosages. The FDA does not authorize or test dietary supplements, and supplements are not required to demonstrate either safety or effectiveness before they are marketed. Although dosage guidelines exist for some of the compounds in dietary supplements, dosages for many are not well established.

Food labels are designed to help consumers make food choices based on the nutrients that are most important to good health. In addition to listing nutrient content by weight, the label puts the information in the context of a daily diet of 2000 calories that includes no more than 65 grams of fat (approximately 30% of total calories). For example, if a serving of a particular product has 13 grams of fat, the label will show that the serving represents 20% of the daily fat allowance. If your daily diet contains fewer or more than 2000 calories, you need to adjust these calculations accordingly (see Table 8.2).

Food labels contain uniform serving sizes. This means that if you look at different brands of salad dressing, for example, you can compare calories and fat content based on the serving amount. Regulations also require that foods meet strict definitions if their packaging includes the terms *light, low-fat,* or *high-fiber* (see below). Health claims such as "good source of dietary fiber" or "low in saturated fat" on packages are signals that those products can wisely be included in your diet. Overall, the food label is an important tool to help you choose a diet that conforms to the Food Guide Pyramid and the Dietary Guidelines.

Selected Nutrient Claims and What They Mean

Healthy A food that is low in fat, is low in saturated fat, has no more than 360–480 mg of sodium and 60 mg of cholesterol, *and* provides 10% or more of the Daily Value for vitamin A, vitamin C, protein, calcium, iron, or dietary fiber.

Light or lite One-third fewer calories or 50% less fat than a similar product.

Reduced or fewer At least 25% less of a nutrient than a similar product; can be applied to fat ("reduced fat"), saturated fat, cholesterol, sodium, and calories.

Extra or added 10% or more of the Daily Value per serving when compared to what a similar product has.

Good source 10–19% of the Daily Value for a particular nutrient.

High, rich in, or excellent source of 20% or more of the Daily Value for a particular nutrient.

Low calorie 40 calories or less per serving.

High fiber 5 g or more of fiber per serving.

Good source of fiber 2.5–4.9 g of fiber per serving.

Fat-free Less than 0.5 g of fat per serving.

Low-fat 3 g of fat or less per serving.

Saturated fat-free Less than 0.5 g of saturated fat and 0.5 g of trans fatty acids per serving.

Low saturated fat 1 g or less of saturated fat per serving and no more than 15% of total calories.

Cholesterol-free Less than 2 mg of cholesterol and 2 g or less of saturated fat per serving.

Low cholesterol 20 mg or less of cholesterol and 2 g or less of saturated fat per serving.

Low sodium 140 mg or less of sodium per serving.

Very low sodium 35 mg or less of sodium per serving.

Lean Cooked seafood, meat, or poultry with less than 10 g of fat, 4.5 g or less of saturated fat, and less than 95 mg of cholesterol per serving.

Extra lean Cooked seafood, meat, or poultry with less than 5 g of fat, 2 g of saturated fat, and 95 mg of cholesterol per serving.

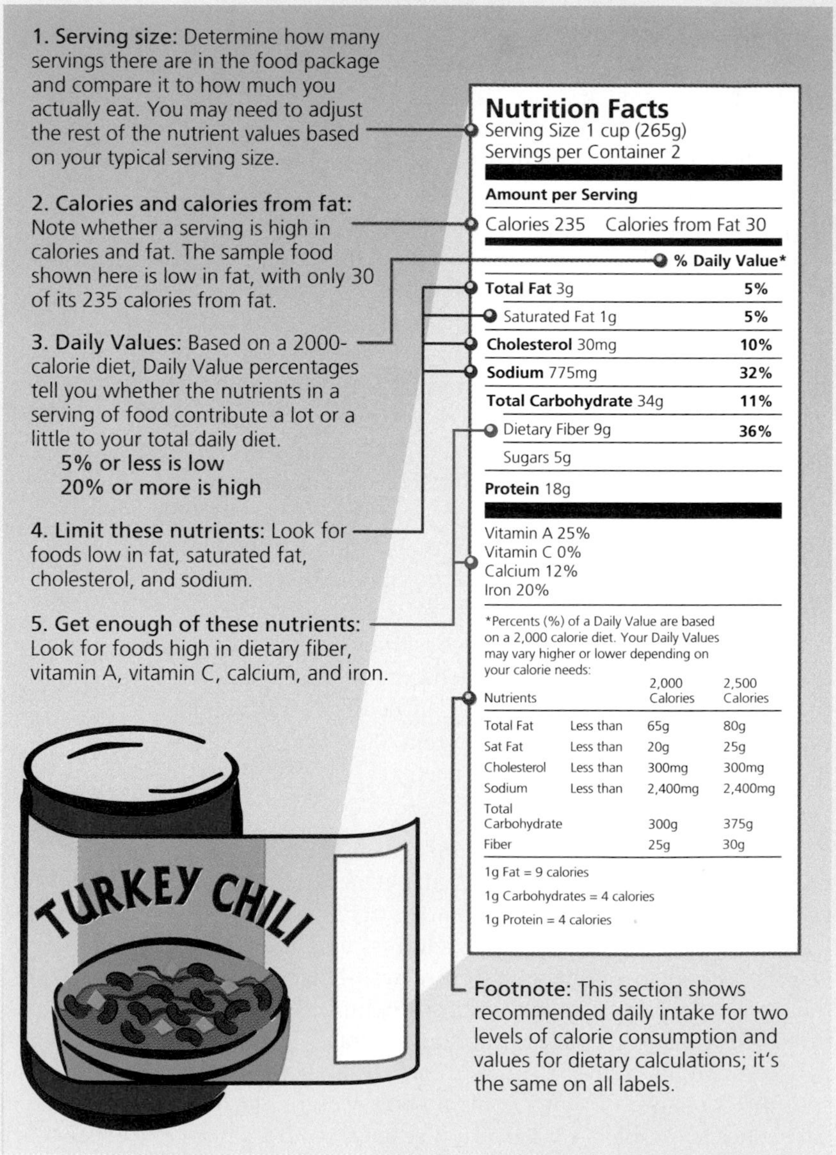

1. Serving size: Determine how many servings there are in the food package and compare it to how much you actually eat. You may need to adjust the rest of the nutrient values based on your typical serving size.
2. Calories and calories from fat: Note whether a serving is high in calories and fat. The sample food shown here is low in fat, with only 30 of its 235 calories from fat.
3. Daily Values: Based on a 2000-calorie diet, Daily Value percentages tell you whether the nutrients in a serving of food contribute a lot or a little to your total daily diet.
5% or less is low
20% or more is high
4. Limit these nutrients: Look for foods low in fat, saturated fat, cholesterol, and sodium.
5. Get enough of these nutrients: Look for foods high in dietary fiber, vitamin A, vitamin C, calcium, and iron.
Nutrition Facts
Serving Size 1 cup (265g)
Servings per Container 2
Amount per Serving
Calories 235 Calories from Fat 30
% Daily Value*
Total Fat 3g 5%
Saturated Fat 1g 5%
Cholesterol 30mg 10%
Sodium 775mg 32%
Total Carbohydrate 34g 11%
Dietary Fiber 9g 36%
Sugars 5g
Protein 18g
Vitamin A 25%
Vitamin C 0%
Calcium 12%
Iron 20%
*Percents (%) of a Daily Value are based on a 2,000 calorie diet. Your Daily Values may vary higher or lower depending on your calorie needs:
Nutrients 2,000 Calories 2,500 Calories
Total Fat Less than 65g 80g
Sat Fat Less than 20g 25g
Cholesterol Less than 300mg 300mg
Sodium Less than 2,400mg 2,400mg
Total Carbohydrate 300g 375g
Fiber 25g 30g
1g Fat = 9 calories
1g Carbohydrates = 4 calories
1g Protein = 4 calories
TURKEY CHILI
Footnote: This section shows recommended daily intake for two levels of calorie consumption and values for dietary calculations; it's the same on all labels.

Many ingredients in dietary supplements are classified by the FDA as "generally recognized as safe," but some have been found to be dangerous on their own or to interact with prescription or over-the-counter drugs in dangerous ways. Garlic supplements, for example, can cause bleeding if taken with anticoagulant ("blood-thinning") medications. Even products that are generally considered safe can have side effects—St. John's wort, for example, increases the skin's sensitivity to sunlight and may decrease the effectiveness of oral contraceptives, drugs used to treat HIV infection, and other medications.

There are also key differences between drugs and supplements in their manufacture. FDA-approved medications are standardized for potency, and quality control and proof of purity are required. Dietary supplement manufacture is not so closely regulated, and there is no guarantee that a product even contains a given ingredient, let alone in the appropriate amount. The potency of herbal supplements can vary widely due to differences in growing and harvesting conditions, preparation methods, and storage. Contamination and misidentification of plant compounds are also potential problems.

In an effort to provide consumers with more reliable and consistent information about supplements, the FDA has developed new labeling regulations. Since March 1999, labels similar to those found on foods have been required for dietary supplements; for more information, see the box "Using Dietary Supplement Labels" on p. 232.

Remember that dietary supplements are no substitute for a healthy diet. Supplements do not provide all the known—or yet-to-be-discovered—benefits of whole foods. Supplements should also not be used as a replacement for medical treatment for serious illnesses.

Food Additives—Benefits and Risks

Today, some 2800 substances are intentionally added to foods for one or more of the following reasons: (1) to maintain or improve nutritional quality, (2) to maintain freshness, (3) to help in processing or preparation, or (4) to alter taste or appearance. Additives make up less than 1% of our food. The most widely used are sugar, salt, and corn syrup; these three, plus citric acid, baking soda, vegetable colors, mustard, and pepper, account for 98% by weight of all food additives used in the United States.

Some additives may be of concern for certain people, either because they are consumed in large quantities or because they cause some type of allergic reaction. Additives having potential health concerns include the following:

- *Nitrates and nitrites:* Used to protect meats from contamination from the microorganism that causes botulism. Consumption of these substances is associated with the synthesis of cancer-causing agents in the stomach, but the cancer risk appears to be low, except for people with low stomach acid output (such as some older people). The use of nitrates or nitrites is allowed in small quantities.
- *BHA and BHT:* Used to help maintain the freshness of foods. Some studies indicate a potential link between BHT and an increased risk of certain cancers. The FDA is reviewing the use of BHT and BHA, but any risk to the diet from these agents is low. Some manufacturers have stopped using BHT and BHA.
- *Sulfites:* Used to keep vegetables from turning brown. They can cause severe reactions in some people. The FDA strictly limits the use of sulfites and requires any foods containing sulfites to be clearly labeled.
- *Monosodium glutamate (MSG):* Typically used as a flavor enhancer. MSG may cause some people to experience episodes of high blood pressure and sweating. If you are sensitive to MSG, check food labels when shopping and ask that it not be added to dishes you order in restaurants.

Food additives pose no significant health hazard to most people because the levels used are well below any that could produce toxic effects. Eat a variety of foods in moderation. If you have any sensitivity to an additive, check food labels when you shop and ask questions when you eat out.

Foodborne Illness—An Increasing Threat

Many people worry about additives or pesticide residues in their food. However, the greatest threat to the safety of the food supply comes from microorganisms that cause foodborne illnesses. Raw or undercooked animal products, such as chicken, hamburger, and oysters, pose the greatest risk for contamination. The CDC estimates that 76 million Americans become sick each year as a result of foodborne illness, 325,000 are hospitalized, and 5200 die. In most cases, foodborne illness produces acute gastroenteritis, characterized by diarrhea, vomiting, fever, and weakness. People often mistake foodborne illness for a bout of the flu. Although the effects of foodborne illness are usually not serious, some groups, such as children and older people, are at risk for severe complications, including rheumatic diseases, kidney failure, seizures, blood poisoning, and death.

Causes of Foodborne Illnesses Most cases of foodborne illness are caused by **pathogens**, disease-causing microorganisms that contaminate food, usually from improper handling. The threats are numerous and varied; among them are the sometimes deadly *Escherichia coli (E. coli)* O157:H7 in meat and water; *Salmonella* in eggs, on vegetables, and on poultry; *Vibrio* in shellfish; *Cyclospora* and hepatitis A virus on fruit; *Cryptosporidium* in drinking water; *Campylobacter jejuni* in meat and

pathogen A microorganism that causes disease.

Terms
Ww

Since 1999, specific types of information have been required on the labels of dietary supplements. In addition to basic information about the product, labels include a "Supplement Facts" panel, modeled after the "Nutrition Facts" panel used on food labels (see the figure). Under the Dietary Supplement Health and Education Act (DSHEA) and food labeling laws, supplement labels can make three types of health-related claims.

- *Nutrient-content claims,* such as "high in calcium," "excellent source of vitamin C," or "high potency." The claims "high in" and "excellent source of" mean the same as they do on food labels. A "high potency" single-ingredient supplement must contain 100% of its Daily Value; a "high potency" multi-ingredient product must contain 100% or more of the Daily Value of at least two-thirds of the nutrients present for which Daily Values have been established.
- *Disease claims,* if they have been authorized by the FDA or another authoritative scientific body. The association between adequate calcium intake and lower risk of osteoporosis is an example of an approved disease claim.
- *Structure-function claims,* such as "antioxidants maintain cellular integrity" or "this product enhances energy levels." Because these claims are not reviewed by the FDA, they must carry a disclaimer (see the sample label).

Tips for Choosing and Using Dietary Supplements

- Check with your physician before taking a supplement. Many are not meant for children, elderly people, women who are pregnant or breastfeeding, people with chronic illnesses or upcoming surgery, or people taking prescription or OTC medications.
- Follow the cautions, instructions for use, and dosage given on the label.
- Look for the *USP* or *NF* designation, indicating that the product meets some minimum safety and purity standard developed by the United States Pharmacopeia. (The United States Pharmacopeia develops standards for purity and potency for pharmaceutical drugs and has also set standards for vitamins, minerals, and some herbal products.) The designation *NNFA* indicates that the manufacturer has met the National Nutritional Foods Association standards for quality control and cleanliness. Other, smaller, associations and labs, including ConsumerLab.Com, also test and rate dietary supplements.
- Choose brands made by nationally known food and drug manufacturers or "house brands" from large retail chains. Due to their size and visibility, such sources are likely to have higher manufacturing standards.
- If you experience side effects, discontinue use of the product and contact your physician. Report any serious reactions to the FDA's MedWatch monitoring program (800-FDA-1088; http://www.fda.gov/medwatch).

For More Information About Dietary Supplements

ConsumerLab.Com: http://www.consumerlab.com

Food and Drug Administration: http://vm.cfsan.fda.gov/~dms/supplmnt.html

National Institutes of Health, Office of Dietary Supplements: http://dietary-supplements.info.nih.gov

National Nutritional Foods Association: http://www.nnfa.org

U.S. Department of Agriculture: http://www.nal.usda.gov/fnic/etext/000015.html

U.S. Pharmacopeia: http://www.usp.org/dietary

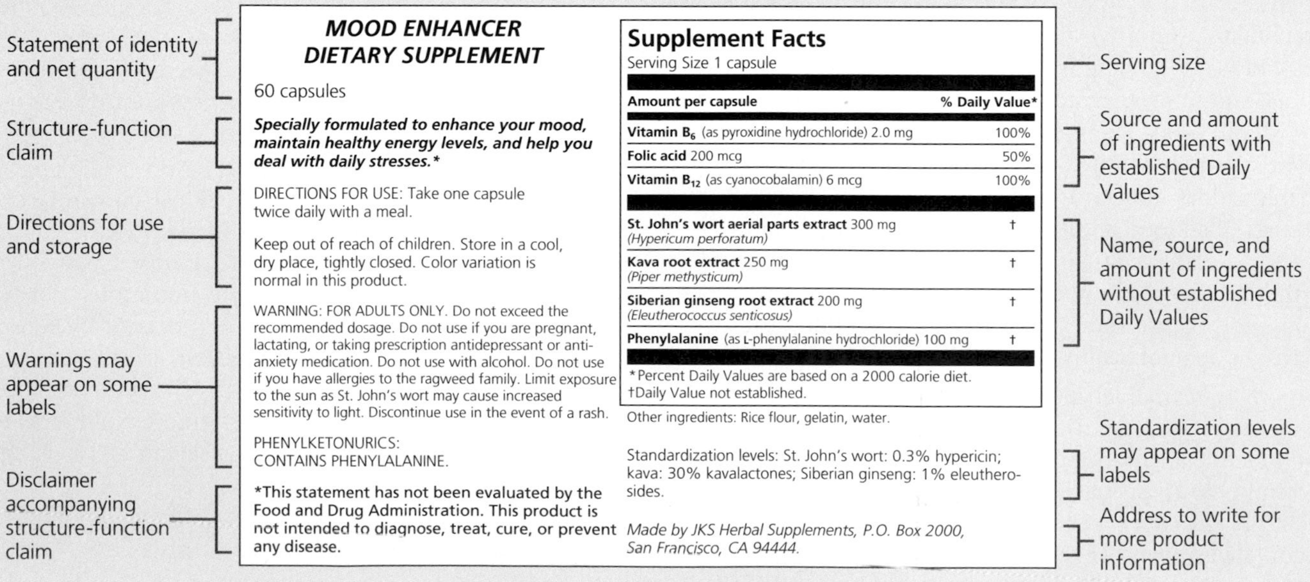

poultry; and *Listeria monocytogenes* in lunch meats, sausages, and hot dogs.

You can't tell by taste, smell, or sight whether a food is contaminated. Some studies have revealed high levels of contamination. In 1998, *Consumer Reports* tested 400 chickens purchased in grocery stores and found that 71% were contaminated with *Campylobacter* and 10% with *Salmonella.*

Although pathogens are usually destroyed during cooking, the U.S. government is taking steps to bring down levels of contamination by improving national testing and surveillance. New tests will not eliminate all contamination, however, and other regulations are designed to help prevent illness from contaminated foods that do make it to consumers. Raw meat and poultry products are now sold with safe handling and cooking instructions, and all packaged, unpasteurized fresh fruit and vegetable juices carry warnings about potential contamination. It is important to note that while foodborne illness outbreaks associated with food-processing plants make headlines, most cases of illness trace back to poor food handling in the home or in food-service establishments.

Preventing and Treating Foodborne Illness The key to protecting yourself from foodborne illness is to handle, cook, and store foods in ways that prevent bacteria from spreading and multiplying. When handling foods, keep these tips in mind:

- Don't buy food in containers that leak, bulge, or are severely dented. Refrigerated foods should be cold, and frozen foods should be solid.
- Refrigerate perishable items as soon as possible after purchase. Use or freeze fresh meats within 3–5 days and fresh poultry, fish, and ground meat within 1–2 days.
- Thaw frozen food in the refrigerator or in the microwave oven, not on the kitchen counter.
- Thoroughly wash your hands with warm soapy water for 20 seconds before and after handling food, especially raw meat, fish, poultry, or eggs.
- Make sure counters, cutting boards, dishes, and other equipment are thoroughly cleaned before and after use. If possible, use separate cutting boards for meat and for foods that will be eaten raw, such as fruits and vegetables. Wash dishcloths and kitchen towels frequently.
- Thoroughly rinse and scrub fruits and vegetables with a brush, if possible, or peel off the skin.
- Cook foods thoroughly, especially beef, poultry, fish, pork, and eggs. Cooking kills most microorganisms, as long as an appropriately high temperature is reached. The USDA now recommends that consumers, especially high-risk individuals, use a food thermometer to verify that hamburgers are cooked to 160° F. When eating out, order red meat cooked "well done."
- Cook stuffing separate from poultry; or wash poultry thoroughly, stuff immediately before cooking, and transfer the stuffing to a clean bowl immediately after cooking.
- Refrigerate foods at or below 40° F and freeze at or below 0° F. Do not leave cooked or refrigerated foods, such as meats or salads, at room temperature for more than 2 hours. Use refrigerated leftovers within 3–4 days.
- Don't eat raw animal products, including raw eggs in Caesar salad, hollandaise sauce, or eggnog. Use only pasteurized milk and juice, and look for pasteurized eggs, which are now available in some states.
- Cook eggs until they're firm and fully cook foods containing eggs. Store eggs in the coldest part of the refrigerator, not on the door, and use them within 3–5 weeks.
- Because of possible contamination with *E. coli* O157:H7 and *Salmonella,* avoid raw sprouts, or eat them only after submerging them in boiling water for 10 seconds.
- According to the USDA, "When in doubt, throw it out."

Additional precautions are recommended for people at particularly high risk for foodborne illness—pregnant women, young children, older persons, and people with weakened immune systems or certain chronic illnesses. If you are a member of one of these groups, don't eat or drink any of the following products: unpasteurized juices; raw sprouts; raw (unpasteurized) milk and products made from unpasteurized milk; raw or undercooked meat, poultry, eggs, fish, and shellfish; and soft cheeses such as feta, Brie, Camembert, or blue-veined varieties. It's also important to avoid ready-to-eat foods such as hot dogs, luncheon meats, and cold cuts unless they are reheated until they are steaming hot.

If you think you may be having a bout of foodborne illness, drink plenty of clear fluids to prevent dehydration and rest to speed recovery. To prevent further contamination, wash your hands often and always before handling food until you recover. A fever higher than 102° F, blood in the stool, or dehydration deserves a physician's evaluation, especially if the symptoms persist for more than 2–3 days. In cases of suspected botulism—characterized by symptoms such as double vision, paralysis, dizziness, and vomiting—consult a physician immediately.

Irradiated Foods— A Technique of Biotechnology

Food irradiation is the treatment of foods with gamma rays, X rays, or high-voltage electrons to kill potentially

food irradiation The treatment of foods with gamma rays, X rays, or high-voltage electrons to kill potentially harmful pathogens and increase shelf life.

Terms

Ww

harmful pathogens, including bacteria, parasites, insects, and fungi that cause foodborne illness. It also reduces spoilage and extends shelf life. Since 1963, the government has allowed the irradiation of certain foods; this growing list includes wheat and flour (1963); white potatoes (1964); pork, herbs and spices, and fruits and vegetables (1986); raw poultry (1992); and red meat (1999). The same irradiation process has also been used for decades on such items as plastic wrap, milk cartons, teething rings, contact lenses, and medical supplies.

Even though irradiation has been generally endorsed by agencies such as the World Health Organization, the Centers for Disease Control and Prevention, and the American Medical Association, few irradiated foods are currently on the market due to consumer resistance and skepticism. Studies haven't conclusively identified any harmful effects of food irradiation, and the newer methods of irradiation involving electricity and X rays do not require the use of any radioactive materials. Studies indicate that when consumers are given information about the process of irradiation and the benefits of irradiated foods, most want to purchase them.

All primary irradiated foods (meat, vegetables, and so on) are labeled with the flowerlike radura symbol and a brief information label; spices and foods that are merely ingredients do not have to be so labeled. It is important to remember that although irradiation kills most pathogens, it does not completely sterilize foods. Proper handling of irradiated foods is still critical for preventing foodborne illness.

Organic Foods—Stricter Standards for a Booming Industry

Some people who are concerned about pesticides and other environmental contaminants choose to buy foods that are **organic.** In December 2000, the USDA enacted a new national standard for organic foods to replace the older system of local, state, and private standards. To be certified as organic, foods must meet strict production, processing, handling, and labeling criteria. Organic crops must meet limits on pesticide residues; for meat, milk, eggs, and other animal products to be certified organic, animals must be given organic feed and access to the outdoors and may not be given antibiotics or growth hormones. The use of genetic engineering, ionizing radiation, and sewage sludge are prohibited. Products can be labeled "100% organic" if they contain all organic ingredients and "organic" if they contain at least 95% organic ingredients; all such products may carry the new USDA organic seal. A product with at least 70% organic ingredients can be labeled "made with organic ingredients" but cannot use the USDA seal.

Foods that are organic are not chemical-free, however. They may be contaminated with pesticides used on neighboring lands or on foods transported in the same train or truck. However, they do tend to have lower levels of pesticide residues than conventionally grown crops. There are strict pesticide limits for all foods—organic and conventional—and the debate about the potential health effects of long-term exposure to small amounts of pesticide residues is ongoing. Supporters of organic foods also note that practices associated with organic farming help maintain biodiversity of crops and are less likely to degrade soil, contaminate water, or expose farm workers to dangerous chemicals. Since 1990, U.S. sales of organic foods have grown by 20% a year, reaching $6.5 billion in 2000. Similarly, sales of organic dairy products are increasing by more than 100% annually.

Terms

organic A designation applied to foods grown and produced according to strict guidelines limiting the use of pesticides, nonorganic ingredients, hormones, antibiotics, genetic engineering, irradiation, and other practices.

A PERSONAL PLAN: APPLYING NUTRITIONAL PRINCIPLES

You've learned the basics of good nutrition, know how to interpret food and supplement labels, and have some guidelines for protecting yourself from foodborne illness. With this foundation, you can now put together a diet that works for you. Based on your particular nutrition and health status, there probably is an ideal diet for you, but there is no single type of diet that provides optimal health for everyone. Many cultural dietary patterns can meet people's nutritional requirements (see the box "Ethnic Foods"). Every individual needs to customize a food plan based on age, gender, weight, activity level, medical risk factors—and, of course, personal tastes.

Assessing and Changing Your Diet

The first step in planning a healthy diet is to examine what you currently eat. Labs 8.1 and 8.2 are designed to help you analyze your current diet and compare it with optimal dietary goals. (This analysis can be completed using Appendix B, a nutritional analysis software program, or one of several Web sites.)

Next, experiment with additions and substitutions to your current diet to bring it closer to your goals. If you are consuming too much fat, for example, try substituting fruit for a calorie-rich dessert. If you aren't getting enough iron, try adding some raisins to your cereal or garbanzo beans to your salad. If you need to plan your diet from the ground up, use the Food Guide Pyramid and the Dietary Guidelines.

To put your plan into action, use the behavioral self-management techniques and tips described in Chapter 1.

There is no one ethnic diet that clearly surpasses all others in providing people with healthful foods. However, every diet has its advantages and disadvantages and, within each cuisine, some foods are better choices. The dietary guidelines described in this chapter can be applied to any ethnic cuisine. For additional guidance, refer to the table below.

	Choose More Often	Choose Less Often
Chinese	Dishes that are steamed, poached (jum), boiled (chu), roasted (kow), barbecued (shu), or lightly stir-fried Hoisin sauce, oyster sauce, wine sauce, plum sauce, velvet sauce, or hot mustard Fresh fish and seafood, skinless chicken, tofu Mixed vegetables, Chinese greens Steamed rice, steamed spring rolls, soft noodles	Fried wontons or egg rolls Crab rangoon Crispy (Peking) duck or chicken Sweet-and-sour dishes made with breaded and deep-fried meat, poultry, or fish Fried rice Fried or crispy noodles
French	Dishes prepared au vapeur (steamed), en brochette (skewered and broiled), or grillé (grilled) Fresh fish, shrimp, scallops, or mussels or skinless chicken, without sauces Clear soups	Dishes prepared à la crème (in cream sauce), au gratin or gratinée (baked with cream and cheese), or en croûte (in pastry crust) Drawn butter, hollandaise sauce, and remoulade (mayonnaise-based sauce)
Greek	Dishes that are stewed, broiled, or grilled, including shish kabobs (souvlaki) Dolmas (grape leaves) stuffed with rice Tzatziki (yogurt, cucumbers, and garlic) Tabouli (bulgur-based salad) Pita bread, especially whole wheat	Moussaka, saganaki (fried cheese) Vegetable pies such as spanakopita and tyropita Baba ghanoush (eggplant and olive oil) Deep-fried falafel (chickpea patties) Gyros stuffed with ground meat Baklava
Indian	Dishes prepared masala (curry), tandoori (roasted in a clay oven), or tikke (pan roasted); kabobs Raita (yogurt and cucumber salad) and other yogurt-based dishes and sauces Dal (lentils), pullao or pilau (basmati rice) Chapati (baked bread)	Ghee (clarified butter) Korma (meat in cream sauce) Samosas, pakoras (fried dishes) Molee and other coconut milk-based dishes Poori, bhatura, or paratha (fried breads)
Italian	Pasta primavera or pasta, polenta, risotto, or gnocchi with marinara, red or white wine, white or red clam, or light mushroom sauce Dishes that are grilled or prepared cacciatore (tomato-based sauce), marsala (broth and wine sauce), or piccata (lemon sauce) Cioppino (seafood stew) Vegetable soup, minestrone or fagioli (beans)	Antipasto (cheese, smoked meats) Dishes that are prepared alfredo, frito (fried), crema (creamed), alla panna (with cream), or carbonara Veal scaloppini Chicken, veal, or eggplant parmigiana Italian sausage, salami, and prosciutto Buttered garlic bread Cannoli
Japanese	Dishes prepared nabemono (boiled), shabu-shabu (in boiling broth), mushimono (steamed), nimono (simmered), yaki (broiled), or yakimono (grilled) Sushi or domburi (mixed rice dish) Steamed rice or soba (buckwheat), udon (wheat), or rice noodles	Tempura (battered and fried) Agemono (deep fried) Katsu (fried pork cutlet) Sukiyaki Fried tofu
Mexican	Soft corn or wheat tortillas Burritos, fajitas, enchiladas, soft tacos, and tamales filled with beans, vegetables, or lean meats Refried beans, nonfat or low-fat, rice and beans Ceviche (fish marinated in lime juice) Salsa, enchilada sauce, and picante sauce Gazpacho, menudo, or black bean soup Fruit or flan for dessert	Crispy, fried tortillas Dishes that are fried, such as chile relleños, chimichangas, flautas, and tostadas Nachos and cheese, chili con queso, and other dishes made with cheese or cheese sauce Guacamole, sour cream, and extra cheese Refried beans made with lard Fried ice cream
Thai	Dishes that are barbecued, sautéed, broiled, boiled, steamed, braised, or marinated Sâté (skewered and grilled meats) Fish sauce, basil sauce, chili or hot sauces Bean thread noodles, Thai salad	Coconut milk soup Peanut sauce or dishes topped with nuts Mee-krob (crispy noodles) Red, green, and yellow curries, which typically contain coconut milk

SOURCES: National Heart, Lung, and Blood Institute. 1998. Tips for Healthy Multicultural Dining Out. In *Clinical Guidelines on the Identification, Evaluation, and Treatment of Overweight and Obesity in Adults.* Bethesda, Md.: National Institutes of Health. Duyff, R. L. 1998. *The American Dietetic Association's Complete Food and Nutrition Guide.* Minneapolis, Minn.: Chronimed. Kirby, J. 1998. *Dieting for Dummies.* Foster City, Calif.: IDG Books.

If you identify several changes you want to make, focus on one at a time. You might start, for example, by substituting nonfat or low-fat milk for whole milk. When you become used to that, you can try substituting whole-wheat bread for white bread. The information on eating behavior in Lab 8.1 will help you identify and change unhealthy patterns of eating.

Staying Committed to a Healthy Diet

Beyond knowledge and information, you also need support in difficult situations. Keeping to your plan is easiest when you choose and prepare your own food at home. Advance planning is the key: mapping out meals and shopping appropriately, cooking in advance when possible, and preparing enough food for leftovers later in the week. A tight budget does not necessarily make it more difficult to eat healthy meals. It makes good health sense and good budget sense to use only small amounts of meat and to have a few meatless meals each week.

In restaurants, keeping to food plan goals becomes somewhat more difficult. Portion sizes in restaurants tend to be larger than serving sizes of the Food Guide Pyramid, but by remaining focused on your goals, you can eat only part of your meal and take the rest home for a meal later in the week. Don't hesitate to ask questions when you're eating in a restaurant. Most restaurant personnel are glad to explain how menu selections are prepared and to make small adjustments, such as serving salad dressings and sauces on the side so they can be avoided or used sparingly. To limit your fat intake, order meat or fish broiled or grilled rather than fried or sauteed, choose rice or a plain baked potato over french fries, and select a clear soup rather than a creamy one. Desserts that are irresistible can, at least, be shared.

Strategies like these can be helpful, but small changes cannot change a fundamentally high-fat, high-calorie meal into a moderate, healthful one. Often, the best advice is to bypass a large steak with potatoes au gratin for a flavorful but low-fat entree. Many of the selections offered in ethnic restaurants are healthy choices (refer to the box on ethnic foods on p. 235 for suggestions).

Fast-food restaurants offer the biggest challenge to a healthy diet. Surveys show that about 70% of 18- to 24-year-olds and 64% of 25- to 34-year-olds visit a fast-food restaurant at least once a week. Fast-food meals are often high in calories, total fat, saturated fat, trans fat, sodium, and sugar; they may be low in fiber and in some vitamins and minerals (see Appendix C). If you do eat at a fast-food restaurant, make sure the rest of your meals that day are low-fat meals rich in fruits and vegetables.

Knowledge of food and nutrition is essential to the success of your program. The information provided in this chapter should give you the tools you need to design and implement a diet that promotes long-term health and well-being. If you need additional information or have questions about nutrition, be sure the source you consult is reliable.

Tips for Today

Eating is one of life's great pleasures. There are many ways to satisfy your nutrient needs so you can create a healthy diet that takes into account your personal preferences and favorite foods. If your current eating habits are not as healthy as they could be, you can choose equally delicious foods that offer both short-term and long-term health benefits. Opportunities to improve your diet present themselves every day, and small changes add up.

Right now you can

- Substitute a healthy snack—an apple, a banana, or plain popcorn—for a bag of chips or cookies.
- Drink a glass of water and put a bottle of water in your backpack for tomorrow.
- Plan to make healthy selections when you go to dinner, such as a baked potato instead of french fries or salmon instead of steak.
- Study the box on ethnic foods in this chapter and plan to order a healthy selection the next time you eat at your favorite ethnic restaurant. Do the same with the fast-food restaurants listed in Appendix C at the end of the book.

SUMMARY

- The six classes of nutrients are carbohydrates, proteins, fats, vitamins, minerals, and water.
- The nutrients essential to humans are released into the body through digestion. Nutrients in foods provide energy, measured in kilocalories (commonly called calories); build and maintain body tissues; and regulate body functions.
- Protein, an important component of body tissue, is composed of amino acids; nine are essential to a diet. Foods from animal sources provide complete proteins; plants provide incomplete proteins.
- Fats, a major source of energy, also insulate the body and cushions the organs; 1 tablespoon of vegetable oil per day supplies the essential fats. For most people, dietary fat should be limited to 30% or less of total calories, and unsaturated fats should be favored over saturated and trans fats.
- Carbohydrates provide energy to the brain, nervous system, and blood and to muscles during high-intensity exercise. Naturally occurring simple carbohydrates and unrefined complex carbohydrates should be favored over added sugars and refined carbohydrates.
- Dietary fiber includes plant substances that are difficult or impossible for the human body to digest. It helps reduce cholesterol levels and promotes the passage of wastes through the intestines.

- The 13 essential vitamins are organic substances that promote specific chemical and cell processes and act as antioxidants. The 17 known essential minerals are inorganic substances that regulate body functions, aid in growth and tissue maintenance, and help in the release of energy from food. Deficiencies in vitamins and minerals can cause severe symptoms over time, but excess doses are also dangerous.
- Water aids in digestion and food absorption, allows chemical reactions to take place, serves as a lubricant or cushion, and helps regulate body temperature.
- Foods contain other substances, such as phytochemicals, that may not be essential nutrients but that may protect against chronic diseases.
- The Dietary Reference Intakes, Food Guide Pyramid, and Dietary Guidelines for Americans provide standards and recommendations for getting all essential nutrients from a varied, balanced diet and for eating in ways that protect against chronic disease.
- Basic recommendations for a healthy diet include aiming for a healthy weight through diet and physical activity; building a healthy base for our diets by following the Pyramid, choosing a variety of plant foods, and handling foods safely; and making sensible choices that consider intake of fat, sugar, salt, and alcohol.
- A vegetarian diet requires special planning but can meet all human nutritional needs.
- Different population groups, such as college students and athletes, face special dietary challenges and should plan their diets to meet their particular needs.
- Consumers can get help applying nutritional principles by reading the standardized labels that appear on all packaged foods and on dietary supplements.
- Other dietary issues of concern include food additives, foodborne illness, food irradiation, and organic foods.
- Although nutritional basics are well established, no single diet provides wellness for everyone. Individuals should focus on their particular needs and adapt general dietary principles to meet them.

COMMON QUESTIONS ANSWERED

Which should I eat—butter or margarine? Both butter and margarine are concentrated sources of fat, containing about 11 grams of fat and 100 calories per tablespoon. Butter is higher in saturated fat, which raises levels of artery-clogging LDL ("bad" cholesterol). Each tablespoon of butter has about 8 grams of saturated fat; margarine has about 2. Butter also contains cholesterol, which margarine does not.

Margarine, on the other hand, contains trans fat, which not only raises LDL but lowers HDL ("good" cholesterol). A tablespoon of stick margarine contains about 2 grams of trans fat. Butter contains a small amount of trans fat as well. Although butter has a combined total of saturated and trans fats that is twice that of stick margarine, the trans fat in stick margarine may be worse for you. Clearly, you should avoid both butter and stick margarine. To solve this dilemma, remember that softer is better. The softer or more liquid a margarine or spread is, the less hydrogenated it is and the less trans fat it contains. Tub and squeeze margarines contain less trans fat than stick margarines; some margarines are modified to be low-trans or trans-free and are labeled as such. Vegetable oils are even better choice for cooking and for table use (such as olive oil for dipping bread) because most are low in saturated fat and completely free of trans fats.

The Food Guide Pyramid seems to recommend such a large number of servings. How can I possibly follow its recommendations without gaining weight? First of all, consider how many servings from each food group are appropriate for you. The suggested number of servings is given as a range, 6–11 servings of grain products, 3–5 of vegetables, and so on. The smaller number of servings is for people who consume about 1600 calories a day, such as many sedentary women. The larger number is for those who consume about 2800 calories a day, such as active men. If the smaller number of servings is appropriate for you, concentrate on choosing nutrient-dense foods—those that are rich in nutrients but relatively low in calories, such as most grains, fruits, and vegetables.

Second, compare the serving sizes of the foods you eat with those used in the Food Guide Pyramid (see pp. 220–221). Some of the Pyramid's serving sizes are smaller than what you might typically eat. For example, many people eat a cup or more of pasta or rice in a meal, which would correspond to 2 or more servings from the grain products group. You'll probably find that your current diet already includes the minimum number of servings from most of the food groups. If not, you may find that you are eating too many servings from one group and not enough from another. Make small changes in your eating habits and food choices to bring your diet into line with the recommendations in the Pyramid, paying particular attention to your consumption of fat and added sugars. The Food Guide Pyramid is designed to help you balance your food choices to ensure good health. Strategies for successful weight management are described in detail in the next chapter.

What are functional foods, and will eating them make me healthier? Functional foods are foods and beverages that contain biologically active compounds that provide health benefits beyond basic nutrition. Technically, this definition covers all healthy whole foods like fruits and vegetables, but the term most often refers to foods with added, modified, or enhanced ingredients. Substances may be added directly to foods, as in the case of calcium added to orange juice; or foods may be modified in other ways, such as when the food of laying hens is manipulated to develop eggs that are high in

(continued)

heart-healthy omega-3 fatty acids. Classical breeding techniques and genetic engineering may also be used. Sales of functional foods have increased rapidly in recent years and now top $10 billion annually.

Like labels for dietary supplements, labels for functional foods may carry disease claims or structure-function claims. Those that carry disease claims have sound science supporting them and so may be used to improve health; good examples are functional foods with added calcium or fiber. One of the most widely marketed and accepted types of functional foods is margarine spreads containing plant sterol or plant stanol esters. In 2000, the FDA approved a disease claim for these compounds, stating that they may reduce the risk of heart disease by reducing LDL.

On the other hand, structure-function claims such as "enhances immunity" or "boosts energy" are not evaluated by the FDA and so must be viewed with skepticism. As in the case of dietary supplements, there may be few studies into the safety, effectiveness, dosages, and interactions of the key ingredient or of the functional food as a whole. In addition, many functional foods contain very low concentrations of their added ingredients and yet may be high in calories—and expensive.

At this point, the best advice for consumers may be to read labels carefully and use common sense. Functional foods cannot take the place of a varied diet rich in fruits, vegetables, and whole grains, which are naturally rich in disease-fighting compounds.

What exactly are genetically modified foods? Are they safe? How can I recognize them on the shelf, and how can I know when I'm eating them? Genetic engineering involves altering the characteristics of a plant, animal, or microorganism by adding, rearranging, or replacing genes in its DNA; the result is a genetically modified (GM) organism. New DNA may come from related species or organisms or from entirely different types of organisms. Many GM crops are already grown in the United States: Over half the current U.S. soybean crop has been genetically modified to be resistant to an herbicide used to kill weeds, and nearly a quarter of the U.S. corn crop carries genes for herbicide resistance or to produce a protein lethal to a destructive type of caterpillar. Products made with GM organisms include juice, soda, nuts, tuna, frozen pizza, spaghetti sauce, canola oil, chips, salad dressing, and soup.

The potential benefits of GM foods cited by supporters include improved yields overall and in difficult growing conditions, increased disease resistance, improved nutritional content, lower prices, and less use of pesticides. Critics of biotechnology argue that unexpected effects may occur: Gene manipulation could elevate levels of naturally occurring toxins or allergens, permanently change the gene pool and reduce biodiversity, and produce pesticide-resistant insects through the transfer of genes. In 2000, a form of GM corn approved for use only in animal feed was found to have comingled with other varieties of corn and to have been used in human foods; this mistake sparked fears of allergic reactions and led to recalls. Opposition to GM foods is particularly strong in Europe; in many developing nations that face food shortages, responses to GM crops have tended to be more positive.

In April 2000, the National Academy of Sciences released a report stating that there is no proof that GM food on the market is unsafe but that changes are needed to better coordinate regulation of GM foods and to assess potential problems. Labeling has been another major concern. Surveys indicate that the majority of Americans want to know if their foods contain GM ingredients. However, under current rules, the FDA requires special labeling only when a food's composition is changed significantly or when a known allergen is introduced. For example, soybeans that contain a gene from a peanut would have to be labeled because peanuts are a common allergen. The only foods guaranteed not to contain GM ingredients are those certified as organic.

How can I tell if I'm allergic to a food? A true food allergy is a reaction of the body's immune system to a food or food ingredient, usually a protein. This immune reaction can occur with minutes of ingesting the food, resulting in symptoms such as hives, diarrhea, difficulty breathing, or swelling of the lips or tongue. The most severe response is a systemic reaction called anaphylaxis, which involves a potentially life-threatening drop in blood pressure. Food allergies affect only about 2% of the adult population and about 4–6% of infants. Just a few foods account for more than 90% of the food allergies in the United States: cow's milk, eggs, peanuts, tree nuts (walnuts, cashews, and so on), soy, wheat, fish, and shellfish.

Many people who believe they have food allergies may actually suffer from a food intolerance, a much more common source of adverse food reactions that typically involves problems with metabolism rather than with the immune system. The body may not be able to adequately digest a food or the body may react to a particular food compound. Food intolerances have been attributed to lactose (milk sugar), gluten (a protein in some grains), tartrazine (yellow food coloring), sulfite (a food additive), MSG, and the sweetener aspartame. Although symptoms of a food intolerance may be similar to those of a food allergy, they are typically more localized and not life-threatening. Many people with food intolerance can safely and comfortably consume small amounts of the food that affects them.

If you suspect you have a food allergy or intolerance, a good first step is to keep a food diary. Note everything you eat or drink, any symptoms you develop, and how long after eating the symptoms appear. Then make an appointment with your physician to go over your diary and determine if any additional tests are needed. People at risk for severe allergic reactions must diligently avoid trigger foods and carry medications to treat anaphylaxis.

FOR FURTHER EXPLORATION

For reliable nutrition advice, talk to a faculty member in the nutrition department on your campus, a registered dietitian (R.D.), or your physician. Many large communities have a telephone service called Dial a Dietitian. By calling this number, you can receive free nutrition information from an R.D.

Experts on quackery suggest that you steer clear of anyone who puts forth any of the following false statements: Most diseases are caused primarily by faulty nutrition, large doses of vitamins are effective against many diseases, hair analysis can be used to determine a person's nutritional state, or a computer-scored nutritional deficiency test is a basis for prescribing vitamins. Any practitioner—licensed or not—who sells supplements in his or her office should be thoroughly scrutinized.

WW *Fit and Well* Online Learning Center (www.mhhe.com/fahey5e)

Use the learning objectives, study guide questions, and glossary flashcards to review key terms and concepts and prepare for exams. You can extend your knowledge of nutrition and gain experience in using the Internet as a resource by completing the activities and checking out the Web links for the topics in Chapter 8 marked with the World Wide Web icon. For this chapter, Internet activities explore specialized food pyramids, food composition analysis, osteoporosis prevention, and dietary supplements; there are Web links for the Vital Statistics table, the Critical Consumer boxes on food labels and dietary supplements, and the chapter as a whole.

Daily Fitness and Nutrition Journal

Review the resources and complete the activities available in the nutrition portion of the journal. Take the portion sizes quiz, complete the preprogram nutrition log, and analyze the results. Based on what you find, set healthy goals for change and complete the contract. Once you put your plan into action, complete the postprogram nutrition log to determine how successful you've been at improving your diet and moving toward the goals you've set.

Health*Quest*

Learn more about your current diet by completing the dietary assessment in the Nutrition and Weight Control module of the Health*Quest* CD-ROM (select How's Your Diet? from the Wellness Activities menu). Your scores will help you pinpoint dietary patterns that you could change to improve wellness. To determine if you are ready to make changes in your diet, complete the Stages of Change quiz (select Stages of Change from the Wellness Activities menu). You'll receive an assessment of your stage plus advice on moving forward toward the action and maintenance stages.

Books

American Dietetic Association. 1999. The *Essential Guide to Nutrition and the Foods We Eat: Everything You Need to Know About the Foods You Eat.* New York: HarperCollins. *An excellent review of current nutrition information and issues.*

Insel, P., R. E. Turner, and D. Ross. 2001. *Nutrition.* Sudbury, Mass.: Jones & Bartlett. *A comprehensive review of major concepts in nutrition.*

Jacobson, M. F., and J. Hurley. 2002. *Restaurant Confidential.* New York: Workman Publishing. Provides information about restaurant foods, including tips for making healthier choices.

Nelson, M. 2000. *Strong Women, Strong Bones: Everything You Need to Know to Prevent, Treat, and Beat Osteoporosis.* New York: Putnam. *A comprehensive, up-to-date guide to preventing and treating osteoporosis through exercise and nutrition.*

Selkowitz, A. 2000. *The College Student's Guide to Eating Well on Campus.* Bethesda, Md.: Tulip Hill Press. *Provides practical advice for students, including how to make healthy choices when eating in a dorm or restaurant and how to stock a first pantry.*

Wardlaw, G. M. 2002. *Perspectives in Nutrition,* 5th ed. New York: McGraw-Hill. *An easy-to-understand review of major concepts in nutrition.*

Williams, M. H. 2001. *Nutrition for Health, Fitness, and Sport,* 6th ed. New York: McGraw-Hill. *An overview of the role of nutrition in enhancing health, fitness, and sport performance.*

Newsletters

Environmental Nutrition (800-829-5384)

Nutrition Action Health Letter (202-332-9110; http://www.cspinet.org)

Tufts University Health and Nutrition Letter (800-274-7581; http://www.healthletter.tufts.edu)

WW Organizations, Hotlines, and Web Sites

American Dietetic Association. Provides a wide variety of educational materials on nutrition.
800-366-1655
http://www.eatright.org

American Heart Association: Delicious Decisions. Provides basic information about nutrition, tips for shopping and eating out, and heart-healthy recipes.
http://www.deliciousdecisions.org

Ask the Dietitian. Questions and answers on many topics relating to nutrition.
http://www.dietitian.com

Consumer Information Center: Food. Provides government publications about dietary fat, fiber, food safety, and other nutrition issues.
http://www.pueblo.gsa.gov/food.htm

CyberDiet. Provides a variety of resources, including a profile that calculates calorie and nutrient needs and a database that provides nutrition information in food label format.
http://www.CyberDiet.com

FDA Center for Food Safety and Applied Nutrition. Offers information about topics such as food labeling, food additives, and foodborne illness.
http://vm.cfsan.fda.gov

Food Safety Hotlines. Provide information on the safe purchase, handling, cooking, and storage of food.
888-SAFEFOOD (FDA)
800-535-4555 (USDA)

Gateways to Government Nutrition Information. Provides access to government resources relating to food safety, including consumer advice and information on specific pathogens.

http://www.nutrition.gov
http://www.foodsafety.gov

Health Canada: Food and Nutrition. Provides information about Canada's Food Guide to Healthy Eating as well as advice for people with special dietary needs.
http://www.hc-sc.gc.ca/english/lifestyles/food_nutr.html

International Food Information Council. Provides helpful information on nutrition and food safety for consumers, journalists, and educators.
http://ific.org/food

Meals.com. A searchable database of more than 10,000 recipes.
http://www.my-meals.com

MedlinePlus: Nutrition. Provides links to information from government agencies and major medical associations on a wide variety of nutrition topics.
http://www.nlm.nih.gov/medlineplus/nutrition.html

National Academies' Food and Nutrition Board. Provides information about the Dietary Reference Intakes and related guidelines.
http://www4.nationalacademies.org/IOM/IOMHome.nsf/Pages/Food+and+Nutrition+Board

National Cancer Institute 5-A-Day Program. Promotes the consumption of five or more servings of fruits and vegetables per day.
http://www.5aday.gov

National Institutes of Health: Osteoporosis and Related Bone Diseases—National Resource Center. Provides information about osteoporosis prevention and treatment; includes a special section on men and osteoporosis.
http://www.osteo.org

National Osteoporosis Foundation. Provides up-to-date information on the causes, prevention, detection, and treatment of osteoporosis.
http://www.nof.org

Tufts University Nutrition Navigator. Provides descriptions and ratings for many nutrition-related Web pages.
http://navigator.tufts.edu

USDA Center for Nutrition Policy and Promotion. Click on Interactive Healthy Eating Index for an online assessment of your diet for one day and a comparison of your diet with the Food Guide Pyramid.
http://www.usda.gov/cnpp

USDA Food and Nutrition Information Center. Provides a variety of materials relating to the Dietary Guidelines, food labels, Food Guide Pyramid, and many other topics.
http://www.nal.usda.gov/fnic

Vegetarian Resource Group. Information and links for vegetarians and people interested in learning more about vegetarian diets.
http://www.vrg.org

You can obtain nutrient breakdowns of individual food items from the following sites:

Nutrition Analysis Tool, University of Illinois, Urbana/Champaign
http://www.nat.uiuc.edu

USDA Food and Nutrition Information Center
http://www.nal.usda.gov/fnic/foodcomp

See also the resources listed in Chapters 9, 11, and 12.

SELECTED BIBLIOGRAPHY

Alberts, D. S., et al. 2000. Lack of effect of a high-fiber cereal supplement on the recurrence of colorectal adenomas. *New England Journal of Medicine* 342(16): 1156–1162.

American College of Sports Medicine, American Dietetic Association, and Dietitians of Canada. 2000. Joint Position Statement: Nutrition and athletic performance. *Medicine and Science in Sports and Exercise* 32(12): 2130–2145.

American Diabetes Association. 2002. Evidence-based nutrition principles and recommendations for the treatment and prevention of diabetes and related complications. *Diabetes Care* 25: 148–198.

American Heart Association Nutrition Committee. 2000. AHA Dietary Guidelines: Revision 2000. *Circulation* 102:2296– 2311.

Bock, S. A., A. Munoz-Furlong, and H. A. Sampson. 2001. Fatalities due to anaphylactic reactions to foods. *Journal of Allergy and Clinical Immunology* 107(1): 191–193.

Bunyard, L. B., K. E. Dennis, and B. J. Nicklas. 2002. Dietary intake and changes in lipoprotein lipids in obese, postmenopausal women placed on an American Heart Association Step 1 diet. *Journal of the American Dietetic Association* 102(1): 52–57.

Capps, O., L. Cleveland, and J. Park. 2002. Dietary behaviors associated with total fat and saturated fat intake. *Journal of the American Dietetic Association* 102(4): 490–502.

Centers for Disease Control and Prevention. 2001. Diagnosis and management of foodborne illnesses. *MMWR Recommendations and Reports* 50(RR-2).

Corle, D. K., et al. 2001. Self-rated quality of life measures: Effect of change to a low-fat, high-fiber, fruit and vegetable enriched diet. *Annals of Behavioral Medicine* 23(3): 198–207.

de Roos, N. M., M. L. Bots, and M. B. Katan. 2001. Replacement of dietary saturated fatty acids by trans fatty acids lowers serum HDL cholesterol and impairs endothelial function in healthy men and women. *Arteriosclerosis, Thrombosis and Vascular Biology* 21(7): 1233–1237.

de Roos, N. M., M. L. Bots, and M. B. Katan. 2001. Replacement of dietary saturated fatty acids by trans fatty acids lowers serum HDL cholesterol and impairs endothelial function in healthy men and women. *Arteriosclerosis, Thrombosis and Vascular Biology* 21(7): 1233–1237.

Feskanich, D., et al. 2002. Vitamin A intake and hips fractures among postmenopausal women. *Journal of the American Medical Association* 287(1): 47–54.

Food and Nutrition Board, National Academies. 2001. *Dietary Reference Intakes for Vitamin A, Vitamin K, Arsenic, Boron, Chromium, Copper, Iodine, Iron, Manganese, Molybdenum, Nickel, Silicon, Vanadium, and Zinc.* Washington, D.C.: National Academy Press.

Formanke, R. 2001. Food allergies: When food becomes the enemy. *FDA Consumer,* July/August.

Fung, T. T., et al. 2001. Association between dietary patterns and plasma biomarkers of obesity and cardiovascular disease risk. *American Journal of Clinical Nutrition* 73:61–67.

Hankinson, S. E., et al., eds. 2001. *Healthy Women, Healthy Lives: A Guide to Preventing Disease from the Landmark Nurses' Health Study.* New York: Simon & Schuster.

Hu, F. B., et al. 2001. Diet, lifestyle, and the risk of type 2 diabetes mellitus in women. *New England Journal of Medicine* 345(11): 790–797.

Insel, P., R. E. Turner, and D. Ross. 2001. *Nutrition.* Sudbury, Mass.: Jones & Bartlett.

Iso, H., et al. 2001. Intake of fish and omega-3 fatty acids and risk of stroke in women. *Journal of the American Medical Association* 285(3): 304–312.

Jacobs, D. R., H. E. Meyer, and K. Solvoll. 2001. Reduced mortality among whole grain bread eaters in men and women in the Norwegian Country Study. *European Journal of Clinical Nutrition* 55(20): 137–143.

Kant, A. K. 2000. Consumption of energy-dense, nutrient-poor foods by adult Americans: Nutritional and health implications. *American Journal of Clinical Nutrition* 72(4): 929–936.

Kaufman, D. W., et al. 2002. Recent patterns of medication use in the ambulatory adult population of the United States. *Journal of the American Medical Association* 287(3): 337–344.

Kennedy, E. T., et al. 2001. Popular diets: Correlation to health, nutrition, and obesity. *Journal of the American Dietetic Association* 101(4): 411–420.

Kleiner, S. M. 1999. Water: An essential but overlooked nutrient. *Journal of the American Dietetic Association* 99(2): 200– 206.

Kris-Etherton, P. M. 1999. AHA Science Advisory: Monounsaturated fatty acids and risk of cardiovascular disease. *Circulation* 100(11): 1253–1258.

Ludwig, D. S. 2002. The glycemic index: Physiological mechanisms relating to obesity, diabetes, and cardiovascular disease. *Journal of the American Medical Association* 287(18): 2414–2423.

National Research Council. 2000. *Genetically Modified Pest-Protected Plants: Science and Regulation.* Washington, D.C.: National Academy Press.

Oomen, C. M., et al. 2001. Association between trans fatty acid intake and 10-year risk of coronary heart disease. *Lancet* 357(9258): 746–751.

Preliminary FoodNet data on the incidence of foodborne illnesses—Selected sites, United States, 2001. 2002. *Morbidity and Mortality Weekly Report* 51(15): 325–329.

Shaw, A., et al. 1997. *Using the Food Guide Pyramid: A Resource for Nutrition Educators.* USDA Center for Nutrition Policy and Promotion (http://www.nal.usda.gov/fnic/Fpyr/guide. pdf; retrieved April 18, 2000).

Tips for the savvy supplement user: Making informed decisions. 2002. *FDA Consumer,* March/April.

Toborek, M., et al. 2002. Unsaturated fatty acids selectively induce an inflammatory environment in human endothelial cells. *American Journal of Clinical Nutrition* 75(1): 119–125.

U.S. Department of Agriculture, Food Safety and Inspection Service. 2000. *Irradiation of Raw Meat and Poultry: Questions and Answers* (http://www.fsis.usda.gov/OA/pubs/qa_irrad. htm; retrieved October 23, 2000).

U.S. Department of Agriculture and U.S. Department of Health and Human Services. 2000. *Nutrition and Your Health: Dietary Guidelines for Americans,* 5th ed. Home and Garden Bulletin No. 232.

Wood, O. B., and C. M. Bruhn. 2000. Position of the American Dietetic Association: Food irradiation. *Journal of the American Dietetic Association* 100(2): 246–253.

Wyshak, G. 2000. Teenaged girls, carbonated beverage consumption, and bone fracture. *Archives of Pediatric and Adolescent Medicine* 154:610–613.

Table 1 *Dietary Reference Intakes (DRIs): Recommended Levels for Individual Intake*

Life Stage	Group	Biotin (μg/day)	Choline (mg/day)[a]	Folate (μg/day)[b]	Niacin (mg/day)[c]	Pantothenic Acid (mg/day)	Riboflavin (mg/day)	Thiamin (mg/day)	Vitamin A (μg/day)[d]	Vitamin B-6 (mg/day)	Vitamin B-12 (μg/day)	Vitamin C (mg/day)[e]	Vitamin D (μg/day)[f]	Vitamin E (mg/day)[g]
Infants	0–6 months	5	125	65	2	1.7	0.3	0.2	400	0.1	0.4	40	5	4
	7–12 months	6	150	80	3	1.8	0.4	0.3	500	0.3	0.5	50	5	5
Children	1–3 years	8	200	**150**	**6**	2	**0.5**	**0.5**	**300**	**0.5**	**0.9**	**15**	5	**6**
	4–8 years	12	250	**200**	**8**	3	**0.6**	**0.6**	**400**	**0.6**	**1.2**	**25**	5	**7**
Males	9–13 years	20	375	**300**	**12**	4	**0.9**	**0.9**	**600**	**1.0**	**1.8**	**45**	5	**11**
	14–18 years	25	550	**400**	**16**	5	**1.3**	**1.2**	**900**	**1.3**	**2.4**	**75**	5	**15**
	19–30 years	30	550	**400**	**16**	5	**1.3**	**1.2**	**900**	**1.3**	**2.4**	**90**	5	**15**
	31–50 years	30	550	**400**	**16**	5	**1.3**	**1.2**	**900**	**1.3**	**2.4**	**90**	5	**15**
	51–70 years	30	550	**400**	**16**	5	**1.3**	**1.2**	**900**	**1.7**	**2.4**[h]	**90**	10	**15**
	>70 years	30	550	**400**	**16**	5	**1.3**	**1.2**	**900**	**1.7**	**2.4**[h]	**90**	15	**15**
Females	9–13 years	20	375	**300**	**12**	4	**0.9**	**0.9**	**600**	**1.0**	**1.8**	**45**	5	**11**
	14–18 years	25	400	**400**[i]	**14**	5	**1.0**	**1.0**	**700**	**1.2**	**2.4**	**65**	5	**15**
	19–30 years	30	425	**400**[i]	**14**	5	**1.1**	**1.1**	**700**	**1.3**	**2.4**	**75**	5	**15**
	31–50 years	30	425	**400**[i]	**14**	5	**1.1**	**1.1**	**700**	**1.3**	**2.4**	**75**	5	**15**
	51–70 years	30	425	**400**[i]	**14**	5	**1.1**	**1.1**	**700**	**1.5**	**2.4**[h]	**75**	10	**15**
	>70 years	30	425	**400**	**14**	5	**1.1**	**1.1**	**700**	**1.5**	**2.4**[h]	**75**	15	**15**
Pregnancy	≤18 years	30	450	**600**[j]	**18**	6	**1.4**	**1.4**	**750**	**1.9**	**2.6**	**80**	5	**15**
	19–30 years	30	450	**600**[j]	**18**	6	**1.4**	**1.4**	**770**	**1.9**	**2.6**	**85**	5	**15**
	31–50 years	30	450	**600**[j]	**18**	6	**1.4**	**1.4**	**770**	**1.9**	**2.6**	**85**	5	**15**
Lactation	≤18 years	35	550	**500**	**17**	7	**1.6**	**1.4**	**1200**	**2.0**	**2.8**	**115**	5	**19**
	19–30 years	35	550	**500**	**17**	7	**1.6**	**1.4**	**1300**	**2.0**	**2.8**	**120**	5	**19**
	31–50 years	35	550	**500**	**17**	7	**1.6**	**1.4**	**1300**	**2.0**	**2.8**	**120**	5	**19**

NOTE: This table includes Dietary Reference Intakes for those nutrients for which DRIs had been set through January 2002. The table includes values for the type of DRI standard—Adequate Intake (AI) or Recommended Dietary Allowance (RDA)—that has been established for that particular nutrient and life stage. RDAs are shown in **bold type.**

[a]Although AIs have been set for choline, there are few data to assess whether a dietary supply of choline is needed at all stages of the life cycle, and it may be that the choline requirement can be met by endogenous synthesis at some of these stages.

[b]As dietary folate equivalents (DFE). 1 DFE = 1 μg food folate = 0.6 μg of folate from fortified food or as a supplement consumed with food = 0.5 μg of a supplement taken on an empty stomach.

[c]As niacin equivalents (NE). 1 mg niacin = 60 mg tryptophan.

[d]As retinol activity equivalents (RAEs): 1 RAE = 1 μg retinol, 12 μg β-carotene, or 24 μg α-carotene or β-cryptoxanthin. Preformed vitamin A (retinol) is abundant in animal-derived foods; provitamin A carotenoids are abundant in some dark-yellow, orange, red, and deep-green fruits and vegetables. For preformed vitamin A and for provitamin A carotenoids in supplements, 1 RE = 1 RAE; for provitamin A carotenoids in foods, divide the REs by 2 to obtain RAEs.

Table 1 **Dietary Reference Intakes (DRIs): Recommended Levels for Individual Intake (continued)**

Life Stage	Group	Vitamin K (µg/day)	Calcium (mg/day)	Chromium (µg/day)	Copper (µg/day)	Fluoride (mg/day)	Iodine (µg/day)	Iron (mg/day)[k]	Magnesium (mg/day)	Manganese (mg/day)	Molybdenum (µg/day)	Phosphorus (mg/day)	Selenium (µg/day)	Zinc (mg/day)[l]
Infants	0–6 months	2.0	210	0.2	200	0.01	110	0.27	30	0.003	2	100	15	2
	7–12 months	2.5	270	5.5	220	0.5	130	11	75	0.6	3	275	20	3
Children	1–3 years	30	500	11	340	0.7	90	7	80	1.2	17	460	20	3
	4–8 years	55	800	15	440	1	90	10	130	1.5	22	500	30	5
Males	9–13 years	60	1300	25	700	2	120	8	240	1.9	34	1250	40	8
	14–18 years	75	1300	35	890	3	150	11	410	2.2	43	1250	55	11
	19–30 years	120	1000	35	900	4	150	8	400	2.3	45	700	55	11
	31–50 years	120	1000	35	900	4	150	8	420	2.3	45	700	55	11
	51–70 years	120	1200	30	900	4	150	8	420	2.3	45	700	55	11
	>70 years	120	1200	30	900	4	150	8	420	2.3	45	700	55	11
Females	9–13 years	60	1300	21	700	2	120	8	240	1.6	34	1250	40	8
	14–18 years	75	1300	24	890	3	150	15	360	1.6	43	1250	55	9
	19–30 years	90	1000	25	900	3	150	18	310	1.8	45	700	55	8
	31–50 years	90	1000	25	900	3	150	18	320	1.8	45	700	55	8
	51–70 years	90	1200	20	900	3	150	8	320	1.8	45	700	55	8
	>70 years	90	1200	20	900	3	150	8	320	1.8	45	700	55	8
Pregnancy	≤18 years	75	1300	29	1000	3	220	27	400	2.0	50	1250	60	13
	19–30 years	90	1000	30	1000	3	220	27	350	2.0	50	700	60	11
	31–50 years	90	1000	30	1000	3	220	27	360	2.0	50	700	60	11
Lactation	≤18 years	75	1300	44	1300	3	290	10	360	2.6	50	1250	70	14
	19–30 years	90	1000	45	1300	3	290	9	310	2.6	50	700	70	12
	31–50 years	90	1000	45	1300	3	290	9	320	2.6	50	700	70	12

[e]Individuals who smoke require an additional 35 mg/day of vitamin C over that needed by nonsmokers; nonsmokers regularly exposed to tobacco smoke should ensure they meet the RDA for vitamin C.

[f]As cholecalciferol: 1 µg cholecalciferol = 40 IU vitamin D. DRI values are based on the absence of adequate exposure to sunlight.

[g]As α-tocopherol. Includes naturally occurring RRR-α-tocopherol and the 2R-stereoisomeric forms from supplements; does not include the 2S-stereoisomeric forms from supplements.

[h]Since 10–30% of older people may malabsorb food-bound B-12, those over age 50 should meet their RDA mainly with supplements or foods fortified with B-12.

[i]In view of evidence linking folate intake with neural tube defects in the fetus, it is recommended that all women capable of becoming pregnant consume 400 µg from supplements or fortified foods in addition to consuming folate from a varied diet.

[j]It is assumed that women will continue consuming 400 µg from supplements or fortified food until their pregnancy is confirmed and they enter prenatal care, which ordinarily occurs after the end of the periconceptional period—the critical time for formation of the neural tube.

[k]Because the absorption of iron from plant foods is low compared to that from animal foods, the RDA for strict vegetarians is approximately 1.8 times higher than the values established for omnivores (14 mg/day for adult male vegetarians; 33 mg/day for premenopausal female vegetarians). Oral contraceptives (OCs) reduce menstrual blood losses, so women taking them need less daily iron; the RDA for premenopausal women taking OCs is 10.9 mg/day. For more on iron requirements for other special situations, refer to *Dietary Reference Intakes for Vitamin A, Vitamin K, Arsenic, Boron, Chromium, Copper, Iodine, Iron, Manganese, Molybdenum, Nickel, Silicon, Vanadium, and Zinc* (visit http://www.nap.edu for the complete report).

[l]Zinc absorption is lower for those consuming vegetarian diets, so the zinc requirement for vegetarians is approximately twofold greater than for those consuming a nonvegetarian diet.

SOURCE: Food and Nutrition Board, Institute of Medicine, National Academies. 2001. *Dietary Reference Intakes Tables* (http://www4.nationalacademies.org/IOM/IOMHome.nsf/Pages/Food+and+Nutrition+Board; retrieved November 15, 2001). The complete Dietary Reference Intake reports are available from the National Academy Press (http://www.nap.edu).

Table 2 Tolerable Nutrient Upper Intake Levels for Adults

Nutrient	Upper Intake Level
Choline	3,500 mg/day
Folate	1,000 μg/day
Niacin	35 mg/day
Vitamin A	3,000 μg/day
Vitamin B-6	100 mg/day
Vitamin C	2,000 mg/day
Vitamin D	50 μg/day
Vitamin E	1,000 mg/day
Boron	20 mg/day
Calcium	2,500 mg/day
Copper	10,000 μg/day
Fluoride	10 mg/day
Iodine	1,100 μg/day
Iron	45 mg/day
Magnesium (nonfood sources)	350 mg/day
Manganese	11 mg/day
Molybdenum	2,000 μg/day
Nickel	1.0 mg/day
Phosphorus	4,000 mg/day
Selenium	400 μg/day
Vanadium	1.8 mg/day
Zinc	40 mg/day

This table includes the adult Tolerable Upper Intake Level (UL) standard of the Dietary Reference Intakes (DRIs). For some nutrients, there is insufficient data on which to develop a UL. This does not mean that there is no potential for adverse effects from high intake, and when data about adverse effects are limited, extra caution may be warranted. In healthy individuals, there is no established benefit from nutrient intakes above the RDA or AI.

SOURCE: Food and Nutrition Board, Institute of Medicine, National Academies. 2001. *Dietary Reference Intakes Tables* (http://www4.nationalacademies.org/IOM/IOMHome.nsf/Pages/Food+and+Nutrition+Board; retrieved November 15, 2001). The complete Dietary Reference Intake reports are available from the National Academy Press (http://www.nap.edu). Reprinted with permission from Dietary Reference Intakes. Copyright © 2001 by the National Academy of Sciences. Courtesy of the National Academy Press, Washington, D.C.

Table 3 Recommended Dietary Allowances, Revised 1989[a,b] (Abridged)

Category	Age (years) or Condition	Protein (g/kg)[c]
Infants	0.0–0.5	2.2
	0.5–1.0	1.6
Children	1–3	1.2
	4–6	1.1
	7–10	1.0
Males	11–14	1.0
	15–18	0.9
	19–24	0.8
	25–50	0.8
	51+	0.8
Females	11–14	1.0
	15–18	0.8
	19–24	0.8
	25–50	0.8
	51+	0.8
Pregnant		+10g
Lactating	1st 6 Months	+15g
	2nd 6 Months	+12g

[a]This table includes RDAs for those nutrients for which DRIs had not yet been established as of May 2002. The allowances, expressed as average daily intakes over time, are intended to provide for individual variations among most normal people as they live in the United States under usual environmental stresses. Diet should be based on a variety of common foods in order to provide other nutrients for which human requirements have been less well defined.

[b]Estimated Minimum Requirements of healthy adults: 500 mg sodium; 750 mg chloride; 2000 mg potassium. (For information on other age groups, see *Recommended Dietary Allowances,* 10th ed.)

[c]The RDA for protein is expressed as grams of protein per kilogram of body weight. To calculate the RDA, multiply body weight in kilograms (1 kilogram = 2.2 pounds) by the appropriate number from the protein column. For example, a 19-year-old male who weighs 165 pounds would calculate his protein RDA as follows: 165 lb ÷ 2.2 kg/lb = 75 kg × 0.8 g/kg (from table) = 60 g protein per day. For pregnant or lactating women, calculate RDA based on age and then add the appropriate number of additional grams listed in the table.

SOURCE: Reprinted with permission from *Recommended Dietary Allowances,* 10th Edition. Copyright © 1989 by the National Academy of Sciences. Courtesy of the National Academy Press, Washington, D.C.

Name ______________________ **Section** ______________ **Date** ______________

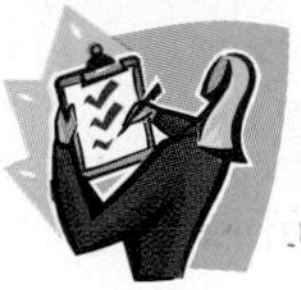

LAB 8.1 *Your Daily Diet Versus the Food Guide Pyramid*

Keep a record of everything you eat for 3 consecutive days. Record all foods and beverages you consume, breaking each food item into its component parts (for example, a turkey sandwich would be listed as 2 slices of bread, 3 oz of turkey, 1 tsp of mayonnaise, and so on). Complete the first two columns of the chart during the course of the day; fill in the remaining information at the end of the day using Figure 8.4 and pp. 220–221 in your text. For fats, oils, and sweets—foods from the tip of the Pyramid—put a star (*) in the Food Group column.

DAY 1

Food	*Portion Size*	*Food Group*	*Number of Servings**

Daily Total

Food Group	*Number of Servings*
Milk, yogurt, cheese	
Meat, poultry, fish, dry beans, eggs, nuts	
Fruits	
Vegetables	
Breads, cereals, rice, pasta	

*Your portion sizes may be smaller or larger than the serving sizes given in the Food Guide Pyramid; list the actual number of Food Guide Pyramid servings contained in the foods you eat.

DAY 2

Food	*Portion Size*	*Food Group*	*Number of Servings**

Daily Total

Food Group	*Number of Servings*
Milk, yogurt, cheese	
Meat, poultry, fish, dry beans, eggs, nuts	
Fruits	
Vegetables	
Breads, cereals, rice, pasta	

*Your portion sizes may be smaller or larger than the serving sizes given in the Food Guide Pyramid; list the actual number of Food Guide Pyramid servings contained in the foods you eat.

DAY 3

Food	*Portion Size*	*Food Group*	*Number of Servings**

Daily Total

Food Group	*Number of Servings*
Milk, yogurt, cheese	
Meat, poultry, fish, dry beans, eggs, nuts	
Fruits	
Vegetables	
Breads, cereals, rice, pasta	

*Your portion sizes may be smaller or larger than the serving sizes given in the Food Guide Pyramid; list the actual number of Food Guide Pyramid servings contained in the foods you eat.

Next, average your serving totals for the 3 days and enter them in the chart below. Fill in the recommended serving totals that apply to you from Figure 8.4 and Table 8.5.

Food Group	*Recommended Number of Servings*	*Actual Number of Servings*
Milk, yogurt, cheese		
Meat, poultry, fish, dry beans, eggs, nuts		
Fruits		
Vegetables		
Breads, cereals, rice, pasta		

Using Your Results

How did you score? How close is your diet to that recommended by the Food Guide Pyramid? Are you at all surprised by the actual number of servings you're consuming from each food group?

What should you do next? If the results of the assessment indicate that you could boost your level of wellness by improving your diet, set realistic goals for change. Do you need to increase or decrease your consumption of any food groups? List any areas of concern below, along with a goal for change and strategies for achieving the goal you've set. If you see that you are falling short in one food group, such as fruits or vegetables, but have many starred items from the fats, oils, and sweets category, you might try decreasing those items in favor of an apple, a bunch of grapes, or some baby carrots. Think carefully about the reasons behind your food choices. For example, if you eat doughnuts for breakfast every morning because you feel rushed, make a list of ways to save time to allow for a healthier breakfast.

Problem: ______________________________

Goal: ______________________________

Strategies for change: ______________________________

____

____

Problem: ______________________________

Goal: ______________________________

Strategies for change: ______________________________

____

____

Problem: ______________________________

Goal: ______________________________

Strategies for change: ______________________________

____

____

Enter the results of this lab in the Preprogram Assessment column in Appendix D. If you've set goals and identified strategies for change, begin putting your plan into action. After several weeks of your program, complete this lab again and enter the results in the Postprogram Assessment column of Appendix D. How do the results compare?

Name ______________________ **Section** ____________ **Date** ______________

LAB 8.2 *Dietary Analysis*

You can complete this activity using either a nutrition analysis software program or the food composition data in Appendix B and the charts printed below. Information about the nutrient content of foods is also available online; see the For Further Exploration section for recommended Web sites. (This lab asks you to analyze one day's diet. For a more complete and accurate assessment of your diet, analyze the results from several different days, including a weekday and a weekend day.)

DATE ______________________ DAY: M Tu W Th F Sa Su

Food	Amount	Calories	Protein (g)	Carbohydrate (g)	Dietary fiber (g)	Fat, total (g)	Saturated fat (g)	Cholesterol (mg)	Sodium (mg)	Vitamin A (RE)	Vitamin C (mg)	Calcium (mg)	Iron (mg)
Recommended totals[a]			10–15%	≥55%	20–35 g	≤30%	<10%	≤300 mg	≤2400 mg	RE	mg	mg	mg
Actual totals[b]		cal	g / %	g / %	g	g / %	g / %	mg	mg	RE	mg	mg	mg

[a]Fill in the appropriate RDA or DRI values for vitamin A, vitamin C, calcium, and iron from Table 1 in the Nutrition Resources section.

[b]Total the values in each column. To calculate the percentage of total calories from protein, carbohydrate, fat, and saturated fat, use the formulas on p. 210. Protein and carbohydrate provide 4 calories per gram; fat provides 9 calories per gram. For example, if you consume a total of 270 grams of carbohydrate and 2000 calories, your percentage of total calories from carbohydrate would be (270 g × 4 cal/g) ÷ 2000 cal = 54%. Do not include data for alcoholic beverages in your calculations. Percentages may not total 100% due to rounding.

Using Your Results

How did you score? How close is your diet to that recommended by the Dietary Guidelines, Dietary Reference Intakes, and other guidelines? Are you surprised by any of the results of this assessment?

What should you do next? Enter the results of this lab in the Preprogram Assessment column in Appendix D. If your daily diet meets all the recommended intakes, congratulations—and keep up the good work. If the results of the assessment pinpoint areas of concern, then work with your food record on the previous page to determine what changes you could make to meet all the guidelines. Make changes, additions, and deletions until it conforms to all or most of the guidelines. Or, if you prefer, start from scratch to create a day's diet that meets the guidelines. Use the chart below to experiment and record your final, healthy sample diet for one day. Then put what you learned from this exercise into practice in your daily life. After several weeks of your program, complete this lab again and enter the results in the Postprogram Assessment column of Appendix D. How do the results compare?

DATE________________________ DAY: M Tu W Th F Sa Su

Food	Amount	Calories	Protein (g)	Carbohydrate (g)	Dietary fiber (g)	Fat, total (g)	Saturated fat (g)	Cholesterol (mg)	Sodium (mg)	Vitamin A (RE)	Vitamin C (mg)	Calcium (mg)	Iron (mg)
Recommended totals			10–15%	≥55%	20–35 g	≤30%	<10%	≤300 mg	≤2400 mg	RE	mg	mg	mg
Actual totals		cal	g / %	g / %	g	g / %	g / %	mg	mg	RE	mg	mg	mg

Name ______________________ Section ______________ Date ______________

LAB 8.3 *Informed Food Choices*

Part I Using Food Labels

Choose three food items to evaluate. You might want to select three similar items, such as regular, low-fat, and nonfat salad dressing, or three very different items. Record the information from their food labels in the table below.

Food Items			
Serving size			
Total calories	cal	cal	cal
Total fat—grams	g	g	g
—% Daily Value	%	%	%
Saturated fat—grams	g	g	g
—% Daily Value	%	%	%
Cholesterol—milligrams	mg	mg	mg
—% Daily Value	%	%	%
Sodium—milligrams	mg	mg	mg
—% Daily Value	%	%	%
Carbohydrates (total)—grams	g	g	g
—% Daily Value	%	%	%
Dietary fiber—grams	g	g	g
—% Daily Value	%	%	%
Sugars—grams	g	g	g
Protein—grams	g	g	g
Vitamin A—% Daily Value	%	%	%
Vitamin C—% Daily Value	%	%	%
Calcium—% Daily Value	%	%	%
Iron—% Daily Value	%	%	%

How do the items you chose compare? You can do a quick nutrient check by totaling the Daily Value percentages for nutrients you should limit (total fat, cholesterol, sodium) and the nutrients you should favor (dietary fiber, vitamin A, vitamin C, calcium, iron) for each food. Which food has the largest percent Daily Value sum for nutrients to limit? For nutrients to favor?

Food Items			
Calories	cal	cal	cal
% Daily Value total for nutrients to limit (total fat, cholesterol, sodium)	%	%	%
% Daily Value total for nutrients to favor (fiber, vitamin A, vitamin C, calcium, iron)	%	%	%

Part II Evaluating Fast Food

Use the information from Appendix C, Nutritional Content of Popular Items from Fast-Food Restaurants, to complete the chart on this page for the last fast-food meal you ate. Add up your totals for the meal. Compare the values for fat, protein, carbohydrate, cholesterol, and sodium content for each food item and for the meal as a whole with the levels suggested by the Dietary Guidelines for Americans. Calculate the percent of total calories derived from fat, saturated fat, protein, and carbohydrate using the formulas given.

If you haven't recently been to one of the restaurants included in the appendix, fill in the chart for any sample meal you might eat. If some of the food items you selected don't appear in Appendix C, ask for a nutrition information brochure when you visit the restaurant, or check out online fast-food information: Arby's (http://www.arbysrestaurant.com), Burger King (http://www.burgerking.com), Domino's Pizza (http://www.dominos.com), Jack in the Box (http://www.jackinthebox.com), KFC (http://www.kfc.com), McDonald's (http://www.mcdonalds.com), Taco Bell (http://www.tacobell.com), Wendy's (http://www.wendys.com).

FOOD ITEMS

	Dietary Guidelines							Total[b]
Serving size (g)		g	g	g	g	g	g	g
Calories		cal	cal	cal	cal	cal	cal	cal
Total fat—grams		g	g	g	g	g	g	g
—% calories[a]	≤30%	%	%	%	%	%	%	%
Saturated fat—grams		g	g	g	g	g	g	g
—% calories[a]	<10%	%	%	%	%	%	%	%
Protein—grams		g	g	g	g	g	g	g
—% calories[a]	10–15%	%	%	%	%	%	%	%
Carbohydrate—grams		g	g	g	g	g	g	g
—% calories[a]	≥55%	%	%	%	%	%	%	%
Cholesterol[c]	100 mg	mg	mg	mg	mg	mg	mg	mg
Sodium[c]	800 mg	mg	mg	mg	mg	mg	mg	mg

[a]To calculate the percent of total calories from each food energy source (fat, carbohydrate, protein), use the following formula:

$$\frac{\text{(number of grams of energy source)} \times \text{(number of calories per gram of energy source)}}{\text{(total calories in serving of food item)}}$$

(*Note:* Fat and saturated fat provide 9 calories per gram; protein and carbohydrate provide 4 calories per gram.) For example, the percent of total calories from protein in a 150-calorie dish containing 10 grams of protein is

$$\frac{\text{(10 grams of protein)} \times \text{(4 calories per gram)}}{\text{(150 calories)}} = \frac{40}{150} = 0.27\text{, or 27\% of total calories from protein}$$

[b]For the Total column, add up the total grams of fat, carbohydrate, and protein contained in your sample meal and calculate the percentages based on the total calories in the meal. (Percentages may not total 100% due to rounding.) For cholesterol and sodium values, add up the total number of milligrams.

[c]Recommended daily limits of cholesterol and sodium are divided by 3 here to give an approximate recommended limit for a single meal.

SOURCE: Insel, P. M., and W. T. Roth. 2002. Wellness Worksheet 57. *Core Concepts in Health,* 9th ed. New York: McGraw-Hill.

Weight Management

9

LOOKING AHEAD

After reading this chapter, you should be able to

- Explain the health risks associated with overweight and obesity
- Explain the factors that may contribute to a weight problem, including genetic, physiological, lifestyle, and psychosocial factors
- Describe lifestyle factors that contribute to weight gain and loss, including the role of food choices, exercise, and emotional factors
- Identify and describe the symptoms of eating disorders and the health risks associated with them
- Design a personal plan for successfully managing body weight

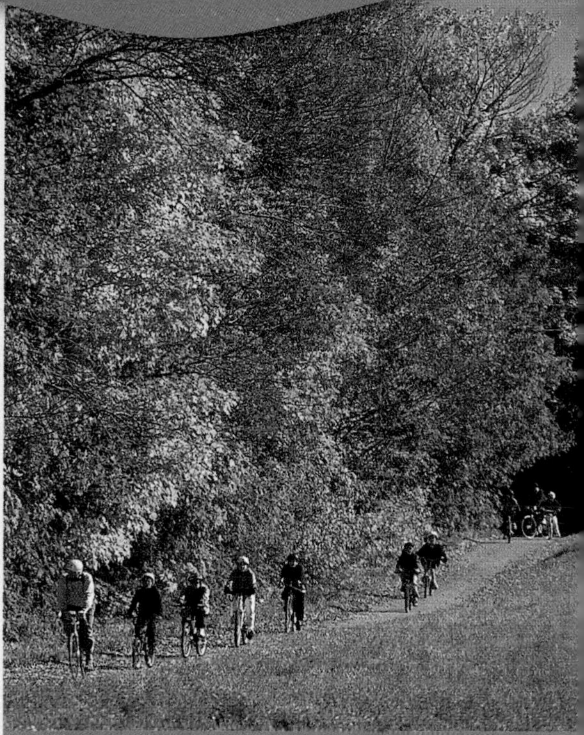

TEST YOUR KNOWLEDGE

1. The consumption of low-calorie sweeteners has helped Americans control their weight.
   True or false?
2. Approximately how many female high school and college students have either anorexia or bulimia?
   a. 1 in 250
   b. 1 in 100
   c. 1 in 30
3. Which of the following snacks contains the fewest calories—about 100 for the serving size listed?
   a. 8 ounces (2/3 can) of soda
   b. 2 fat-free sandwich cookies
   c. 4 pretzel twists
   d. 2 cups strawberries
   e. 20 baby carrots

TEST YOUR KNOWLEDGE ANSWERS

1. FALSE. Since the introduction of low-calorie sweeteners, both total calorie intake and total sugar intake have increased, as has the proportion of Americans who are overweight.

2. C. About 2–4% of female students suffer from bulimia or anorexia, and many more occasionally engage in behaviors associated with these disorders.

3. ALL FIVE ARE EQUAL. Each of these snacks provides about 100 calories; however, the servings of strawberries and carrots are much larger because they are lower in energy (calorie) density.

Fit and Well Online Learning Center

www.mhhe.com/fahey5e

Visit the *Fit and Well* Online Learning Center for study aids, additional information about weight management, links, Internet activities that explore the role of weight management in wellness, and much more.

Achieving and maintaining a healthy body weight is a serious public health challenge in the United States and a source of distress for many Americans. Under standards developed by the National Institutes of Health, about 60% of American adults are overweight, including more than 20% who are obese (Table 9.1). The rate of obesity has nearly doubled since 1960, and it continues to rise. If current rates of weight gain continue, *all* American adults will be overweight by 2030.

Controlling body weight is really a matter of controlling body fat. As explained in Chapter 6, the most important consideration for health is not total weight but body composition—the proportion of fat to fat-free mass. Many people who are "overweight" are also "overfat," and the health risks they face are due to the latter condition. Although this chapter uses the common terms *weight management* and *weight loss,* the goal for wellness is to adopt healthy behaviors and achieve an appropriate body composition, not to conform to rigid standards of total body weight.

Although not completely understood, managing body weight is not a mysterious process. The "secret" is balancing calories consumed with calories expended in daily activities—in other words, eating a moderate diet and getting regular physical activity. Unfortunately, this formula is not as exciting as the latest fad diet or "scientific breakthrough" that promises slimness without effort. Many people fail in their efforts to manage their weight because they emphasize short-term weight loss rather than permanent changes in lifestyle. Dieting is not part of a wellness lifestyle. Successful weight management requires the long-term coordination of many aspects of a wellness lifestyle, including proper nutrition, adequate physical activity, and stress management. The goal is the adoption of healthy and sustainable habits that maximize energy and well-being and reduce the risk of chronic diseases.

Body image is a related area of concern. More and more people are becoming unhappy with their bodies and obsessed with their weight. In recent surveys, more than half of Americans have stated that they are dissatisfied with their weight; only about 10% report being completely satisfied with their bodies. Dissatisfaction with body weight and shape is associated with dangerous eating patterns such as binge eating or self-starvation and with eating disorders.

VITAL STATISTICS

Table 9.1 *The Prevalence of Obesity: Populations of Special Concern*

Group	Estimated Prevalence of Obesity*	*Healthy People 2010* Target
Children (age 6–11)	11%	5%
Adolescents (age 12–19)	10	5
Adults (age 20–74)	23	15
Men	20	15
Women	25	15
Low-income people	29	15
Mexican American women	35	15
Black women	38	15

*Children and adolescents are classified as obese if they have a BMI at or above the appropriate 95th percentile for body mass index (BMI); adults are classified as obese if they have a BMI of 30 or above.

SOURCE: Department of Health and Human Services, 2000. *Healthy People 2010,* 2d ed. Washington, D. C.: DHHS.

This chapter explores the factors that contribute to the development of overweight and obesity as well as to eating disorders. It also takes a closer look at weight management through lifestyle and suggests specific strategies for reaching and maintaining a healthy weight. This information is designed to provide the tools necessary for integrating effective weight management into a wellness lifestyle.

HEALTH IMPLICATIONS OF OVERWEIGHT AND OBESITY

As rates of **overweight** and **obesity** have risen in the United States, so has the prevalence of the health conditions associated with overweight—including a more than 33% rise in the rate of diabetes in just the past decade. It's estimated that inactivity and overweight account for more than 300,000 premature deaths annually in the United States, second only to tobacco-related deaths. Overweight and obesity are one of the most serious and widespread challenges to wellness.

As described in Chapter 6, excess body fat increases a person's risk of developing numerous diseases and unhealthy conditions. Obesity is one of six major controllable risk factors for heart disease; it also increases risk for other forms of cardiovascular disease (CVD), hypertension, certain forms of cancer, diabetes, gallbladder disease, respiratory problems, joint diseases, skin problems, impaired immune function, and sleep disorders. Obese people have an overall mortality rate almost twice that of

Terms

overweight Characterized by a body weight that falls above the range associated with minimum mortality: weighing 10% or more over recommended weight or having a BMI over 25.

obesity Severely overweight, with an excess of body fat: weighing 20% or more over recommended weight or having a BMI over 30.

resting metabolic rate (RMR) The energy required (in calories) to maintain vital body functions, including respiration, heart rate, body temperature, and blood pressure, while the body is at rest.

nonobese people. Gaining weight over the years has also been found dangerous; in one study, women who gained more than 22 pounds since they were 18 years old had a sevenfold increase in the risk of heart disease. Many studies have confirmed that overweight and obesity shorten lives.

At the same time, research has shown that even modest weight loss can have a significant positive impact on health. A weight loss of just 5–10% in obese individuals can reduce the risk of coronary heart disease, hypertension, stroke, diabetes, and other weight-related conditions and increase life expectancy.

FACTORS CONTRIBUTING TO EXCESS BODY FAT

Much research has been done in an effort to pinpoint the cause of overweight and obesity. It appears, however, that body weight and body composition are determined by multiple factors that may vary with each individual. These factors can be grouped into genetic, physiological, lifestyle, and psychosocial factors.

Genetic Factors

Estimates of the genetic contribution to obesity vary widely, from about 5% to 40%. More than 20 genes have been linked to obesity, but their actions are still under study. Genes influence body size and shape, body fat distribution, and metabolic rate. Genetic factors also affect the ease with which weight is gained as a result of overeating and where on the body extra weight is added. If both parents are overweight, their children are twice as likely to be overweight as children who have only one overweight parent. In studies that compared adoptees and their biological parents, the weights of the adoptees were found to be more like those of the biological parents than the adoptive parents, again indicating a strong genetic link.

Research thus suggests a genetic component in the determination of body weight. However, hereditary influences must be balanced against the contribution of environmental factors. Not all children of obese parents become obese, and normal-weight parents also have overweight children. The incidence of obesity is rising rapidly in the United States, but not in all parts of the world. In a study comparing men born and raised in Ireland with their biological brothers who lived in the United States, the American men were found to weigh, on average, 6% more than their Irish brothers. Environmental factors like diet and exercise are probably responsible for this difference in weight. Thus, the *tendency* to develop obesity may be inherited, but the expression of this tendency is affected by environmental influences.

The message you should take from this research is that genes are not destiny. It is true that some people have a harder time losing weight and maintaining weight loss than others. However, with increased exercise and attention to diet, even those with a genetic tendency toward obesity can maintain a healthy body weight. And regardless of genetic factors, lifestyle choices remain the cornerstone of successful weight management.

Physiological Factors

Metabolism is a key physiological factor in the regulation of body fat and body weight; hormones also play a role. Another physiological factor that has been proposed as contributing to obesity is weight cycling.

Metabolism and Energy Balance Metabolism is the sum of all the vital processes by which food energy and nutrients are made available to and used by the body. The largest component of metabolism, **resting metabolic rate (RMR)**, is the energy required to maintain vital body functions, including respiration, heart rate, body temperature, and blood pressure, while the body is at rest. As shown in Figure 9.1 (p. 256), RMR accounts for 55–75% of daily energy expenditure. The energy required to digest food accounts for an additional 5–15% of daily energy expenditure. The remaining 10–40% is expended during physical activity.

Both heredity and behavior affect metabolic rate. Men, who have a higher proportion of muscle mass than women, have a higher RMR (muscle tissue is more metabolically active than fat). Also, some individuals inherit a higher or lower RMR than others. A higher RMR means that a person burns more calories while at rest and can therefore take in more calories without gaining weight.

Exercise has a positive effect on metabolism. When people exercise, they slightly increase their RMR—the number of calories their bodies burn at rest. They also increase their muscle mass, which is associated with a higher metabolic rate. The exercise itself also burns calories, raising total energy expenditure. The higher the energy expenditure, the more the person can eat without gaining weight. Weight loss or gain also affects metabolic rate. When a person loses weight, both RMR and the energy required to perform physical tasks decrease. The reverse occurs when weight is gained. (To determine your own RMR, complete Lab 9.1.)

The two parts of the energy balance equation over which you have the most control are the energy you take in as food and the energy you burn during physical activity. To lose weight and body fat, you can increase the amount of energy you burn by increasing your level of physical activity and/or decrease the amount of energy you take in by consuming fewer calories. Specific strategies for altering energy balance are discussed later in the chapter.

Hormones Hormones clearly play a role in the accumulation of body fat, especially for females. Hormonal

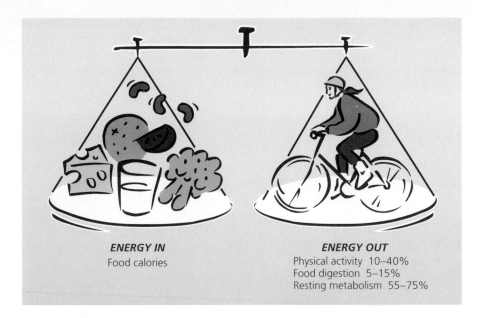

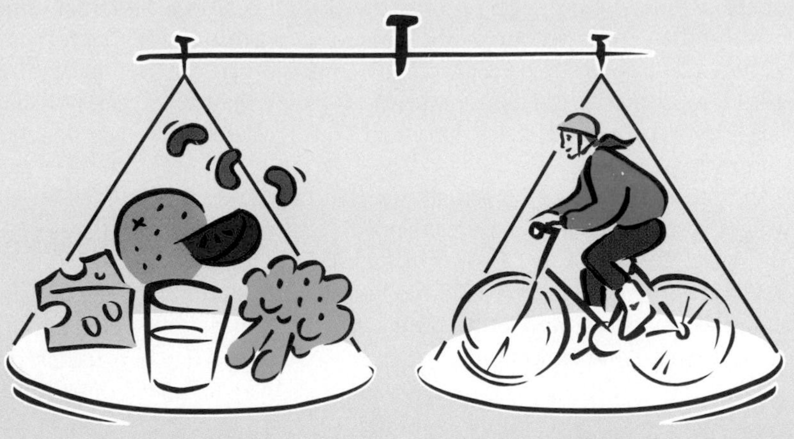
ENERGY IN
Food calories
ENERGY OUT
Physical activity 10–40%
Food digestion 5–15%
Resting metabolism 55–75%

Figure 9.1 The energy-balance equation. To maintain your current weight, you must burn up as many calories as you take in as food each day.

changes at puberty, during pregnancy, and at menopause contribute to the amount and location of fat accumulation. For example, during puberty, hormones cause the development of secondary sex characteristics, including larger breasts, wider hips, and a fat layer under the skin. This addition of body fat at puberty is normal and healthy.

One hormone thought to be linked to obesity is leptin. Secreted by the body's fat cells, leptin is carried to the brain, where it appears to let the brain know how big or small the body's fat stores are. With this information, the brain can regulate appetite and metabolic rate accordingly. Other hormones that may be involved in the regulation of appetite are cholecystokinin (CCK), peptide YY, and gluconlike peptide-1 (GLP-1). Researchers hope to use these hormones to develop treatments for obesity based on appetite control; however, as most of us will admit, hunger is often *not* the primary reason we overeat. Cases of obesity based solely or primarily on hormone abnormalities do exist, but they are rare. Lifestyle choices still account for the largest proportion of the differences in body weight and body composition among individuals.

Weight Cycling It has been hypothesized that repeatedly losing and regaining weight, known as weight cycling or yo-yo dieting, might be harmful to both overall health and to efforts at weight loss. Weight cycling, it was thought, might make the body more efficient at extracting and storing calories from food; thus, with each successive diet, it would become more difficult to lose weight. Most studies, however, have not supported this idea. Other studies have explored whether weight cycling might change body fat distribution, increase the body's preference for dietary fat, contribute to gallbladder disease and death from CVD, or lead to disordered eating habits. Studies have not yet conclusively shown weight cycling to be harmful to the health of an obese person, and most researchers believe that obese individuals should continue to try to control their weight. Losing even a few pounds brings substantial health benefits that appear to exceed any potential risks that might be incurred from weight loss or weight cycling.

Lifestyle Factors

Genetic and physiological factors may increase risk for excess body fat, but they are not sufficient to explain the increasingly high rate of obesity seen in the United States. The gene pool has not changed dramatically in the past 40 years, during which time the rate of obesity among Americans has doubled. Clearly, other factors are at work—particularly lifestyle factors such as increased energy intake and decreased physical activity.

Eating Americans have access to an abundance of highly palatable and calorie-dense foods, and many have eating habits that contribute to weight gain. Most overweight adults will admit to eating more than they should of high-fat, high-sugar, high-calorie foods. Americans eat out more frequently now than in the past, and we rely more heavily on fast food and packaged convenience foods. Restaurant and convenience food portion sizes tend to be very large, and the foods themselves are more likely to be high in fat, sugar, and calories and low in nutrients. Studies have consistently found that people underestimate portion sizes by as much as 25%.

Terms

binge eating A pattern of eating in which normal food consumption is interrupted by episodes of high consumption.

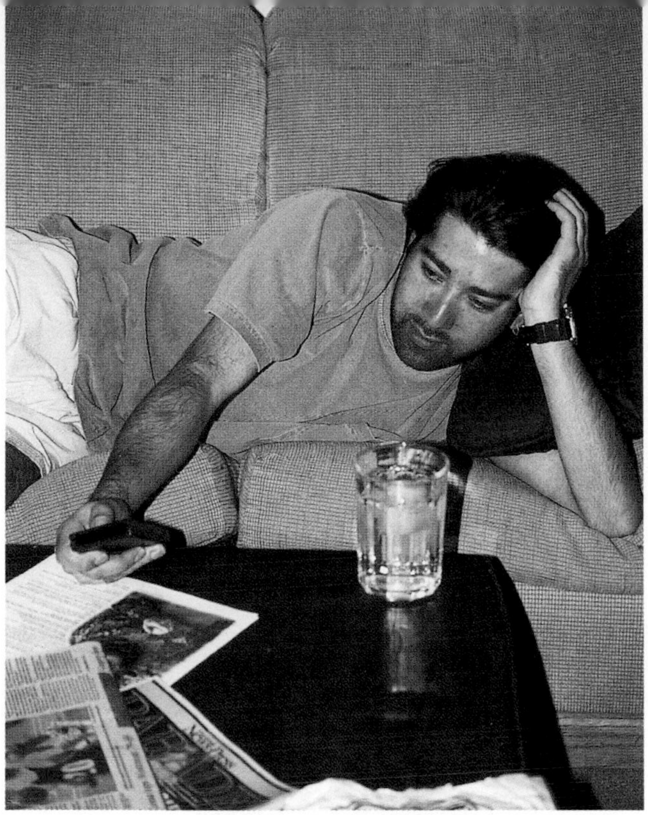

College living often makes it difficult to maintain a healthy weight. Fast foods and sedentary habits can lead to weight problems in both the short and the long term.

According to the CDC, the average calorie intake by Americans has increased by 100–300 calories per day over the past two decades. Levels of physical activity declined during this period; the net result has been a substantial increase in the number of Americans who are overweight. Healthy eating habits that are part of successful weight management are described later in this chapter.

Physical Activity Activity levels among Americans are declining, beginning in childhood and continuing throughout the life cycle. Most adults drive to work, sit all day, and then relax in front of the TV at night. During leisure time, both children and adults surf the Internet, play video games, or watch TV rather than bicycle, participate in sports, or just do yardwork or chores around the house. One study found that 60% of the incidence of overweight can be linked to excessive television viewing. On average, Americans exercise 15 minutes per day and watch 150 minutes of TV. Modern conveniences such as remote controls, elevators, and power mowers have also reduced daily physical activity.

Psychosocial Factors Many people have learned to use food as a means of coping with stress and negative emotions. Eating can provide a powerful distraction from difficult feelings—loneliness, anger, boredom, anxiety, shame, sadness, inadequacy. It can be used to combat low moods, low energy levels, and low self-esteem. When food and eating become the primary means of regulating emotions, **binge eating** or other disturbed eating patterns can develop.

Obesity is strongly associated with socioeconomic status. The prevalence of obesity goes down as income level goes up. More women are obese at lower income levels than men, but men are somewhat more obese at higher levels. These differences may reflect the greater sensitivity and concern for a slim physical appearance among upper-income women, as well as greater access to information about nutrition and to low-fat and low-calorie foods. It may also reflect the greater acceptance of obesity among certain ethnic groups, as well as different cultural values related to food choices.

In some families and cultures, food is used as a symbol of love and caring. It is an integral part of social gatherings and celebrations. In such cases, it may be difficult to change established eating patterns because they are linked to cultural and family values.

ADOPTING A HEALTHY LIFESTYLE FOR SUCCESSFUL WEIGHT MANAGEMENT

When all the research has been assessed, it is clear that most weight problems are lifestyle problems. Looking at these problems in a historical context reveals why fad diets and other quick-fix approaches are not effective in reversing overweight. About 100 years ago, Americans consumed a diet very different from today's diet and got much more exercise as well. Americans now eat more calories, fat, and refined sugars and fewer complex carbohydrates. Americans today also get far less exercise than their great-grandparents did. Walking, bicycling, and farm and manual labor have all declined, resulting in a decrease in daily energy expenditure of about 200 calories.

Permanent weight loss is not something you start and stop. You need to adopt healthy behaviors that you can maintain throughout your life. Lifestyle factors that are critical for successful long-term weight management include diet and eating habits, physical activity and exercise, an ability to think positively and manage your emotions effectively, and the coping strategies you use to deal with the stresses and challenges in your life.

Ww Diet and Eating Habits

In contrast to "dieting," which involves some form of food restriction, "diet" refers to your daily food choices. Everyone has a diet, but not everyone is dieting. You need to develop a diet that you enjoy and that enables you to maintain a healthy body composition.

Use the Food Guide Pyramid as the basis for planning a healthy diet (see Chapter 8). For weight management, you may need to pay special attention to total calories, portion sizes, energy density, fat and sugar intake, and eating habits.

Total Calories The Food Guide Pyramid suggests the following approximate daily energy intakes:

- 1600 calories: Many sedentary women and some older adults
- 2200 calories: Most children, teenage girls, active women, and many sedentary men
- 2800 calories: Teenage boys, many active men, and some very active women

However, energy balance may be a more important consideration for weight management than total calories consumed. To maintain your current weight, the total number of calories you eat must equal the number you burn (refer to the energy-balance equation in Figure 9.1). To lose weight, you must decrease your calorie intake and/or increase the number of calories you burn; to gain weight, the reverse is true. To calculate your daily caloric needs, complete the calculations in Lab 9.1.

The best approach for weight loss is probably combining an increase in physical activity with moderate calorie restriction. Don't go on a "crash diet." You need to consume enough food to meet your need for essential nutrients. Also, to maintain weight loss, you will probably have to maintain some degree of the calorie restriction you used to lose the weight. Therefore, it is important that you adopt a level of food intake that you can live with over the long term. To identify weight-loss goals and ways to meet them, complete Lab 9.2.

Portion Sizes Overconsumption of total calories is closely tied with portion sizes. Many Americans are unaware that the portion sizes of packaged foods and of foods served at restaurants have increased in size, and most of us significantly underestimate the amount of food we eat. Limiting portion sizes to those recommended in the Food Guide Pyramid is critical for weight management. For many people, concentrating on portion sizes is also a much easier method of monitoring and managing total food intake than counting calories.

To counteract portion distortion, weigh and measure your food at home for a few days every now and then. In addition, check the serving sizes listed on packaged foods. With practice, you'll learn to judge portion sizes more accurately. Refer to Chapter 8 for more information and hints on choosing appropriate portion sizes.

Energy (Calorie) Density Experts also recommend that you pay attention to "energy density"—the number of calories per ounce or gram of weight in a food. Studies suggest that it isn't consumption of a certain amount of fat or calories in food that reduces hunger and leads to feelings of fullness and satisfaction; rather, it is consumption of a certain weight of food. Foods that are low in energy density have more volume and bulk—that is, they are relatively heavy but have few calories. For example, for the same 100 calories, you could consume 21 baby carrots or 4 pretzel twists; you are more likely to feel full after eating the serving of carrots because it weighs 10 times that of the serving of pretzels (10 ounces versus 1 ounce).

To cut back on calories and still feel full, then, you should favor foods with a low energy density. Fresh fruits and vegetables, with their high water and fiber content, are low in energy density, as are whole-grain foods. Meat, ice cream, potato chips, croissants, crackers, and low-fat cakes and cookies are examples of foods high in energy density. Strategies for lowering the energy density of your diet include the following:

- Eat fruit with breakfast and for dessert.
- Add extra vegetables to sandwiches, casseroles, stir-fry dishes, pizza, pasta dishes, and fajitas.
- Start meals with a bowl of broth-based soup; include a green salad or fruit salad.
- Snack on fresh fruits and vegetables rather than crackers, chips, or other energy-dense snack foods.
- Limit serving sizes of energy-dense foods such as butter, mayonnaise, cheese, chocolate, fatty meats, croissants, and snack foods that are fried or high in added sugars (including reduced-fat products).

Fat Calories Although some fat is needed in the diet to provide essential nutrients, you should avoid overeating fatty foods. There is some evidence that fat calories are more easily converted to body fat than calories from protein or carbohydrate. Limiting fat in the diet can also help you limit your total calories. As described in Chapter 8, most people should consume no more than 30% of their average total daily calories from fat, which translates into no more than 66 grams of fat in a 2000-calorie diet each day. Foods rich in fat include oils, margarine, butter, cream, and lard, which are almost pure fat; meat, processed foods, and fast foods, which contain a great deal of "hidden" fat; and nuts, seeds, and avocados, which are plant sources of fats.

Some people are better fat burners than others; that is, they burn more of the fat they take in as calories and therefore have less fat to store. Low fat burners convert more dietary fat to stored body fat. This tendency to hoard fat calories may be an important part of the genetic tendency toward obesity. For low fat burners, restricting fat calories to a level even below 30% may be helpful in weight control.

As Chapter 8 made clear, then, moving toward a diet strong in complex carbohydrates and fresh fruits and vegetables, and away from a reliance on meat, processed foods, and fast foods is an effective approach to reducing fat consumption. Watch out for processed foods labeled "fat-free" or "reduced-fat" because they may be high in calories (see the box "Evaluating Fat and Sugar Substitutes"). In addition, researchers have found that many Americans compensate for a lower-fat diet by consuming more calories overall.

CRITICAL CONSUMER Evaluating Fat and Sugar Substitutes

For successful weight management, some people find it helpful to limit their intake of foods high in fat and simple sugars. Foods made with fat and sugar substitutes are often promoted for weight loss. But just what are fat and sugar substitutes? And can they really contribute to weight management?

Fat Substitutes

A variety of substances are used to replace fats in processed foods and other products. Some contribute calories, protein, fiber, and/or other nutrients; others do not. Fat replacers can be classified into three general categories:

- *Carbohydrate-based fat replacers* include starch, fibers, gums, cellulose, polydextrose, and fruit purees. They are the oldest and most widely used form of fat replacer and are found in dairy and meat products, baked goods, salad dressing, and many other prepared foods. Newer types such as Oatrim, Z-trim, and Nu-trim are made from types of dietary fiber that may actually lower cholesterol levels. Carbohydrate-based fat replacers contribute 0–4 calories per gram.
- *Protein-based fat replacers* are typically made from milk, egg whites, soy, or whey; trade names include Simplesse, Dairy-lo, and Supro. They are used in cheese, sour cream, mayonnaise, margarine spreads, frozen desserts, salad dressings, and baked goods. Protein-based fat replacers typically contribute 1–4 calories per gram.
- *Fat-based fat replacers* include glycerides, olestra, and other types of fatty acids. Some of these compounds are not absorbed well by the body and so provide fewer calories per gram (5 calories compared with the standard 9 for fats); others are impossible for the body to digest and so contribute no calories at all. Olestra, marketed under the trade name Olean and used in fried snack foods, is an example of the latter type of compound. Concerns have been raised about the safety of olestra because it reduces the absorption of fat-soluble nutrients and certain antioxidants and because it causes gastrointestinal distress in some people.

Nonnutritive Sweeteners

Sugar substitutes are often referred to as nonnutritive sweeteners because they provide no calories or essential nutrients. By 2001, four types of nonnutritive sweeteners had been approved for use in the United States: acesulfame-K (Sunett, Sweet One), aspartame (NutraSweet, Equal, Natra Taste), saccharin (Sweet 'N Low), and sucralose (Splenda). They are used in beverages, desserts, baked goods, yogurt, chewing gum, and products such as toothpaste, mouthwash, and cough syrup. Other nonnutritive sweeteners currently under review include alitame, cyclamate, neotame, and stevia.

Fat and Sugar Substitutes in Weight Management

Whether fat and sugar substitutes help you achieve and maintain a healthy weight depends on your lifestyle—your overall eating and activity habits. When evaluating foods containing fat and sugar substitutes, consider these issues:

- *Is the food lower in calories or just lower in fat?* Reduced-fat foods often contain extra sugar to improve the taste and texture lost when fat is removed, so such foods may be as high or even higher in total calories than their fattier counterparts. Limiting fat intake is an important goal for weight management, but so is controlling total calories.
- *Are you choosing foods with fat and/or sugar substitutes* instead of *foods you typically eat or* in addition to *foods you typically eat?* If you consume low-fat, no-sugar-added ice cream instead of regular ice cream, you may save calories. But if you add such ice cream to your daily diet simply because it is lower in fat and sugar, your overall calorie consumption—and your weight—may increase.
- *How many foods containing fat and sugar substitutes do you consume each day?* Although the FDA has given at least provisional approval to all the fat and sugar substitutes currently available, health concerns about some of these products linger. One way to limit any potential adverse effects is to read labels and monitor how much of each product you consume. Remember that fat and sugar substitutes are found in a wide variety of products.
- *Is an even healthier choice available?* Many of the foods containing fat and sugar substitutes are low-nutrient snack foods. Although substituting a lower-fat or lower-sugar version of the same food may be beneficial, fruits, vegetables, and whole grains are healthier snack choices.

Complex Carbohydrates It has long been the fashion among dieters to cut back on bread and pasta to control weight. But complex carbohydrates from these sources, as well as from vegetables, legumes, and whole grains, are precisely the nutrients that can help you achieve and maintain a healthy body weight. They help provide a feeling of satiety, or fullness, that can keep you from overeating. Carbohydrates should make up about 55–65% of your total daily calories.

Simple Sugars and Refined Carbohydrates Foods high in added simple sugars provide calories but few nutrients. There is also some evidence that foods high in sugar and/or refined carbohydrates may trigger overeating in some people by affecting the rate of glucose absorption and the levels of hormones that influence appetite. Choose fresh fruits, whole grains, and legumes instead of foods high in added sugars and refined carbohydrates. Avoid or minimize consumption of regular (nondiet) soft drinks and fruit drinks (not juices), which are often high in simple sugars but low in other nutrients.

Protein The typical American consumes more than an adequate amount of protein. Dietary supplements with extra protein are unnecessary for most people, and protein not needed by the body for growth and tissue repair will be stored as fat. Foods high in protein are often also high in fat. Stick to the recommended protein intake of 10–15% of total daily calories.

Periodically, new diet books hit the market proclaiming a "scientific breakthrough" involving a high-protein, low-carbohydrate diet. Such diets usually cause an immediate and rather dramatic loss of body fluid, which may inaccurately be interpreted as fat loss. They typically involve significant calorie restriction, which is what actually causes any fat loss that does occur. A high-protein, low-carbohydrate diet does not conform to the Dietary Guidelines for Americans and is difficult to maintain. Most authorities recommend diets high in complex carbohydrates and moderate in protein consumption. Fad diets are discussed later in the chapter.

Eating Habits Equally important to weight management is eating small, frequent meals—three or more a day plus snacks—on a dependable, regular schedule. Skipping meals leads to excessive hunger; feelings of deprivation; and increased vulnerability to binge eating or snacking on high-calorie, high-fat, or sugary foods. A regular pattern of eating, along with some personal "decision rules" governing food choices, is a way of thinking about and then internalizing the many details that go into a healthy, low-fat diet. Decision rules governing breakfast might be these, for example: Choose a sugar-free, high-fiber cereal with nonfat milk most of the time; once in a while (no more than once a week), have a hard-boiled egg; save pancakes and waffles for special occasions.

Decreeing some foods "off-limits" generally sets up a rule to be broken. The better principle is "everything in moderation." No foods need to be entirely off-limits, though some should be eaten judiciously. Making the healthier choice more often than not is the essence of moderation.

Table 9.2 *Calorie Costs of Selected Physical Activities**

To determine how many calories you burn when you engage in a particular activity, multiply the calorie multiplier given below by your body weight (in pounds) and then by the number of minutes you exercise.

Activity	Cal/lb/ min ×	Body Weight ×	Min =	Total Calories
Cycling (13 mph)	.071	______	____	______
Digging	.062	______	____	______
Driving a car	.020	______	____	______
Housework	.029	______	____	______
Painting a house	.034	______	____	______
Shoveling snow	.052	______	____	______
Sitting quietly	.009	______	____	______
Sleeping and resting	.008	______	____	______
Standing quietly	.012	______	____	______
Typing or writing	.013	______	____	______
Walking briskly (4.5 mph)	.048	______	____	______

*See Chapter 7 for the energy costs of fitness activities.

SOURCE: Adapted from Kusinitz, I., and M. Fine. 1995. *Your Guide to Getting Fit*, 3d ed. Mountain View, Calif.: Mayfield.

Physical Activity and Exercise

Regular physical activity is another important lifestyle factor in weight management. Physical activity and exercise burn calories and keep the metabolism geared to using food for energy instead of storing it as fat.

Physical Activity The first step in becoming more active is to incorporate more physical activity into your daily life. Follow the recommendations in the Surgeon General's report by accumulating 30 minutes or more of moderate-intensity physical activity—walking, gardening, housework, and so on—on most, or preferably all, days of the week, for a total of 150 minutes or more per week. Take advantage of routine opportunities to be more active. Take the stairs instead of the elevator, walk or bike instead of driving. In the long term, even a small increase in activity level can help maintain your current weight or help you lose a moderate amount of weight (Table 9.2). In fact, research suggests that fidgeting—stretching, squirming, standing up, and so on—may help prevent weight gain in some people.

If you are overweight and want to lose weight, a greater amount of physical activity can help. Researchers have found that people who lose weight and don't regain it typically burn about 2800 calories per week in physical activity—the equivalent of about 1 hour of brisk walking per day.

Exercise Once you become more active every day, begin a formal exercise program that includes cardiorespiratory endurance exercise, resistance training, and stretching exercises. (Consult Chapter 7 for advice on creating a complete, personalized exercise program.) Moderate-intensity endurance exercise, if performed frequently for a relatively long duration, can burn a significant number of calories. Endurance training also increases the rate at which your body uses calories after your exercise session is over—burning an additional 5–180 extra calories, depending on the intensity of exercise. Resistance training builds muscle mass, and more muscle translates into a higher metabolic rate. Resistance training can also help you maintain your muscle mass during a period of weight loss, helping you avoid the significant drop in RMR associated with weight loss.

The body's fuel-use patterns vary with exercise intensity and change during recovery. During low-intensity exercise, a higher proportion of energy comes from fat (50%) than is true during high-intensity exercise (40%). However, high-intensity exercise burns more calories overall, so even though a lower proportion of those calories comes from fat, high-intensity exercise tends to burn more fat than low-intensity exercise. Intense exercise also causes the body to use more fat as fuel during the recovery period. However, high-intensity exercise is not necessarily the best strategy for controlling weight. All physical activity will help you manage your weight, and most people find that a program of moderate-intensity exercise is easier to maintain over the long term.

Regular physical activity, maintained throughout life, makes weight management easier. The sooner you establish good habits, the better. The key to success is making exercise an integral part of a lifestyle you can enjoy now and will enjoy in the future.

Thoughts and Emotions

The way you think about yourself and your world influences, and is influenced by, how you feel and how you act. In fact, research on people who have a weight problem indicates that low self-esteem and the negative emotions that accompany it are significant problems. People with low self-esteem mentally compare the actual self to an internally held picture of the "ideal self," an image based on perfectionistic goals and beliefs about how they and others should be. The more these two pictures differ, the larger the impact on self-esteem and the more likely the presence of negative emotions.

Besides the internal picture we carry of ourselves, all of us carry on a internal dialogue about events happening to us and around us. This **self-talk** can be either self-deprecating or positively motivating, depending on our beliefs and attitudes. Having realistic beliefs and goals and engaging in positive self-talk and problem solving support a healthy lifestyle. (Chapter 10 and Activity 11 in the Behavior Change Workbook at the end of the text include strategies for developing realistic self-talk.)

Coping Strategies

Adequate and appropriate coping strategies for dealing with the stresses and challenges of life are another lifestyle factor in weight management. One strategy that many people adopt for coping is eating. (Others may cope by turning to drugs, alcohol, smoking, or gambling.) Those who overeat might use food to alleviate loneliness, as a pickup for fatigue, as an antidote to boredom, or as a distraction from problems. Some people even overeat to punish themselves for real or imagined transgressions.

Those who recognize that they are using food in these ways can analyze their eating habits with fresh eyes. They can consciously attempt to find new coping strategies and begin to use food appropriately—to fuel life's activities, to foster growth, and to bring pleasure, *not* to manage stress. For a summary of the components of weight management through healthy lifestyle choices, see the box "Lifestyle Strategies for Successful Weight Management" on p. 262.

APPROACHES TO OVERCOMING A WEIGHT PROBLEM

Now you know the factors that contribute to a weight problem, and you understand the importance of diet and physical activity in successful weight management. If you are overweight, you may already be planning how to go about losing weight and keeping it off. There are many options available to you.

Doing It Yourself

Research indicates that people are far more successful than was previously thought at losing weight and keeping it off. One study found that about 64% of the subjects achieved long-term success without joining a formal program or getting special help. Supporting these findings, a U.S. Public Health Service survey indicated that nearly 50% of the general public succeed with long-term weight management.

Other researchers investigated the characteristics that distinguished those who lost at least 20% of their body weight and maintained this loss for 2 years or more. Although some had used diet alone to lose weight, some had used exercise alone, and others had used a combination of diet and exercise, virtually all maintained their success by making exercise a permanent part of their lifestyle. They also kept tabs on their weight and habits. In addition, they learned to develop their own diet, exercise, and maintenance plans, and they became more involved in and excited by activities other than eating—such as careers, projects, and special interests. Long-term success depends on maintaining the lifestyle changes that helped you lose the weight in the first place.

If you need to lose weight, focus on adopting the healthy lifestyle described throughout this book. The "right" weight for you will naturally evolve, and you won't

self-talk A person's internal comments and discussion; instrumental in shaping self-image.

Terms

Ww

Food Choices

- Follow the recommendations in the Food Guide Pyramid for eating a moderate, varied diet.
- Pay attention to the energy density and nutrient density of your food choices. Favor foods with a low energy density and a high nutrient density.
- Check food labels for serving sizes, calories, and nutrient levels.
- Watch for hidden calories. Reduced-fat foods often have as many calories as their full-fat versions. Fat-based condiments like butter, margarine, mayonnaise, and salad dressings provide about 100 calories per tablespoon; added sugars such as jams, jellies, and syrup are also packed with calories.
- Drink fewer calories. Many Americans consume high-calorie beverages such as soda, fruit drinks, sports drinks, alcohol, and specialty coffees and teas. (People who get extra calories from solid food tend to compensate by eating less later; those whose extra calories come in liquid form don't compensate and consume more calories overall.)
- For problem foods, try eating small amounts under controlled conditions. Go out for a scoop of ice cream, for example, rather than buying half a gallon for your freezer.

Planning and Serving

- Keep a log of what you eat. Before you begin your program, your log will provide a realistic picture of your current diet and what changes you can make. Once you start your program, a log will keep you focused on your food choices and portion sizes. Consider tracking the following:
  food eaten
  hunger level
  circumstances (location, other activities)
  outside influences (environment, other people)
  thoughts and emotions
- Eat three meals a day, including breakfast. Replace impulse snacking with planned, healthy snacks. Keep low-calorie snacks on hand to combat the "munchies": baby carrots, popcorn, and fresh fruits and vegetables are good choices.
- When shopping for food, make a list and stick to it. Don't shop when you're hungry. Avoid aisles that contain problem foods.
- In a cafeteria, examine all the possible food choices before you begin making selections. This will help you avoid overloading your plate. Don't take dessert during your first trip through the line: What seems like an appropriate choice and portion size for dessert may look very different *after* you've eaten a meal.
- Pay special attention to portion sizes. Use measuring cups and spoons and a food scale to become more familiar with appropriate portion sizes.
- Serve meals on small plates and in small bowls to help you eat smaller portions without feeling deprived.
- Eat only in specifically designated spots. Remove food from other areas of your house or apartment.
- When you eat, just eat—don't do anything else, such as read or watch TV.
- Eat more slowly. It takes time for your brain to get the message that your stomach is full. Take small bites and chew food thoroughly. Pay attention to every bite, and enjoy your food. Between bites, try putting your fork or spoon down and taking sips of water or another beverage.
- When you're done eating, remove your plate. Cue yourself that the meal is over—drink a glass of water, suck on a mint, chew gum, or brush your teeth.

Special Occasions

- When you eat out, choose a restaurant where you can make healthy food choices. Ask the server not to put bread and butter on the table before the meal and request that sauces and salad dressings be served on the side. If portion sizes are large, take half your food home for a meal later in the week.
- If you cook a large meal for friends, send leftovers home with your guests.
- If you're eating at a friend's, eat a little and leave the rest. Don't eat to be polite; if someone offers you food you don't want, thank the person and decline firmly: "No thank you, I've had enough" or "It's delicious, but I'm full."
- Take care during the winter holidays. Research indicates that people gain less than they think during the winter holidays (about a pound) but that the weight isn't lost during the rest of the year, leading to slow, steady weight gain.

Physical Activity and Stress Management

- Increase your level of daily physical activity. If you have been sedentary for a long time or are seriously overweight, increase your level of activity slowly. Start by walking 10 minutes at a time, and work toward 30 minutes or more of moderate physical activity per day.
- Begin a formal exercise program that includes cardiorespiratory endurance exercise, strength training, and stretching.
- Develop techniques for handling stress—go for a walk or use a relaxation technique. Practice positive self-talk. See Chapter 10 for more on stress management.
- Develop strategies for coping with nonhunger cues to eat, such as boredom, sleepiness, or anxiety. Try calling a friend, taking a shower, or reading a magazine.
- Tell family members and friends that you're making some changes in your eating and exercise habits. Ask them to be supportive.

have to diet. However, if you must diet, do so in combination with exercise and avoid very-low-calorie diets. Don't try to lose more than 0.5–2 pounds per week. Realize that most low-calorie diets cause a rapid loss of body water at first. When this phase passes, weight loss declines. As a result, dieters are often misled into believing that their efforts are not working. They give up, not realizing that smaller losses later in the diet are actually better than the initial big losses, because later loss is mostly fat loss, whereas initial loss was primarily fluid.

For more tips on losing weight on your own, refer to the section later in the chapter on creating an individual weight-management plan.

Diet Books

Many people who try to lose weight by themselves fall prey to one or more of the dozens of diet books on the market. Although a very few of these do contain useful advice and tips for motivation, most make empty promises. Here are some guidelines for evaluating and choosing a diet book:

1. Reject books that advocate an unbalanced way of eating, such as a high-carbohydrate-only diet or low-carbohydrate, high-protein diets. Also reject books promoting a single food, such as cabbage or grapefruit.
2. Reject books that claim to be based on a "scientific breakthrough" or to have the "secret" to success.
3. Reject books that use gimmicks, like matching eating to blood type, hyping insulin resistance as the single cause of obesity, combining foods in special ways to achieve weight loss, rotating levels of calories, or purporting that a weight problem is due to food allergies, food sensitivities, yeast infections, or hormone imbalances.
4. Reject books that promise quick weight loss or that limit the selection of foods.
5. Accept books that advocate a balanced approach to diet plus exercise and sound nutrition advice.

A recent crop of popular books has promoted diets high in protein, low in carbohydrate, and relatively high in fat. Weight loss on low-carbohydrate diets comes mainly from loss of water and protein, not fat, and weight is usually quickly regained when dieting ends. Low-carbohydrate diets may be high in unhealthy saturated fats, and they often limit or eliminate foods such as grains, fruits, and vegetables that are rich in nutrients and fiber. The American College of Sports Medicine, the American Dietetic Association, the Cooper Institute for Aerobics Research, and the Women's Sports Foundation released a joint statement saying that such diets are not a good weight-loss strategy, will not improve athletic performance, and can be harmful in some cases. The only reason such plans help some people lose weight is that the diets they advocate provide so few calories; but they are difficult to maintain over any period of time, and they do not focus on basic strategies such as portion control or a healthy balance among food groups. (See the January 1999 issue of *Environmental Nutrition* and the May 2000 issue of *Nutrition Action Healthletter* for reviews of many top-selling diet books; For Further Exploration at the end of the chapter lists additional resources.)

Dietary Supplements and Diet Aids

The number of dietary supplements and other weight loss aids on the market has also increased in recent years. Promoted in advertisements, magazines, direct mail campaigns, infomercials, and Web sites, these products typically promise a quick and easy path to weight loss. Most of these products are marketed as dietary supplements and so are subject to fewer regulations than over-the-counter medications. If you are considering one of these products, use your critical thinking skills and the information in the box "Over-the-Counter Diet Pills and Diet Aids" (p. 264).

Ww Weight-Loss Programs

Weight-loss programs come in a variety of types, including noncommercial support organizations, commercial programs, Web sites, and medically supervised clinical programs.

Noncommercial Weight-Loss Programs Noncommercial programs such as TOPS (Take Off Pounds Sensibly) and Overeaters Anonymous (OA) mainly provide group support. They do not advocate any particular diet, but they do recommend seeking professional advice for creating an individualized diet and exercise plan. Like Alcoholics Anonymous, OA is a 12-step program with a spiritual orientation that promotes "abstinence" from compulsive overeating. These types of programs are generally free. Your physician or a registered dietitian can also provide information and support for weight loss.

Commercial Weight-Loss Programs Commercial programs such as Weight Watchers, Jenny Craig, Diet Workshop, and Richard Simmons Slimmons typically provide group support, nutrition education, physical activity recommendations, and behavior modification advice. Some also make available packaged foods to assist in following dietary advice. Many commercial programs voluntarily belong to the Partnership for Healthy Weight Management established by the Federal Trade Commission in 1999. By doing so, they agree to provide clients with information on staff training and education, the risks associated with overweight and obesity, the risks associated with each program or product, the costs of the program, and the expected outcomes of the program, including rates of success. A responsible and safe weight-loss program should have the following features:

1. The recommended diet should be safe and balanced, include all the food groups, and meet the DRIs for all nutrients. Physical activity and exercise should be strongly encouraged.

Over-the-Counter Diet Pills and Diet Aids

Many over-the-counter (OTC) products are promoted for appetite control and fat loss, but few have evidence supporting their effectiveness. Testimonials and anecdotes are not good substitutes for scientific research findings. With herbs and other products marketed as dietary supplements, safety and cost are also a concern. In addition, use of OTC products doesn't help in the adoption of lifestyle behaviors that can help people achieve and maintain a healthy weight over the long term.

Formula Drinks and Food Bars

Canned diet drinks, powders used to make shakes, and diet food bars and snacks are designed to achieve weight loss by substituting for some or all of a person's daily food intake. However, most people find it difficult to use these products for long periods as a substitute for more satisfying "real" food, and serious health problems may result if they are used as the sole source of nutrition for extended periods of time. Use of such products can result in rapid weight loss for those who can stick with them, but such weight loss is accompanied by loss of muscle mass, and the weight is typically regained because users have not learned to change the eating and lifestyle behaviors that caused the weight problem in the first place.

Herbs and Herbal Products

Although many people believe that because herbs are "natural" they are safe, it is important to remember that herbs contain biologically active compounds that can be dangerous, especially if taken in large doses. As described in Chapter 8, herbs are marketed as dietary supplements, so there is little information about effectiveness, proper dosage, drug interactions, and side effects. In addition, labels may not accurately reflect the ingredients and dosages present, and safe manufacturing practices are not guaranteed. For example, the substitution of a toxic herb for another compound during the manufacture of a Chinese herbal weight-loss preparation caused more than 100 cases of kidney damage and cancer among users in Europe.

Ephedra, also known as ma huang or desert herb, is a popular herb found in weight-loss aids. Its active ingredient, ephedrine, is structurally similar to amphetamine. As a stimulant, ephedra may suppress appetite and increase body temperature and basal metabolic rate, causing calories to be burned at a faster rate. However, few studies have been done to identify safe and effective uses of ephedra, and long-term use is not recommended. In addition, many products containing ephedra also contain other stimulants—caffeine or herbal products that contain caffeine such as guarana seeds or kola nuts. There have been many reports of adverse effects from use of ephedra, including elevated blood pressure, panic attacks, seizures, insomnia, headache, and nausea; it may also increase the risk of heart attack or stroke in some people, particularly if combined with another stimulant. The FDA is considering new regulations for ephedra, including dosage guidelines and warnings.

Herbal "dieter's teas" often contain a variety of strong botanical laxatives and diuretics such as senna, aloe, buckthorn, rhubarb root, cascara, and castor oil. These stimulate the colon and, if used in excess, can cause extreme diarrhea, nausea, vomiting, dehydration, fainting, and electrolyte imbalances that can lead to heart rhythm problems. If used regularly, the colon may become dependent on the laxative effect, resulting in chronic constipation. Any weight loss that occurs is due to fluid loss, not fat loss.

Other Dietary Supplements and Diet Aids

Supplements containing specific amino acids and proteins are also marketed for weight loss. Promoters claim that amino acids may ward off cravings and the impulse to binge-eat by affecting levels of neurotransmitters such as dopamine or hormones such as cholecystokinin (CCK) that are involved in appetite. However, there is little research to support these claims. In addition, even if such products do affect appetite, they may not be very helpful in weight management. Hunger is often not the reason that people consume high-calorie foods or overeat. The use of so-called "fat burners" or "fat inhibitors" such as carnitine, hydroxycitrate, chromium, or pyruvate is also not currently supported by research findings.

Fiber is another common ingredient in OTC diet aids. Manufacturers claim that fiber can swell in the stomach and control appetite by making people feel full. However, dietary fiber acts as a bulking agent in the large intestine, not in the stomach. The FDA has found no data to warrant classifying any type of fiber as an aid in weight control. In addition, most diet aids contain a mere 1–3 grams of fiber, which do not contribute much toward the recommended daily intake of 20–35 grams.

Until 2000, the synthetic compound phenylpropanolamine (PPA) was a common ingredient in OTC diet pills. Like ephedra, PPA acts as a mild stimulant and appetite suppressant. Although originally approved for short-term use, reports of increased risk for stroke led the FDA in 2000 to ask manufacturers to stop marketing products containing PPA.

The bottom line on nonprescription diet aids is *caveat emptor*—let the buyer beware. There is no quick and easy way to lose weight. The most effective approach is to develop healthy diet and exercise habits and make them a permanent part of your lifestyle.

2. The program should promote slow, steady weight loss averaging ½–2 pounds per week. (There may be rapid weight loss initially due to fluid loss.)
3. If a participant plans to lose more than 20 pounds, has any health problems, or is taking medication on a regular basis, physician evaluation and monitoring should be recommended. The staff of the program should include qualified counselors and health professionals.
4. The program should include plans for weight maintenance after the weight-loss phase is over.
5. The program should provide information on all fees and costs, including those of supplements and prepackaged

foods, as well as data on risks and expected outcomes of participating in the program.

In addition, you should consider whether a program fits your lifestyle and whether you are truly ready to make a commitment to it. A strong commitment and a plan for maintenance are especially important because studies indicate that only 10–15% of program participants maintain their weight loss—the rest gain back all or more than they had lost. One study of participants found that regular exercise was the best predictor of maintaining weight loss, whereas frequent television viewing was the best predictor of weight gain. This reinforces the idea that successful weight management requires long-term life-style changes.

Online Weight-Loss Programs A recent addition to the weight-loss program scene is the Internet-based program. Most such Web sites include a cross between self-help and group support through chat rooms, bulletin boards, and e-newsletters. Many sites offer online self-assessment for diet and physical activity habits as well as a meal plan; some provide access to a staff professional for individualized help. Many are free but some charge a small weekly or monthly fee. Preliminary research suggests that this type of program provides an alternative to in-person diet counseling and can lead to weight loss for some people. The criteria used to evaluate commercial programs can also be applied to Internet-based programs. In addition, check whether a program offers member-to-member support and access to staff professionals.

Clinical Weight-Loss Programs Medically supervised clinical programs are usually located in a hospital or other medical setting. Designed to help those who are severely obese, these programs typically involve a closely monitored very-low-calorie diet. The cost of a clinical program is usually high, but insurance often covers part of the fee.

Prescription Drugs

The medications most often prescribed for weight loss are appetite suppressants that reduce feelings of hunger or increase feelings of fullness. Appetite suppressants usually work by increasing levels of catecholamine or serotonin, two brain chemicals that affect mood and appetite. All prescription weight-loss drugs have potential side effects. Those that affect catecholamine levels, including phentermine (Ionamin), diethylpropion (Tenuate), and mazindol (Sanorex), may cause sleeplessness, nervousness, and euphoria. Sibutramine (Meridia) acts on both the serotonin and catecholamine systems; it may trigger increases in blood pressure and heart rate.

A newer medication for obesity is orlistat (Xenical), which lowers calorie consumption by blocking fat absorption in the intestines; it prevents about 30% of the fat in food from being digested. Similar to the fat substitute olestra, orlistat reduces the absorption of fat-soluble vitamins and antioxidants. Side effects include diarrhea, cramping, and other gastrointestinal problems if users do not follow a low-fat diet.

Studies have generally found that appetite suppressants produce modest weight loss—about 5–22 pounds above the loss expected with nondrug obesity treatments. Unfortunately, weight loss tends to level off or reverse after 4 to 6 months on a medication, and many people regain the weight they've lost if they stop taking the drugs. Because most weight-loss medications are approved for only short-term use, regaining weight is a serious problem.

Side effects and risks are other concerns. In 1997, the FDA removed from the market two prescription weight-loss drugs, fenfluramine (Pondimin) and dexfenfluramine (Redux), after their use was linked to potentially life-threatening heart valve problems. (Fenfluramine was used most often in combination with phentermine, an off-label combination referred to as "fen/phen.") It appears that people who took these drugs over a long period or at high dosages are at greatest risk for problems, but the FDA recommends that anyone who has taken either of these drugs be examined by a physician.

Prescription weight-loss drugs are not for people who want to lose a few pounds to wear a smaller size of jeans. The latest federal guidelines advise people to try lifestyle modification for at least 6 months before trying drug therapy. Prescription drugs are recommended—in conjunction with lifestyle changes—only in certain cases: for people who have been unable to lose weight with non-drug options and who have a BMI over 30 (or over 27 if two or more additional risk factors such as diabetes and high blood pressure are present).

Surgery

About 3% of Americans are severely obese, meaning they have a BMI of 40 or higher or are 100 pounds or more over recommended weight. Surgical intervention may be necessary as a treatment of last resort for those who have not been successful in permanently reducing weight through other methods. For surgery to treat extreme obesity, an expert panel from the National Institutes of Health has recommended a procedure called the *Roux-en-Y gastric bypass,* in which the stomach is divided in two with staples to form a small (1-ounce) stomach pouch. Gastric bypass works primarily by restricting the amount of food that can be consumed at any one time, and it requires permanent lifestyle changes.

Psychological Help

Many people can lose weight just by increasing their physical activity level and moderately restricting total calories, especially fat calories. When concern about body weight and shape have developed into an eating disorder, the help of a professional is recommended. A therapist should have experience working with weight management, body image issues, eating disorders, addictions, and abuse issues. Your physician may be able to provide a referral.

BODY IMAGE

The collective picture of the body as seen through the mind's eye, **body image** consists of perceptions, images, thoughts, attitudes, and emotions. A negative body image is characterized by dissatisfaction with the body in general or some part of the body in particular. Recent surveys indicate that the majority of Americans, many of whom are not actually overweight, are unhappy with their body weight or with some aspect of their appearance. Developing a positive body image is an important aspect of psychological wellness.

Severe Body Image Problems

Poor body image can cause significant psychological distress. A person can become preoccupied by a perceived defect in appearance, thereby damaging self-esteem and interfering with relationships. Adolescents and adults who have a negative body image are more likely to diet restrictively, eat compulsively, or develop some other form of disordered eating.

When dissatisfaction becomes extreme, the condition is called body dysmorphic disorder (BDD). BDD can begin in adolescence or adulthood, with complaints often focusing on slight "flaws" of the face or head—things that are not obvious to others. Individuals with BDD may spend hours every day thinking about their defect and looking at themselves in mirrors; they may desire and seek repeated cosmetic surgeries. BDD is related to obsessive-compulsive disorder and can lead to depression, social phobia, and suicide if left untreated. Medication and psychotherapy can help people with BDD.

In some cases, body image may bear little resemblance to fact. A person suffering from the eating disorder anorexia nervosa typically has a severely distorted body image—she believes herself to be fat even when she has become emaciated (see the next section for more on anorexia). Distorted body image is also a hallmark of muscle dysmorphia, a disorder experienced by some body builders in which they see themselves as small and out of shape despite being very muscular. Those who suffer from muscle dysmorphia may let obsessive bodybuilding interfere with their work and relationships.

Terms

body image The mental representation a person holds about her or his body at any given moment in time, consisting of perceptions, images, thoughts, attitudes, and emotions about the body.

The image of the "ideal" female body promoted by the fashion and fitness industries doesn't reflect the wide range of body shapes and sizes that are associated with good health. An overconcern with body image can contribute to low self-esteem and the development of eating disorders.

To assess your own body image, complete the body image self-test in Lab 9.3.

Acceptance and Change

Most Americans, young and old, are unhappy with some aspect of their appearance and often their weight. The "can-do" attitude of Americans, together with the belief that there is a solution to this dissatisfaction, leads to even more problems with body image, as well as to dieting, disordered eating, and the desire for cosmetic surgery to "fix" perceived defects.

In fact, there are limits to the changes that can be made to body weight and body shape, both of which are influenced by heredity. The changes that can and should be made are lifestyle changes—engaging in regular physical activity, obtaining adequate nutrition, and maintaining healthy eating habits. With these changes, the body weight

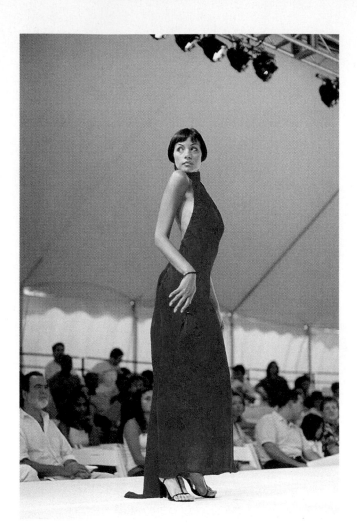

DIMENSIONS OF DIVERSITY Gender, Ethnicity, and Body Image

Body Image and Gender

Women are much more likely than men to be dissatisfied with their bodies, often wanting to be thinner than they are. In one study, only 30% of eighth-grade girls reported being content with their bodies, while 70% of their male classmates expressed satisfaction with their looks. Girls and women are much more likely than boys and men to diet, develop eating disorders, and be obese.

One reason that girls and women are dissatisfied with their bodies is that they are influenced by the media—particularly advertisements and women's fashion magazines. Most teen girls report that the media influence their idea of the perfect body and their decision to diet. In a study of adult women, viewing pictures of thin models in magazines had an immediate negative effect on their mood. Clearly, media images affect women's self-image and self-esteem. For American women of all ages, success is still too often equated with how we look rather than who we are.

It is important to note that the image of the "perfect" woman presented in the media is often unrealistic and even unhealthy. In a review of BMI data for Miss America pageant winners since 1922, researchers noted a significant decline in BMI over time, with an increasing number of recent winners having BMIs in the "underweight" category. The average fashion model is 4–7 inches taller and 20 pounds lighter than the average American woman.

Our culture may be promoting an unattainable masculine ideal as well. Researchers studying male action figures such as GI Joe from the past 40 years noted that they have become increasingly muscular. A recent Batman action figure, if projected onto a man of average height, would result in someone with a 30-inch waist, 57-inch chest, and 27-inch biceps. Such media messages can be demoralizing; and although not as commonly, boys and men also suffer from body image problems.

Body Image and Ethnicity

The thin, toned look as a feminine ideal is just a fashion, one that is not shared by all cultures. Although some groups espouse thinness as an "ideal" body type, others do not. In many traditional African societies, for example, full-figured women's bodies are seen as symbols of health, prosperity, and fertility. African American teenage girls have a much more positive body image than white girls; in one survey, two-thirds of them defined beauty as "the right attitude," whereas white girls were more preoccupied with weight and body shape. Nevertheless, recent evidence indicates that African American women are as likely to engage in disordered eating behavior, especially binge eating and vomiting, as their Latina, Native American, and white counterparts. This finding underscores the complex nature of eating disorders and body image.

Avoiding Body Image Problems

To minimize your risk of developing a body image problem, keep the following strategies in mind:

- Focus on healthy habits and good physical health. Eat a moderate, balanced diet and choose physical activities you enjoy. Avoid chronic or repetitive dieting.
- Focus on good psychological health and put concerns about physical appearance in perspective. Your worth as a human being does not depend on how you look.
- Practice body acceptance. You can influence your body size and type through lifestyle to some degree, but the basic fact is that some people are genetically designed to be bigger or heavier than others. Focus on healthy lifestyle behaviors and accept your body as it is.
- Find things to appreciate in yourself besides an idealized body image. Men and women whose self-esteem is based primarily on standards of physical attractiveness can find it difficult to age gracefully. Those who can learn to value other aspects of themselves are more accepting of the physical changes that occur naturally with age.
- View eating as a morally neutral activity. Don't make food choices a moral issue—eating dessert isn't "bad" and doesn't make you a bad person. Adopting healthy eating habits is an important part of a wellness lifestyle, but the things you really care about and do are more important in defining who you are.
- Don't judge yourself or others based on appearance. Watch your attitudes toward people of differing body sizes and shapes, and don't joke about someone's body type. Take people seriously for what they say and do, not for their appearance. Body size is just one external characteristic; there are millions of happy and successful people who just also happen to have a weight problem.
- See the beauty and fitness industries for what they are. Realize that one of their goals is to prompt dissatisfaction with yourself so that you will buy their products.

and shape that develop will be natural and appropriate for an individual's particular genetic makeup.

Knowing when the limits to healthy change have been reached—and learning to accept those limits—is crucial for overall wellness. Women in particular tend to measure self-worth in terms of their appearance; when they don't measure up to an unrealistic cultural ideal, they see themselves as defective and their self-esteem falls. The result can be negative body image, disordered eating, or even a full-blown eating disorder (see the box "Gender, Ethnicity, and Body Image").

Obesity is a serious health risk, but weight management needs to take place in a positive and realistic atmosphere. For an obese person, losing as few as 10 pounds can reduce blood pressure and improve mood. The hazards of excessive dieting and overconcern about body weight need to be countered by a change in attitude about what constitutes the perfect body and a reasonable body weight. A reasonable weight must take into account a person's weight history, social circumstances, metabolic profile, and psychological well-being.

EATING DISORDERS

Problems with body weight and weight control are not limited to excessive body fat. A growing number of people, especially adolescent girls and young women, experience **eating disorders,** characterized by severe disturbances in eating patterns and eating-related behavior. The major eating disorders are anorexia nervosa, bulimia nervosa, and binge-eating disorder. More than 8 million Americans, most of them women, suffer from eating disorders. Many more people have abnormal eating habits and attitudes about food that, although not meeting the criteria for a full-blown eating disorder, do disrupt their lives (see the box "Borderline Disordered Eating"). To assess your eating habits, complete the eating disorder checklist in Lab 9.3.

Although many different explanations for the development of eating disorders have been proposed, they share one central feature: a dissatisfaction with body image and body weight. Such dissatisfaction is created by distorted thinking, including perfectionistic beliefs, unreasonable demands for self-control, and excessive self-criticism. Dissatisfaction with body weight leads to dysfunctional attitudes about eating, such as fear of fat, preoccupation with food, and problematic eating behaviors.

Anorexia Nervosa

A person suffering from **anorexia nervosa** does not eat enough food to maintain a reasonable body weight. Anorexia affects 1–3 million Americans, 95% of them female. Although it can occur later, anorexia typically develops between the ages of 12 and 18. People suffering from anorexia have an intense fear of gaining weight or becoming fat. Their body image is distorted so that even when emaciated, they think they are fat. People with anorexia may engage in compulsive behaviors or rituals that help keep them from eating; they also commonly use vigorous and prolonged physical activity to reduce body weight. Although they may express a great interest in food, their own diet becomes more and more extreme. Anorexic people are typically introverted, emotionally reserved, and socially insecure. Their entire sense of self-esteem may be tied up in their evaluation of their body shape and weight.

Anorexia nervosa has been linked to a variety of medical complications, including disorders of the cardiovascular, gastrointestinal, and endocrine systems. Because of extreme weight loss, females with anorexia often stop menstruating. When body fat is virtually gone and muscles are severely wasted, the body turns to its own organs in a desperate search for protein. Death can occur from heart failure caused by electrolyte imbalances. Depression and suicide are also serious risks. As many as 16% of people with anorexia die of disease-related complications.

Bulimia Nervosa

A person suffering from **bulimia nervosa** engages in recurrent episodes of binge eating followed by **purging.** Although bulimia usually begins in adolescence or young adulthood, it has recently begun to emerge at increasingly younger (11–12 years) and older (40–60 years) ages. During a binge, a bulimic person may consume anywhere from 1000 to 60,000 calories within a few hours. This is followed by an attempt to get rid of the food by purging, usually by vomiting or using laxatives or diuretics. During a binge, people with bulimia feel as though they have lost control and cannot stop or limit how much they eat. Some binge and purge only occasionally; others do so many times every day. Binges may be triggered by a major life change or other stressful event. Binge eating and purging may become a way of dealing with difficult feelings such as anger and disappointment.

The binge-purge cycle of bulimia places a tremendous strain on the body and can have serious health effects, including tooth decay, esophageal damage and chronic hoarseness, menstrual irregularities, depression, liver and kidney damage, and cardiac arrhythmia. Bulimia is often difficult to recognize because sufferers conceal their eating habits and usually maintain a normal weight, although they may experience fluctuations of 10–15 pounds. About 1–3% of Americans suffer from bulimia.

Binge-Eating Disorder

Binge-eating disorder is characterized by uncontrollable eating without any compensatory purging behaviors. Common eating patterns are eating more rapidly than normal, eating until uncomfortably full, eating when not hungry, and preferring to eat alone. Uncontrolled eating is usually

Terms

eating disorder A serious disturbance in eating patterns or eating-related behavior, characterized by a negative body image and concerns about body weight or body fat.

anorexia nervosa An eating disorder characterized by a refusal to maintain body weight at a minimally healthy level and an intense fear of gaining weight or becoming fat; self-starvation.

bulimia nervosa An eating disorder characterized by recurrent episodes of binge eating and purging: overeating and then using compensatory behaviors such as vomiting and excessive exercise to prevent weight gain.

purging The use of vomiting, laxatives, excessive exercise, restrictive dieting, enemas, diuretics, or diet pills to compensate for food that has been eaten and that the person fears will produce weight gain.

binge-eating disorder An eating disorder characterized by binge eating and a lack of control over eating behavior in general.

WELLNESS CONNECTION Borderline Disordered Eating

For every person diagnosed with a full-blown eating disorder, there are many more who don't meet all the criteria but who have eating problems that significantly disrupt their lives. People with borderline disordered eating have some symptoms of eating disorders but do not meet the full diagnostic criteria for anorexia, bulimia, or binge-eating disorder. Behaviors such as excessive dieting, occasional bingeing or purging, or the inability to control eating turn food into the enemy and create havoc in the lives of millions of American children and adults.

Eating habits and body image run a continuum from healthy to seriously disordered. Where we fall along that continuum can change depending on life stresses, illnesses, and many other factors. Meaningful statistics about borderline disordered eating are hard to come by, in part because it is difficult to define exactly when eating habits cross the line between normal and disordered. However, many experts feel that the majority of Americans, particularly women, have at least some unhealthy attitudes and behaviors in relation to food and self-image. About 80% of American women are dissatisfied with their appearance, and concerns about weight and dieting are so common as to be considered culturally "normal" for the majority of Americans.

Ideally, our relationship to food should be a happy one. The biological urge to satisfy hunger is one of our most basic drives, and eating is associated with many pleasurable sensations. For some of us, food triggers pleasant memories of good times, family, holidays, and fun. But for too many people, food is a source of anguish rather than pleasure. Eating results in feelings of guilt and self-loathing rather than satisfaction. Borderline eating problems may not be as immediately life threatening as full-blown eating disorders, but they cause tremendous disruption in the lives of the affected individuals. And experts estimate that as many as one-quarter of people with borderline disordered eating will eventually develop a full eating disorder.

How do you know if you have disordered eating habits? When thoughts about weight and food dominate your life, you have a problem. If you're convinced that your worth as a person hinges on how you look and how much you weigh, it's time to get help. We've all overeaten at a delicious holiday meal, but if you habitually eat until your stomach hurts, and if you feel guilty after a meal or a snack, you may have borderline disordered eating. Self-induced vomiting or laxative use after meals, even if only once in a while, is reason for concern. Do you feel compelled to overexercise to compensate for what you've eaten? Do you routinely restrict your food intake and sometimes eat nothing in an effort to feel more in control? These are all danger signs and could mean that you are developing a serious problem.

What can you do if you suspect you have an eating problem? Don't try to go it alone. Eating problems tend to become worse when you cloak them in secrecy. Check with your student health or counseling center—nearly all colleges have counselors and medical personnel who can help you or refer you to a specialist if needed. If you are initially intimidated about asking for help, an easy first step is to learn more about eating problems online by visiting a reliable Web site; several good resources are listed in the For Further Exploration section at the end of the chapter. These Web sites include information on disordered eating, local counseling resources, and online support groups. Don't hesitate to get help, even if you think your problem is "not that bad." Problem eating is about more than just food. It can be a serious threat to your health and happiness—and even your life.

followed by weight gain and feelings of guilt, shame, and depression. Many people with binge-eating, disorder mistakenly see rigid dieting as the only solution to their problem. However, rigid dieting usually causes feelings of deprivation and a return to overeating. Compulsive overeaters rarely eat because of hunger. Instead, they use food to cope with stress, conflict, and other difficult emotions or to provide solace or entertainment. Binge eaters are almost always obese, so they face all the health risks associated with obesity. In addition, binge eaters may have higher-than-average rates of depression and anxiety. Binge-eating disorder may affect 2–5% of all adults and 8% of those who are obese.

Treating Eating Disorders

The treatment of eating disorders must address both problematic eating behaviors and the misuse of food to manage stress and emotions. Treatment for anorexia nervosa first involves averting a medical crisis by restoring adequate body weight; then the psychological aspects of the disorder can be addressed. The treatment of bulimia nervosa or binge-eating disorder involves first stabilizing the eating patterns, then identifying and changing the patterns of thinking that lead to disordered eating. Treatment usually involves a combination of psychotherapy, medication, and medical management. Researchers have found that antidepressants such as Prozac are effective for some people with bulimia nervosa or body dysmorphic disorder. Friends and family members often want to know what they can do to help someone with an eating disorder. For suggestions, see the box "If Someone You Know Has an Eating Disorder . . ." (p. 270).

People with milder patterns of disordered eating may benefit from getting a nutrition checkup with a registered dietitian. A professional can help determine appropriate body weight and calorie intake and offer advice on how to budget calories into a balanced, healthy diet.

Eating disorders can be seen as the logical extension of the concern with weight that pervades American society. The challenge is to achieve a healthy body weight through sensible eating habits and an active lifestyle.

TAKE CHARGE If Someone You Know Has an Eating Disorder . . .

Secrecy and denial are two hallmarks of eating disorders, making these conditions potentially difficult to identify and treat. Signs that a friend may suffer from an eating disorder include sudden weight loss, extreme weight fluctuations, excessive dieting or exercise, excessive eating without weight gain, claiming to feel fat while at a normal weight, guilt or preoccupation with food and eating, frequent weighing, wearing of baggy and/or layered clothing, avoidance of food-related social events, evidence of binge eating (hoarding food, food wrappers), evidence of self-induced vomiting (bathroom visits following a meal, sores or calluses on the back of the hand), and use of laxatives, diuretics, or diet pills to control weight. Approaching a friend with your concerns can be difficult, but the following strategies may help.

- Educate yourself about eating disorders and their risks and about treatment resources in your community. (See For Further Exploration at the end of this chapter for suggestions.) Consider consulting a professional about the best way to approach the situation. Obtain information about how and where your friend can get help.
- Realize that your friend may not admit to having a problem or needing help. You may see your friend's disordered eating as unhealthy, but for your friend, disordered eating habits may be an important coping mechanism for problems in her or his life.
- Arrange to speak privately with the person. Plan ahead so that you have enough time to talk in a place where you won't be interrupted.
- Express your caring for your friend. Offer specific incidents or observations about your friend's psychological state and behavior. For example, "I'm worried about you because you seem anxious and unhappy. I've noticed that you've been skipping meals and that you often talk about feeling fat."
- Even if your friend becomes angry or denies there is a problem, remain calm and nonjudgmental and continue to express your concern. Give your friend information about where she or he can get help; offer to go along. Tell your friend that you believe she or he needs and deserves help.
- After you raise your concerns, give your friend time to think and respond. Listen to your friend and express your support and understanding. Emphasize your friend's good characteristics, successes, and strengths. Help maintain the person's sense of personal responsibility and decision making.
- Avoid giving simplistic advice about eating habits and making comments about how someone looks. Many people with eating disorders are very sensitive to comments about appearance and do not want to discuss the details of their disorder with friends.
- If an emergency situation arises—if the person has fainted or attempted suicide, for example—take immediate action. Call 911 for help.

If a friend is in treatment for an eating disorder, be patient and realistic. Recovery is a long process. If you feel very upset about the situation, seek professional help for yourself. Remember that you are not to blame for another person's eating disorder.

CREATING AN INDIVIDUAL WEIGHT-MANAGEMENT PLAN

Would you like to lose weight on your own? Here are some strategies for creating a program of weight management that will last a lifetime.

Assess Your Motivation and Commitment

Before embarking on your chosen weight-management program, it's important that you take a fresh look within and assess your motivation and commitment. The point is not only to achieve success but also to guard against frustration, negative changes in self-esteem, and the sense of failure that attends broken resolves or "yo-yo dieting." Think about the reasons you want to lose weight. Self-focused reasons, such as to feel good about yourself or to have a greater sense of well-being, can often lead to success. Trying to lose weight for others or out of concern for how others view you is a poor foundation for a weight-management program. Make a list of your reasons for wanting to manage your weight and post it in a prominent place.

Set Reasonable Goals

Choose a goal weight or body fat percentage that is both healthy and reasonable. The 2000 Dietary Guidelines for Americans recommend that people who are overweight aim to lose about 10% of their weight over about 6 months. Refer to the calculations you completed in Lab 6.2 to arrive at a goal. Subdivide your long-term goal into a series of short-term goals. Be willing to renegotiate your final goal as your program moves along.

Assess Your Current Energy Balance

Your energy balance is the balance between calories consumed and calories used in physical activity. When your weight is constant, you are burning approximately the same number of calories you are taking in. To tip your energy balance toward weight loss, you must either consume fewer calories or burn more through physical activity. To lose the recommended ½–2 pounds a week, you'll need to create a negative energy balance of between 1750 and 7000 calories a week, or 250–1000 calories a day. (No diet should reduce calorie intake below 1500 a day for men or 1200 a day for women.) Complete Labs 9.1 and 9.2 to assess your current daily expenditure and to develop strategies for achieving a negative energy balance that will lead to gradual, moderate weight loss. (See pp. 272–273 for guidelines for altering your energy balance to *gain* weight.)

Increase Your Level of Physical Activity

To generate a negative energy balance, it's usually best to exercise more rather than eat less. One reason is that dieting reduces RMR, whereas exercise raises it. Furthermore, studies have shown that being physically fit is even more important than weight loss in reducing your mortality risk (see Chapter 6). The key is keeping fit with moderate exercise.

Table 9.2 lists the calorie costs of selected physical activities; refer to Table 7.1 for the calorie costs of different types of sports and fitness activities.

Make Changes in Your Diet and Eating Habits

If you can't generate a large enough negative calorie balance solely by increasing physical activity, you may want to supplement exercise with some dietary strategies. Don't think of this as "going on a diet"; your goal is to make small changes in your diet that you can maintain for a lifetime. Don't try skipping meals, fasting, or a very-low-calorie diet. These strategies seldom work, and they can have negative effects on your ability to manage your weight and on your overall health. Instead, try monitoring calories or fat grams, or simply cutting portion sizes. Refer back to the box "Lifestyle Strategies for Successful Weight Management" for suggestions.

Another strategy is to limit your intake of certain foods, such as those high in fat, sugar, or refined carbohydrates. The strategy of simply eating more vegetables, fruits, and dietary fiber has helped others achieve and maintain a healthy weight.

Put Your Plan into Action

Be systematic in your efforts to change your behavior, both what you eat and how you exercise. Many of those who are successful at controlling their weight track their progress in writing, enlist the support of others, and think positively. Here are tips gleaned from studies of people who have succeeded in long-term weight management.

Write Daily Write down everything you eat, including how many calories it contains. (See Figure 1.5 for one example of a food journal.) Researchers have found that writing down the food choices you make every day increases your commitment and helps you stick to your diet, especially during high-risk times such as holidays, parties, and family gatherings. Writing every day also serves as a reminder to you that losing weight is important.

Besides keeping track of what you eat, keep track of your formal exercise program and other daily physical activities so you can begin increasing either their intensity or duration. People who succeed in their health program expend lots of energy in physical activity—according to one study, an average of 2700 calories a week. Popular activities are walking, cycling, aerobic dance, and stair climbing.

Keeping a journal is an excellent way to keep track of your calorie intake—the foods you eat each day—and expenditure—your daily physical activities. You can also write down your thoughts and feelings to make sure you're maintaining a positive self-image and a realistic attitude about weight management.

Get Others to Help Enlist friends and family members to help and give them specific suggestions about what you would find helpful. You might, for instance, ask someone to leave you an encouraging voice mail once a day or twice a week, or ask someone to send you reminders by e-mail or phone. Besides asking for regular moral support, find a buddy to work out with you regularly and to be there as an emergency support.

Think Positively Remember to give yourself lots of praise and rewards. Think about your accomplishments each day, and congratulate yourself. You can write these positive thoughts in your food journal. If you do slip, stay objective and don't waste time on self-criticism. If you are keeping a food journal, you can see the slip for what it is—an easily contained lapse rather than a catastrophic relapse that ends in your losing confidence and control. Remember that as weight loss slows, the weight loss at this slower rate is more permanent than earlier, more dramatic losses.

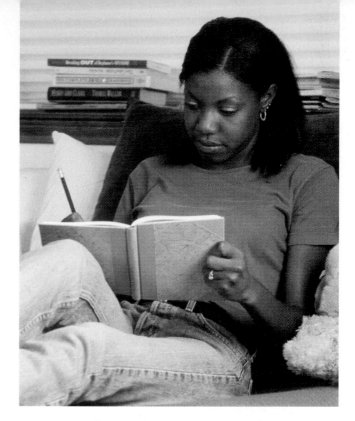

Tips for Today

Maintaining a healthy weight means balancing calories in with calories out. Many forces and factors in contemporary society work against a healthy balance, so it's imperative that individuals take active control of managing their weight. Many approaches work, but the simplest formula is moderate food intake coupled with regular exercise.

Right now you can

- Drink a glass of water instead of a soda.
- Throw away any high-calorie, low-nutrient snack foods in your kitchen or room and start a list of fruits and vegetables you can buy as snacks instead.
- Put a sign on your refrigerator reminding you of your weight-management goals.
- Go outside and walk or jog for 15 minutes or take a 15-minute bike ride.
- Review the information on portion sizes in Chapter 8 and consider whether the portions you usually take at meals are larger than they need to be.

SUMMARY

- Excess body weight increases the risk of numerous diseases, particularly cardiovascular disease, cancer, and diabetes.
- Although genetic factors help determine a person's weight, the influence of heredity can be overcome.
- Physiological factors involved in the regulation of body weight and body fat include metabolic rate and hormones.
- Energy-balance components that an individual can control are calories taken in and calories expended in physical activity.
- Nutritional guidelines for weight management and wellness include controlling consumption of total calories, fat, sugar, and protein; monitoring portion sizes and calorie density; increasing consumption of complex carbohydrates; and developing an eating schedule based on decision rules.
- Activity guidelines for weight control emphasize engaging in moderate-intensity physical activity for 150 minutes or more per week; regular, prolonged endurance exercise and weight training can burn a significant number of calories while maintaining muscle mass.
- The sense of well-being that results from a well-balanced, low-fat diet can reinforce commitment to weight control; improve self-esteem; and lead to realistic, as opposed to negative, self-talk. Successful weight management results in not using food as a way to cope with stress.
- In cases of extreme obesity, weight loss requires medical supervision; otherwise, people can set up individual programs, perhaps getting guidance from reliable books, or they can get help by joining a formal weight-loss program.
- Dissatisfaction with body image and body weight can lead to physical problems and serious eating disorders, including anorexia nervosa, bulimia nervosa, and binge-eating disorder.
- A successful personal plan assesses motivation, sets reasonable and healthy goals, and emphasizes increased activity rather than decreased calories.

COMMON QUESTIONS ANSWERED

How can I safely gain weight? Although for most of us the focus of a weight-management program is losing weight, some people face the opposite challenge. Just as for losing weight, a program for weight gain should be gradual and should include both exercise and dietary changes. The foundation of a successful and healthy program for weight gain is a combination of strength training and a high-carbohydrate, high-calorie diet. Strength training is critical because it will help you add weight as muscle rather than fat.

Energy balance is also important in a program for gaining weight. You need to consume more calories than your body needs in order to gain weight, but you need to choose those extra calories wisely. Fatty, high-calorie foods may seem like an obvious choice, but consuming additional calories as fat can jeopardize your health and your weight-management program. A diet high in fat carries health risks, including increased risk of cardiovascular disease and certain types of cancer. Furthermore, your body is more likely to convert dietary fat into fat tissue than into muscle mass. A better strategy is to consume additional calories as complex carbohydrates from whole grains, fruits, and vegetables. Experts recommend that a diet for weight gain should contain about 60–65% of total daily calories from carbohydrates. You probably do not need to be concerned with protein: Although protein requirements increase when you exercise, the protein consumption of most Americans is already well above the RDA.

In order to gain primarily muscle weight instead of fat, a gradual program of weight gain is your best bet. Try these strategies for consuming extra calories:

COMMON QUESTIONS ANSWERED

- Don't skip any meals.
- Add two or three snacks to your daily eating routine.
- Try a sports drink or supplement that has at least 60% of calories from carbohydrates, as well as significant amounts of protein, vitamins, and minerals. (But don't use supplements to replace meals, because they don't contain all food components.)

How can I achieve a "perfect" body? The current cultural ideal of an ultrathin, ultrafit body is impossible for most people to achieve. A reasonable goal for body weight and body shape must take into account an individual's heredity, weight history, social circumstances, metabolic rate, and psychological well-being. Don't set goals based on movie stars or fashion models. Modern photographic techniques can make people look much different on film or in magazines than they look in person. Many of these people are also genetically endowed with body shapes that are impossible for most of us to emulate. The best approach is to work with what you've got. Adopting a wellness lifestyle that includes regular exercise and a healthy diet will naturally result in the best possible body shape for you. Obsessively trying to achieve unreasonable goals can lead to problems such as eating disorders, overtraining, and injuries.

FOR FURTHER EXPLORATION

WW *Fit and Well* Online Learning Center (www.mhhe.com/fahey5e)

Use the learning objectives, study guide questions, and glossary flashcards to review key terms and concepts and prepare for exams. You can extend your knowledge of weight management and gain experience in using the Internet as a resource by completing the activities and checking out the Web links for the topics in Chapter 9 marked with the World Wide Web icon. For this chapter, Internet activities explore eating habits, online weight-loss programs, and body image; there are Web links for the Vital Statistics table, the Critical Consumer box on dietary supplements, and the chapter as a whole.

Daily Fitness and Nutrition Journal

Review the resources and complete the activities in the weight management portion of the journal. Complete the program plan by setting goals and examining your activities and eating habits for ways to tip the energy balance equation in the appropriate direction. Once you put your plan into action, continue to monitor your behavior using a daily log.

Health*Quest*

Learn more about your personal energy balance equation by completing the Energy Balance activity on the Health*Quest* CD-ROM (choose Energy Balance from the Wellness Activities menu in the Nutrition and Weight Control module). By selecting foods and entering your daily physical activities, you can determine your current energy balance and see what it would take to change it.

Books

King, J. E., ed. 2002. *Mayo Clinic on Healthy Weight.* Broomall, PA: Macon Crest. *Presents basic information on determining and achieving a healthy body weight.*

Kirby, J., and the American Dietetic Association. 1998. *Dieting for Dummies.* Indianapolis, Ind.: IDG Books. *Presents basic facts about all facets of weight loss, including strategies for evaluating commercial programs and diet books.*

Levenkorn, S. 2000. *Anatomy of Anorexia.* New York: Norton. *An up-to-date work on the symptoms, diagnosis, and treatment of anorexia for patients, families, and therapists.*

Nash, J. D. 1999. *Binge No More: Your Guide to Overcoming Disordered Eating.* Oakland, Calif.: New Harbinger. *Provides information and techniques for overcoming binge eating in the context of all types of disordered eating.*

Pope, H. G., K. A. Phillips, and R. Olivardia. 2000. *Adonis Complex: The Secret Crisis of Male Body Obsession.* New York: Free Press. *Provides a historical review of the changing fashions in male body type and information about male problems with body image.*

Rolls, B. J., and R. A. Barnett. 2001. *Volumetrics: Feel Full on Fewer Calories.* New York: HarperCollins. *Presents a research-based weight-management plan centering on the concept of energy density.*

WW Organizations and Web Sites

Cyberdiet. Provides a variety of assessment and planning tools as well as practical tips for eating a healthy diet and being physically active.
  http://www.cyberdiet.com

FDA Consumer: Ways to Win at Weight Loss. Includes guidelines for a variety of weight-loss strategies and special tips for using food labels to aid in weight management.
  http://www.fda.gov/fdac/reprints/weight.html

Frontline: Fat. Information from a PBS Frontline special that looked at how society, genetics, and biology have influenced our relationship with food and at current problems with obesity and eating disorders.
  http://www.pbs.org/wgbh/pages/frontline/shows/fat

Go Ask Alice. Sponsored by Columbia University Health Service, provides answers to a wide variety of students' questions, including many about weight management, diet, and exercise.
  http://www.goaskalice.columbia.edu

MedlinePlus: Obesity and Weight Loss. Provides news and links to reliable information from government agencies and key professional associations; includes separate listings.
  http://www.nlm.nih.gov/medlineplus/obesity.html
  http://www.nlm.nih.gov/medlineplus/weightlossdieting.html

National Heart, Lung, and Blood Institute (NHLBI): Aim for a Healthy Weight. Provides information and tips on diet and physical activity, as well as a BMI calculator.
  http://www.nhlbi.nih.gov/health/public/heart/obesity/lose_wt

National Institute of Diabetes and Digestive and Kidney Diseases (NIDDK). Health Information: Nutrition and Obesity. Provides information and referrals for problems related to obesity, weight control, and nutritional disorders.
877-946-4627
http://www.niddk.nih.gov/health/nutrit/nutrit.htm

Partnership for Healthy Weight Management. Provides information on evaluating weight-loss programs and advertising claims.
http://www.consumer.gov/weightloss

Shape Up America! Provides materials about safe dietary and physical fitness strategies for successful weight management. Web site includes an online BMI calculator and a physical activity IQ quiz.
http://shapeup.org

U.S. Consumer Gateway: Health—Dieting and Weight Control. Provides links to government sites with advice on evaluating claims about weight-loss products and programs.
http://www.consumer.gov/health.htm

USDA Food and Nutrition Information Center: Reports and Studies on Obesity. Provides links to recent reports and studies on the issue of obesity among Americans; includes links to ongoing USDA studies on popular diets.
http://www.nal.usda.gov/fnic/reports/obesity.html

There are also many resources for people concerned about eating disorders:

Eating Disorders Shared Awareness
http://www.something-fishy.org

Harvard Eating Disorders Center
http://www.hedc.org

MedlinePlus: Eating Disorders
http://www.nlm.nih.gov/medlineplus/eastingdisorders.html

National Association of Anorexia Nervosa and Associated Disorders
847-831-3438
http://www.anad.org

National Eating Disorders Association
800-931-2237
http://www.nationaleatingdisorders.org

See also the listings in Chapters 1, 6, and 8.

SELECTED BIBLIOGRAPHY

American College of Sports Medicine. 2001. Position Stand: Appropriate intervention strategies for weight loss and prevention of weight regain for adults. *Medicine and Science in Sports and Exercise* 33(12): 2145–2156.

American Dietetic Association. 2001. Nutrition intervention in the treatment of anorexia nervosa, bulimia nervosa, and eating disorders not otherwise specified (EDNOS). *Journal of the American Dietetic Association* 101(7): 810–819.

American Dietetic Association. 1998. Fat replacers. Position paper. *Journal of the American Dietetic Association* 98:463–468.

American Dietetic Association. 1998. Use of nutritive and non-nutritive sweeteners. Position paper. *Journal of the American Dietetic Association* 98:580–587.

American Institute for Cancer Research. 2000. Fad diets versus Dietary Guidelines (http://www.aicr.org/faddiets.htm; retrieved March 1, 2000).

Blanck, H. M., L. K. Khan, and M. K. Serdula. 2001. Use of nonprescription weight loss products. *Journal of the American Medical Association* 286(8): 930–935.

Chemistry of fat substitutes: Can you stomach it? 2001. *Discover,* March.

Crespo, C. J., et al. 2001. Television watching, energy intake, and obesity in U.S. children. *Archives of Pediatric and Adolescent Medicine* 155(3): 360–365.

Dwyer, J. T., et al. 2001. Adolescents' eating patterns influence their nutrient intakes. *Journal of the American Dietetic Association* 101(7): 798–802.

Food and Drug Administration. 2001. FDA issues public health advisory on phenylpropanolamine in drug products. *FDA Consumer,* January/February.

Guide to rating weight-loss Web sites. 2000. *Tufts University Health and Nutrition Letter,* July Special Supplement.

Harvack, L. J., R. W. Jeffery, and K. N. Boutelle. 2000. Temporal trends in energy intake in the United States: An ecological perspective. *American Journal of Clinical Nutrition* 71:1478–1484.

Harvard Eating Disorders Center. 2001. *Helping Yourself, Helping Your Friend* (http://www.hedc.org; retrieved November 20, 2001).

Heffernan, D. D., S. M. Harper, and D. McWilliam. 2002. Women's perceptions of the outcome of weight loss diets: A signal detection approach. *International Journal of Eating Disorders* 31(3): 339–343.

Kernan, W. N., et al. 2000. Phenylpropanolamine and the risk of hemorrhagic stroke. *New England Journal of Medicine* 343(25): 1826–1832.

Kimm, S. Y., et al. 2002. Racial differences in the relation between uncoupling protein genes and resting energy expenditure. *American Journal of Clinical Nutrition* 75(4): 714–719.

Leit, R. A., J. J. Gray,a nd H. G. Pope, Jr. 2002. The media's representation of the ideal male body: A cause for muscle dysmorphia? *International Journal of Eating Disorders* 31(3): 334–338.

Loos, R. J., et al. 2002. Birth weight and body composition in young women: A prospective twin study. *American Journal of Clinical Nutrition* 75(4): 676–682.

Losing weight: More than counting calories. 2002. *FDA Consumer,* January/February.

McInnis, K. J. 2000. Exercise for obese clients. *ACSM's Health and Fitness Journal* 4(1): 25–31.

McLaren, L., and L. Gauvin. 2002. Neighbourhood level versus individual level correlates of women's body dissatisfaction: Toward a multilevel understanding of the role of affluence. *Journal of Epidemiology and Community Health* 56(3): 193–199.

McManus, K., L. Antinoro, and F. Sacks. 2001. A randomized controlled trial of a moderate-fat, low-energy diet compared with a low fat, low-energy diet for weight loss in overweight adults. *International Journal of Obesity and Related Metabolic Disorders* 25(10): 1503–1511.

Mitka, M. 2001. Magazine ideals wrong. *Journal of the American Medical Association* 286(4): 409.

Mokdad, A. H., et al. 2001. The continuing epidemics of obesity and diabetes in the United States. *Journal of the American Medical Association* 286(10): 1195–2000.

National Institute of Diabetes and Digestive and Kidney Disorders. 2001. *Prescription Medications for the Treatment of Obesity* (http://www.niddk.nih.gov/health/nutrit/pubs/presmeds.htm; retrieved April 19, 2001).

Phillips, K. A., R. S. Albertini, and S. A. Rasmussen. 2002. A randomized placebo-controlled trial of fluoxetine in body dysmorphic disorder. *Archives of General Psychiatry* 59(4): 381–388.

Pope, H. G., Jr., et al. 1999. Evolving ideals of male body image as seen through action toys. *International Journal of Disorders* 26(1): 65–72.

Rubinstein, S., and B. Caballero. 2000. Is Miss America an undernourished role model? *Journal of the American Medical Association* 283(12): 1569.

Stevens, V. J., et al. 2001. Long-term weight loss and changes in blood pressure. *Annals of Internal Medicine* 134:1–11.

Tate, D. F., R. R. Wing, and R. A. Winett. 2001. Using Internet technology to deliver a behavioral weight loss program. *Journal of the American Medical Association* 285(9): 1172–1777.

Treuth, M. S., et al. 2001. Familial resemblance of body composition in prepubertal girls and their biological parents. *American Journal of Clinical Nutrition* 74(4): 529–533.

Wirth, A., and J. Krause. 2001. Long-term weight loss with sibutramine. *Journal of the American Medical Association* 286(11): 1331–1339.

Ziccardi, P., et al. 2002. Reduction of inflammatory cytokine concentrations and improvement of endothelial functions in obese women after weight loss over one year. *Circulation* 105(7): 804–809.

Name ______________________ Section ______________ Date ______________

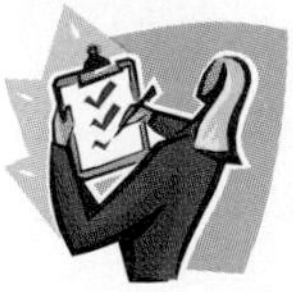

LAB 9.1 *Calculating Daily Energy Balance*

Ww

Part I Resting Metabolic Rate

Resting metabolic rate varies depending on age, gender, and weight. Use the equations below to calculate your approximate RMR.

World Health Organization Equations

1. Convert body weight to kilograms:

   ______________ lb ÷ 2.2 lb/kg = ______________ kg

2. Find the appropriate formula in the table below, and calculate your RMR. (For example, a 19-year-old male weighing 80 kg would have an RMR of approximately (15.3 × 80) + 679 = 1224 + 679 = 1903 calories a day.)

	Equation to Derive RMR in cal/day	
Age Range (years)	Males	Females
10–18	(17.5 × wt) + 651	(12.2 × wt) + 746
18–30	(15.3 × wt) + 679	(14.7 × wt) + 496
30–60	(11.6 × wt) + 879	(8.7 × wt) + 829
Over 60	(13.5 × wt) + 487	(10.5 × wt) + 596

RMR = (______________ × ______________ kg) + ______________ = ______________ **cal/day**

(factor from table) (body weight) (factor from table)

Harris Benedict Equations

1. Convert body weight to kilograms: ______________ lb ÷ 2.2 lb/kg = ______________ kg
2. Convert height to centimeters: 68 in. × 2.54 cm/in. = 160.02 cm
3. Use the appropriate equation to calculate RMR. (For example, a 20-year-old female 160 cm tall, weighing 60 kg, would have an RMR of approximately 655 + (9.56 × 60) + (1.85 × 160) − (4.68 × 20) = 1431 calories a day.)

   Women: RMR = 655 + (9.56 × weight ______________ kg) + (1.85 × height ______________ cm)
   − (4.68 × age ______________ yr) = ______________ **cal/day**

   Men: RMR = 66.5 + (13.8 × weight ______________ kg) + (5 × height ______________ cm)
   − (6.76 × age ______________ yr) = ______________ **cal/day**

Approximate Resting Metabolic Rate

Average the values you obtained from these equations to determine your approximate RMR.

World Health Organization Equation: ______________ cal/day

Harris Benedict Equation: ______________ cal/day

Average value for RMR: ______________ **cal/day**

Part II Daily Energy Expenditures

List all your activities for a 3-day period and classify them according to the categories listed in the table below. (Representative values of the calorie costs of different types of activities are presented below as multiples of resting metabolic rate.) Table 7.1 provides general guidelines for how to classify your sports and fitness activities: Activities with high cardiorespiratory endurance ratings probably fall in the heavy category, those with medium CRE ratings in the moderate category, and those with low CRE ratings in the light category. Take your intensity into account when classifying fitness activities; basketball, for example, can be played at an easy pace or intensely.

Your total daily energy expenditure can be estimated by calculating a daily activity factor based on the amount of time you engage in activities in each category of intensity. By adding up weighted activity factors and finding the average, you can calculate total daily energy requirements. Since your activity levels probably vary widely from day to day, it's more accurate to calculate energy output for several days to come up with an average daily range of calorie output.

Activity Categorty	*Representative Value for Activity Factor per Unit Time of Activity*
Resting: Sleeping, lying down	RMR × 1.0
Very light: Seated and standing activities such as driving, lab work, writing, typing, cooking, playing cards, or playing a musical instrument	RMR × 1.5
Light: Walking on a level surface 2.5–3.0 mph, house cleaning, child care, carpentry, restaurant trades, and sports/activities with low fitness ratings such as golf, bowling, and sailing	RMR × 2.5
Moderate: Walking 3.5–4.0 mph, gardening, carrying a load, and sports/activities with medium fitness ratings such as baseball and volleyball	RMR × 5.0
Heavy: Walking with a load uphill, heavy manual labor, sports/activities with high fitness ratings such as aerobic dance and cross-country skiing	RMR × 7.0

For each day, add up the total number of hours for each activity category. Then multiply the total duration for each category by the category's activity factor. Add the weighted activity factors, then divide the total weighted activity factor by 24 to get an average daily activity factor. A sample of completed calculations for one day is shown below.

SAMPLE

Activity	*Duration*	*Category*
sleeping	8 hours	resting
eating in dorm	1-1/2	very light
class	5	very light
bicycling to class, lab...	1	moderate
job in library	2-1/2	very light
cleaning room/laundry	1	light
basketball	1	heavy
studying in library	4	very light

Category	*Activity Factor*	*Duration*	*Weighted Activity Factor*
Resting	1.0	8	8.0
Very light	1.5	13	19.5
Light	2.5	1	2.5
Moderate	5.0	1	5.0
Heavy	7.0	1	7.0
Total		24 hours	42.0
Average daily activity factor (Total of weighted factors ÷ 24)			1.75

RECORDS FOR 3 DAYS

Day 1

Activity	*Duration*	*Category*

Day 1

Category	*Activity Factor*	*Duration*	*Weighted Activity Factor*
Resting	1.0		
Very light	1.5		
Light	2.5		
Moderate	5.0		
Heavy	7.0		
Total		24 hours	
Average daily activity factor (Total of weighted factors ÷ 24)			

Day 2

Activity	*Duration*	*Category*

Day 2

Category	*Activity Factor*	*Duration*	*Weighted Activity Factor*
Resting	1.0		
Very light	1.5		
Light	2.5		
Moderate	5.0		
Heavy	7.0		
Total		24 hours	
Average daily activity factor (Total of weighted factors ÷ 24)			

Day 3

Activity	*Duration*	*Category*

Day 3

Category	*Activity Factor*	*Duration*	*Weighted Activity Factor*
Resting	1.0		
Very light	1.5		
Light	2.5		
Moderate	5.0		
Heavy	7.0		
Total		24 hours	
Average daily activity factor (Total of weighted factors ÷ 24)			

Day 1 average daily activity factor ___________

Day 2 average daily activity factor ___________

Day 3 average daily activity factor ___________

Finally, use the middle or average of your three daily activity factors to calculate your average daily energy output. For RMR, use the value you calculated in the first part of this lab. (For example, a person with an average daily activity factor of 1.75 and an RMR of 1450 calories a day would have an approximate daily energy expenditure of 1.75 × 1450 = 2540 calories per day.)

Average of three daily activity factors ___________ × RMR ___________ cal/day
(from Part 1)

= approximate daily energy expenditure: ___________ cal/day

Using Your Results

How did you score? Are you surprised by the values you calculated for your resting metabolic rate and approximate daily energy expenditure? If so, are the values higher or lower than you expected?

If you completed Lab 8.2, how does your daily energy expenditure compare with the approximate number of calories you consume daily? (If your weight is holding steady, the values should be approximately equal.)

What should you do next? Enter the results of this lab in the Preprogram Assessment column in Appendix D. If you wish to change your energy balance to lose weight, complete Lab 9.2 to set goals and develop specific strategies for change. (If your goal is weight gain, see pp. 272–273 for basic guidelines.) One of the best ways to tip your energy balance toward weight loss is to increase your daily physical activity. If you include increases in activity as part of your program, then you can use the results of this lab to chart changes in your daily energy expenditure. Look for ways to increase the amount of time you spend in activities with a higher intensity and corresponding activity factor. After several weeks of your program, complete this lab again, and enter the results in the Postprogram Assessment column of Appendix D. How do the results compare? Did your program for boosting physical activity show up as an increase in your daily activity factor and daily energy expenditure?

SOURCES: National Research Council. 1989. *Recommended Dietary Allowances*, 10th ed. Washington, D.C.: National Academy Press. World Health Organization. 1985. *Energy and Protein Requirements: Report of a Joint FAO/WHO/UNO Expert Consultation*. Geneva: World Health Organization, Technical Report Series 724.

Name ______________________ Section ____________ Date ______________

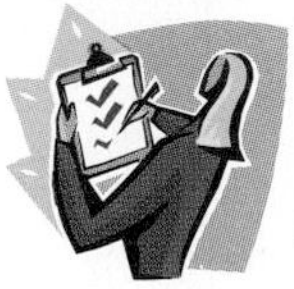

LAB 9.2 *Identifying Weight-Loss Goals and Ways to Meet Them*

Negative Calorie Balance

Complete the following calculations to determine your weekly and daily negative calorie balance goals and the number of weeks to achieve your target weight.

Current weight ________ lb − target weight (from Lab 6.2) ________ lb

= total weight to lose ________ lb

Total weight to lose ________ lb ÷ weight to lose each week ________ lb

= time to achieve target weight ______ weeks

Weight to lose each week ________ lb × 3500 cal/lb = weekly negative calorie balance ________ cal/week

Weekly negative calorie balance ________ cal/week ÷ 7 days/week

= daily negative calorie balance ________ cal/day

To keep your weight-loss program on schedule, you must achieve the daily negative calorie balance by either decreasing your calorie consumption (eating less) or increasing your calorie expenditure (being more active). A combination of the two strategies will probably be most successful.

Changes in Activity Level

Adding a few minutes of exercise every day is a good way of expending calories. Use the calorie costs for different activities listed in Table 7.1 and Table 9.2 to plan ways for raising your calorie expenditure level.

Activity	Duration	Calories Used
	Total calories expended:	

Changes in Diet

Look closely at your diet from one day, as recorded in Lab 8.2. Identify ways to cut calorie consumption by eliminating certain items or substituting lower-calorie choices. Be realistic in your cuts and substitutions; you need to develop a plan you can live with.

Food Item	Substitute Food Item	Calorie Savings
	Total calories cut:	

Total calories expended ________ **+ total calories cut** ________ **= Total negative calorie balance** ________

Have you met your required negative energy balance? If not, revise your dietary and activity changes to meet your goal.

Common Problem Eating Behaviors

For each of the groups of statements that appear below, check those that are true for you. If you check several statements for a given pattern or problem, it will probably be a significant factor in your weight-management program. One possible strategy for dealing with each type of problem is given. For those eating problems you identify as important, add your own ideas to the strategies listed.

1. _____ I often skip meals.

   _____ I often eat a number of snacks in place of a meal.

   _____ I don't have a regular schedule of meal and snack times.

   _____ I make up for missed meals and snacks by eating more at the next meal.

   Problem: Irregular eating habits

   Possible solutions:

   - Write out a plan for each day's meals in advance. Carry it with you and stick to it.
   - ____
   - ____

2. _____ I eat more than one sweet dessert or snack each day.

   _____ I usually snack on foods high in calories and fat (chips, cookies, ice cream).

   _____ I drink regular (not sugar-free) soft drinks.

   _____ I choose types of meat that are high in fat.

   _____ I consume more than one alcoholic beverage a day.

   Problem: Poor food choices

   Possible solutions:

   - Keep a supply of raw fruits or vegetables handy for snacks.
   - ____
   - ____

3. _____ I always eat everything on my plate.

   _____ I often go back for seconds and thirds.

   _____ I take larger helpings than most people.

   _____ I eat up leftovers instead of putting them away.

   Problem: Portion sizes too large

   Possible solutions:

   - Measure all portions with a scale or measuring cup.
   - ____
   - ____

Name ______________________ Section ______________ Date ______________

LAB 9.3 *Checking for Body Image Problems and Eating Disorders*

Assessing Your Body Image

	Never	Sometimes	Often	Always
1. I dislike seeing myself in mirrors.	0	1	2	3
2. When I shop for clothing, I am more aware of my weight problem, and consequently I find shopping for clothes somewhat unpleasant.	0	1	2	3
3. I'm ashamed to be seen in public.	0	1	2	3
4. I prefer to avoid engaging in sports or public exercise because of my appearance.	0	1	2	3
5. I feel somewhat embarrassed about my body in the presence of someone of the other sex.	0	1	2	3
6. I think my body is ugly.	0	1	2	3
7. I feel that other people must think my body is unattractive.	0	1	2	3
8. I feel that my family or friends may be embarrassed to be seen with me.	0	1	2	3
9. I find myself comparing myself with other people to see if they are heavier than I am.	0	1	2	3
10. I find it difficult to enjoy activities because I am self-conscious about my physical appearance.	0	1	2	3
11. Feeling guilty about my weight problem preoccupies most of my thinking.	0	1	2	3
12. My thoughts about my body and physical appearance are negative and self-critical.	0	1	2	3
Now add up the number of points you have circled in each column:_____	0	+_____	+_____	+_____

Score Interpretation

The lowest possible score is 0, and this indicates a positive body image. The highest possible score is 36, and this indicates an unhealthy body image. A score higher than 14 suggests a need to develop a healthier body image.

SOURCE: Nash, J. D. 1997. *The New Maximize Your Body Potential*. Palo Alto, Calif.: Bull Publishing. Reprinted with permission of the publisher.

Eating Disorder Checklist

	Always	Very Often	Often	Sometimes	Rarely	Never
1. I like eating with other people.	0	0	0	1	2	3
2. I like my clothes to fit tightly.	0	0	0	1	2	3
3. I enjoy eating meat.	0	0	0	1	2	3
4. I have regular menstrual periods.	0	0	0	1	2	3
5. I enjoy eating at restaurants.	0	0	0	1	2	3
6. I enjoy trying new rich foods.	0	0	0	1	2	3
7. I prepare foods for others, but do not eat what I cook.	3	2	1	0	0	0
8. I become anxious prior to eating.	3	2	1	0	0	0
9. I am terrified about being overweight.	3	2	1	0	0	0
10. I avoid eating when I am hungry.	3	2	1	0	0	0
11. I find myself preoccupied with food.	3	2	1	0	0	0.
12. I have gone on eating binges where I feel that I may not be able to stop.	3	2	1	0	0	0
13. I cut my food into small pieces.	3	2	1	0	0	0

	Statement	Always	Very Often	Often	Sometimes	Rarely	Never
14.	I am aware of the calorie content of foods that I eat.	3	2	1	0	0	0
15.	I particularly avoid foods with a high carbohydrate content (bread, potatoes, rice, etc.).	3	2	1	0	0	0
16.	I feel bloated after meals.	3	2	1	0	0	0
17.	I feel others would prefer me to eat more.	3	2	1	0	0	0
18.	I vomit after I have eaten.	3	2	1	0	0	0
19.	I feel extremely guilty after eating.	3	2	1	0	0	0
20.	I am preoccupied with a desire to be thinner.	3	2	1	0	0	0
21.	I exercise strenuously to burn off calories.	3	2	1	0	0	0
22.	I weight myself several times a day.	3	2	1	0	0	0
23.	I wake up early in the morning.	3	2	1	0	0	0
24.	I eat the same foods day after day.	3	2	1	0	0	0
25.	I think about burning up calories when I exercise.	3	2	1	0	0	0
26.	Other people think I am too thin.						
27.	I am preoccupied with the thought of having fat on my body.	3	2	1	0	0	0
28.	I take longer than others to eat my meals.	3	2	1	0	0	0
29.	I take laxatives.	3	2	1	0	0	0
30.	I avoid foods with sugar in them.						
31.	I eat diet foods.	3	2	1	0	0	0
32.	I feel that food controls my life.	3	2	1	0	0	0
33.	I display self-control around foods.	3	2	1	0	0	0
34.	I feel that others pressure me to eat.	3	2	1	0	0	0
35.	I give too much time and thought to food.	3	2	1	0	0	0
36.	I suffer from constipation.	3	2	1	0	0	0
37.	I feel uncomfortable after eating sweets.	3	2	1	0	0	0
38.	I engage in dieting behavior.	3	2	1	0	0	0
39.	I like my stomach to be empty.						
40.	I have the impulse to vomit after meals.	3	2	1	0	0	0
	Now add up the number of points in each column for statements 1 through 40: _____	_____ +	_____ +	_____ +	_____ +	_____ +	_____

Score Interpretation

The possible range is 0–120. A score higher than 50 suggests an eating disorder. A score between 30 and 50 suggests a borderline eating disorder. A score less than 30 is within the normal range. Among those with normal eating habits, the average score is 15.4.

SOURCE: Nieman, D. 1999. *Exercise Testing and Prescription: A Health-Related Approach,* 4th ed. Mountain View, Calif.: Mayfield. Reproduced with permission from The McGraw-Hill Companies.

Using Your Results

How did you score? Are you surprised by your scores? Do the results of either assessment indicate that you may have a problem with body image or disordered eating?

What should you do next? If your results are borderline, consider trying some of the self-help strategies suggested in the chapter. If body image or disordered eating is a significant problem for you, get professional advice; a physician, therapist, and/or registered dietitian can help. Make an appointment today.

Stress

10

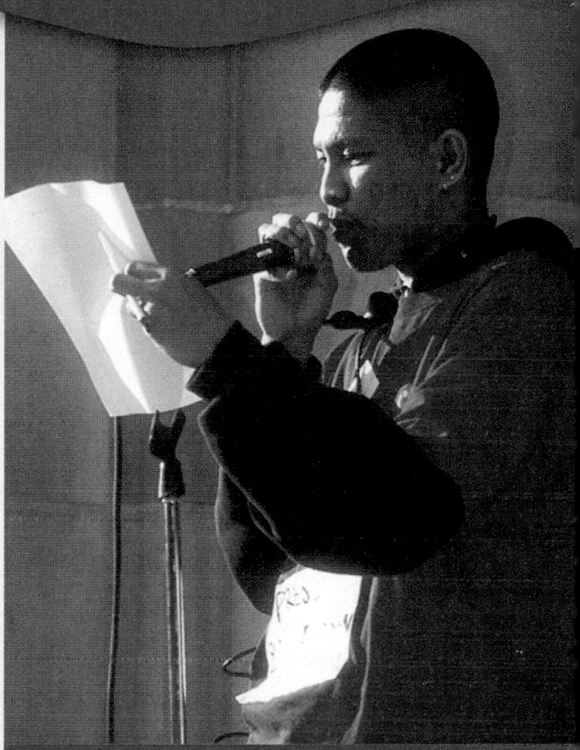

LOOKING AHEAD

After reading this chapter, you should be able to

- Explain what stress is and how people react to it—physically, emotionally, and behaviorally
- Describe the relationship between stress and disease
- List common sources of stress
- Describe techniques for preventing and managing stress
- Put together a plan for successfully managing the stress in your life

TEST YOUR KNOWLEDGE

1. Which of the following events can cause stress?
   a. taking out a loan
   b. failing a test
   c. graduating from college
   d. watching a hockey game
2. About twice as many male college students as female college students report feeling frequently overwhelmed.
   True or false?
3. High levels of stress can impair memory and cause physical changes in the brain.
   True or false?

TEST YOUR KNOWLEDGE ANSWERS

1. ALL FOUR. Stress-producing factors can be pleasant or unpleasant and can include physical challenges and goal achievement as well as what are perceived as negative events.

2. FALSE. In recent surveys, about 20% of male and 40% of female college students report feeling frequently overwhelmed. Female college students are more likely to report financial worries, and they spend more time in activities such as volunteer work, housework, and child care.

3. TRUE. Low levels of stress may improve memory, but high stress levels impair learning and memory and, over the long term, may shrink an area of the brain called the hippocampus.

Fit and Well Online Learning Center

www.mhhe.com/fahey5e

Visit the *Fit and Well* Online Learning Center for study aids, additional information about stress, links, Internet activities that explore the role of stress management in wellness, and much more.

Like the term *fitness*, *stress* is a word many people use without really understanding its precise meaning. Stress is popularly viewed as an uncomfortable response to a negative event, which probably describes *nervous tension* more than the cluster of physical and psychological responses that actually constitute stress. In fact, stress is not limited to negative situations; it is also a response to pleasurable physical challenges and the achievement of personal goals. Whether stress is experienced as pleasant or unpleasant depends largely on the situation and the individual. Because learning effective responses to whatever induces stress can enhance psychological health and help prevent a number of serious diseases, stress management is an important component in any wellness program.

This chapter explains the physiological and psychological reactions that make up the stress response and describes how these reactions can be risks to good health. The chapter also presents ways of managing stress with a personal program or with the help of others.

Terms

stressor Any physical or psychological event or condition that produces stress.

stress response The physiological changes associated with stress.

stress The collective physiological and emotional responses to any stimulus that disturbs an individual's homeostasis.

autonomic nervous system The branch of the peripheral nervous system that, largely without conscious thought, controls basic body processes; consists of the sympathetic and parasympathetic divisions.

parasympathetic division A division of the autonomic nervous system that moderates the excitatory effect of the sympathetic division, slowing metabolism and restoring energy supplies.

sympathetic division A division of the autonomic nervous system that reacts to danger or other challenges by almost instantly accelerating body processes.

endocrine system The system of glands, tissues, and cells that secrete hormones into the bloodstream to influence metabolism and other body processes.

hormone A chemical messenger produced in the body and transported in the bloodstream to target cells or organs for specific regulation of their activities.

cortisol A steroid hormone secreted by the cortex (outer layer) of the adrenal gland; also called *hydrocortisone*.

epinephrine A hormone secreted by the inner core of the adrenal gland; also called *adrenaline*, the "fear hormone."

norepinephrine A hormone secreted by the inner core of the adrenal gland; also called *noradrenaline*, the "anger hormone."

endorphins Brain secretions that have pain-inhibiting effects.

fight-or-flight reaction A defense reaction that prepares an individual for conflict or escape by triggering hormonal, cardiovascular, metabolic, and other changes.

homeostasis A state of stability and consistency in an individual's physiological functioning.

WHAT IS STRESS?

In common usage, *stress* refers to two different things: situations that trigger physical and emotional reactions *and* the reactions themselves. In this text, we'll use the more precise term **stressor** for a situation that triggers physical and emotional reactions and the term **stress response** for those reactions. A final exam, then, is a stressor; sweaty palms and a pounding heart are symptoms of the stress response. We'll use the term **stress** to describe the general physical and emotional state that accompanies the stress response. A person taking a final exam experiences stress.

Physical Responses to Stressors

Imagine a near miss: As you step off the curb, a car careens toward you. With just a fraction of a second to spare, you leap safely out of harm's way. In that split second of danger and in the moments following it, you experience a predictable series of physical reactions. Your body goes from a relaxed state to one prepared for physical action to cope with a threat to your life. Two major control systems in your body are responsible for your physical response to stressors: the nervous system and the endocrine system.

Actions of the Nervous System The nervous system consists of the brain, spinal cord, and nerves. Part of the nervous system is under voluntary control, as when you tell your arm to reach for a chocolate. The part that is not under conscious supervision, such as what controls the digestion of the chocolate, is known as the **autonomic nervous system.** In addition to digestion, it controls your heart rate, breathing, blood pressure, and hundreds of other functions you normally take for granted. The autonomic nervous system consists of two divisions. The **parasympathetic division** is in control when you are relaxed; it aids in digesting food, storing energy, and promoting growth. In contrast, the **sympathetic division** is activated when there is an emergency, such as severe pain, anger, or fear. Sympathetic nerves act on many targets—on nearly every organ, sweat gland, blood vessel, and muscle, in fact—to enable your body to handle an emergency. In general, the sympathetic division commands your body to stop storing energy and instead to mobilize all energy resources to respond to the crisis.

Actions of the Endocrine System One important target of the sympathetic nervous system is the activation of the **endocrine system.** This system of glands, tissues, and cells helps control body functions by releasing **hormones** and other chemical messengers into the bloodstream. These chemicals act on a variety of targets throughout the body. Along with the nervous system with which it closely interacts, the endocrine system helps prepare the body to respond to a stressor.

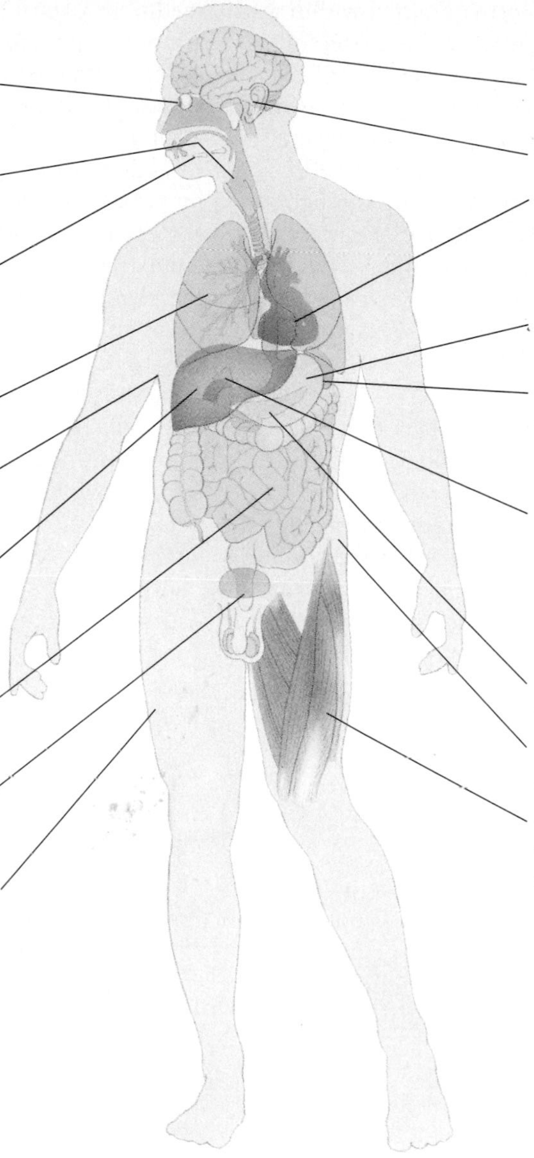

Pupils dilate to admit extra light for more sensitive vision.
Mucous membranes of nose and throat shrink, while muscles force a wider opening of passages to allow easier air flow.
Secretion of saliva and mucus decreases; digestive activities have a low priority in an emergency.
Bronchi dilate to allow more air into lungs.
Perspiration increases, especially in armpits, groin, hands, and feet, to flush out waste and cool overheating system by evaporation.
Liver releases sugar into bloodstream to provide energy for muscles and brain.
Muscles of intestines stop contracting because digestion has halted.
Bladder relaxes. Emptying of bladder contents releases excess weight, making it easier to flee.
Blood vessels in skin and viscera contract; those in skeletal muscles dilate. This increases blood pressure and delivery of blood to where it is most needed.
Endorphins are released to block any distracting pain.
Hearing becomes more acute.
Heart accelerates rate of beating, increases strength of contraction to allow more blood flow where it is needed.
Digestion, an unnecessary activity during an emergency, halts.
Spleen releases more red blood cells to meet an increased demand for oxygen and to replace any blood lost from injuries.
Adrenal glands stimulate secretion of epinephrine and norepinephrine, increasing blood sugar, blood pressure, and heart rate; also spur increase in amount of fat in blood. These changes provide an energy boost.
Pancreas decreases secretions because digestion has halted.
Fat is removed from storage and broken down to supply extra energy.
Voluntary (skeletal) muscles contract throughout the body, readying them for action.

Figure 10.1 The fight-or-flight reaction. In response to a stressor, the autonomic nervous system and the endocrine system cause physical changes that prepare the body to deal with an emergency.

The Two Systems Together How do both systems work together in an emergency? Let's go back to your near collision with a car. As the car travels toward you, you feel only fear, but outside your awareness, things happen to prepare you to meet the danger. Chemical messages cause the release of key hormones, including **cortisol**, **epinephrine**, and **norepinephrine.** These hormones trigger a series of profound physiological changes (Figure 10.1):

- Hearing and vision become more acute.
- The heart rate accelerates to pump more oxygen through the body.
- The liver releases extra sugar into the bloodstream to provide an energy boost.
- Perspiration increases to cool the skin.
- **Endorphins** are released to relieve pain in case of injury.

Taken together, these almost-instantaneous physical changes are called the **fight-or-flight reaction.** They give you the heightened reflexes and strength you need to dodge the car or deal with other stressors. Although these physical changes may vary in intensity, the same basic set of physical reactions occurs in response to any type of stressor, positive or negative.

The Return to Homeostasis Once a stressful situation ends, the parasympathetic division of your autonomic nervous system takes command and halts the reaction. It initiates the adjustments necessary to restore **homeostasis,** a state in which blood pressure, heart rate, hormone levels, and other vital functions are maintained within a narrow range of normal. Your parasympathetic nervous system calms your body down, slowing a rapid heartbeat, drying sweaty palms, and returning breathing to normal. Gradually, your body resumes its normal "housekeeping" functions, such as digestion and temperature regulation. Damage that may have been sustained during the fight-or-flight reaction is repaired. The day after you narrowly dodge the car, you wake up feeling fine. In this way, your body can grow, repair itself, and acquire reserves of energy. When the next crisis comes, you'll be ready to respond—instantly—again.

The Fight-or-Flight Reaction in Modern Life The fight-or-flight reaction is a part of our biological heritage, and it's a survival mechanism that has served humankind well. In modern life, however, it is often absurdly inappropriate. Many of the stressors we face in everyday life do not require a physical response—for example, an exam, a mess left by a roommate, or a red traffic light. The fight-or-flight reaction prepares the body for physical action regardless of whether such action is a necessary or appropriate response to a particular stressor.

Emotional and Behavioral Responses to Stressors

The physical response to a stressor may vary in intensity from person to person and situation to situation, but we all experience a similar set of physical changes—the fight-or-flight reaction. Emotionally and behaviorally, however, individuals respond in very different ways to stressors.

Effective and Ineffective Responses Common emotional responses to stressors include anxiety, depression, and fear. Although emotional responses are determined in part by inborn personality or temperament, we often can moderate or learn to control them. Coping techniques are discussed later in the chapter.

Behavioral responses to stressors—controlled by the **somatic nervous system,** which manages our conscious actions—are entirely under our control. Effective behavioral responses such as talking, laughing, exercising, meditating, learning time-management skills, and finding a more compatible roommate can promote wellness and enable us to function at our best. Ineffective behavioral responses to stressors include overeating and using tobacco, alcohol, or other drugs.

Let's consider the individual variations demonstrated by two students, David and Amelia, responding to the same stressor—the first exam of the semester. David enters the exam with a feeling of dread and, as he reads the exam questions, responds to his initial anxiety with more anxiety. The more emotionally upset he gets, the less he can remember and the more anxious he becomes. Soon he's staring into space, imagining what will happen if he fails the course. Amelia, on the other hand, takes a deep breath to relax before she reads the questions, wills herself to focus on the answers she knows, and then goes back over the exam to deal with those questions she's not sure of. She leaves the room feeling calm, relaxed, and confident that she has done well.

It's not difficult to see that avoiding destructive responses to stress and adopting effective and appropriate ones can have a direct effect on emotional and physical well-being.

Factors Influencing How We Respond to Stressors A complex set of factors—temperament, health, life experiences, values, and coping skills—can influence an individual's response to a stressful situation. Personality, the sum of emotional and behavioral tendencies, plays a role in enabling people to cope more or less successfully with stress. People who are ultracompetitive, controlling, impatient, aggressive, and hostile (so-called Type A personalities) tend to react more explosively to stressors and have more problems coping with stress. In contrast, people with "hardy" personalities—those who view potential stressors as challenges and opportunities for growth and learning, rather than as burdens—tend to perceive fewer situations as stressful and to react more mildly to the stressors in their lives. (See p. 301 for more on personality and stress.)

Past experiences can profoundly influence the evaluation of a potential stressor. Consider an individual who has had a bad experience giving a speech in the past. He or she is much more likely to perceive an upcoming speech assignment as stressful than someone who has had positive public speaking experiences. Gender and cultural background also influence our response to stressors. For example, some behavioral responses to stressors, such as crying or expressing anger, may be deemed more appropriate for one gender than the other.

The Stress Experience as a Whole

Physical, emotional, and behavioral responses to stressors are intimately interrelated. The more intense the emotional response, the stronger the physical response. Effective behavioral responses can lessen stress; ineffec-

Terms

Ww

somatic nervous system The branch of the peripheral nervous system that governs motor functions and sensory information, largely under our conscious control.

general adaptation syndrome (GAS) A pattern of stress responses consisting of three stages: alarm, resistance, and exhaustion.

eustress Stress resulting from a pleasant stressor.

distress Stress resulting from an unpleasant stressor.

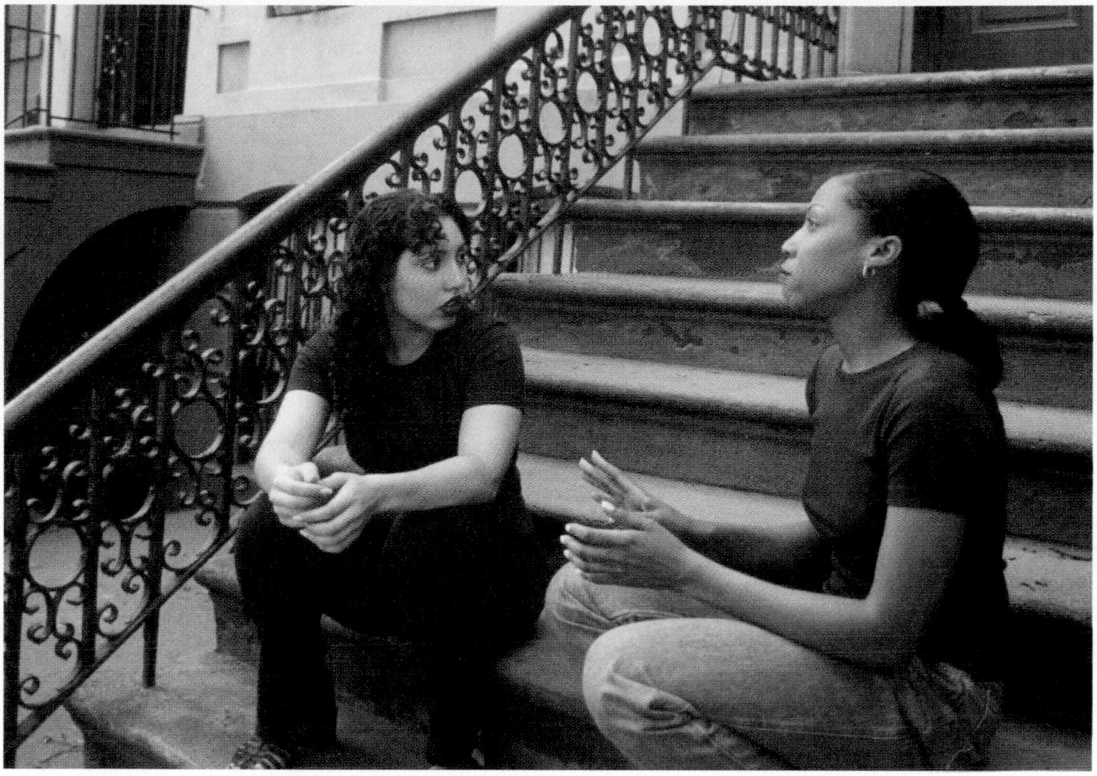

A person's emotional and behavioral responses to stressors depend on many different factors, including personality, gender, and cultural background. Research suggests that women are more likely than men to respond to stressors by seeking social support.

tive ones only worsen it. Sometimes people have such intense responses to stressors or such ineffective coping techniques that they need professional help. (Table 10.1 on p. 288 highlights some of the signals of excess stress.) More often, however, people can learn to handle stressors on their own.

STRESS AND WELLNESS

The role of stress in health and disease is complex, and much remains to be learned about the exact mechanisms by which stress influences health. However, mounting evidence suggests that stress—interacting with a person's genetic predisposition, personality, social environment, and health-related behaviors—can increase vulnerability to numerous illnesses and ailments. Several theories have been proposed to explain the relationship between stress and disease.

The General Adaptation Syndrome

Biologist Hans Selye was one of the first scientists to develop a comprehensive theory of stress and disease. Based on his work in the 1930s and 1940s, Selye coined the term **general adaptation syndrome (GAS)** to describe what he believed is a universal and predictable response pattern to all stressors. He recognized that stressors could be pleasant, such as attending a party, or unpleasant, such as a bad grade. He called stress triggered by a pleasant stressor **eustress** and stress triggered by an unpleasant stressor **distress.** The sequence of physical responses associated with GAS is the same for both eustress and distress and occurs in three stages: alarm, resistance, and exhaustion.

Alarm The alarm stage includes the complex sequence of events brought on by the activation of the sympathetic nervous system and the endocrine system—the fight-or-flight reaction. During this stage, the body is more susceptible to disease or injury because it is geared up to deal with a crisis. A person in this phase may experience headaches, indigestion, anxiety, and disrupted sleeping and eating patterns.

Resistance Selye theorized that with continued stress, the body develops a new level of homeostasis in which it is more resistant to disease and injury than normal. During the resistance stage, a person can cope with normal life and added stress.

Table 10.1 *Symptoms of Excess Stress*

Physical Symptoms	Emotional Symptoms	Behavioral Symptoms
Dry mouth	Anxiety or edginess	Crying
Excessive perspiration	Depression	Disrupted eating habits
Frequent illnesses	Fatigue	Disrupted sleeping habits
Gastrointestinal problems	Hypervigilance	Harsh treatment of others
Grinding of teeth	Impulsiveness	Problems communicating
Headaches	Inability to concentrate	Sexual problems
High blood pressure	Irritability	Social isolation
Pounding heart	Trouble remembering things	Increased use of tobacco, alcohol, or other drugs
Stiff neck or aching lower back		

Exhaustion Both the mobilization of forces during the alarm reaction and the maintenance of homeostasis during the resistance stage require a considerable amount of energy. If a stressor persists, or if several stressors occur in succession, general exhaustion results. This is not the sort of exhaustion people complain of after a long, busy day. It's a life-threatening type of physiological exhaustion characterized by such symptoms as distorted perceptions and disorganized thinking.

Allostatic Load

While Selye's model of GAS is still viewed as a key contribution to modern stress theory, some aspects are now discounted. For example, increased susceptibility to disease after repeated or prolonged stress is now thought to be due to the effects of the stress response itself rather than to a depletion of resources (Selye's exhaustion stage). In particular, long-term overexposure to stress hormones such as cortisol has been linked with a variety of health problems.

Researchers have termed the long-term wear and tear of the stress response the *allostatic load.* An individual's allostatic load depends on many factors, including genetics, life experiences, and emotional and behavioral responses to stressors. A high allostatic load may be due to frequent stressors, poor adaptation to common stressors, an inability to shut down the stress response, or imbalances in the stress response of different body systems. Researchers have linked high allostatic load with heart disease, high blood pressure, obesity, and reduced brain and immune system functioning. In other words, when your allostatic load exceeds your ability to cope, you are more likely to get sick.

Terms

Vw

psychoneuroimmunology (PNI) The study of the interactions among the nervous system, the endocrine system, and the immune system.

Psychoneuroimmunology

One of the most fruitful areas of current research into the relationship between stress and disease is **psychoneuroimmunology (PNI).** PNI is the study of the interactions among the nervous system, the endocrine system, and the immune system. The underlying premise of PNI is that stress, through the actions of the nervous and endocrine systems, impairs the immune system and thereby affects health.

Researchers have discovered a complex network of nerve and chemical connections between the nervous and endocrine systems and the immune system. We have already seen the profound physical effects of the hormones and other chemical messengers released during the stress response. These compounds also influence the immune system by affecting the number and efficiency of immune system cells, or lymphocytes.

The nervous, endocrine, and immune systems share other connections. Scientists have identified hormone-like substances called neuropeptides that appear to translate emotions into physiological events. Neuropeptides are produced and received by both brain and immune cells, so that the brain and the immune system share a biochemical "language," which also happens to be the language of emotions. The biochemical changes accompanying particular emotions can strongly influence the functioning of the immune system.

Links Between Stress and Specific Conditions

Although much remains to be learned, it is clear that people who have unresolved chronic stress in their lives or who handle stressors poorly are at risk for a wide range of health problems. In the short term, the problem might just be a cold, a stiff neck, or a stomachache. Over the long term, the problems can be more severe—cardiovascular disease or impairment of the immune system.

Cardiovascular Disease The stress response profoundly affects the cardiovascular system, and these changes have

TAKE CHARGE Overcoming Insomnia

At some time in their lives, most people have trouble falling asleep or staying asleep. This condition is known as insomnia. Most people can overcome insomnia by discovering the cause of poor sleep and taking steps to remedy it. Insomnia that lasts for more than 6 months and interferes with daytime functioning requires consultation with a physician. Sleeping pills are not recommended for chronic insomnia because they can be habit-forming; they also lose their effectiveness over time.

If you're bothered by insomnia, here are some tips for getting a better night's sleep:

- Determine how much sleep you need to feel refreshed the next day, and don't sleep longer than that (but do make sure you get enough).
- Go to bed at the same time every night and, more important, get up at the same time every morning, 7 days a week. Don't nap during the day.
- Exercise every day, but not too close to bedtime. Your metabolism takes up to 6 hours to slow down after exercise.
- Avoid tobacco (nicotine is a stimulant), caffeine in the later part of the day, and alcohol before bedtime (it causes disturbed, fragmented sleep).
- Have a light snack before bedtime; you'll sleep better if you're not hungry.
- Deal with worries before bedtime. Try writing them down, along with some possible solutions, and then allow yourself to forget about them until the next day.
- Use your bed only for sleep. Don't eat, read, study, or watch television in bed.
- Relax before bedtime with a warm bath (again, not too close to bedtime—allow about 2 hours for your metabolism to slow down afterward), a book, music, or some relaxation exercises. Don't lie down in bed until you're sleepy.
- If you don't fall asleep in 15–20 minutes, or if you wake up and can't fall asleep again, get out of bed, leave the room if possible, and do something monotonous until you feel sleepy.
- Keep a perspective on your plight. Losing a night's sleep isn't the end of the world. Getting upset only makes it harder to fall asleep. Relax, and trust in your body's natural ability to drift off to sleep.

important implications for cardiovascular health, especially over the long term. During the stress response, heart rate increases and blood vessels constrict, causing blood pressure to rise. Chronic high blood pressure is a major cause of atherosclerosis, a disease in which the lining of the blood vessels becomes damaged and caked with fatty deposits. These deposits can block arteries, causing heart attacks and strokes (see Chapter 11).

Recent research suggests that certain types of emotional responses increase a person's risk of cardiovascular disease. So-called "hot reactors," people who exhibit extreme increases in heart rate and blood pressure in response to emotional stressors, may face an increased risk of cardiovascular problems.

Altered Functioning of the Immune System Sometimes you seem to get sick when you can least afford it—during exam week, when you're going on vacation, or when you have a job interview. As described earlier regarding PNI, research suggests that this is more than mere coincidence. Some of the health problems linked to stress-related changes in immune function include vulnerability to colds and other infections, asthma and allergy attacks, susceptibility to cancer, and flare-ups of chronic diseases such as genital herpes and HIV infection.

Other Health Problems Many other health problems may be caused or worsened by uncontrolled stress, including the following:

- Digestive problems such as stomachaches, diarrhea, constipation, irritable bowel syndrome, and ulcers
- Tension headaches and migraines
- Insomnia and fatigue (see the box "Overcoming Insomnia")
- Injuries, including on-the-job injuries caused by repetitive strain
- Menstrual irregularities, impotence, and pregnancy complications
- Psychological problems, including depression, anxiety, panic attacks, eating disorders, and post-traumatic stress disorder (PTSD), which afflicts people who have suffered or witnessed severe trauma

COMMON SOURCES OF STRESS

We are surrounded by stressors—at home, at school, on the job, and within ourselves. Being able to recognize potential sources of stress is an important step in successfully managing the stress in our lives.

Major Life Changes

Any major change in your life that requires adjustment and accommodation can be a source of stress. Early adulthood and the college years are typically associated with many significant changes, such as moving out of the family home, establishing new relationships, setting educational and career goals, and developing a sense of identity and purpose. Even changes typically thought of as positive—graduation, job promotion, marriage—can be stressful.

Researchers have hypothesized that clusters of life changes, particularly those that are perceived negatively, may be linked to health problems. Personality and coping skills are important moderating influences, however. People with a strong support network and a stress-resistant personality are less likely to become ill in response to major life changes than people with fewer internal and external resources.

Daily Hassles

Although major life changes are undoubtedly stressful, they seldom occur regularly. Researchers have proposed that minor problems—life's daily hassles—can be an even greater source of stress because they occur much more often. Daily hassles might include:

- Misplacing your keys, wallet, or an assignment
- Having an argument with a troublesome neighbor, coworker, or customer
- Waiting in a long line
- Being stuck in traffic or having another problem with transportation
- Worrying about money
- Being upset about the weather

People who perceive hassles negatively are likely to experience a moderate stress response every time they are faced with one. Over time, this can take a significant toll on health. Studies indicate that for some people, daily hassles contribute to a general decrease in overall wellness.

Ww College Stressors

College is a time of major life changes and abundant minor hassles. You are learning new information and skills and making major decisions about your future. You may be away from home for the first time, or you may be adding extra responsibilities to a life already filled with job and family.

- *Academic stressors:* Exams, grades, and choosing a major are among the many academic stressors faced by college students. In addition to an increased workload compared to that in high school, high-quality efforts are expected of college students, so earning good grades takes more effort and dedication. Careful planning and preparation can help make academic stressors more predictable and manageable.

- *Interpersonal stressors:* The college years often involve such potential stressors as establishing new relationships and balancing multiple roles—student, employee, friend, spouse, parent, and so on. You'll have the opportunity to meet new people and make new friends at the start of every term and in every new class and activity. Viewed as an exciting challenge or a painful necessity, interacting with others involves attention, on-the-spot decision making, and energy expenditure. Be yourself and try not to be overly concerned with being liked by everyone you meet.

- *Time-related pressures:* Time pressures are a problem for most students, but they may be particularly acute for those who also have job and family responsibilities. Most people do have enough time to fulfill all of their key responsibilities, but they don't manage their time or their priorities effectively. For these people, it's important to make a plan and stick to it. Effective time-management strategies are described in the next section.

- *Financial concerns:* Many students live off savings from full-time summer jobs and part-time jobs during the school year, and many take out loans to pay tuition. Some students work full-time and support a family while taking college courses. Regardless of your situation, avoid extravagant spending and excessive worry about finances. Instead, use your resources to pursue academic achievements that will help enhance your future financial picture.

Job-Related Stressors

In recent surveys, Americans rate their jobs as one of the key sources of stress in their lives. Tight schedules and overtime leave less time to exercise, socialize, and engage in other stress-proofing activities. More than one-third of Americans report that they always feel rushed, and nearly half say they would give up a day's pay for a day off. Worries about job performance, salary, and job security and interactions with bosses, coworkers, and customers can contribute to stress. High levels of job stress are also common for people who are left out of important decisions relating to their jobs. When workers are given the opportunity to shape how their jobs are performed, job satisfaction goes up and stress levels go down.

If job-related (or college-related) stress is severe or chronic, the result can be **burnout,** a state of physical, mental, and emotional exhaustion. Burnout occurs most often in highly motivated and driven individuals who come to feel that their work is not recognized or that they are not accomplishing their goals. People in the helping professions—teachers, social workers, caregivers, police officers, and so on—are also prone to burnout. For some people who suffer from burnout, a vacation or leave of absence may be appropriate. For others, a reduced work schedule, better communication with superiors, or a change in job goals may be necessary. Improving time-management skills can also help.

Terms Ww

burnout A state of physical, mental, and emotional exhaustion.

Interpersonal and Social Stressors

Although social support is a key buffer against stress, your interactions with others can themselves be a source of stress. Your relationships with family members and old friends may change during your college years as you develop new interests and a new course for your life. You will be meeting new people and establishing new relationships.

The community and society in which you live can also be major sources of stress. Social stressors include prejudice and discrimination. You may feel stress as you try to relate to people of other ethnic or socioeconomic groups. As a member of a particular ethnic group, you may feel pressure to assimilate into mainstream society. If English is not your first language, you face the added burden of conducting many daily activities in a language with which you may not be completely comfortable.

Other Stressors

Other stressors are found in the environment and in ourselves. Environmental stressors—external conditions or events that cause stress—include loud noises, unpleasant smells, industrial accidents, violence, and natural disasters. Internal stressors are found not in our interactions with our environment but within ourselves. We put pressure on ourselves to reach personal goals and then evaluate our progress and performance. Physical and emotional states such as illness and exhaustion are other examples of internal stressors.

MANAGING STRESS

What can you do about all this stress? A great deal. By shoring up your social support systems; improving your communication skills; developing and maintaining healthy exercise, eating, and sleeping habits; and mastering simple techniques to identify and moderate individual stressors, you can learn to control the stress in your life—instead of allowing it to control you. The effort is well worth the time: People who manage stress effectively not only are healthier, they also have more time to enjoy life and accomplish their goals.

Ww Social Support

People need people. Sharing fears, frustrations, and joys not only makes life richer but also seems to contribute—indirectly but significantly—to the well-being of body and mind. Research supports this conclusion: One study of college students living in overcrowded apartments, for example, found that those with a strong social support system were less distressed by their cramped quarters than were the "loners" who navigated life's challenges on their own. Other studies have shown that married people live longer than single people and have lower death rates from a wide range of conditions. And people infected with HIV remain symptom-free longer if they have a strong social support network. The crucial common denominator in all these findings is the meaningful connection with others. For more on developing and maintaining your social network, see the box "Building Social Support" on p. 292.

Communication

Do you often find yourself angry at others? Some people express their anger directly by yelling or being aggressive; others express anger indirectly by excessively criticizing others or making cynical comments. A person who is angry with others often has difficulty forming and maintaining successful social relationships. Better communication skills can help. To learn strategies for managing anger, see the box "Dealing with Anger" on pp. 294–295.

At the other extreme, you may suppress your feelings and needs entirely. You may have trouble saying no and allow people to take advantage of you. Many businesses encourage employees to take assertiveness training workshops to help them overcome shyness and resistance to communicating their needs. Such communication skills are also valuable in social relationships.

Exercise

One recent study found that taking a long walk can be effective at reducing anxiety and blood pressure. Another study showed that a brisk walk of as little as 10 minutes' duration can leave people feeling more relaxed and energetic for up to 2 hours. Regular exercise has even more benefits. Researchers have found that people who exercise regularly react with milder physical stress responses before, during, and after exposure to stressors, and that their overall sense of well-being increases as well. Although even light exercise—a brisk walk, an easy bike outing—can have a beneficial effect, an integrated fitness program like the one recommended in this book can have a significant impact on stress.

One warning: For some people, exercise can become just one more stressor in a highly stressed life. People who exercise compulsively risk overtraining, a condition characterized by fatigue, irritability, depression, and diminished athletic performance. An overly strenuous exercise program can even make a person sick by compromising immune function. For the details of a safe and effective exercise program, refer to Chapter 7.

Nutrition

As discussed in Chapter 8, a healthy, balanced diet will supply the energy needed to cope with stress. Two additional nutrition tips for stress management are to limit or avoid caffeine and to avoid the high-potency vitamin compounds and amino acid supplements designated as "stress formulas." (These supplements are worthless for reducing tension or anxiety.)

Meaningful connections with others can play a key role in stress management and overall wellness. A sense of isolation can lead to chronic stress, which in turn can increase one's susceptibility to temporary illnesses like colds and to chronic illnesses like heart disease. Although the mechanism isn't clear, social isolation can be as significant to mortality rates as factors like smoking, high blood pressure, and obesity.

There is no single best pattern of social support that works for everyone. However, research suggests that having a variety of types of relationships may be important for wellness. To help determine whether your social network measures up, circle whether each of the following statements is true or false for you.

T F **1.** If I needed an emergency loan of $100, there is someone I could get it from.

T F **2.** There is someone who takes pride in my accomplishments.

T F **3.** I often meet or talk with family or friends.

T F **4.** Most people I know think highly of me.

T F **5.** If I needed an early morning ride to the airport, there's no one I would feel comfortable asking to take me.

T F **6.** I feel there is no one with whom I can share my most private worries and fears.

T F **7.** Most of my friends are more successful making changes in their lives than I am.

T F **8.** I would have a hard time finding someone to go with me on a day trip to the beach or country.

To calculate your score, add the number of true answers to questions 1–4 and the number of false answers to questions 5–8. If your score is 4 or more, you should have enough support to protect your health. If your score is 3 or less, you may need to reach out. There are a variety of things you can do to strengthen your social ties:

- *Foster friendships.* Keep in regular contact with your friends. Offer respect, trust, and acceptance, and provide help and support in times of need. Express appreciation for your friends.
- *Keep your family ties strong.* Stay in touch with the family members you feel close to. Participate in family activities and celebrations. If your family doesn't function well as a support system for its members, create a second "family" of people with whom you have built meaningful ties.
- *Get involved with a group.* Do volunteer work, take a class, attend a lecture series, join a religious group. These types of activities can give you a sense of security, a place to talk about your feelings or concerns, and a way to build new friendships. Choose activities that are meaningful to you and that include direct involvement with other people.
- *Build your communication skills.* The more you share your feelings with others, the closer the bonds between you will become. When others are speaking, be a considerate and attentive listener.

Individual relationships change over the course of your life, but it's never too late to build friendships or become more involved in your community. Your investment of time and energy in your social network will pay off—in a brighter outlook now, and in better health and well-being for the future.

SOURCES: Friends can be good medicine. 1998. *Mind/Body Newsletter* 7(1): 3–6. Quiz from Japenga, A. 1995. A family of friends. *Health,* November/December, 94. Adapted with permission.

Sleep

Lack of sleep can be both a cause and an effect of excess stress. As described in Chapter 7, without sufficient sleep, our mental and physical processes steadily deteriorate. We get headaches, feel irritable, are unable to concentrate, forget things, and may be more susceptible to illness. Fatigue and sleep deprivation are major factors in many fatal car, truck, and train crashes. Adequate sleep, on the other hand, improves mood, fosters feelings of competence and self-worth, and supports optimal mental and emotional functioning. Make time in your busy schedule to obtain adequate sleep; if insomnia is a problem for you, refer to the tips in the box on p. 289.

Time Management

Learning to manage your time successfully can be crucial to coping with everyday stressors. Overcommitment, procrastination, and even boredom are significant stressors for many people. Along with gaining control of nutrition and exercise to maintain a healthy energy balance, time management is an important element in a wellness program. Try these strategies for improving your time-management skills:

- *Set priorities.* Divide your tasks into three groups: essential, important, and trivial. Focus on the first two. Ignore the third.
- *Schedule tasks for peak efficiency.* You've undoubtedly noticed you're most productive at certain times of the day (or night). Schedule as many of your tasks for those hours as you can and stick to your schedule.
- *Set realistic goals and write them down.* Attainable goals spur you on. Impossible goals, by definition, cause frustration and failure. Fully commit yourself to achieving your goals by putting them in writing.
- *Budget enough time.* For each project you undertake, calculate how long it will take to complete. Then tack on another 10–15%, or even 25%, as a buffer.

- *Break up long-term goals into short-term ones.* Instead of waiting for or relying on large blocks of time, use short amounts of time to start a project or keep it moving.
- *Visualize the achievement of your goals.* By mentally rehearsing your performance of a task, you will be able to reach your goal more smoothly.
- *Keep track of the tasks you put off.* Analyze the reasons why you procrastinate. If the task is difficult or unpleasant, look for ways to make it easier or more fun. For example, if you find the readings for one of your classes particularly difficult, choose an especially nice setting for your reading and then reward yourself each time you complete a section or chapter.
- *Consider doing your least-favorite tasks first.* Once you have the most unpleasant ones out of the way, you can work on the projects you enjoy more.
- *Consolidate tasks when possible.* For example, try walking to the store so that you run your errands and exercise in the same block of time.
- *Identify quick transitional tasks.* Keep a list of 5- to 10-minute tasks you can do while waiting or between other tasks, such as watering your plants, doing the dishes, or checking a homework assignment.
- *Delegate responsibility.* Asking for help when you have too much to do is no cop-out; it's good time management. Just don't delegate to others the jobs you know you should do yourself.
- *Say no when necessary.* If the demands made on you don't seem reasonable, say no—tactfully, but without guilt or apology.
- *Give yourself a break.* Allow time for play—free, unstructured time when you ignore the clock. Don't consider this a waste of time. Play renews you and enables you to work more efficiently.
- *Stop thinking or talking about what you're going to do, and just do it!* Sometimes the best solution for procrastination is to stop waiting for the right moment and just get started. You will probably find that things are not as bad as you feared, and your momentum will keep you going.

For more help with time management, complete Activity 10 in the Behavior Change Workbook at the end of the text.

Cognitive Techniques

Certain thought patterns and ways of thinking, including ideas, beliefs, and perceptions, can contribute to stress and have a negative impact on health. But other habits of mind, if practiced with patience and consistency, can help break unhealthy thought patterns. Below are some suggestions for changing destructive thinking.

- Modify expectations; they often restrict experience and lead to disappointment. Try to accept life as it comes.

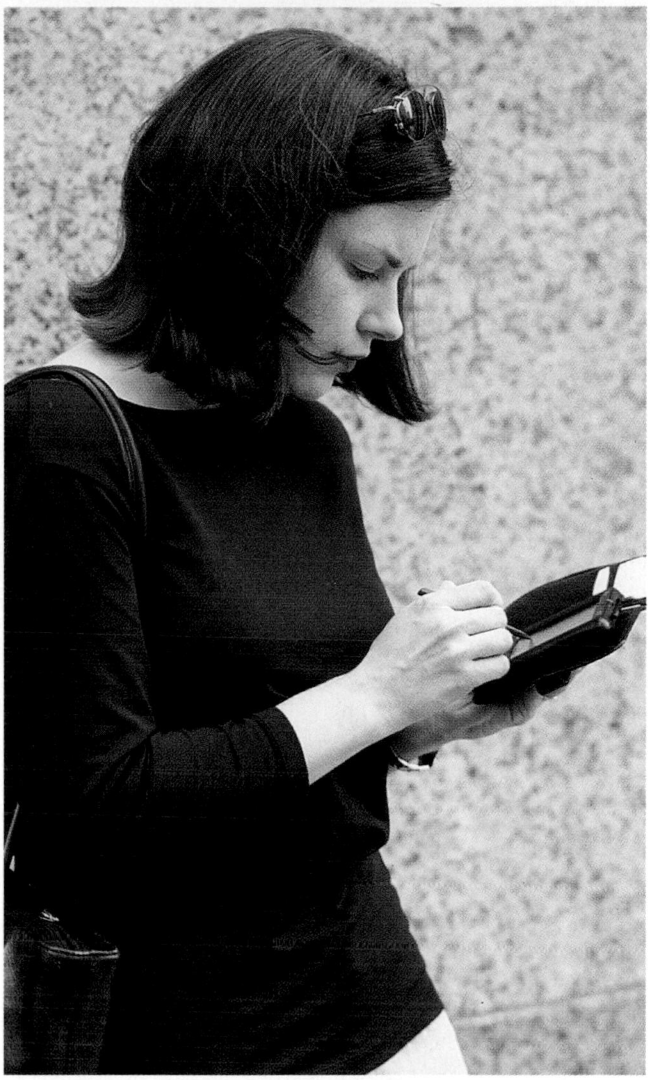

Managing the many commitments of adult life—including work, school, and relationships—can sometimes feel overwhelming and produce a great deal of stress. Time-management skills, including careful scheduling with a date book or handheld computer, can help people cope with busy days.

- Monitor your self-talk and attempt to minimize hostile, critical, suspicious, and self-deprecating thoughts (see the box "Realistic Self-Talk," p. 296).
- Problem-solve if you find yourself stewing over a task. State the problem in one or two sentences, identify its causes, consider alternative solutions, weigh the pros and cons for each alternative, choose a particular solution, and then act on your choice.
- Live in the present; clear your mind of old debris and fears for the future so you can enjoy life as it is now.
- "Go with the flow." Accept what you can't change; forgive faults; be flexible.
- Laugh. Seek out therapeutic humor (not dark or offensive humor, which is an unconscious means of dealing with fears). Laughter can temporarily elevate the heart rate, aid digestion, relax muscles, ease pain, and trigger the release of endorphins.

TAKE CHARGE Dealing with Anger

Anger is a natural response to something we perceive as a betrayal, injustice, threat, or other wrong—whether real or imagined. Angry responses include both emotions and physiological changes. Angry emotions can range from mild irritation to boiling mad, out-of-control rage. The body responds with faster heart and breathing rates, muscle tension, a "knot" in the stomach, trembling, or a red face. We can be angry with a person, a situation or condition, or ourselves. Anger is a useful emotion when it alerts us that something is wrong, and we respond with constructive action. But when anger gets out of control, it causes problems for ourselves and for others.

Managing Your Own Anger

How should you deal with anger? Popular wisdom has said that you should express rather than suppress anger to maintain psychological and physical wellness. However, recent studies have questioned this idea by showing that people who are overtly hostile seem to be at higher risk for heart attacks. Furthermore, angry words or actions won't contribute to wellness if they damage important personal or professional relationships or produce feelings of guilt or loss of control.

At one extreme are people who never express anger or any opinion that might offend others, even when their own rights and needs are being jeopardized. They may be chronically deprived of satisfaction at work and at home, and may find themselves stuck in unhealthy relationships. At the other extreme are people whose anger is explosive or misdirected. Explosive anger, or rage, renders people temporarily unable to think straight or act in their own best interest; in the long run, frequent expressions of rage increase the risk for heart disease.

What is the best approach to anger, then? Try looking at each situation and distinguishing between a gratuitous expression of anger and a reasonable level of self-assertiveness. If you feel your anger building, ask yourself whether the situation is really important enough to get angry about, whether you are truly justified in getting angry, and whether expressing your anger is going to make a positive difference. If you can answer "yes" to all three questions, then calm but assertive communication may be an appropriate response.

If your anger isn't reasonable, try distracting or calming yourself rather than expressing anger. First, try to reframe what you're thinking at that moment. You'll be less angry at another person if there is a possibility that his or her behavior was not intentionally directed against you. Did the driver who cut into your lane on the freeway do it deliberately to spite you, or did he simply fail to see you? Look for possible mitigating factors that would make you less likely to blame him: Maybe he's late for a job interview and preoccupied with worries. If you're angry because you've just been criticized, avoid mentally replaying scenes from the past when you received similar unjust criticisms. Think about what is happening now and act analytically rather than defensively. Why are you taking it personally? Why are you acting like a jerk just because she did?

Second, try to distract yourself to calm down. Use the old trick of counting to 10 before you respond, or start concentrating on your breathing. Imagine yourself in a peaceful place. If needed, take a longer cooling-off period by leaving the situation until your anger has subsided.

These techniques do not mean that you should permanently avoid issues and people who make you angry. If you've decided that an expression of anger is the best response, return to the issue when you've had a chance to think about it more clearly and are ready to express yourself calmly and clearly. Use "I"

Relaxation Techniques

First identified and described by Herbert Benson of Harvard Medical School, the **relaxation response** is a physiological state characterized by a feeling of warmth and quiet mental alertness. This response is the opposite of the fight-or-flight reaction. When the relaxation response is triggered by a relaxation technique, heart rate, breathing, and metabolism slow down; blood flow to the brain and skin increases; and brain waves shift from an alert beta rhythm to a relaxed alpha rhythm.

The techniques described in this section and in the box "Stress-Management Techniques from Around the World" (p. 297) are among the most popular techniques and the easiest to learn. All these techniques take practice, so it may be several weeks before the benefits become noticeable in everyday life.

Progressive Relaxation In this simple relaxation technique, you tense, then relax the muscles of the body one by one. Also known as deep muscle relaxation, this technique addresses the muscle tension that occurs when the body is experiencing stress. Consciously relaxing tensed muscles sends a message to other body systems to reduce the stress response.

To practice progressive relaxation, begin by inhaling as you contract your right fist. Then exhale as you release your fist. Repeat. Contract and relax your right bicep. Repeat. Do the same using your left arm. Then, working from forehead to feet, contract and relax other muscles. Repeat each contraction at least once, inhaling as you tense and exhaling as you relax. To speed up the process, tense and relax more muscles at one time—for example, both arms simultaneously. With practice you'll be able to relax quickly by simply clenching and releasing only your fists.

Terms

Vw

relaxation response A physiological state characterized by a feeling of warmth and quiet mental alertness.

statements ("I would like . . ." "I feel . . .") when expressing your feelings, and listen carefully to the other person's point of view. Negotiate a constructive solution; don't attack verbally and make demands. If you decide it's not appropriate to express your anger, don't stay stuck in the feeling by fuming, dwelling on the injustice of the situation, or thinking how to get back at the person indirectly later. Express your feelings in a constructive manner or move on.

If you have trouble expressing anger, you might explore training in assertiveness to help you learn to express your needs, desires, and opinions constructively. If, on the other hand, your anger is out of control, consider counseling. With counseling, a highly angry person can move closer to a middle range of anger in about two to three months.

Dealing with Anger in Other People

If someone you're with becomes very angry, respond "asymmetrically" by reacting not with anger but with calm. Try to validate the other person by acknowledging that he or she had some reason to be angry. This does not mean apologizing, if you don't think you're to blame, or accepting verbal abuse, which is always inappropriate. Try to focus on solving the problem by allowing the individual to explain why he or she is so angry and what can be done to alleviate the situations. For instance, instead of "Quit yelling at me!" you might say, "I realize you're upset because I erased your messages. Is there anything I can do to help you find out who called?" Finally, if the person cannot be calmed, it may be best to disengage, at least temporarily. After a time-out, a rational problem-solving approach may be more successful.

Warning Signs of Violence

It's normal to feel angry or frustrated when you've been let down or betrayed. But anger and frustration don't justify violent action. If you notice the following signs over a period of time, the potential for violence exists: a history of making threats and engaging in aggressive behavior; serious drug or alcohol use; gang membership; access to or fascination with weapons; feeling rejected or alone; withdrawal from friends and usual activities; poor school performance; having been a victim of bullying; feeling constantly disrespected; and failing to acknowledge the rights of others. If you see these immediate warning signs, violence is a serious possibility:

- Daily loss of temper or frequent physical fighting
- Significant vandalism or property damage
- Increased risk-taking behavior or use of drugs or alcohol
- Threats or detailed plans to commit acts of violence
- Pleasure in hurting animals
- Carrying a weapon

If you or someone you know shows warning signs of violence, get help. Don't spend time alone with people who show warning signs. If you are worried about being a victim of violence, get someone in authority to help you. Do not resort to violence or use a weapon to protect yourself. Instead, ask an experienced professional for help.

Visualization Visualization, also known as using imagery, is so effective in enhancing sports performance that it has become part of the curriculum at training camps for U.S. Olympic athletes. This same technique can be used to induce relaxation, to help change habits, or to improve performance on an exam, on stage, or on a playing field.

To practice visualization, imagine yourself floating on a cloud, sitting on a mountaintop, or lying in a meadow. Try to identify all the perceptible qualities of the environment—sight, sound, temperature, smell, and so on. Your body will respond as if your imagery were real.

An alternative is to close your eyes and imagine a deep purple light filling your body. Then change the color into a soothing gold. As the color lightens, so should your distress. Imagery can also enhance performance: Visualize yourself succeeding at a task that worries you.

Deep Breathing Your breathing pattern is closely tied to your stress level. Deep, slow breathing is associated with relaxation. Rapid, shallow, often irregular breathing occurs during the stress response. With practice, you can learn to slow and quiet your breathing pattern, thereby also quieting your mind and relaxing your body. Try one of the breathing techniques described in the box "Breathing for Relaxation" (p. 298) for on-the-spot tension relief, as well as for long-term stress reduction.

Listening to Music Music can relax us. It has been shown to influence pulse, blood pressure, and the electrical activity of muscles. Studies of newborns and those hospitalized because of stroke have shown that listening to soothing, lyrical music can lessen depression, anxiety, and stress levels.

To experience the stress-management benefits of music yourself, set aside a time to listen. Choose music you enjoy and selections that make you feel relaxed.

Other Techniques

Other stress-management techniques, such as biofeedback, hypnosis and self-hypnosis, and massage, require a

TAKE CHARGE Realistic Self-Talk

Do your patterns of thinking make events seem worse than they truly are? Do negative beliefs about yourself become self-fulfilling prophecies? Substituting realistic self-talk for negative self-talk can help you build and maintain self-esteem and cope better with the challenges in your life. Here are some examples of common types of distorted, negative self-talk, along with suggestions for more accurate and rational responses.

Cognitive Distortion	Negative Self-Talk	Realistic Self-Talk
Focusing on negatives	School is so discouraging—nothing but one hassle after another.	School is pretty challenging and has its difficulties, but there certainly are rewards. It's really a mixture of good and bad.
Expecting the worst	Why would my boss want to meet with me this afternoon if not to fire me?	I wonder why my boss wants to meet with me. I guess I'll just have to wait and see.
Overgeneralizing	(After getting a poor grade on a paper) Just as I thought—I'm incompetent at everything.	I'll start working on the next paper earlier. That way, if I run into problems, I'll have time to consult with the TA.
Minimizing	I won the speech contest, but none of the other speakers was very good. I wouldn't have done as well against stiffer competition.	It may not have been the best speech I'll ever give, but it was good enough to win the contest. I'm really improving as a speaker.
Blaming others	I wouldn't have eaten so much last night if my friends hadn't insisted on going to that restaurant.	I overdid it last night. Next time I'll make different choices.
Expecting perfection	I should have scored 100% on this test. I can't believe I missed that one problem through a careless mistake.	Too bad I missed one problem through carelessness, but overall I did very well on this test. Next time I'll be more careful.

SOURCE: Excerpt from *Stress Management for Wellness,* 3d ed., by Walt Schafer. Copyright © 1996 by Holt, Rinehart, and Winston. Reprinted by permission of the publisher.

partner or professional training or assistance. As with the relaxation techniques presented, all take practice, and it may be several weeks before the benefits are noticeable.

Biofeedback Biofeedback helps people reduce their response to stress by enabling them to become more aware of their level of physiological arousal. In biofeedback some measure of stress—perspiration, heart rate, skin temperature, or muscle tension—is mechanically monitored, and feedback is given using sound (a tone or music), light, or a meter or dial. With practice, people begin to exercise conscious control over their physiological stress responses. The point of biofeedback training is to develop the ability to transfer the skill to daily life without the use of electronic equipment. Biofeedback initially requires the help of a therapist, stress counselor, or technician.

Hypnosis and Self-Hypnosis Hypnosis, a mental focusing technique that can profoundly affect the body, has been a part of healing since ancient times. Today hypnosis is being used to help correct eating disorders, help people stop smoking, alleviate cancer pain, and hasten recovery from surgery. Many people have misconceptions about hypnosis and may associate it with sleep. But in sleep one's focus of attention dissolves, whereas in hypnosis it intensifies. A pioneer of medical hypnosis describes hypnosis as an "attentive perception and concentration, which leads to controlled imagination." Using that controlled imagination lets participants choose to feel something other than anxiety or stress or pain. Hypnosis works well for the subset of people who respond easily to being hypnotized. That same subset can be trained in self-hypnosis. In a sense, all hypnosis can be seen as self-hypnosis.

Massage Massage, the manipulation of the body's tissues, is a time-honored part of health and medicine. Massage is known to subdue the stress response, diminish depression, and even increase alertness, though no one knows exactly how. Nowadays many workers are taking a few minutes at their office for a weekly back rub as a way of reducing stress. In a study of English medical workers, those who got 10 weekly rubdowns outscored their colleagues on timed math tests.

Although there are many ways in which massage helps our minds and bodies, the effects can be most dramatic with diseases that have stress as a small or even major component. Massage has been used successfully with premature

The origins of techniques for relaxation span many continents and many centuries. Three techniques that are growing in popularity in the United States are meditation, hatha yoga, and tai chi. Although you may not choose to adopt the philosophical bases of these techniques, all of them can help you manage stress by promoting the relaxation response.

Meditation

At its most basic level, meditation, or self-reflective thought, involves quieting or emptying the mind to achieve deep relaxation. Some practitioners of meditation view it on a deeper level as a means of focusing concentration, increasing self-awareness, and bringing enlightenment to their lives. The origins of meditation can be traced back to the sixth century B.C. in Asia. Meditation has been integrated into the practices of several religions—Buddhism, Hinduism, Confucianism, Taoism—but it is not a religion itself, nor does its practice require any special knowledge, belief, or background.

There are two general styles of meditation, centered around different ways of quieting the mind. In exclusive meditation, one focuses on a single word or thought, eliminating all others. In inclusive meditation, the mind is allowed to wander uncontrolled from thought to thought, but one must observe these thoughts in a detached way, without judgment or emotion. Exclusive meditation tends to be easier to learn. Several years ago, Herbert Benson developed a simple, practical technique for eliciting the relaxation response using exclusive meditation:

1. Pick a word, phrase, or object to focus on. You can choose a word or phrase that has a deep meaning for you, but any word or phrase will work. In Zen meditation, the word *mu* (literally, "absolutely nothing") is often used. Some meditators prefer to focus on their breathing.
2. Sit comfortably in a quiet place. Close your eyes if you're not focusing on an object.
3. Relax your muscles.
4. Breathe slowly and naturally. If you're using a focus word or phrase, silently repeat it each time you exhale. If you're using an object, focus on it as you breathe.
5. Keep your attitude passive. Disregard thoughts that drift in.
6. Continue for 10–20 minutes once or twice a day.
7. After you've finished, sit quietly for a few minutes with your eyes closed, then open. Then stand up.

Allow relaxation to occur at its own pace, don't try to force it. Don't be surprised if you can't tune your mind out for more than a few seconds at a time. It's nothing to get angry about. The more you ignore the intrusions, the easier it will become. If you want to time your session, peek at a watch or clock occasionally, but don't set a jarring alarm.

The technique works best on an empty stomach, before a meal or about 2 hours after eating. Avoid times of day when you're tired, unless you want to fall asleep.

Although you'll feel refreshed even after the first session, it may take a month or more to get noticeable results. Be patient. Eventually the relaxation response will become so natural that it will occur spontaneously or on demand when you sit quietly for a few moments.

Hatha Yoga

Yoga is an ancient Sanskrit word meaning "union"; it refers specifically to the union of mind, body, and soul and for some serves as a preliminary to meditation. The development and practice of yoga are rooted in the Hindu philosophy of spiritual enlightenment. The founders of yoga developed a system of physical postures, called *asanas,* designed to cleanse the body, unlock energy paths, and raise the level of consciousness.

Although there are many kinds of yoga, the one most commonly practiced in the Western world is hatha yoga. It emphasizes physical balance and breathing control. It also integrates components of flexibility, muscular strength and endurance, and muscle relaxation.

A session of hatha yoga typically involves a series of *asanas* held for a few seconds to several minutes. The combination of stretching and *asanas* can be very relaxing, as long as one stretches to the point of relaxation and not to the point of pain or injury. There are hundreds of different *asanas,* and they must be performed correctly to be beneficial. For this reason, qualified instruction is recommended, particularly for beginners. Yoga classes are offered through many community recreation centers, YMCAs and YWCAs, and private clubs. Regardless of whether you accept the philosophy and symbolism of different *asanas,* the practice of yoga can induce the relaxation response as well as develop flexibility, muscular strength and endurance, and body awareness.

Tai Chi Chuan

A martial art that developed in China, tai chi chuan (pronounced "tie JEE choo-on" and often called simply "tai chi") has in recent years become a popular form of exercise in the United States. Its movements, called forms, resemble a slow, graceful dance that mimics animals such as the snake and the crane. At its core is the Taoist belief that good health results from balanced *chi,* an energy force that surrounds and permeates all things. The forms, which can be practiced almost anywhere, are performed to help balance the body's chi to promote health and spiritual growth. The goal is to become calm and centered and to conserve and concentrate energy. Tai chi's slow, graceful movements reinforce the idea of moving *with* rather than *against* the stressors of everyday life. Researchers have found that tai chi is an appropriate activity for people of all ages and that it helps older adults safely boost their level of physical functioning.

The practice of tai chi promotes relaxation and concentration as well as the development of body awareness, balance, muscular strength and endurance, and flexibility. It usually takes some time and practice to reap the stress-management benefits of tai chi, and, as with yoga, it's best to begin with some qualified instruction.

SOURCES: Adapted from Li, F., et al. 2001. An evaluation of the effects of tai chi exercise on physical function among older persons: A randomized controlled trial. *Annals of Behavioral Medicine* 23:139–146. Seaward, B. L. 1999: *Managing Stress: Principles and Strategies for Health and Wellbeing,* Web-enhanced 2d ed. Boston: Jones and Bartlett. Can yoga make you fit? 1997. *University of California, Berkeley Wellness Letter,* May. Benson, H., with W. Proctor. 1984. *Beyond the Relaxation Response.* New York: Times Books.

TAKE CHARGE Breathing for Relaxation

Diaphragmatic Breathing

1. Lie on your back with your body relaxed.
2. Place one hand on your chest and one on your abdomen. (You will use your hands to monitor the depth and location of your breathing.)
3. Inhale slowly and deeply through your nose into your abdomen. Your abdomen should push up as far as is comfortable. Your chest should expand only a little and only in conjunction with the movement of your abdomen.
4. Exhale gently through your mouth.
5. Continue for about 5–10 minutes per session. Focus on the sound and feel of your breathing.

Breathing In Relaxation, Breathing Out Tension

1. Assume a comfortable position, lying on your back or sitting in a chair.
2. Inhale slowly and deeply into your abdomen. Imagine the inhaled, warm air flowing to all parts of your body. Say to yourself, "Breathe in relaxation."
3. Exhale from your abdomen. Imagine tension flowing out of your body. Say to yourself. "Breathe out tension."
4. Pause before you inhale.
5. Continue for 5–10 minutes or until no tension remains.

Chest Expansion

1. Sit in a comfortable chair or stand.
2. Inhale slowly and deeply into your abdomen as you raise your arms out to the sides. Pull your shoulders and arms back and lift your chin slightly so that your chest opens up.
3. Exhale gradually as you lower your arms and chin and return to the starting position.
4. Repeat five to ten times or until your breathing is deep and regular and your body feels relaxed and energized.

Quick Tension Release

1. Inhale into your abdomen slowly and deeply as you count slowly to 4.
2. Exhale slowly as you again count slowly to 4. As you exhale, concentrate on relaxing your face, neck, shoulders, and chest.
3. Repeat several times. With each exhalation, feel more tension leaving your body.

SOURCES: Stop stress with a deep breath. 1996. *Health*, October, 53. Breathing for health and relaxation. 1995. *Mental Medicine Update* 4(2): 3–6. When you're stressed, catch your breath. 1995. *Mayo Clinic Health Letter,* December, 5.

infants to help them gain weight and with asthmatics to improve lung functioning and lessen their anxiety. It has also been used successfully with men who have HIV to strengthen their immune systems and significantly reduce their anxiety.

Counterproductive Coping Strategies

College is a time when you'll learn to adapt to new and challenging situations and gain skills that will last a lifetime. It is also a time when many people develop habits, in response to stress, that are counterproductive and unhealthy and that may also last well beyond graduation.

- *Tobacco:* The nicotine in cigarettes and other tobacco products can make you feel relaxed and even increase your ability to concentrate, but it is highly addictive. Smoking causes cancer, heart disease, impotence, and many other health problems and is the leading preventable cause of death in the United States.
- *Alcohol:* Having a few drinks might make you feel temporarily at ease, and drinking until you're intoxicated may help you forget your current stressors. However, using alcohol to deal with stress places you at risk for all the short-term and long-term problems associated with alcohol abuse. It also does nothing to address the actual causes of stress in your life.
- *Other drugs:* Altering your body chemistry in order to cope with stress is a strategy that has many pitfalls and does not directly address your stressors. For example, caffeine raises cortisol levels and blood pressure and disrupts sleep. Marijuana can elicit panic attacks with repeated use, and some research suggests that it enhances the stress response.
- *Binge eating:* The feelings of satiation and sedation that follow eating produce a relaxed state that reduces stress. However, regular use of eating as a means of coping with stress may lead to binge eating, a risky behavior associated with weight gain and eating disorders.

For more on these unhealthy coping techniques, refer to Chapters 9 and 13.

GETTING HELP

You can use the principles of behavioral self-management described in Chapter 1 to create a stress-management program tailored specifically to your needs. The starting

CRITICAL CONSUMER Choosing and Evaluating Mental Health Professionals

College students are usually in a good position to find convenient, affordable mental health care. Larger schools typically have both health services that employ psychiatrists and psychologists and counseling centers staffed by professionals and peer counselors. Resources in the community may include a school of medicine, a hospital, and a variety of professionals who work independently. It's a good idea to get recommendations from physicians, clergy, friends who have been in therapy, or community agencies rather than to pick a name at random.

Financial considerations are also important. Find out how much different services will cost and what your health insurance will cover. If you're not adequately covered by a health plan, don't let that stop you from getting help; investigate low-cost alternatives on campus and in your community. The cost of treatment is linked to how many therapy sessions will be needed, which in turn depends on the type of therapy and the nature of the problem. Psychological therapies focusing on specific problems may require eight or ten sessions at weekly intervals. Therapies aiming for psychological awareness and personality change can last months or years.

Deciding whether a therapist is right for you will require meeting the therapist in person. Before or during your first meeting, find out about the therapist's background and training:

- Does she or he have a degree from an appropriate professional school and a state license to practice?
- Has she or he had experience treating people with problems similar to yours?
- How much will therapy cost?

You have a right to know the answers to these questions and should not hesitate to ask them. After your initial meeting, evaluate your impressions:

- Does the therapist seem like a warm, intelligent person who would be able to help you and is interested in doing so?
- Are you comfortable with the personality, values, and beliefs of the therapist?
- Is he or she willing to talk about the techniques in use? Do these techniques make sense to you?

If you answer yes to these questions, this therapist may be satisfactory for you. If you feel uncomfortable—and you're not in need of emergency care—it's worthwhile to set up one-time consultations with one or two others before you make up your mind. Take the time to find someone who feels right for you.

Later in your treatment, evaluate your progress:

- Are you being helped by the treatment?
- If you are displeased, is it because you aren't making progress or because therapy is raising difficult, painful issues you don't want to deal with?
- Can you express dissatisfaction to your therapist? Such feedback can improve your treatment.

If you're convinced your therapy isn't working or is harmful, thank your therapist for her or his efforts and find another.

point of a successful program is to listen to your body. When you learn to recognize the stress response and the emotions and thoughts that accompany it, you'll be in a position to take charge of how you handle stress. Labs 10.1 and 10.2 can guide you in identifying and finding ways to cope with stress-inducing situations. (Appendix A has some specific guidelines for coping after terrorism or mass violence.)

If you feel you need guidance beyond the information in this text, excellent self-help guides can be found in bookstores or the library; helpful Web sites are listed in For Further Exploration at the end of the chapter. Some people also find it helpful to express their feelings in a journal. Grappling with a painful experience in this way provides an emotional release and can help you develop more constructive ways of dealing with similar situations in the future.

Peer Counseling and Support Groups

If you have attempted to fashion a stress-management program to cope with the stressors in your life but still feel overwhelmed, you may want to seek outside help. Peer counseling, often available through the student health center or student affairs office, is usually staffed by volunteer students with special training that emphasizes maintaining confidentiality. Peer counselors can steer those seeking help to appropriate campus and community resources or just offer sympathetic listening.

Support groups are typically organized around a particular issue or problem: all group members might be entering a new school, reentering school after an interruption, struggling with single parenting, experiencing eating disorders, or coping with particular kinds of trauma. Simply voicing concerns that others share can relieve stress.

Professional Help

Psychotherapy, especially a short-term course of sessions, can also be tremendously helpful in dealing with stress-related problems. Not all therapists are right for all people, so it's a good idea to shop around for a compatible psychotherapist with reasonable fees. (See the box "Choosing and Evaluating Mental Health Professionals.")

Is It Stress or Something More Serious?

Most of us have had periods of feeling down when we become pessimistic, anxious, less energetic, and less able to enjoy life. Such feelings and thoughts can be normal responses to the ordinary challenges of life. Symptoms that may indicate a more serious problem that requires professional help include the following:

- Depression, anxiety, or other emotional problems begin to interfere seriously with school or work performance or in getting along with others.
- Suicide is attempted or is seriously considered (see below).
- Symptoms such as hallucinations, delusions, incoherent speech, or loss of memory occur.
- Alcohol or drugs are used to the extent that they impair normal functioning; finding or taking drugs occupies much of the week; or reducing the dosage leads to psychological or physical withdrawal symptoms.

Depression is of particular concern because severe depression is linked to suicide, one of the leading causes of death among college students. In some cases, depression, like severe stress, is a clear-cut reaction to a specific event, such as the loss of a loved one or failing in school or work. In other cases, no trigger event is obvious. Symptoms of depression include the following:

- Negative self-concept
- Pervasive feelings of sadness and hopelessness
- Loss of pleasure in usual activities
- Poor appetite and weight loss
- Insomnia or disturbed sleep
- Restlessness or fatigue
- Thoughts of worthlessness and guilt
- Trouble concentrating or making decisions
- Thoughts of death or suicide

Not all of these symptoms are present in everyone who is depressed, but most do experience a loss of interest or pleasure in their usual activities. Warning signs of suicide include expressing the wish to be dead; revealing contemplated suicide methods; increasing social withdrawal and isolation; and a sudden, inexplicable lightening of mood (which can indicate the person has finally decided to commit suicide). If you are severely depressed or know someone who is, expert help from a mental health professional is essential. Most communities have emergency help available, often in the form of a hotline telephone counseling service, and many colleges have health services and counseling centers that can provide help. Treatments for depression and many other psychological disorders are highly effective.

Tips for Today

Some stress is unavoidable in life. How you respond to it is what determines whether you become "stressed out" or maintain your serenity. For the stress you can't avoid, develop a range of stress-management techniques and strategies.

Right now you can

- Sit in a comfortable chair and practice deep breathing for 5 to 10 minutes.
- Visualize a relaxing, peaceful place and imagine yourself experiencing it as vividly as possible; you might "feel" a gentle breeze on your skin or "hear" the soothing sound of a waterfall. Stay there as long as you can.
- Stand up and do some stretching exercises, such as gently rolling your head from side to side, stretching your arms out in front of your body and over your head, and slowly bending over and letting your arms hang toward the floor.
- Get out your datebook and schedule what you'll be doing the rest of today and tomorrow. Pencil in a short walk and a conversation with a friend. Plan to go to bed 15 minutes earlier than usual.

SUMMARY

- Stress is the collective physiological and emotional response to any stressor. Physiological responses to stressors are the same for everyone.
- The autonomic nervous system and the endocrine system are responsible for the body's physical response to stressors. The sympathetic nervous system mobilizes the body and activates key hormones of the endocrine system, causing the fight-or-flight reaction. The parasympathetic system returns the body to homeostasis.
- Behavioral responses to stress are controlled by the somatic nervous system and fall under a person's conscious control.
- The general adaptation syndrome model and research in psychoneuroimmunology contribute to our understanding of the links between stress and disease. People who have many stressors in their lives or handle stress poorly are at risk for cardiovascular disease, impairment of the immune system, and many other problems.
- Potential sources of stress include major life changes, daily hassles, college- and job-related stressors, and interpersonal and social stressors.
- Positive ways of managing stress include support from other people, clear communication, regular exercise, good nutrition, effective time management, cognitive techniques, and other relaxation techniques.
- If a personal program for stress management doesn't work, peer counseling, support groups, and psychotherapy are available.

COMMON QUESTIONS ANSWERED

Are there any relaxation techniques I can use in response to an immediate stressor? There are various strategies for dealing with stressors on the spot. In addition to the deep breathing techniques described in the chapter, try some of the following to see which ones work best for you:

- Do a full-body stretch while standing or sitting. Stretch your arms out to the sides and then reach them as far as possible over your head. Rotate your body from the waist. Bend over as far as is comfortable for you.
- Do a partial session of progressive muscle relaxation. Tense and then relax some of the muscles in your body. Focus on the muscles that are stiff or tense. Shake out your arms and legs.
- Take a short, brisk walk (3–5 minutes). Breathe deeply.
- Engage in realistic self-talk about the stressor. Mentally rehearse dealing successfully with the stressor. As an alternative, focus your mind on some other activity.

Can stress cause headaches? Stress is one possible cause of the most common type of headache, the tension headache. About 90% of all headaches are tension headaches, characterized by a dull, steady pain, usually on both sides of the head. It may feel as though a band of pressure is tightening around the head, and the pain may extend to the neck and shoulders. Acute tension headaches may last from hours to days, while chronic tension headaches may occur almost every day for months or even years. Stress, poor postures, and immobility are leading causes of tension headaches. There is no cure, but the pain can be relieved with over-the-counter painkillers; many people also try such therapies as massage, relaxation, hot or cold showers, and rest. Stress is also one possible trigger of migraine headaches, which are typically characterized by throbbing pain (often on one side of the head), heightened sensitivity to light, visual disturbances such as flashing lights, nausea, and fatigue.

If your headaches are frequent, keep a journal with details about the events surrounding each one. Are your tension headaches associated with late nights, academic deadlines, or long periods spent sitting at a computer? Are migraines associated with certain foods, stress, fatigue, specific sounds or odors, or (in women) menstruation? If you can identify the stressors or other factors that are consistently associated with your headaches, you can begin to gain more control over the situation. If you suffer persistent tension headaches, you should consult your physician.

What is Type A personality, and how does it relate to stress? While investigating links between personality and heart disease, cardiologists Meyer Friedman and Ray Rosenman reported that people with certain personality characteristics had a higher incidence of heart disease than others. They describe people with "Type A" personalities as ultracompetitive, controlling, impatient, aggressive, and hostile. "Type B" individuals, on the other hand, are relaxed, contemplative, and much less hurried; they tend to be less frustrated by the flow of daily events and more tolerant of the behavior of others. Recent evidence has suggested that only certain characteristics of the Type A pattern—anger, hostility, and cynicism—increase heart disease risk (see Chapter 11). However, Type A people tend to react more explosively to stressors, and they are upset by events that others would consider only mild annoyances.

People with a "hardy" personality, as described by psychologist Suzanne Kobasa, have a particular form of optimism that helps them deal more successfully with stress. They view potential stressors as challenges and opportunities for growth and learning, rather than as burdens. Hardy people tend to perceive fewer situations as stressful, and their reaction to stressors tend to be less intense. They typically have an internal locus of control and feel at least partly in control of events in their lives.

Is there anything you can do to change your personality and become more stress-resistant? It is unlikely that you can change your basic personality. However, you can change your typical behaviors and patterns of thinking and develop positive techniques for coping with stress.

FOR FURTHER EXPLORATION

Fit and Well Online Learning Center (www.mhhe.com/fahey5e)

Use the learning objectives, study guide questions, and glossary flash cards to review key terms and concepts and prepare for exams. You can extend your knowledge of stress and gain experience in using the Internet as a resource by completing the activities and checking out the Web links for the topics in Chapter 10 marked with the World Wide Web icon. For this chapter, Internet activities explore college stressors, social support, and sleep; there are Web links for the Critical Consumer box on mental health professionals and the chapter as a whole.

Daily Fitness and Nutrition Journal

Engaging in regular physical activity and eating a healthy diet are two important strategies for successful stress management. Continue to use your journal to monitor your exercise program and, if needed, to keep records of your diet. You can also use your fitness and nutrition journal as a model for creating a stress-management journal. The Online Learning Center has samples of other types of journals you might choose to keep during a behavior change program.

Health*Quest*

Learn more about your current stress level and techniques for managing stress by reviewing the resources and completing the activities in the stress-management module of the HealthQuest CD-ROM. You'll find assessments that evaluate your current stressors and mental wellness status. The Cyberstress exploration evaluates how you deal with the stressors encountered in a sample day and provides tips on a variety of stress-management techniques, including social support, time management, yoga, relaxation techniques, and conflict resolution. To determine if you're ready to make changes in your stress-related behavior, complete the Stages of Change quiz. You'll receive an assessment of your stage plus advice on moving forward toward the action and maintenance stages.

Books

Benson, H. 2000. *The Relaxation Response*. New York: Avon, Wholecare. *An expanded and updated edition of the 1975 classic on relaxation techniques and their physical benefits.*

Dement, W. C. 1999. *The Promise of Sleep*. New York: Delacorte. *An exploration of sleep and its effects on wellness by a prominent sleep researcher; for more information on Dement's research, go to* http://www.SleepQuest.com.

Justice, B. 2000. *Who Gets Sick: How Beliefs, Moods and Thoughts Affect Health*. Los Angeles, Calif.: Jeremy Tarcher. *Explores what is known today about the role of thought and emotion in health and illness.*

Sapolsky, R. M. 1998. *Why Zebras Don't Get Ulcers: An Updated Guide to Stress-Related Diseases, and Coping*. New York: W. H. Freeman. *An entertaining look at the effects of stress on the body and the relationship between stress and disease.*

Smith, J. C. 2002. *Stress Management: A Comprehensive Handbook of Techniques and Strategies*. New York: Springer. A guide to all types of techniques for managing stress.

WW Organizations and Web Sites

American Psychological Association. Provides information on stress management and psychological disorders.
202-336-5500; 800-964-2000 (referrals)
http://www.apa.org; http://helping.apa.org

Association for Applied Psychophysiology and Biofeedback. Provides information and links about biofeedback.
http://www.aapb.org

Center for Anxiety and Stress Treatment. A commercial site that includes an anxiety symptom checklist and stress-busting tips for work stress.
http://www.stressrelease.com

The Humor Project. A clearinghouse for information and practical ideas related to humor.
518-587-8770
http://www.humorproject.com

National Institute of Mental Health (NIMH). Offers information about stress and stress management as well as other aspects of psychological health, including anxiety, depression, and eating disorders.
800-421-4211; 301-443-4513
http://www.nimh.nih.gov

National Institute for Occupational Safety and Health (NIOSH). Provides information and links on job stress.
http://www.cdc.gov/niosh/stresshp.html

National Sleep Foundation. Provides information about sleep and how to overcome sleep problems such as insomnia and jet lag; brochures are available from the Web site or via fax.
202-347-3471; 202-347-3472
http://www.sleepfoundation.org

Student Counseling Virtual Pamphlet Collection. Links to online pamphlets from student counseling centers at colleges and universities across the country; topics include stress, sleep, and time management.
http://counseling.uchicago.edu/vpc

SELECTED BIBLIOGRAPHY

American Psychological Association. 1999. *Warning Signs: A Violence Prevention Guide for Youth from MTV and APA* (http://helping.apa.org/warningsigns; retrieved October 10, 1999).

Bremner, J. D. 1999. Does stress damage the brain? *Biological Psychiatry* 45(7): 797–805.

Cerbone, F. G., and C. L. Larison. 2000. A bibliographic essay: The relationship between stress and substance use. *Substance Use and Misuse* 35(5): 757–786.

Clements, K., and G. Turpin. 2000. Life event exposure, physiological reactivity, and psychological strain. *Journal of Behavioral Medicine* 23(1): 73–94.

Danner, D. D., D. A. Snowdon, and W. W. Friesen. 2001. Positive emotions in early life and longevity: Findings from the nun study. *Journal of Personality and Social Psychology* 80(5): 804–813.

de Quervain, D. J., et al. 2000. Acute cortisone administration impairs retrieval of long-term declarative memory in humans. *Nature Neuroscience* 3(4): 313–314.

Field, T. 1999. Massage therapy: More than a laying on of hands. *Contemporary Pediatrics* 16(5): 77.

Gang, A., et al. 2001. Psychological stress perturbs epidermal permeability barrier homeostasis: Implications for the pathogenesis of stress-associated skin disorders. *Archives of Dermatology* 137(1): 53–59.

Higher Education Research Institute. 2000. *An Overview of the 1999 Freshman Norms* (http://www.gseis.ucla.edu/heri/test/ executive.htm).

Kimata, H. 2001. Effect of humor on allergen-induced wheal reactions. *Journal of the American Medical Association* 285(6): 738.

Lacey, K., et al. 2000. A prospective study of neuroendocrine and immune alterations associated with the stress of an oral academic examination among graduate students. *Psychoneuroendocrinology* 25(4): 339–356.

Laitinen, J., E. Ek, and U. Sovio. 2002. Stress-related eating and drinking behavior and body mass index and predictors of this behavior. *Preventive Medicine* 34(1): 29–39.

Lucini, D., et al. 2002. Hemodynamic and autonomic adjustments to real life stress conditions in humans. *Hypertension* 39(1): 184–188.

McEwen, B. S. 1998. Protective and damaging effects of stress mediators. *New England Journal of Medicine* 338(3): 171–179.

McKinney, C. H., et al. 1997. Effects of guided imagery and music (GIM) therapy on mood and cortisol in healthy adults. *Health Psychology* 16(4): 390–400.

Nordstrom, C. K., et al. 2001. Work-related stress and early atherosclerosis. *Epedemiology* 12(2): 180–185.

Pashkow, F. J. 1999. Is stress linked to heart disease? The evidence grows stronger. *Cleveland Clinic Journal of Medicine* 66(2): 75–77.

Rothwell, J. D. 2000. *In the Company of Others: An Introduction to Communication*. Mountain View, Calif.: Mayfield.

Scheufele, P. M. 2000. Effects of progressive relaxation and classical music on measurements of attention, relaxation, and stress responses. *Journal of Behavioral Medicine* 23(2): 207–228.

Shepard, J. D., et al. 2000. Additive pressure effects of caffeine and stress in male medical students at risk for hypertension. *American Journal of Hypertension* 13(5 Pt. 1): 475–481.

Siegman, A. W., et al. 2000. Antagonistic behavior, dominance, hostility, and coronary heart disease. *Psychosomatic Medicine* 62(2): 248–257.

Skirka, N. 2000. The relationship of hardiness, sense of coherence, sports participation, and gender to perceived stress and psychological symptoms among college students. *Journal of Sports Medicine and Physical Fitness* 40(1): 63–70.

Steptoe, A., M. Cropley, and K. Joekes. 2000. Task demands and the pressures of everyday life: Associations between cardiovascular reactivity and work blood pressure and heart rate. *Healthy Psychology* 19(1): 46–54.

Takkouche, B., C. Regueira, and J. J. Gestal-Otero. 2001. A cohort study of stress and the common cold. *Epidemiology* 12(3): 345–349.

Taylor, S. E., et al. 2000. Biobehavioral responses to stress in females. Tend-and-befriend, not fight-or-flight. *Psychological Review* 107(3): 411–429.

Name ______________________ Section ______________ Date ______________

LAB 10.1 *Identifying Your Stress Level and Key Stressors*

How Stressed Are You?

To help determine how much stress you experience on a daily basis, answer the following questions.

How many of the symptoms of excess stress in the list below do you experience frequently? __________

Symptoms of Excess Stress

Physical Symptoms
Dry mouth
Excessive perspiration
Frequent illnesses
Gastrointestinal problems
Grinding of teeth
Headaches
High blood pressure
Pounding heart
Stiff neck or aching lower back

Emotional Symptoms
Anxiety or edginess
Depression
Fatigue
Hypervigilance
Impulsiveness
Inability to concentrate
Irritability
Trouble remembering things

Behavioral Symptoms
Crying
Disrupted eating habits
Disrupted sleeping habits
Harsh treatment of others
Problems communicating
Sexual problems
Social isolation
Increased use of tobacco, alcohol, or other drugs

Yes	No	
_____	_____	1. Are you easily startled or irritated?
_____	_____	2. Are you increasingly forgetful?
_____	_____	3. Do you have trouble falling or staying asleep?
_____	_____	4. Do you continually worry about events in your future?
_____	_____	5. Do you feel as if you are constantly under pressure to produce?
_____	_____	6. Do you frequently use tobacco, alcohol, or other drugs to help you relax?
_____	_____	7. Do you often feel as if you have less energy than you need to finish the day?
_____	_____	8. Do you have recurrent stomachaches or headaches?
_____	_____	9. Is it difficult for you to find satisfaction in simple life pleasures?
_____	_____	10. Are you often disappointed in yourself and others?
_____	_____	11. Are you overly concerned with being liked or accepted by others?
_____	_____	12. Have you lost interest in intimacy or sex?
_____	_____	13. Are you concerned that you do not have enough money?

Experiencing some of the stress-related symptoms or answering "yes" to a few questions is normal. However, if you experience a large number of stress symptoms or you answered "yes" to a majority of the questions, you are likely experiencing a high level of stress. Take time out to develop effective stress-management techniques. Many coping strategies that can aid you in dealing with your college stressors are described in this chapter. Additionally, your school's counseling center can provide valuable support.

Weekly Stress Log

Now that you are familiar with the signals of stress, complete the weekly stress log to map patterns in your stress levels and identify sources of stress. Enter a score for each hour of each day according to the ratings listed below.

	A.M.							P.M.												
	6	7	8	9	10	11	12	1	2	3	4	5	6	7	8	9	10	11	12	*Average*
Monday																				
Tuesday																				
Wednesday																				
Thursday																				
Friday																				
Saturday																				
Sunday																				
Average																				

Ratings: 1 = No anxiety; general feeling of well-being
2 = Mild anxiety; no interference with activity
3 = Moderate anxiety; specific signal(s) of stress present
4 = High anxiety; interference with activity
5 = Very high anxiety and panic reactions; general inability to engage in activity

To identify daily or weekly patterns in your stress level, average your stress rating for each hour and each day. For example, if your scores for 6:00 A.M. are 3, 3, 4, 3, and 4, with blanks for Saturday and Sunday, your 6:00 A.M. rating would be 17 ÷ 5, or 3.4 (moderate to high anxiety). Finally, calculate an average weekly stress score by averaging your daily average stress scores. Your weekly average will give you a sense of your overall level of stress.

Using Your Results

How did you score? How high are your daily and weekly stress scores? Are you at all surprised by your score for average stress level?

Are you satisfied with your stress rating? If not, set a specific goal: ______________________________

What should you do next? Enter the results of this lab in the Preprogram Assessment column in Appendix D. If you've set a goal for improvement, begin by using your log to look for patterns and significant time periods in order to identify key stressors in your life. Below, list any stressors that caused you a significant amount of discomfort this week; these can be people, places, events, or recurring thoughts or worries. For each, enter one strategy that would help you deal more successfully with the stressor; examples of strategies might include practicing an oral presentation in front of a friend or engaging in positive self-talk.

Next, begin to put your strategies into action. In addition, complete Lab 10.2 to help you incorporate lifestyle stress-management techniques into your daily routine.

Name ______________________ Section ______________ Date ______________

LAB 10.2 *Stress-Management Techniques*

Part I Lifestyle Stress Management

For each of the areas listed in the table below, describe your current lifestyle as it relates to stress management. For example, do you have enough social support? How are your exercise and nutrition habits? Is time management a problem for you? For each area, list two ways that you could change your current habits to help you manage your stress. Sample strategies might include calling a friend before a challenging class, taking a short walk before lunch, and buying and using a datebook to track your time.

	Current lifestyle	Lifestyle change #1	Lifestyle change #2
Social support system			
Exercise habits			
Nutrition habits			
Time-management techniques			
Self-talk patterns			
Sleep habits			

Part II Relaxation Techniques

Choose two relaxation techniques described in this chapter (progressive relaxation, visualization, deep breathing, meditation, yoga, tai chi, massage, listening to music). If a taped recording is available for progressive relaxation or visualization, these techniques can be performed by your entire class as a group.

List the techniques you tried.

1. ______________________________

2. ______________________________

How did you feel before you tried these techniques?

____

____

____

What did you think or how did you feel during each of the techniques you tried?

1. ______________________________

____

____

2. ______________________________

____

____

How did you feel after you tried these techniques?

____

____

____

Cardiovascular Health

11

LOOKING AHEAD

After reading this chapter, you should be able to

- Describe the controllable and uncontrollable risk factors associated with cardiovascular disease
- Discuss the major forms of cardiovascular disease and how they develop
- List the steps you can take now to lower your personal risk of developing cardiovascular disease

TEST YOUR KNOWLEDGE

1. Women are about as likely to die of cardiovascular disease as they are to die of breast cancer.
   True or false?
2. How much earlier, on average, do sedentary people develop heart disease compared with people who exercise?
   a. 6 months
   b. 2 years
   c. 6 years
3. Which of the following foods would be a good choice for promoting heart health?
   a. tofu
   b. salmon
   c. bananas

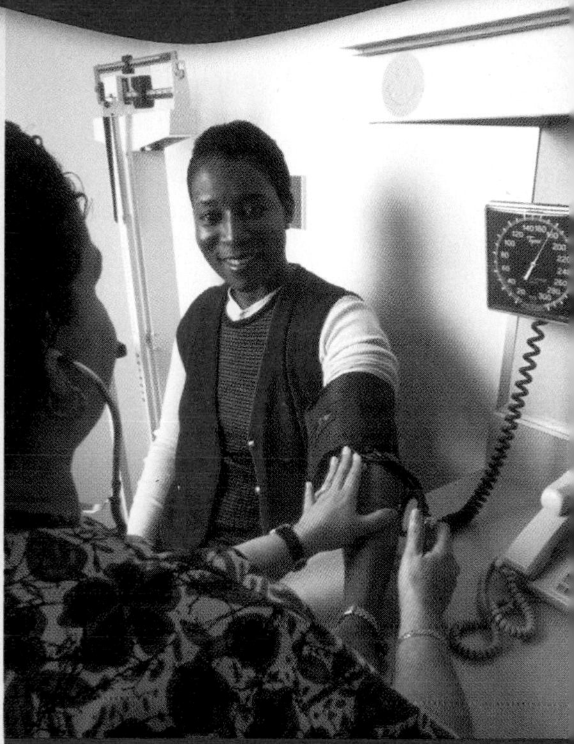

TEST YOUR KNOWLEDGE ANSWERS

1. FALSE. Cardiovascular disease kills far more. Among American women, about 1 in 2 deaths is due to CVD and about 1 in 23 is due to breast cancer.

2. C. Both endurance exercise and strength training significantly improve cardiovascular health.

3. ALL THREE. Soy protein (tofu), foods with omega-3 fatty acids (salmon), and foods high in potassium and low in sodium (bananas) all improve cardiovascular health.

Fit and Well Online Learning Center

www.mhhe.com/fahey5e

Visit the *Fit and Well* Online Learning Center for study aids, additional information about cardiovascular health, links, Internet activities that explore the prevention of cardiovascular disease, and much more.

Cardiovascular disease (CVD) is the leading cause of death in the United States; nearly half of all Americans alive today will die from CVD. If all major forms of CVD were eliminated, U.S. life expectancy would rise by almost 7 years. As discussed in Chapter 1, much of the incidence of CVD is attributable to the American way of life. Too many Americans eat a high-fat diet, are overweight and sedentary, smoke cigarettes, manage stress ineffectively, have uncontrolled high blood pressure or high cholesterol levels, and don't know the signs of CVD. Not all risk factors for CVD are controllable—some people have an inherited tendency toward high cholesterol levels, for example—but many are within the control of the individual.

This chapter explains the major forms of CVD, including hypertension, atherosclerosis, and stroke. It also considers the factors that put people at risk for CVD. Most important, it explains the steps individuals can take to protect their hearts and promote cardiovascular health throughout their lives.

Ww RISK FACTORS FOR CARDIOVASCULAR DISEASE

Researchers have identified a variety of factors associated with an increased risk of developing cardiovascular disease. They are grouped into two categories: major risk factors and contributing risk factors. Some major risk factors, such as diet, exercise habits, and use of tobacco, are linked to controllable aspects of lifestyle and can therefore be changed. Others, such as age, sex, and heredity, are beyond an individual's control. (You can evaluate your personal CVD risk factors in Part I of Lab 11.1.)

Major Risk Factors That Can Be Changed

The American Heart Association (AHA) has identified six major risk factors for CVD that can be changed. These are tobacco use, high blood pressure, unhealthy blood cholesterol levels, physical inactivity, obesity, and diabetes.

Tobacco Use People who smoke a pack of cigarettes a day have twice the risk of heart attack that nonsmokers have; smoking two or more packs a day triples the risk. And when smokers do have heart attacks, they are two to four times more likely than nonsmokers to die from them. Women who smoke and use oral contraceptives are up to 39 times more likely to have a heart attack and up to 22 times more likely to have a stroke than women who don't smoke and take the pill. About one in five deaths from CVD can be attributed to smoking.

Smoking harms the cardiovascular system in several ways. Smoking damages the linings of arteries, and it contributes to unhealthy blood fat levels by reducing levels of **high-density lipoproteins (HDL)**, "good" cholesterol, and raising levels of triglycerides and **low-density lipoproteins (LDL)**, "bad" cholesterol. The psychoactive drug in tobacco, nicotine, is a central nervous system stimulant, causing increased blood pressure and heart rate. The carbon monoxide in cigarette smoke displaces oxygen in the blood, reducing the amount of oxygen available to the heart and other parts of the body. Cigarette smoking also causes the **platelets** in blood to become sticky and cluster, promoting clotting. Smoking also permanently accelerates the rate at which fatty deposits are laid down in arteries. All these effects increase a person's risk of heart attack and other forms of CVD.

You don't have to smoke to be affected. **Environmental tobacco smoke (ETS)** in high concentrations has been linked to the development of cardiovascular disease. ETS and high cholesterol levels act together to damage the cells that line artery walls. Researchers estimate that 50,000 nonsmokers die from heart attacks each year as a result of exposure to ETS.

High Blood Pressure High blood pressure, or **hypertension**, is a risk factor for many forms of CVD but is also considered a disease itself. High blood pressure occurs when too much force or pressure is exerted against the walls of the arteries. If your blood pressure is high, your heart has to work harder to push the blood forward. Over time, a strained heart weakens and tends to enlarge, which weakens it further. Increased blood pressure also scars and hardens arteries, making them less elastic. Heart attacks, strokes, **atherosclerosis**, and kidney failure can result.

Terms Ww

cardiovascular disease (CVD) Disease of the heart and blood vessels.

high-density lipoproteins (HDL) Blood fats that help transport cholesterol out of the arteries, thereby protecting against heart disease; "good" cholesterol.

low-density lipoproteins (LDL) Blood fats that transport cholesterol to organs and tissues; excess amounts result in the accumulation of deposits on artery walls; "bad" cholesterol.

platelets Microscopic disk-shaped cell fragments in the blood that disintegrate on contact with foreign objects and release chemicals necessary for the formation of blood clots.

environmental tobacco smoke (ETS) Smoke that enters the atmosphere from the burning end of a cigarette, cigar, or pipe, as well as smoke that is exhaled by smokers; also called *secondhand smoke.*

hypertension Sustained abnormally high blood pressure.

atherosclerosis Cardiovascular disease in which the inner layers of artery walls are made thick and irregular by deposits of a fatty substance; the internal channels of the arteries thus become narrowed, and blood supply is reduced.

lipoproteins Blood fats formed in the liver that carry cholesterol throughout the body.

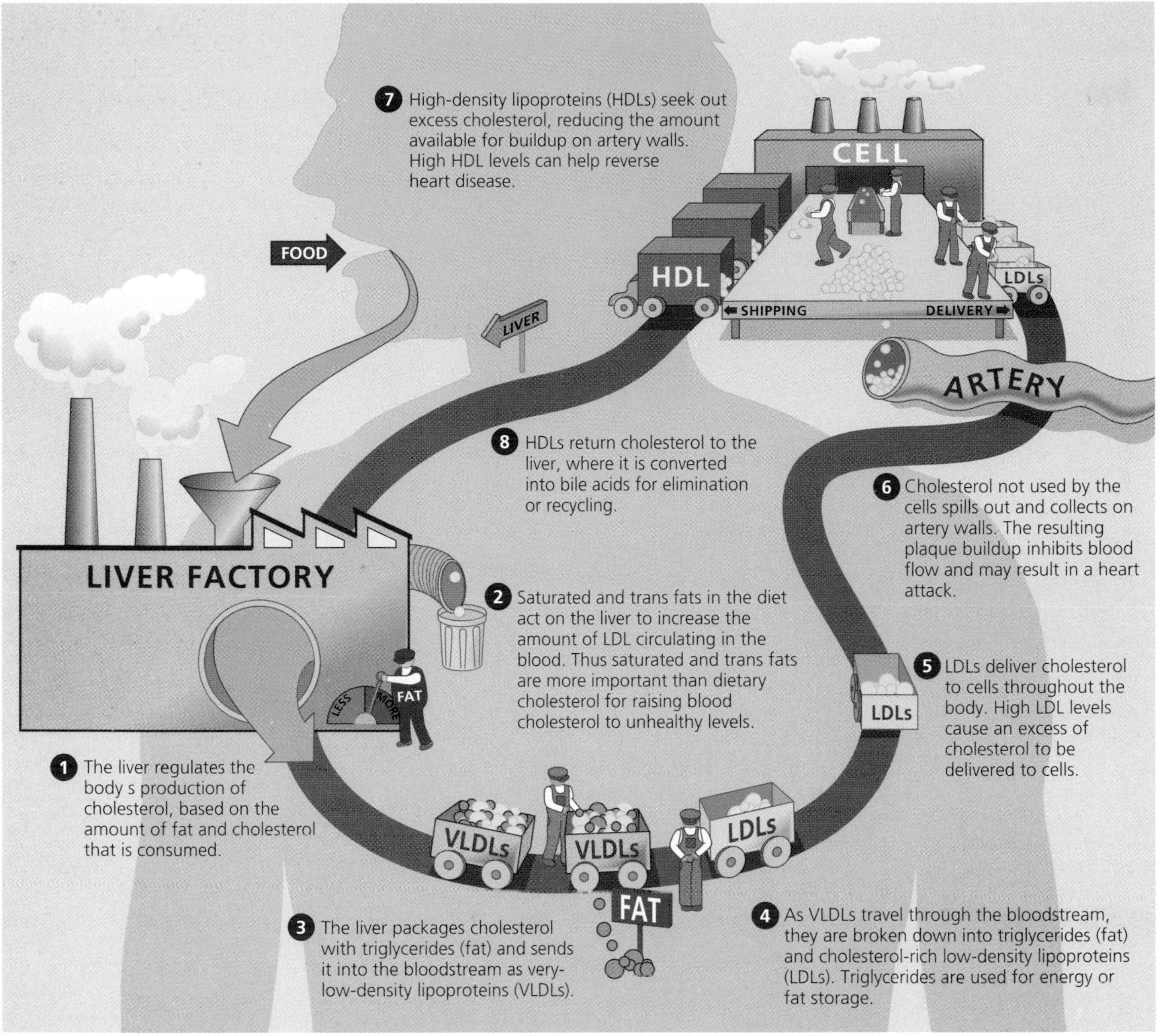

7 High-density lipoproteins (HDLs) seek out excess cholesterol, reducing the amount available for buildup on artery walls. High HDL levels can help reverse heart disease.
CELL
FOOD
HDL
SHIPPING
DELIVERY
LDLs
LIVER
ARTERY
8 HDLs return cholesterol to the liver, where it is converted into bile acids for elimination or recycling.
6 Cholesterol not used by the cells spills out and collects on artery walls. The resulting plaque buildup inhibits blood flow and may result in a heart attack.
LIVER FACTORY
2 Saturated and trans fats in the diet act on the liver to increase the amount of LDL circulating in the blood. Thus saturated and trans fats are more important than dietary cholesterol for raising blood cholesterol to unhealthy levels.
LESS
MORE
FAT
LDLs
5 LDLs deliver cholesterol to cells throughout the body. High LDL levels cause an excess of cholesterol to be delivered to cells.
1 The liver regulates the body s production of cholesterol, based on the amount of fat and cholesterol that is consumed.
VLDLs
VLDLs
LDLs
FAT
3 The liver packages cholesterol with triglycerides (fat) and sends it into the bloodstream as very-low-density lipoproteins (VLDLs).
4 As VLDLs travel through the bloodstream, they are broken down into triglycerides (fat) and cholesterol-rich low-density lipoproteins (LDLs). Triglycerides are used for energy or fat storage.

Figure 11.1 Travels with cholesterol.

Hypertension usually has no early warning signs, so it's important to have your blood pressure tested at least once every two years—more often if you have CVD risk factors. (High blood pressure and atherosclerosis are discussed later in the chapter.)

Unhealthy Cholesterol Levels Cholesterol is a fatty, waxlike substance that circulates through the bloodstream and is an important component of cell membranes, sex hormones, vitamin D, the fluid that coats the lungs, and the protective sheaths around nerves. Adequate cholesterol is essential for the proper functioning of the body. However, excess cholesterol can clog arteries and increase the risk of CVD (Figure 11.1).

Our bodies obtain cholesterol in two ways: from the liver, which manufactures it, and from the foods we eat. Cholesterol levels vary depending on diet, age, sex, heredity, and other factors.

GOOD VERSUS BAD CHOLESTEROL Cholesterol is carried in protein-lipid packages called **lipoproteins.** Lipoproteins can be thought of as shuttles that transport cholesterol to and from the liver through the circulatory system. Low-density lipoproteins (LDLs) shuttle cholesterol from the liver to the organs and tissues that require it. LDL is known as "bad" cholesterol because if there is more than the body can use, the excess is deposited in the blood vessels. LDL that accumulates and becomes trapped in artery walls may be oxidized by free radicals, speeding inflammation and damage to artery walls and increasing the likelihood that an artery will become blocked, causing a heart attack or stroke. High-density lipoproteins (HDLs),

Table 11.1 Cholesterol Guidelines

LDL cholesterol (mg/dl)	
Less than 100	Optimal
100–129	Near optimal/above optimal
130–159	Borderline high
160–189	High
190 or more	Very high
Total cholesterol (mg/dl)	
Less than 200	Desirable
200–239	Borderline high
240 or more	High
HDL cholesterol (mg/dl)	
Less than 40	Low
60 or more	High
Triglycerides (mg/dl)	
Less than 150	Normal
150–199	Borderline high
200–499	High
500 or more	Very high

SOURCE: Expert Panel on Detection, Evaluation, and Treatment of High Blood Cholesterol in Adults. 2001. Executive Summary of the Third Report of the National Cholesterol Education Program (NCEP) Expert Panel on Detection, Evaluation, and Treatment of High Blood Cholesterol in Adults (Adult Treatment Panel III). *Journal of the American Medical Association* 285(19).

Bad cholesterol

Good cholesterol

or "good" cholesterol, shuttle unused cholesterol back to the liver for recycling.

RECOMMENDED BLOOD CHOLESTEROL LEVELS The risk for CVD increases with increasing blood cholesterol levels, especially LDL. The National Cholesterol Education Program (NCEP) recommends testing at least once every 5 years for all adults, beginning at age 20. The recommended test is a lipoprotein profile that measures total cholesterol, LDL cholesterol, HDL cholesterol, and triglycerides (another blood fat). General cholesterol and triglyceride guidelines are given in Table 11.1. In general, high LDL levels and low HDL levels are associated with a high risk for CVD; low levels of LDL and high levels of HDL are associated with lower risk. HDL is important because a high HDL level seems to offer protection from CVD even in cases where total cholesterol is high.

As shown in Table 11.1, LDL levels below 100 mg/dl (milligrams per deciliter) and total cholesterol levels below 200 mg/dl are desirable. An estimated 100 million American adults—over half the population—have total cholesterol levels of 200 mg/dl or higher. The CVD risk associated with elevated cholesterol levels also depends on other factors. For example, an above optimal level of LDL would be of more concern for an individual who also smoked and had high blood pressure than for an individual without these additional CVD risk factors.

IMPROVING CHOLESTEROL LEVELS Your primary goal should be to reduce LDL to healthy levels. Important dietary changes for reducing LDL levels include substituting unsaturated for saturated and trans fats and increasing soluble fiber intake. Decreasing your intake of saturated and trans fats is particularly important because they promote the production and excretion of cholesterol by the liver. Exercising regularly and eating more fruits, vegetables, and whole grains also help. You can raise your HDL levels by exercising regularly, losing weight if you are overweight, quitting smoking, and altering the amount and type of fat you consume. These and other lifestyle changes promoting heart health are discussed in greater detail later in this chapter.

Physical Inactivity An estimated 35–50 million Americans are so sedentary that they are at high risk for developing CVD. Exercise is thought to be the closest thing we have to a "magic bullet" against heart disease. It lowers CVD risk by helping decrease blood pressure, increase HDL levels, maintain desirable weight, improve the condition of the blood vessels, and prevent or control diabetes. One recent study found that women who accumulated at least 3 hours of brisk walking each week cut their risk of heart attack and stroke by more than half. (See Chapter 3 for more information on the physical and psychological effects of exercise.)

Obesity A person whose body weight is more than 30% above the recommended level is at higher risk for heart disease and stroke, even if no other risk factors are present. Excess weight increases the strain on the heart by contributing to high blood pressure and high cholesterol. It can also lead to diabetes, another CVD risk factor (see below). As discussed in Chapter 6, distribution of body fat is also significant: Fat that collects in the torso is more dangerous than fat that collects around the hips. A sensible diet and regular exercise are the best ways to achieve and maintain a healthy body weight. For someone who is overweight, even modest weight reduction can reduce CVD risk by lowering blood pressure, improving cholesterol levels, and reducing diabetes risk.

Diabetes As described in Chapter 6, diabetes is a disorder in which the metabolism of glucose is disrupted, causing a buildup of glucose in the bloodstream. People with diabetes are at increased risk for CVD, partly because elevated blood glucose levels can damage the lining of arteries, making them more vulnerable to atherosclerosis; diabetics also often have other risk factors, including hypertension, obesity, unhealthy cholesterol and triglyceride

Stress and social isolation can increase risk of cardiovascular disease. A strong social support network improves both heart health and overall wellness.

levels, and platelet and blood coagulation abnormalities. Even people whose diabetes is under control face an increased risk of CVD; therefore, careful control of other risk factors is critical for people with diabetes.

Contributing Risk Factors That Can Be Changed

Various other factors that can be changed have been identified as contributing to CVD risk, including triglyceride levels and psychological and social factors.

High Triglyceride Levels Like cholesterol, triglycerides are blood fats that are obtained from food and manufactured by the body. High triglyceride levels are a reliable predictor of heart disease, especially if associated with other risk factors, such as low HDL levels, obesity, and diabetes. Factors contributing to elevated triglyceride levels include excess body fat, physical inactivity, cigarette smoking, excess alcohol intake, very high carbohydrate diets, and certain diseases and medications.

A full lipid profile should include testing and evaluation of triglyceride levels (see Table 11.1). For people with borderline high triglyceride levels, increased physical activity and weight reduction can help bring levels down into the healthy range; for people with high triglycerides, drug therapy may be recommended. Being moderate in the use of alcohol and quitting smoking are also important.

Psychological and Social Factors Many of the psychological and social factors that influence other areas of wellness are also important risk factors for CVD.

- *Stress.* Excessive stress can strain the heart and blood vessels over time and contribute to CVD. A full-blown stress response causes blood vessels to constrict and blood pressure to rise. Blood platelets become more likely to cluster, possibly enhancing the formation of artery-clogging clots. Stress can trigger abnormal heart rhythms, with potentially fatal consequences. People sometimes also adopt unhealthy habits such as smoking or overeating as a means of dealing with severe stress.
- *Chronic hostility and anger.* Certain traits in the hard-driving "Type A" personality—hostility, cynicism, and anger—are associated with increased risk of heart disease. People who are prone to chronic hostility experience the stress response more intensely and frequently than more relaxed individuals. When they encounter the irritations of daily life, their blood pressure increases and their blood vessels constrict much more than is the case for their relaxed counterparts. In a 10-year study of young adults age 18–30 years, those with high hostility levels were more than twice as likely to develop coronary artery calcification (a marker of early atherosclerosis) as those with low hostility levels. (Part II of Lab 11.1 includes a hostility self-assessment and tips for managing anger.)
- *Suppressing psychological distress.* Consistently suppressing anger and other negative emotions may also be hazardous to a healthy heart. People who hide psychological distress tend to have a higher rate of heart disease than people who experience similar distress but share it with others. People with so-called Type D personalities tend to be pessimistic, negative, and unhappy and to suppress these feelings.

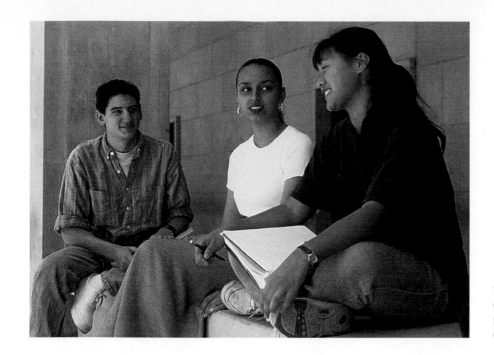

WELLNESS CONNECTION Religion and Wellness

In the past decade, numerous observational studies have shown a link between religious or spiritual factors and health. Evidence connects religion and wellness along several dimensions:

- *Reduced risk of disease and faster recovery.* Researchers have found that regular churchgoers have especially low rates of heart disease, lung disease, cirrhosis of the liver, and some kinds of cancer. Elderly church attendees have healthier immune systems and recover from surgery more quickly.
- *Improved emotional health.* Religion also seems to aid in recovery from depression. Participating in church activities, listening to religious programs on the radio, and watching religious programs on television are all associated with fewer symptoms of depression.
- *Longer life expectancy.* One study found that people who attend religious services one or more times a week live about 8 years longer than people who never attend services. How involved people are in their faith may be more important than was previously believed.

Although researchers are not sure how or why religion or spirituality seems to improve health, several explanations have been offered:

- *Social support.* Attending religious services helps people feel they are part of a community with similar values. It promotes social support and caring.
- *Healthy habits.* Religion may encourage healthy habits—such as eating less meat, drinking less alcohol, or eating a vegetarian diet—and also discourage behavior that is harmful to health, such as smoking and indiscriminate sex.
- *Positive attitude.* Having a sense of meaning and purpose in life results in a positive attitude. This outlook may help patients be cooperative and participate in their own care.
- *Moments of relaxation.* Deep relaxation during prayer or meditation may invoke benefits by eliciting the relaxation response.

Anyone, with or without religious beliefs, can help improve wellness by focusing on these positive behaviors.

SOURCES: Strawbridge, W. J., et al. 2001. Religious attendance increases survival by improving and maintaining good health behaviors, mental health, and social relationships. *Annals of Behavioral Medicine* 23(1): 68–74. Hummer, R. A., et al. 1999. Religious involvement and U.S. adult mortality. *Demography* 36:273–285.

- *Depression and anxiety.* Both mild and severe depression are linked to an increased risk of CVD. Researchers have also found a strong association between anxiety disorders and an increased risk of death from heart disease, particularly sudden death from heart attack.
- *Social isolation.* People with little social support are at higher risk of dying from CVD than people with close ties to others. Studies suggest that religious commitment has a positive effect on heart health, perhaps because of the strong community provided by church membership. A strong social support network is a major antidote to stress. Friends and family members can also promote and support a healthy lifestyle. See the box "Religion and Wellness."
- *Low socioeconomic status.* Low socioeconomic status and low educational attainment also increase risk for CVD, probably because of a variety of factors, including lifestyle, response to stress, and access to health care.

Major Risk Factors That Can't Be Changed

A number of major risk factors for CVD cannot be changed: heredity, aging, being male, and ethnicity.

Heredity The tendency to develop CVD seems to be inherited. High cholesterol levels, hypertension, abnormal blood-clotting problems, diabetes, and obesity are other CVD risk factors that have genetic links. People who inherit a tendency for CVD are not destined to develop it, but they may have to work harder than other people to prevent it.

Aging The risk of heart attack increases dramatically after age 65. About 70% of all heart attack victims are age 65 or older, and more than four out of five who suffer fatal heart attacks are over 65. For people over 55, the incidence of stroke more than doubles in each successive decade. However, many people in their thirties and forties, especially men, have heart attacks.

Being Male Although CVD is the leading killer of both men and women in the United States, men face a greater risk of heart attack than women, especially earlier in life (Figure 11.2). Until age 55, men also have a greater risk of hypertension than women. The incidence of stroke is higher for males than females until age 65. Estrogen production, which is highest during the childbearing years, may offer premenopausal women some protection against CVD.

Ethnicity Death rates from heart disease vary among ethnic groups in the United States, with African Americans having much higher rates of hypertension, heart disease, and stroke than other groups (see the box "African Americans and CVD," p.314). Puerto Rican Americans,

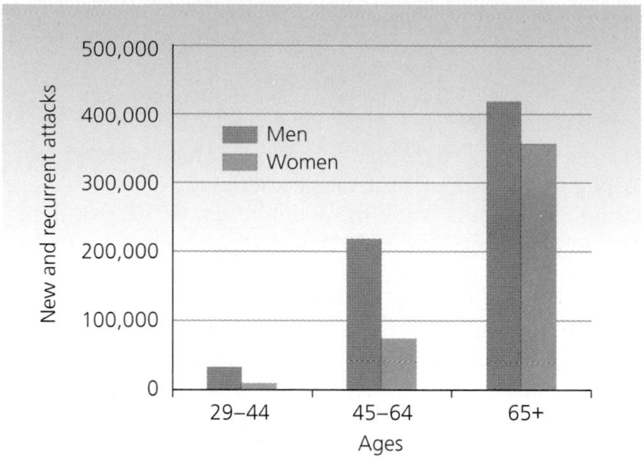

VITAL STATISTICS

Figure 11.2 Annual incidence of heart attack. Among heart attack victims under age 65, men significantly outnumber women; after age 65, women start to catch up. SOURCE: American Heart Association. 2002. *2002 Heart and Stroke Facts Statistical Update.* Dallas, Tex.: American Heart Association.

Cuban Americans, and Mexican Americans are also more likely to suffer from high blood pressure and angina than non-Hispanic white Americans. Asian Americans historically have had far lower rates of CVD than white Americans. However, cholesterol levels among Asian Americans appear to be rising, presumably because of the adoption of a high-fat American diet.

Possible Risk Factors Currently Being Studied

In recent years, a number of other possible risk factors for cardiovascular disease have been identified.

Elevated blood levels of homocysteine, an amino acid that may damage the lining of blood vessels, are associated with an increased risk of CVD. Men generally have higher homocysteine levels than women, as do individuals with diets low in folic acid, vitamin B-12, and vitamin B-6. Most people can lower homocysteine levels easily by adopting a healthy diet rich in fruits, vegetables, and grains and by taking supplements if needed.

High levels of a specific type of LDL called lipoprotein(a), or Lp(a), have been identified as a possible risk factor for coronary heart disease (CHD), especially when associated with high LDL or low HDL levels. Lp(a) levels have a strong genetic component and are difficult to treat. LDL particles differ in size and density, and people with a high proportion of small, dense LDL particles—a condition called LDL pattern B—also appear to be at greater risk for CVD. Exercise, a low-fat diet, and certain lipid-lowering drugs may help lower CVD risk in people with LDL pattern B.

Several infectious agents, including *Chlamydia pneumoniae, cytomegalovirus,* and *Helicobacter pylori,* have also been identified as possible risk factors. Infections may damage arteries and lead to chronic inflammation, another potential risk factor for CVD. When an artery is injured by smoking, cholesterol, infectious agents, or other factors, the body responds with inflammation. A substance called C-reactive protein is released into the bloodstream during the inflammatory response; high levels of C-reactive protein may indicate an elevated risk of heart attack and stroke. Another marker for higher risk is fibrinogen, a protein involved in blood clotting. Aspirin, which reduces both clotting and inflammation, is often recommended for people at high risk for heart attacks and strokes.

Researchers have found that certain CVD risk factors are often found in a cluster. As a group, these risk factors—abdominal obesity, high blood pressure, high triglycerides, low HDL, and insulin resistance—are called metabolic syndrome or syndrome X. A recent survey found that about 47 million Americans have metabolic syndrome, defined as the presence of three or more of the risk factors associated with the condition; metabolic syndrome becomes more common with increasing age, and U.S. prevalence rises from 7% among those in their twenties to 40% among those in their sixties. The underlying causes are not well understood, but metabolic syndrome is thought to have a genetic basis. Because people with metabolic syndrome have insulin resistance and often diabetes, some experts recommend a diet somewhat different from that recommended in the *Dietary Guidelines for Americans*—slightly higher in unsaturated fats and lower in carbohydrates—to help keep glucose and insulin levels under control. The glycemic load of carbohydrate foods is another consideration for people with metabolic syndrome; see the box "Glycemic Index and Glycemic Load" (p. 315). The NCEP recommends weight control and physical activity to reduce all of the risk factors associated with metabolic syndrome.

MAJOR FORMS OF CARDIOVASCULAR DISEASE

Collectively, the various forms of CVD kill more Americans than the next four leading causes of death combined. The financial burden of CVD, including the costs of medical treatments and lost productivity, exceeds $300 billion annually. Although the main forms of CVD are interrelated and have elements in common, we treat them separately here for the sake of clarity.

Hypertension

Blood pressure, the force exerted by the blood on blood vessel walls, is created by the pumping action of the heart. When the heart contracts (systole), blood pressure increases; when the heart relaxes (diastole), pressure decreases. Short periods of high blood pressure are normal, but blood pressure that is continually at an abnormally high level is known as hypertension.

African Americans have higher rates of coronary heart disease, stroke, and hypertension than any other group of Americans. The prevalence of hypertension among African Americans is among the highest in the world. What accounts for these rates? Contributing factors can be grouped into three areas: genetic factors, low income and discrimination, and lifestyle factors.

Genetic Factors

A number of genetic factors may contribute to CVD in African Americans, including heightened sensitivities to lead and salt, which can lead to high blood pressure. Heredity may also play a role in higher cholesterol levels among blacks. And sickle-cell disease, a genetic disorder that occurs mainly in blacks, can lead to impaired blood flow and heart failure. Blacks also respond to stress differently in that their blood vessels don't dilate as readily. This response can lead to hypertension.

Low Income and Discrimination

About 25% of African Americans live below the official poverty line. Economic deprivation usually means reduced access to adequate health care and health insurance. Associated with low income are poorer educational opportunities and less information about preventive health measures, such as diet and stress management.

Discrimination may also play a role. Many physicians and hospitals treat the medical problems of African Americans differently from those of whites. Discrimination, along with low income, may also increase stress, which is linked with CVD.

Lifestyle Factors

Lifestyle factors may be the key in explaining high CVD rates among African Americans. A large-scale study determined that birthplace, not ethnicity, is the key indicator of CVD risk among African Americans. The study found that among New Yorkers born in the Northeast, blacks and whites have nearly identical risk for CVD. But black New Yorkers who were born in the South have a sharply higher risk, and black New Yorkers born in the Caribbean have a significantly lower risk. In fact, blacks who were born in the South and moved to New York City were twice as likely to die of heart disease as blacks or whites born in the Northeast. Researchers speculate that some risk factors for CVD, including smoking and a high-fat diet, may be more common in the South. When combined with urban stress, these factors create a lifestyle that is far from heart-healthy. And people with low incomes, who are disproportionately African American, tend to smoke more, use more salt, and exercise less than those with higher incomes. In addition, half of black women and one-third of black men are significantly overweight.

General CVD prevention strategies may be particularly critical for blacks: regular blood pressure checks, exercise, healthy diet, stress management, and avoidance of tobacco. In addition, recent research has identified several specific dietary factors that may be of special importance for blacks. Studies have found that diets high in potassium and calcium improve blood pressure in African Americans. Fruits, vegetables, grains, and nuts are rich in potassium, dairy products are high in calcium.

Blood pressure is measured with a stethoscope and an instrument called a sphygmomanometer. It is expressed as two numbers—for example, 120 over 80—and measured in millimeters of mercury. The first and larger number is the systolic blood pressure; the second is the diastolic blood pressure. Average blood pressure readings for young adults in good physical condition are 110–120 systolic over 70–80 diastolic. High blood pressure in adults is defined as equal to or greater than 140 over 90 (Table 11.2).

High blood pressure results from either an increased output of blood by the heart or, most often, increased resistance to blood flow in the arteries. In those with high blood pressure, the heart must work harder than normal

Table 11.2 *Blood Pressure Classification for Healthy Adults*

Category[a]	Systolic (mm Hg)		Diastolic (mm Hg)
Optimal[b]	below 120	and	below 80
Normal	below 130	and	below 85
High-normal	130–139	or	85–89
Hypertension[c]			
Stage 1	140–159	or	90–99
Stage 2	160–179	or	100–109
Stage 3	180 and above	or	110 and above

[a]When systolic and diastolic pressure fall into different categories, the higher category should be used to classify blood pressure status.

[b]Optimal blood pressure with respect to cardiovascular risk is below 120/80 mm Hg; however, unusually low readings should be evaluated.

[c]Based on the average of two or more readings taken at different physician visits.

SOURCE: *The Sixth Report of the Joint National Committee on Prevention, Detection, Evaluation, and Treatment of High Blood Pressure*. 1997. Bethesda, Md.: National Heart, Lung, and Blood Institute. National Institutes of Health (NIH Publication No. 98-4080).

Terms

glycemic index (GI) A measure of how high and how fast a particular food raises blood glucose levels.

glycemic load A measure of how a particular food affects blood glucose levels, calculated by multiplying the glycemic index of a food by its carbohydrate content

IN FOCUS Glycemic Index and Glycemic Load

"Eat a high-carbohydrate, low-fat diet" has been the nutritionists' refrain for the last few decades. Now, nutritionists are speculating on whether that advice may have been too simple. Recent research has shown that eating the right types of carbohydrates may help protect against coronary heart disease, diabetes, and obesity, while eating the wrong carbohydrates may actually increase the risk of health problems.

As described in Chapter 8, all carbohydrate foods are broken down in the body into simple sugars that are absorbed into the bloodstream, causing blood glucose and insulin levels to rise. Some carbohydrates are broken down very quickly, resulting in a large and rapid increase in blood sugar; others are digested more slowly, causing a more gradual change in blood sugar level. **Glycemic index (GI)** is a measure of how fast and high blood sugar rises after eating a particular food. When you eat high-GI foods, your blood sugar spikes rapidly, followed by a steep fall a little while later. Rapidly falling blood sugar levels may increase appetite. Foods with low GIs take longer to digest and cause a lower, longer-lasting rise in blood sugar; hunger tends to return much more slowly after eating low-GI foods. High-GI foods may also contribute to insulin resistance and oxidative stress, risk factors associated with diabetes and CVD.

The GI of a food is not always easy to predict. In general, rapidly digestible starchy or sugary foods such as white bread, white potatoes, and sweets tend to have relatively high GIs, while foods higher in fiber and fat are digested more slowly and have lower GIs. The GI values for some foods are surprising—bread has a higher GI than table sugar, for example, and raisins have a higher GI than grapes.

Some experts have recommended using a slightly different measure, called **glycemic load**, to get a better picture of how the body responds to particular foods. Glycemic load is calculated by measuring the carbohydrate content of a specific amount of food and multiplying it by the GI. For example, carrots have a relatively high GI, yet the glycemic load of a serving consisting of one raw carrot is quite low. Why? The type of carbohydrate in carrots is rapidly digestible, resulting in a high glycemic *index*, but the total amount of carbohydrate in one serving of raw carrots is very small, resulting in a low glycemic *load*. In other words, eating a single serving of raw carrots is not going to raise your blood sugar very much, despite the high-GI value of carrots.

Why does any of this matter? Evidence is mounting that eating a diet rich in low-GI foods reduces the risk of developing Type 2 diabetes and coronary heart disease, particularly among people who are overweight or who have the cluster of risk factors known as metabolic syndrome. The diet industry has also recognized glycemic index and its possible effects on hunger, and a number of popular weight-loss diets have been devised around the concept. Unfortunately, some of these diets are high in saturated fat, which actually increases the risk of CVD. It is also important to note that glycemic index should not be the sole criterion for selecting foods: Low-GI hard cheese isn't a healthier choice than high-GI carrots, and diets high in carbohydrate-rich fruits, vegetables, and grain are linked to reduced risk of many diseases.

Some experts feel we don't yet understand enough about glycemic load to make specific diet recommendations. Limitations of the glycemic load concept include the fact that GI measurements vary from one study to another. How a food is prepared also changes the GI; for example, instant white rice and instant oatmeal have much higher GI values than regular white rice and old-fashioned oatmeal. Even factors such as ripeness can make a difference: The GI of a relatively ripe banana can be twice that of a less ripe one. Also, GI gives us information about what can happen to blood sugar when a given food is eaten by itself; estimating the glycemic load of a typical mixed meal is more complicated. Given the confusion and complexities, some experts are skeptical about whether glycemic index will ever be really useful in daily practice.

Despite all the uncertainty, the basic idea of glycemic index can be helpful if it is kept simple. Eating more low-GI foods can be one way to improve your health, especially if you have a family history of diabetes or heart disease, are overweight, or suspect you have metabolic syndrome. Rather than worrying about the exact GI of foods, keep in mind that certain classes of foods such as whole grains, nonstarchy vegetables, and fruits tend to have lower GIs than starchy or highly refined foods. Most of the carbohydrates in the current American diet come from refined or starchy foods, including soft drinks, sweets, white potatoes (including those served as french fries), white bread, and refined ready-to-eat cereals. Focus on choosing healthier sources of carbohydrate. In general, this translates to eating more of the fruits, vegetables, and whole-grain foods that nutrition experts have been recommending for a long time!

to force blood through the arteries, thereby straining both the heart and the arteries. High blood pressure is often called a "silent killer" because it usually has no symptoms. A person may have hypertension for years without realizing it. But during that time, it damages vital organs and increases the risk of heart attack, congestive heart failure, stroke, kidney failure, and blindness.

Hypertension is common, occurring in about 1 in 4 adults. In most cases, hypertension cannot be cured, but it can be controlled. The key to avoiding the complications of hypertension is to have your blood pressure checked regularly and to follow your physician's advice about lifestyle changes and medication.

People with mild hypertension can frequently lower their blood pressure through lifestyle changes, including quitting smoking, exercising regularly, and improving diet. Controlling total calorie intake is important for achieving and maintaining a healthy body weight. Increasing intake of fruits, vegetables, and whole grains is recommended because these foods are rich in potassium and fiber, both of which may reduce blood pressure. About half of all people with hypertension are "salt-

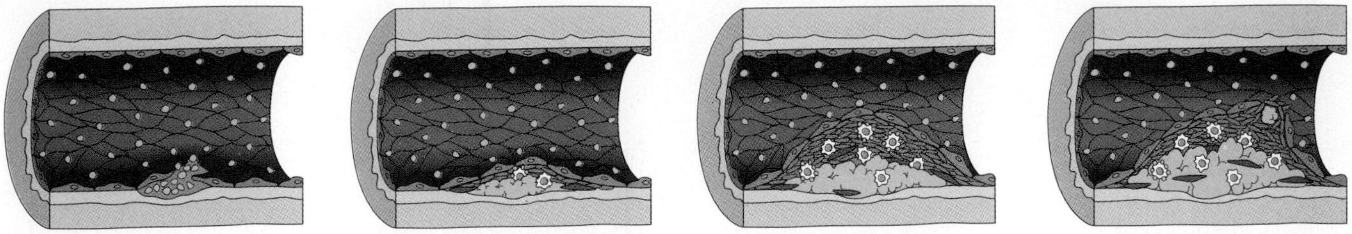

Plaque buildup begins when endothelial cells lining the arteries are damaged by smoking, high blood pressure, oxidized LDL, and other causes; excess cholesterol particles collect beneath these cells.

In response to the damage, platelets and other types of cells collect at the site; a fibrous cap forms, isolating the plaque within the artery wall. An early-stage plaque is called a fatty streak.

Chemicals released by cells in and around the plaque cause further inflammation and buildup; an advanced plaque contains LDL, white blood cells, connective tissue, smooth muscle cells, platelets, and other compounds.

The narrowed artery is vulnerable to blockage by clots. The risk of blockage and heart attack rises if the fibrous cap cracks (probably due to destructive enzymes released by white blood cells within the plaque).

Figure 11.3 Stages of plaque development.

sensitive," meaning that their blood pressure will decrease significantly when salt intake is restricted. Most experts feel that restricting sodium intake to about 2400 mg per day is a good strategy for all people—whether they have hypertension or not. Recent research has shown that lowering your blood pressure through healthy lifestyle changes improves cardiovascular health even if your current blood pressure is already below 140 over 90. For people whose blood pressure isn't adequately controlled with lifestyle changes, many different types of antihypertensive drugs are available.

Atherosclerosis

Atherosclerosis is a form of arteriosclerosis, or thickening and hardening of the arteries. In atherosclerosis, arteries become narrowed by deposits of fat, cholesterol, and other substances. The process begins when the cells lining the arteries (endothelial cells) become damaged, often through a combination of factors such as smoking, high blood pressure, and deposits of oxidized LDL particles. The body's response to this damage results in inflammation and changes in the artery lining. Deposits, called **plaques,** accumulate on artery walls; the arteries lose their elasticity and their ability to expand and contract, restricting blood flow. Once narrowed by a plaque, an artery is vulnerable to blockage by blood clots (Figure 11.3). Atherosclerosis often begins in childhood.

If the heart, brain, and/or other organs are deprived of blood, and thus the vital oxygen it carries, the effects of atherosclerosis can be deadly. Coronary arteries, which supply the heart with blood, are particularly susceptible to plaque buildup, a condition called **coronary heart disease (CHD),** or *coronary artery disease.* The blockage of a coronary artery causes a heart attack. If a cerebral artery (leading to the brain) is blocked, the result is a stroke. The main risk factors for atherosclerosis are cigarette smoking, physical inactivity, high levels of blood cholesterol, high blood pressure, and diabetes.

Heart Disease and Heart Attacks

Although a **heart attack,** or myocardial infarction (MI), often comes without warning, it is usually the end result of a long-term disease process. The heart requires a steady supply of oxygen-rich blood to function properly (Figure 11.4). If one of the coronary arteries that supplies blood to the heart becomes blocked by a blood clot, a heart attack results. A heart attack caused by a clot is called a coronary thrombosis. During a heart attack, part of the heart muscle (myocardium) may die from lack of oxygen. If an MI is not fatal, the heart muscle may partially repair itself.

Chest pain called **angina pectoris** is a signal that the heart isn't getting enough oxygen to supply its needs. Although not actually a heart attack, angina—felt as an extreme tightness in the chest and heavy pressure behind the breastbone or in the shoulder, neck, arm, hand, or back—is a warning that the heart is overloaded.

If the electrical impulses that control heartbeat are disrupted, the heart may beat too quickly, too slowly, or in an irregular fashion, a condition known as **arrhythmia.** The symptoms of arrhythmia range from imperceptible to severe and even fatal. **Sudden cardiac death** is most often caused by an arrythmia called ventricular fibrillation, a kind of "quivering" of the ventricle that makes it ineffective in pumping blood. If ventricular fibrillation continues for more than a few minutes, it is fatal. Cardiac defribillation, in which an electrical shock is delivered to the heart, can jolt the heart into a more efficient rhythm.

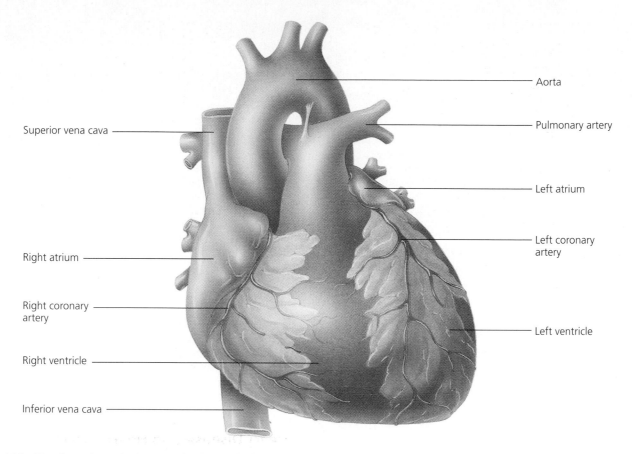

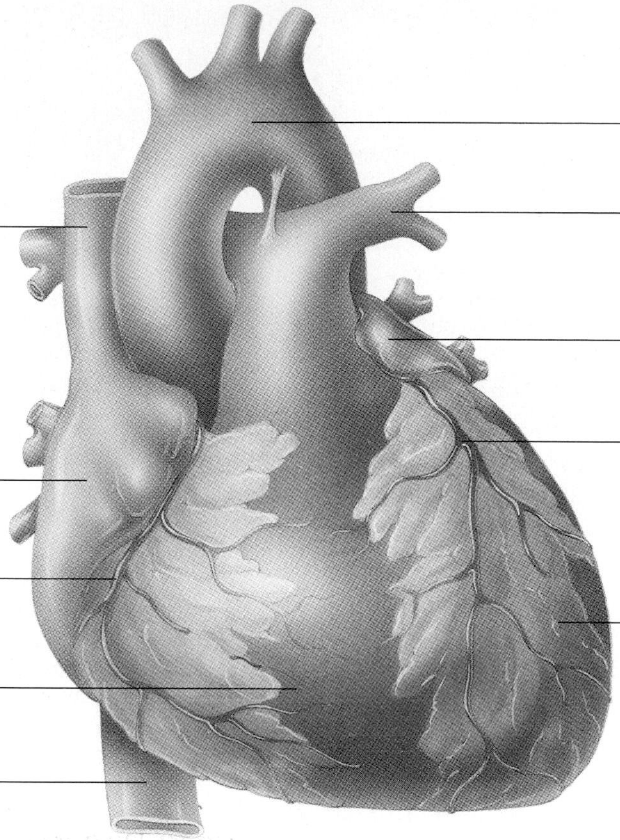

Figure 11.4 Blood supply to the heart. Blood is supplied to the heart from the right and left coronary arteries, which branch off the aorta. If a coronary artery becomes blocked by plaque buildup and a blood clot, a heart attack occurs; part of the heart muscle may die due to lack of oxygen.

If symptoms of heart trouble do occur, it is critical to contact the emergency medical service or go immediately to the nearest hospital or clinic with a 24-hour emergency cardiac facility (see the box "What to Do in Case of a Heart Attack or Stroke," p. 318). One additional step recommended by many experts is for the affected individual to chew and swallow one adult aspirin tablet (325 mg); aspirin has an immediate anticlotting effect. If someone having a heart attack gets to the emergency room quickly enough, a clot-dissolving agent can be injected to dissolve a clot in the coronary artery, reducing the amount of damage to the heart muscle.

Physicians have a variety of diagnostic tools and treatments for heart disease. A patient may undergo a stress or exercise test, in which he or she runs on a treadmill or pedals a stationary cycle while being monitored with an electrocardiogram (ECG or EKG). Certain characteristic changes in the heart's electrical activity while it is under stress can reveal particular heart problems, such as restricted blood flow to the heart muscle. Tools that allow the physician to visualize a patient's heart and arteries include magnetic resonance imaging (MRI), electron-beam computed tomography (EBC), echocardiograms, and angiograms.

If tests indicate a problem or if a person has already had a heart attack, several treatments are possible. Along

Terms
VW

plaque A deposit of fatty (and other) substances on the inner wall of the arteries.

coronary heart disease (CHD) Heart disease caused by hardening of the arteries that supply oxygen to the heart muscle; also called *coronary artery disease*.

heart attack Damage to, or death of, heart muscle, sometimes resulting in a failure of the heart to deliver enough blood to the body; also known as myocardial infarction (MI).

angina pectoris A condition in which the heart muscle does not receive enough blood, causing severe pain in the chest and often in the left arm and shoulder.

arrhythmia An irregularity in the force or rhythm of the heartbeat.

sudden cardiac death A nontraumatic, unexpected death from sudden cardiac arrest, most often due to arrhythmia; in most instances, victims have underlying heart disease.

TAKE CHARGE What to Do in Case of a Heart Attack or Stroke

Heart Attack Warning Signs

Some heart attacks are sudden and intense—the "movie heart attack," in which a person dramatically gasps, clutches her or his heart, and drops to the ground, and no one doubts what's happening. But most heart attacks start slowly, with mild pain or discomfort. Often the people affected aren't sure what's wrong and wait too long before getting help. Here are some signs that can mean a heart attack is happening:

- Chest discomfort. Most heart attacks involve discomfort in the center of the chest that lasts more than a few minutes, or that goes away and comes back. It can feel like uncomfortable pressure, squeezing, fullness, or pain.
- Discomfort in other areas of the upper body. Symptoms can include pain or discomfort in one or both arms, the back, neck, jaw, or stomach.
- Shortness of breath. This feeling often comes with chest discomfort, but it can occur before the chest discomfort.
- Other signs may include breaking out in a cold sweat, nausea, or lightheadedness.

If you or someone you're with has chest discomfort, especially with one or more of the other signs, don't wait longer than a few minutes (no more than 5) before calling for help. Call 911. Get to a hospital right away.

Stroke Warning Signs

- Sudden numbness or weakness of the face, arm, or leg, especially on one side of the body.
- Sudden confusion or trouble speaking or understanding.
- Sudden trouble seeing in one or both eyes.
- Sudden trouble walking, dizziness, or loss of balance or coordination.
- Sudden, severe headache with no known cause.

Not all these warning signs occur in every stroke. If some start to occur, don't wait. Get help immediately. Stroke is a medical emergency—call 911.

SOURCE: American Heart Association. 2002. *2002 Heart and Stroke Facts Statistical Supplement.* Dallas, Tex.: American Heart Association. Reproduced with permission from American Heart Association World Wide Web Site www.americanheart.org/presenter.jhtml?identifier=3053.

with a low-fat diet, regular exercise, and smoking cessation, many patients are also advised to take half an aspirin tablet daily to reduce clotting and inflammation. Prescription drugs can also help reduce the strain on the heart. *Balloon angioplasty*, a common surgical treatment, involves threading a catheter with an inflatable balloon tip through a coronary artery until it reaches the area of blockage; the balloon is then inflated, flattening the plaque and widening the arterial opening. Many surgeons permanently implant coronary stents—flexible stainless steel tubes—to prop the artery open and prevent reclogging after angioplasty. In *coronary bypass surgery,* healthy blood vessels are grafted to coronary arteries to bypass blockages.

Stroke

For brain cells to function as they should, they must have a continuous and ample supply of oxygen-rich blood. If brain cells are deprived of blood for more than a few minutes, they die. A **stroke,** also called a *cerebrovascular accident (CVA),* occurs when the blood supply to the brain is cut off. Prompt treatment of stroke can greatly decrease the risk of permanent disability.

A stroke may be caused by a blood clot that blocks an artery (ischemic stroke) or by a ruptured blood vessel (hemorrhagic stroke). Ischemic strokes are often caused by atherosclerosis or certain types of arrhythmia; hemorrhagic strokes may occur if there is a weak spot in an artery wall or following a head injury. The interruption of the blood supply to any area of the brain prevents the nerve cells there from functioning—in some cases, causing death. Nerve cells control sensation and most body movements; depending on the area of the brain that is affected, a stroke may cause paralysis, walking disability, speech impairment, or memory loss. Of the 600,000 or more Americans who have strokes each year, nearly one-third die within a year; those who survive usually have some lasting disability.

Effective treatment requires the prompt recognition of symptoms and correct diagnosis of the type of stroke that has occurred. Treatment may involve the use of clot-dissolving and antihypertensive drugs. Even if brain tissue has been damaged or destroyed, nerve cells in the brain can make new pathways, and some functions can be taken over by other parts of the brain.

Congestive Heart Failure

A number of conditions—high blood pressure, heart attack, atherosclerosis, **rheumatic fever,** birth defects—can damage the heart's pumping mechanism. When the heart cannot maintain its regular pumping rate and force, fluids begin to back up. When extra fluid seeps through capillary walls, edema (swelling) results, usually in the legs and ankles, but sometimes in other parts of the body as well. Fluid can collect in the lungs and interfere with breathing, particularly when a person is lying down. This condition is called *pulmonary edema,* and the entire process is known as **congestive heart failure.** Treatment includes reducing the workload on the heart, modifying

Do More

- Eat a diet rich in fruits, vegetables, whole grains, and low-fat or fat-free dairy products. Eat 5–9 servings of fruits and vegetables each day.
- Eat several servings of high-fiber foods each day.
- Eat 2 or more servings of fish per week; try a few servings of nuts and soy foods each week.
- Choose unsaturated fats rather than saturated and trans fats.
- Be physically active; do both endurance exercise and strength training on a regular basis.
- Achieve and maintain a healthy weight.
- Develop effective strategies for handling stress and anger. Nurture old friendships and family ties, and make new friends; pay attention to your spiritual side.
- Obtain recommended screening tests and follow your physician's recommendations.

Do Less

- Don't use tobacco in any form: cigarettes, spit tobacco, cigars, pipes, bidis, or clove cigarettes.
- Avoid exposure to environmental tobacco smoke.
- Limit consumption of fats, especially trans fats and saturated fats.
- Limit consumption of cholesterol, added sugars, and refined carbohydrates.
- Avoid excessive alcohol consumption—no more than one drink per day for women and two drinks per day for men.
- Limit consumption of salt to no more than 2400 mg of sodium per day.
- Avoid excess stress, anger, and hostility.

Figure 11.5 Strategies for reducing your risk of cardiovascular disease.

salt intake, and using drugs that help the body eliminate excess fluid.

PROTECTING YOURSELF AGAINST CARDIOVASCULAR DISEASE

You can take several important steps right now to lower your risk of developing CVD in the future (Figure 11.5). Reducing CVD risk factors when you are young can pay off with many extra years of life and health.

Eat Heart-Healthy

For most Americans, changing to a heart-healthy diet involves cutting total fat intake, substituting unsaturated fats for saturated and trans fats, and increasing fiber.

Decreased Fat and Cholesterol Intake The National Cholesterol Education Program (NCEP) recommends that all Americans over the age of 2 adopt a diet in which total fat consumption is no more than 30% of total daily calories, with no more than one-third of those fat calories (10% of total daily calories) coming from saturated fat. For people with heart disease or high LDL levels, the NCEP recommends a total fat intake of 25–35% of total daily calories and a saturated fat intake of less than 7% of total calories. This higher total fat allowance is helpful for people who also have high triglyceride and low HDL levels. (Diets rich in high-glycemic-index carbohydrates may lower HDL levels and raise levels of triglycerides and glucose in some people, including those with metabolic syndrome. For this group, then, a diet slightly higher in unsaturated fats is allowed, while saturated fats are further restricted.)

Saturated fat is found in animal products, palm and coconut oil, and hydrogenated vegetable oils, which are also high in trans fats. Saturated and trans fats influence the production and excretion of cholesterol by the liver, so decreasing intake of these fats is the most important dietary change you can make to improve cholesterol levels. Animal products contain cholesterol as well as saturated fat, and the NCEP recommends that most Americans limit dietary cholesterol intake to no more than 300 mg per day; for people with heart disease or high LDL levels, the suggested daily limit is 200 mg.

Increased Fiber Intake Soluble fiber traps the bile acids the liver needs to manufacture cholesterol and carries them to the large intestine, where they are excreted. It also slows the production of proteins that promote blood clotting. Insoluble fiber may interfere with the absorption of dietary fat and may also help you cut

Terms

stroke An impeded blood supply to some part of the brain resulting in the destruction of brain cells; also called *cerebrovascular accident (CVA).*

rheumatic fever A disease, mainly of children, characterized by fever, inflammation, and pain in the joints; often damages the heart muscle, a condition called rheumatic heart disease.

congestive heart failure A condition resulting from the heart's inability to pump out all the blood that returns to it. Blood backs up in the veins leading to the heart, causing an accumulation of fluid in various parts of the body.

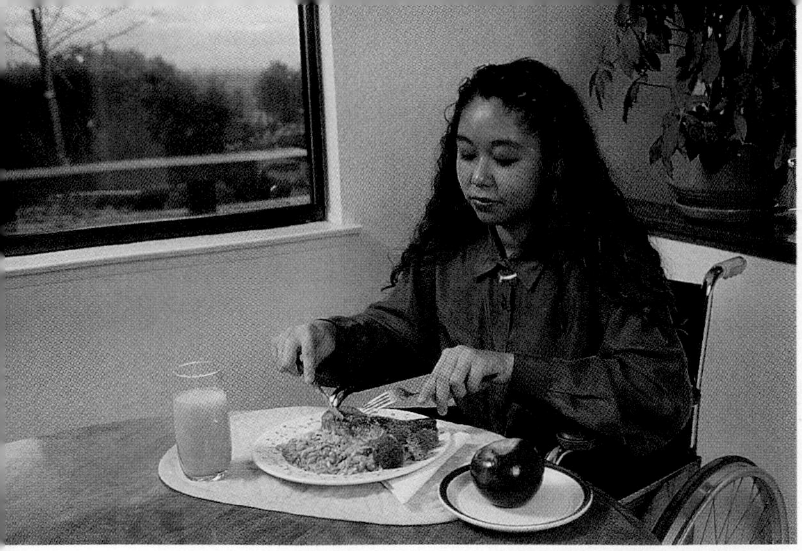

A diet high in fiber and low in saturated and trans fats can help lower levels of total cholesterol and LDL. This young woman is enjoying a healthy dinner of baked chicken, broccoli, rice, fruit, and juice.

total food intake because foods rich in insoluble fiber tend to be filling. To obtain the recommended 20–35 grams of dietary fiber a day, choose a diet rich in whole grains, fruits, and vegetables. Good sources of fiber include oatmeal, some breakfast cereals, barley, legumes, and most fruits and vegetables.

Alcohol The *Dietary Guidelines for Americans* state that moderate alcohol consumption may lower the risk of CHD among men over 45 and women over 55. (Moderate means no more than one drink per day for women and two drinks per day for men.) For most people under age 45, however, the risks of alcohol use probably outweigh any health benefit. If you do drink, do so moderately, with food and at times when drinking will not put you or others at risk.

DASH A dietary plan that reflects many of the suggestions described here was released as part of a study called Dietary Approaches to Stop Hypertension, or DASH. This is the DASH diet plan:

- 7–8 servings a day of grains and grain products
- 4–5 servings a day of vegetables
- 4–5 servings a day of fruits
- 2–3 servings a day of low-fat or nonfat dairy products
- 2 or fewer servings a day of meats, poultry, and fish
- 4–5 servings a *week* of nuts, seeds, and legumes
- 2–3 servings a day of added fats, oils, and salad dressings
- 5 servings a *week* of snacks and sweets

The DASH diet also follows the dietary recommendations for lowering one's risk of cancer, osteoporosis, and heart disease.

Exercise Regularly

You can significantly reduce your risk of CVD with a moderate amount of physical activity. Try to accumulate at least 30 minutes of moderate-intensity physical activity each day through such activities as brisk walking and stair climbing. A formal exercise program can provide even greater benefits. The American Heart Association recently recommended strength training in addition to aerobic exercise for building and maintaining cardiovascular health.

Avoid Tobacco

Remember: The number-one risk factor for CVD that you can control is smoking. If you smoke, quit. If you don't, don't start. The majority of people who start don't believe they will become hooked, but most do. If you live or work with people who smoke, encourage them to quit—for their sake and yours. Regular exposure to ETS in social settings, at home, or at work raises your risk of CVD. If you find yourself breathing in smoke, take steps to prevent or stop this exposure. Quitting smoking will significantly reduce your CVD risk, but studies show that smoking and exposure to ETS may permanently increase the rate of plaque formation in arteries. Quitting smoking is highly beneficial, but abstaining from smoking and avoiding ETS throughout your life is even better.

Know and Manage Your Blood Pressure

Currently, only about 27% of Americans with hypertension have their blood pressure under control. If you have no CVD risk factors, have your blood pressure measured at least once every 2 years; yearly tests are recommended if you have other risk factors. If your blood pressure is high, follow your physician's advice on how to lower it.

Know and Manage Your Cholesterol Levels

Everyone age 20 and over should have a lipoprotein profile—which measures total cholesterol, HDL, LDL, and triglyceride levels—at least once every five years. Your goal for LDL depends in part on how many of the following major risk factors you have: cigarette smoking, high blood pressure, low HDL cholesterol (less than 40 mg/dl), a family history of heart disease, and age above 45 years for men and 55 years for women. (An HDL level of 60 mg/dl or higher is protective and removes one risk factor from your total count of risk factors.)

If you have two or fewer risk factors, the NCEP sets an LDL goal of less than 160 mg/dl. If your LDL is above that level, begin the "Therapeutic Lifestyle Changes," or TLC, recommended by the NCEP, including weight management, increased physical activity, and the TLC diet, which suggests total fat intake of 25–35% of total daily calories, saturated fat intake less than 7% of daily calories, and, for some people, 10–25 grams per day of soluble fiber and 2 grams per day of plant stanols and sterols (see p. 322). If your LDL level is 190 mg/dl or higher, medication may also be recommended.

If you have two or more risk factors for heart disease, the NCEP sets an LDL goal of less than 130 mg/dl. If your LDL level is 130 or above, you should begin TLC. Depending on other factors, your physician may also suggest drug therapy.

If you have CVD or diabetes, your goal for LDL is less than 100 mg/dl. TLC is recommended for all people in this risk category, and a variety of medications is available to lower LDL and improve other blood fat levels.

Develop Ways to Handle Stress and Anger

To reduce the psychological and social risk factors for CVD, develop effective strategies for handling the stress in your life. Shore up your social support network, and try some of the techniques described in Chapter 10 for managing stress and anger. If anger and hostility are problems for you, refer to Chapter 10 for tips on diffusing your anger.

Know Your Risk Factors

Know your CVD risk factors and follow your physician's advice for testing, lifestyle changes, and any drug treatments. Consider the possible use of hormone replacement therapy (for postmenopausal women) and regular small doses of aspirin (for men and women to treat some types of CVD). Aspirin has side effects, however, and should be used only after consulting a physician.

Tips for Today

Risk factors for cardiovascular disease fall into two categories—those you can do something about, such as physical activity and levels of stress, and those you can't, such as age and ethnicity. Because cardiovascular disease is a long-term process that can begin when you're young, it's important to develop heart-healthy habits early in life.

Right now you can

- Plan to have fish for dinner two times this week.
- Go to the gym or fitness facility on your campus and get started on an aerobic exercise program.
- Practice time management by prioritizing your day's activities; work on accomplishing the most important tasks first.
- Resolve to address any nagging interpersonal issue that's been causing you stress.

SUMMARY

- The major controllable risk factors for CVD are smoking, hypertension, unhealthy cholesterol levels, a sedentary lifestyle, obesity, and diabetes.
- Contributing factors for CVD that can be changed include high triglyceride levels, inadequate stress management, a hostile personality, depression, anxiety, lack of social support, and poverty.
- Major risk factors that can't be changed are heredity, aging, being male, and ethnicity.
- Hypertension weakens the heart and scars and hardens arteries, causing resistance to blood flow. It is defined as blood pressure equal to or higher than 140 over 90.
- Atherosclerosis is a progressive hardening and narrowing of arteries that can lead to restricted blood flow and even complete blockage; high blood pressure and high levels of blood cholesterol are contributing factors.
- Heart attacks, strokes, and congestive heart failure are the results of a long-term disease process; hypertension and atherosclerosis are usually involved.
- Reducing heart disease risk involves eating a heart-healthy diet, exercising regularly, avoiding tobacco, managing blood pressure and cholesterol levels, handling stress and anger, and knowing your risk factors.

COMMON QUESTIONS ANSWERED

Do women have a lower risk for cardiovascular disease than men, and, if so, why? Until about age 65, women have a significant advantage over men when it comes to CVD. Women who develop CVD tend to be about 10 years older than men when they first have symptoms and about 20 years older when they have a heart attack. Before age 60, 1 in 3 men develop some form of CVD, but the odds for women are 1 in 10.

What explains this difference? Research thus far has focused on the beneficial effects of estrogen, which, prior to menopause, circulates in high concentrations in a woman's body. Estrogen improves blood cholesterol levels by raising the concentration of HDL and lowering levels of LDL. Women, on average, have much better blood cholesterol profiles than men. Estrogen also seems to prevent blood clots from forming and

(continued)

to dissolve clots that do form. This is significant because clots can lead to heart attacks and strokes. And estrogen may also lower blood concentrations of homocysteine, high levels of which may be linked with heart attacks and strokes. Lifestyle factors may also help explain lower rates of CVD among women.

Women should not be complacent about their risk for cardiovascular disease, however. CVD is the leading cause of death among women. Nearly 1 in 2 women dies of CVD, whereas only 1 in 27 dies of breast cancer. After menopause, estrogen levels fall, and LDL levels begin to rise. By age 65, heart attack risk for women is almost equal to that of men. Women are less likely to survive a heart attack, in part because they tend to have them at an older age. Diagnosis can also be more difficult: A recent study found that about one-third of heart attack victims do not complain of chest pain and that women are more likely than men to have a heart attack without experiencing chest pain. More than 60% of women who die suddenly of heart disease have no earlier symptoms.

As more studies of CVD among women are completed, scientists may learn more about how female biochemistry affects the development of CVD. In the meantime, the general advice for preventing CVD presented in this chapter—exercising regularly, managing stress, limiting fat in the diet, and so on—is appropriate for everyone.

I know what foods to avoid to prevent CVD, but are there any foods I should eat to protect myself from CVD? The most important dietary change for CVD prevention is a negative one: cutting back on foods high in saturated and trans fat. However, research indicates that certain foods can be helpful. The positive effects of unsaturated fats, soluble fiber, and alcohol on heart health were discussed earlier in the chapter. Other potentially beneficial foods include those rich in the following:

- *Omega-3 fatty acids.* Found in fish, shellfish, and some nuts and seeds, omega-3 fatty acids reduce clotting and inflammation and may lower the risk of fatal arrhythmia.
- *Folic acid, vitamin B-6, and vitamin B-12.* These vitamins may affect CVD risk by lowering homocysteine levels; see Table 8.2 for a list of food sources.
- *Plant stanols and sterols.* Plant stanols and sterols, found in some types of trans-free margarines and other products, reduce the absorption of cholesterol in the body and help lower LDL levels.
- *Vitamin E.* The antioxidant vitamin E—found in nuts, vegetable oils, wheat germ, margarine, avocados, and leafy green vegetables—may inhibit the buildup of fatty plaques on artery walls.
- *Soy protein.* Replacing some animal protein with soy protein can lower LDL cholesterol. Soy-based foods include tofu, tempeh, and soy-based beverages.
- *Potassium and calcium.* Diets rich in potassium and calcium may be helpful in preventing and treating hypertension; they may also decrease the risk of stroke. The best way to ensure adequate intake of these minerals is to consume the recommended number of servings of fruits, vegetables, and low-fat or nonfat dairy products.

The advice I hear from the news about protecting myself from CVD seems to be changing all the time. What am I supposed to believe? Health-related research is now described in popular newspapers and magazines rather than just medical journals, meaning that more and more people have access to the information. Researchers do not deliberately set out to mislead or confuse people. However, news reports may oversimplify the results of research studies, leaving out some of the qualifications and questions the researchers present with their findings. In addition, news reports may not differentiate between a preliminary finding and a result that has been verified by a large number of long-term studies. And researchers themselves must strike a balance between reporting promising preliminary findings to the public, thereby allowing people to act on them, and waiting 10–20 years until long-term studies confirm (or disprove) a particular theory.

Although you cannot become an expert on all subjects, there are some general strategies you can use to better assess the health advice that appears in the media; see the box "Evaluating Health News."

What's a heart murmur, and is it dangerous? A heart murmur is an extra or altered heart sound heard during a routine medical exam. The source is often a problem with one of the heart valves that separate the chambers of the heart. Congenital defects and certain infections can cause abnormalities in the valves. The most common heart valve disorder is mitral valve prolapse (MVP), which occurs in about 4% of the population. MVP is characterized by a "billowing" of the mitral valve, which separates the left ventricle and left atrium, during ventricular contraction; in some cases, blood leaks from the ventricle into the atrium. Most people with MVP have no symptoms; they have the same ability to exercise and live as long as people without MVP.

MVP can be confirmed with echocardiography. Treatment is usually unnecessary, although surgery may be needed in the rare cases where leakage through the faulty valve is severe. Experts disagree over whether patients with MVP should take antibiotics prior to dental procedures, a precautionary step used to prevent bacteria, which may be dislodged into the bloodstream during some types of dental and surgical procedures, from infecting the defective valve. Most often, only those patients with significant blood leakage are advised to take antibiotics.

Although MVP usually requires no treatment, more severe heart valve disorders can impair blood flow through the heart. Treatment depends on the location and severity of the problem. More serious defects may be treated with surgery to repair or replace a valve.

CRITICAL CONSUMER Evaluating Health News

Americans face an avalanche of health information from newspapers, magazines, books, and television programs. It's not always easy to decide what to believe. The following questions can help you evaluate health news:

1. *Is the report based on research or on an anecdote?* Information or recommendations based on one or more carefully designed research studies has more validity than one person's experiences.
2. *What is the source of the information?* A study in a respected publication has been reviewed by editors and other researchers in the field—people who are in a position to evaluate the merits of a study and its results. Information put forth by government agencies and national research organizations is also usually considered fairly reliable.
3. *How big was the study?* A study that involves many subjects is more likely to yield reliable results than a study involving only a few people. Another indication that a finding is meaningful is if several different studies yield the same results.
4. *Who were the people involved in the study?* Research findings are more likely to apply to you if you share important characteristics with the subjects of the study. For example, the results of a study on men over age 50 who smoke may not be particularly meaningful for a 30-year-old nonsmoking woman. Even less applicable are studies done in test tubes or on animals.
5. *What kind of study was it?* Epidemiological studies involve observation or interviews in order to trace the relationships among lifestyle, physical characteristics, and diseases. Although epidemiological studies can suggest links, they cannot establish cause-and-effect relationships. Clinical or interventional studies involve testing the effects of different treatments on groups of people who have similar lifestyles and characteristics. They are more likely to provide conclusive evidence of a cause-and-effect relationship. The best interventional studies share the following characteristics:
   - *Controlled.* A group of people who receive the treatment is compared with a matched group who do not receive the treatment.
   - *Randomized.* The treatment and control groups are selected randomly.
   - *Double-blind.* Researchers and participants are unaware of who is receiving the treatment.
   - *Multicenter.* The experiment is performed at more than one institution.
6. *What do the statistics really say?* First, are the results described as "statistically significant"? If a study is large and well designed, its results can be deemed statistically significant, meaning there is less than a 5% chance that the findings resulted from chance. Second, are the results stated in terms of relative or absolute risk? Many findings are reported in terms of relative risk—how a particular treatment or condition affects a person's disease risk. Consider the following examples of relative risk:
   - According to some estimates, taking estrogen without progesterone can increase a postmenopausal woman's risk of dying from endometrial cancer by 233%.
   - Giving AZT to HIV-infected pregnant women reduces prenatal transmission of HIV by 90%.

   The first of these two findings seems far more dramatic than the second—until one also considers absolute risk, the actual risk of the illness in the population being considered. The absolute risk of endometrial cancer is 0.3%; a 233% increase based on the effects of estrogen raises it to 1%, a change of 0.7%. Without treatment, about 25% of infants born to HIV-infected women will be infected with HIV; with treatment, the absolute risk drops to about 2%, a change of 23%. Because the absolute risk of an HIV-infected mother passing the virus to her infant is so much greater than a woman's risk of developing endometrial cancer (25% compared with 0.3%), a smaller change in relative risk translates into a much greater change in absolute risk.
7. *Is new health advice being offered?* If the media report new guidelines for health behavior or medical treatment, examine the source. Government agencies and national research foundations usually consider a great deal of evidence before offering health advice. Above all, use common sense, and check with your physician before making a major change in your health habits based on news reports.

FOR FURTHER EXPLORATION

Fit and Well Online Learning Center (www.mhhe.com/fahey5e)

Use the learning objectives, study guide questions, and glossary flashcards to review key terms and concepts and prepare for exams. You can extend your knowledge of cardiovascular health and gain experience in using the Internet as a resource by completing the activities and checking out the Web links for the topics in Chapter 11 marked with the World Wide Web icon. For this chapter, Internet activities explore CVD risk factors, major forms of CVD, and prevention; there are Web links for the Vital Statistics figure, the Critical Consumer box on evaluating health news, and the chapter as a whole.

Daily Fitness and Nutrition Journal

Engaging in regular physical activity and eating a healthy diet are two important strategies for preventing CVD. Continue to use your journal to monitor your exercise program and, if needed, to keep records of your diet. You may want to use the nutrition journal to focus on a specific dietary factor related to CVD, such as saturated fat.

Health*Quest*

Learn more about your personal CVD risk and how you can prevent CVD by reviewing the resources and completing the activities in the cardiovascular health module of the Health*Quest* CD-ROM. You'll find an assessment that evaluates your current risk for heart attack. Cardiovascular Exploration takes a closer look at the cardiovascular system and risk factors for CVD. To determine if you're ready to make changes in your lifestyle as it affects your CVD risk, complete the Stages of Change quiz. You'll receive an assessment of your stage plus advice on moving forward toward the action and maintenance stages.

Books

American Heart Association and American Cancer Society. 1999. *Living Well, Staying Well: The Ultimate Guide to Help Prevent Heart Disease and Cancer.* New York: Times Books. *Provides practical, easy-to-follow guidelines to help you reduce your risk of developing CVD and cancer.*

Cohen, B. 2002. *Coronary Heart Disease: A Guide to Diagnosis and Treatment.* Omaha, Nebr.: Addicus Books. *Provides information about heart disease treatment and recovery for patients and their families.*

Gersh, B. J., ed. 2000. *The Mayo Clinic Heart Book.* New York: Morrow. *Covers risk factors, major forms of CVD, diagnosis, and treatment.*

Reaven, G. M. 2000. *Syndrome X: Overcoming the Silent Killer That Can Give You a Heart Attack.* New York: Simon & Schuster. *Provides information about syndrome X and insulin resistance, including lifestyle strategies for affected individuals.*

WW Organizations and Web Sites

American Heart Association. Provides information on hundreds of topics relating to the prevention and control of CVD.
800-AHA-USA1; 888-MY-HEART
http://www.americanheart.org (general information)
http://www.deliciousdecisions.org (dietary advice)
http://www.justmove.org (fitness advice)

Cardiology Compass. An index and links to cardiovascular information on the Internet.
http://www.cardiologycompass.com

Franklin Institute Science Museum/The Heart: An On-Line Exploration. An online museum exhibit containing information on the structure and function of the heart, how to monitor your heart's health, and how to maintain a healthy heart.
http://www.fi.edu/biosci/heart.html

HeartInfo—Heart Information Network. Provides information for heart patients and others interested in identifying and reducing their risk factors for heart disease; includes links to many related sites.
http://www.heartinfo.org

National Heart, Lung, and Blood Institute. Provides information on a variety of topics relating to cardiovascular health and disease, including cholesterol, smoking, obesity, and hypertension.
800-575-WELL
http://www.nhlbi.nih.gov; http://rover.nhlbi.nih.gov/chd

National Stroke Association. Provides information and referrals for stroke victims and their families; the Web site has a stroke risk assessment.
800-STROKES
http://www.stroke.org

See also the listings for Chapters 9 and 10.

SELECTED BIBLIOGRAPHY

American Heart Association. 2002. *Heart and Stroke Statistical Update, 2002.* Dallas, Tex.: American Heart Association.

American Heart Association. 2000. *An Eating Plan for Healthy Americans: The New 2000 Food Guidelines.* Dallas, Tex.: American Heart Association.

Aranow, W., et al. 2000. Aiming for lower than 140/90 mm Hg. *Patient Care* 34(7): 60–176.

Burke, A. P., et al. 2002. Elevated C-reactive protein values and atherosclerosis in sudden coronary death. *Circulation* 105(17): 2019–2023.

Canto, J. 2000. Prevalence, clinical characteristics, and mortality among patients with myocardial infarction presenting without chest pain. *Journal of the American Medical Association* 283(24): 3223–3229.

Cardillo, C. et al. 2000. Racial differences in nitric oxide-mediated vasodilator responses to mental stress in the forearm circulation. *Hypertension* 31(6): 1235–1239.

Carney, R. M., et al. 2001. Depression, heart rate variability, and acute myocardial infarction. *Circulation* 104(17): 2024–2028.

Centers for Disease Control and Prevention. 2002. State-specific mortality from sudden cardiac death. *Morbidity and Mortality Weekly* Report 51(6): 123–6.

Chang, P. P., et al. 2002. Anger in young men and subsequent premature cardiovascular disease. *Archives of Internal Medicine* 162(8): 901–906.

Djousse, L., et al. 2002. Alcohol consumption and risk of ischemic stroke: The Framingham Study. *Stroke* 33(4): 907–912.

Ford, E. S., W. H. Giles, and W. H. Dietz. 2002. Prevalence of metabolic syndrome among U.S. adults. *Journal of the American Medical Association* 287(3): 356–359.

Gibler, W. B., et al. 2002. Persistence of delays in presentation and treatment for patients with acute myocardial infarction. *Annals of Emergency Medicine* 39(2): 123–130.

Hayden, M., et al. 2002. Aspirin for the primary prevention of cardiovascular events: A summary of the evidence for the U.S. Preventive Services Task Force. *Annals of Internal Medicine* 136(2): 161–172.

Hu, F. B., et al. 2002. Fish and omega-3 fatty acid intake and risk of coronary heart disease in women. *Journal of the American Medical Association* 287(14): 1815–1821.

Joshipura, K. J., et al. 2001. The effect of fruit and vegetable intake on risk for coronary heart disease. *Annals of Internal Medicine* 134(12): 1106–1114.

Lee, I-M., et al. 2001. Physical activity and coronary heart disease in women. *Journal of the American Medical Association* 285(11): 1447–1254.

Ludwig, D. S. 2002. The glycemic index: Physiological mechanisms relating to obesity, diabetes, and cardiovascular disease. *Journal of the American Medical Association* 287(18): 2414–2423.

Marchioli, R., et al. 2002. Early protection against sudden death by n-3 polyunsaturated fatty acids after myocardial infarction. *Circulation* 105(16): 1897–1903.

Pollock, M., et al. 2000. AHA Science Advisory: Resistance exercise in individuals with and without cardiovascular disease. *Circulation* 101(7): 828–833.

Reid, I. R., et al. 2002. Effects of calcium supplementation on serum lipid concentrations in normal older women: A randomized controlled trial. *American Journal of Medicine* 112(5): 343–347.

Rutledge, T., et al. 2001. Effects on blood pressure of reduced dietary sodium and the Dietary Approaches to Stop Hypertension (DASH) diet. *New England Journal of Medicine* 344(1): 3–10.

Sheps, D. S., et al. 2002. Mental stress-induced ischemia and all-cause mortality in patients with coronary artery disease. Circulation 105(15): 1780–1784.

Vaccarino, V., et al. 2001. Sex differences in 2-year mortality after hospital discharge for myocardial infarction. *Annals of Internal Medicine* 134(2): 173–181.

Name ______________________ Section ______________ Date ______________

LAB 11.1 *Cardiovascular Health*

Part I CVD Risk Assessment

Your chances of suffering a heart attack or stroke before age 55 depend on a variety of factors, many of which are under your control. To help identify your risk factors, circle the response for each risk category that best describes you.

1. Sex and Age
   - 0 Female age 55 or younger; male age 45 or younger
   - 2 Female over age 55; male over age 45
2. Heredity
   - 0 Neither parent suffered a heart attack or stroke before age 60.
   - 3 One parent suffered a heart attack or stroke before age 60.
   - 7 Both parents suffered a heart attack or stroke before age 60.
3. Smoking
   - 0 Never smoked
   - 3 Quit more than 2 years ago and lifetime smoking is less than 5 pack-years*
   - 6 Quit less than 2 years ago and/or lifetime smoking is greater than 5 pack-years*
   - 8 Smoke less than ½ pack per day
   - 13 Smoke more than ½ pack per day
   - 15 Smoke more than 1 pack per day
4. Environmental Tobacco Smoke
   - 0 Do not live or work with smokers
   - 2 Exposed to ETS at work
   - 3 Live with smoker
   - 4 Both live and work with smokers
5. Blood Pressure

   The average of the last three readings:
   - 0 130/80 or below
   - 1 131/81–140/85
   - 5 141/86–150/90
   - 9 151/91–170/100
   - 13 Above 170/100
6. Total Cholesterol

   The average of the last three readings:
   - 0 Lower than 190
   - 1 190–210
   - 2 Don't know
   - 3 211–240
   - 4 241–270
   - 5 271–300
   - 6 Over 300
7. HDL Cholesterol

   The average of the last three readings:
   - 0 Over 65 mg/dl
   - 1 55–65
   - 2 Don't know HDL
   - 3 45–54
   - 5 35–44
   - 7 25–34
   - 12 Lower than 25
8. Exercise
   - 0 Exercise three times a week
   - 1 Exercise once or twice a week
   - 2 Occasional exercise less than once a week
   - 7 Rarely exercise
9. Diabetes
   - 0 No personal or family history
   - 2 One parent with diabetes
   - 6 Two parents with diabetes
   - 9 Type 2 diabetes
   - 13 Type 1 diabetes
10. Weight
    - 0 Near ideal weight
    - 1 6 pounds or less above ideal weight
    - 3 7–19 pounds above ideal weight
    - 5 20–40 pounds above ideal weight
    - 7 More than 40 pounds above ideal weight
11. Stress
    - 0 Relaxed most of the time
    - 1 Occasionally stressed and angry
    - 2 Frequently stressed and angry
    - 3 Usually stressed and angry

Scoring

Total your risk factor points. Refer to the list below to get an approximate rating of your risk of suffering an early heart attack or stroke.

Score	*Estimated Risk*
Less than 20	Low risk
20–29	Moderate risk
30–45	High risk
Over 45	Extremely high risk

*Pack-years can be calculated by multiplying the number of packs you smoked per day by the number of years you smoked. For example, if you smoked a pack and a half a day for 5 years, you would have smoked the equivalent of 1.5 × 5 = 7.5 pack-years.

LABORATORY ACTIVITIES

Part II Hostility Assessment

Current research indicates that three aspects of hostility are particularly harmful to cardiovascular health: cynicism (a mistrusting attitude regarding other people's motives), anger (an emotional response to other people's "unacceptable" behavior), and aggression (behaviors in response to negative emotions such as anger and irritation). To get an idea of how hostile you are, check any of the following statements that are true for you.

____ 1. Stuck in a long line at the express checkout in the grocery store, I often count the number of items the people in front of me have to see if anyone is over the limit.

_X_ 2. I am often irritated by other people's incompetence.

____ 3. If a cashier gives me the wrong change, I assume he or she is probably trying to cheat me.

_X_ 4. I've been so angry at someone that I've thrown things or slammed a door.

____ 5. If someone is late, I plan the angry words I'm going to say.

____ 6. I tend to remember irritating incidents and get mad all over again.

____ 7. If someone cuts me off in traffic, I honk my horn, flash my lights, pound the steering wheel, or shout.

_X_ 8. Little annoyances have a way of adding up during the day, leaving me frustrated and impatient.

____ 9. If the person who cuts my hair trims off more than I want, I fume about it for days afterward.

_X_ 10. When I get into an argument, I feel my jaw clench and my pulse and breathing rate climb.

____ 11. If someone mistreats me, I look for an opportunity to pay them back, just for the principle of the thing.

____ 12. I find myself getting annoyed at little things my spouse or significant other does that get under my skin.

Add up the number of items you checked. A score of 3 or less indicates a generally cool head. A score between 4 and 8 indicates that your level of hostility could be raising your risk of heart disease. A score of 9 or more indicates a hothead—a level of cynicism, anger, and aggression high enough to endanger both heart health and interpersonal relationships.

Using Your Results

How did you score? (1) What is your CVD risk assessment score? Are you at all surprised by your score?

-yep

Are you satisfied with your CVD risk rating? If not, set a specific goal: ________

(2) What is your hostility assessment score? Are you at all surprised by the result?

4 - no

Are you satisfied with your hostility rating? If not, set a specific goal: ________ -yes

What should you do next? Enter the results of this lab in the Preprogram Assessment column in Appendix D. (1) If you've set a goal for the overall CVD risk assessment score, identify a risk area that you can change, such as smoking, exercise, and stress. Then list three steps or strategies for changing the risk area you've chosen.

Risk area: ________________________________

Strategies for change:

(2) If you've set a goal for the hostility assessment score, begin by keeping a log of your hostile responses to people and situations. Familiarize yourself with the patterns of thinking that lead to hostile feelings and try to head them off before they develop into full-blown anger. Review the anger management strategies in Chapter 10 (p. 294) and select several that you will try to use to manage your own angry responses. Strategies for anger management:

Next, begin to put your strategies into action. After several weeks of a program to reduce CVD risk or hostility, do this lab again and enter the results in the Postprogram Assessment column of Appendix D. How do the results compare?

SOURCES: CVD risk assessment from Insel, P. M., and W. T. Roth. 2002. *Core Concepts in Health,* 9th ed. New York: McGraw-Hill. Hostility quiz from *Anger Kills*, by Redford B. Williams, M.D., and Virginia Williams, Ph.D. Copyright © 1993 by Redford B. Williams, M.D., and Virginia Williams, Ph.D. Adapted with permission of Times Books, a division of Random House, Inc.

Injury Prevention and Personal Safety

APPENDIX

A

Unintentional injuries are the fifth leading cause of death among Americans overall and the leading killer of young people. Injuries affect all segments of the population, but they are particularly common among minorities and people with low incomes, primarily due to social, environmental, and economic factors. The economic cost of injuries in the United States is high, with more than $500 billion spent each year for medical care and rehabilitation of injured people, employer losses, vehicle-damage costs, and fire losses.

Injuries are generally classified into four categories, based on where they occur: motor vehicle injuries, home injuries, leisure injuries, and work injuries.

MOTOR VEHICLE INJURIES

Incidents involving motor vehicles are the leading cause of death for people between the ages of 1 and 29, the leading cause of paralysis due to spinal injury, and the leading cause of severe brain injury.

Factors in Motor Vehicle Injuries

Driving Habits Nearly two-thirds of all motor vehicle injuries are caused by bad driving, especially speeding. As speed increases, momentum and force of impact increase and the time available for the driver to react decreases. Speed limits are posted to establish the safest *maximum* speed limit for a given area under *ideal* conditions. Anything that distracts a driver—sleepiness, bad mood, children or pets in the car, use of a cellular phone—can increase the risk of a crash.

Safety Belts and Air Bags A person who doesn't wear a safety belt is twice as likely to be injured in a crash as a person who does wear a safety belt. Safety belts not only prevent occupants from being thrown from the car at the time of the crash but also provide protection from the "second collision," which occurs when the occupant of the car hits something inside the car, such as the steering column or windshield. The safety belt also spreads the stopping force of a collision over the body.

Since 1998, all new cars have been equipped with dual air bags—one for the driver and one for the front passenger seat. Although air bags provide some supplemental protection in the event of a collision, most are useful only in head-on collisions. They also deflate immediately after inflating and so do not provide protection in collisions involving multiple impacts. To ensure that air bags work as intended, always follow these basic guidelines: Place infants in rear-facing infant seats in the back seat, transport children age 12 and under in the back seat, always use safety belts or appropriate safety seats, and keep 10 inches between the air bag cover and the breastbone of the driver or passenger. In the rare event that a person cannot comply with these guidelines, he or she can apply to the National Highway Traffic Safety Administration for permission to install an on-off switch that temporarily disables the air bag.

Alcohol and Other Drugs Alcohol is involved in about half of all fatal crashes. Alcohol-impaired driving, defined by blood alcohol concentration (BAC), is illegal. The legal BAC limit varies from 0.08% to 0.10%, but driving ability is impaired at much lower BACs. All psychoactive drugs have the potential to impair driving ability.

Preventing Motor Vehicle Injuries

About 75% of all motor vehicle collisions occur within 25 miles of home and at speeds lower than 40 mph. These crashes often occur because the driver believes safety measures are not necessary for short trips. Clearly, the statistics prove otherwise.

To prevent motor vehicle injuries:

- Obey the speed limit. If you have to speed to get to your destination on time, you're not allowing enough time. Try leaving 10–15 minutes earlier.
- Always wear a safety belt. Strap infants and toddlers into government-approved car seats in the back seat of the vehicle.
- Never drive under the influence of alcohol or other drugs. Never ride with a driver who has been drinking or using drugs.
- Keep your car in good working order. Regularly inspect tires, oil and fluid levels, windshield wipers, spare tire, and so on.
- Always allow enough following distance. Follow the "3-second rule": When the vehicle ahead passes a reference point, count out 3 seconds. If you pass the reference point before you finish counting, drop back and allow more following distance.
- Always increase following distance and slow down if weather or road conditions are poor.
- Choose interstate highways rather than rural roads. Highways are much safer because of better visibility, wider lanes, fewer surprises, and other factors.
- Always signal before turning or changing lanes.
- Stop completely at stop signs. Follow all traffic laws.
- Take special care at intersections. Always look left, right, and then left again. Make sure you have plenty of time to complete your maneuver in the intersection.
- Don't pass on two-lane roads unless you're in a designated passing area and have a clear view ahead.

A

Motorcycles and Mopeds

About one out of every ten traffic fatalities among people age 15–34 involves someone riding a motorcycle. Injuries from motorcycle collisions are generally more severe than those involving automobiles because motorcycles provide little, if any, protection. Moped riders face additional challenges. Mopeds usually have a maximum speed of 30–35 mph and have less power for maneuverability.

To prevent motorcycle and moped injuries:

- Make yourself easier to see by wearing light-colored clothing, driving with your headlights on, and correctly positioning yourself in traffic.
- Develop the necessary skills. Lack of skill, especially when evasive action is needed to avoid a collision, is a major factor in motorcycle and moped injuries. Skidding from improper braking is the most common cause of loss of control.
- Wear a close-fitting helmet, one marked with the symbol DOT (for Department of Transportation).
- Protect your eyes with goggles, a face shield, or a windshield.
- Drive defensively and never assume that other drivers see you.

Pedestrians and Bicycles

Injuries to pedestrians and bicyclists are considered motor vehicle related because they are usually caused by motor vehicles. About one in seven motor vehicle deaths each year involves a pedestrian; more than 90,000 pedestrians are injured each year.

To prevent injuries when walking or jogging:

- Walk or jog in daylight.
- Make yourself easier to see by wearing light-colored, reflective clothing.
- Face traffic when walking or jogging along a roadway, and follow traffic laws.
- Avoid busy roads or roads with poor visibility.
- Cross only at marked crosswalks and intersections.
- Don't listen to a radio, tape, or CD on headphones while walking or jogging.
- Don't hitchhike; it places you in a potentially dangerous situation.

Bicycle injuries result primarily from not knowing or understanding the rules of the road, failing to follow traffic laws, and not having sufficient skill or experience to handle traffic conditions. Bicycles are considered vehicles; bicycle riders must obey all traffic laws that apply to automobile drivers, including stopping at traffic lights and stop signs.

To prevent injuries when riding a bike:

- Wear safety equipment, including a helmet, eye protection, gloves, and proper footwear. Secure the bottom of your pant legs with clips and secure your shoelaces so they don't get tangled in the chain.
- Make yourself easier to see by wearing light-colored, reflective clothing. Equip your bike with reflectors and use lights, especially at night or when riding in wooded or other dark areas.
- Ride with the flow of traffic, not against it, and follow traffic laws. Use bike paths when they are available.
- Ride defensively; never assume that drivers see you. Be especially careful when turning or crossing at corners and intersections. Watch for cars turning right.
- Stop at all traffic lights and stop signs. Know and use hand signals.
- Continue pedaling at all times when moving (don't coast) to help keep the bike stable and to maintain your balance.
- Properly maintain your bike in working condition.

Aggressive Driving

Aggressive driving, known as road rage, has increased more than 50% since 1990. Aggressive drivers increase the risk of crashes for themselves and others. They further increase the risk of injuries if they stop their vehicles and confront each other. Even if you are successful at controlling your own aggressive driving impulses, you may still encounter an aggressive driver.

To avoid being the victim of an aggressive driver:

- *Always keep distance between your car and others.* If you are behind a very slow driver and can't pass, slow down to increase distance in case that driver does something unexpected. If you are being tailgated, do not increase your speed; instead, let the other driver pass you. If you are in the left lane when being tailgated, signal and pull over to let the other driver go by, even if you are traveling at the speed limit. When you are merging, make sure you have plenty of room. If you are being cut off by a merging driver, slow down to make room.
- *Be courteous, even if the other driver is not.* Use your horn rarely, if ever. Avoid making gestures of irritation, even shaking your head. When parking, let the other driver have the space that you both found.
- *Refuse to join in a fight.* Avoid eye contact with an angry driver. If someone makes a rude gesture, ignore it. If you think another car is following you and you have a cellular phone, call the police. Otherwise, drive to a public place and honk your horn to get someone's attention.
- *If you make a mistake while driving, apologize.* Raise or wave your hand or touch or knock your head with the palm of your hand to indicate "What was I thinking?" You can also mouth the words "I'm sorry."

HOME INJURIES

Contrary to popular belief, home is one of the most dangerous places to be. The most common fatal home injuries are caused by falls, poisoning, fires, suffocation and choking, and incidents involving firearms.

Falls

Falls are second only to motor vehicle injuries in terms of causing deaths. They are the fifth leading cause of unintentional death for people under age 25. Most deaths occurring from falls involve falling on stairs or steps or from one level to another. Falls also occur on the same level, from tripping, slipping, or stumbling. Alcohol is a contributing factor in many falls.

To prevent injuries from falls:

- Place skidproof backing on rugs and carpets.
- Install handrails and nonslip applications in the shower and bathtub.
- Keep floors clear of objects or conditions that could cause slipping or tripping, such as heavy wax coating, electrical cords, and toys.
- Put a light switch by the door of every room so that no one has to walk across a room to turn on a light. Use night-lights in bedrooms, halls, and bathrooms.
- Outside the house, clear dangerous surfaces created by ice, snow, fallen leaves, or rough ground.
- Install handrails on stairs. Keep stairs well lit and clear of objects.
- When climbing a ladder, use both hands. Never stand higher than the third step from the top. When using a stepladder, make sure the spreader brace is in the locked position. Don't stand on chairs to reach things.
- If there are small children in the home, place gates at the top and bottom of stairs. Never leave a baby unattended on a bed or table.

Poisoning

More than 2 million poisonings occur every year in the United States.

To prevent poisoning:

- Store all medicines out of the reach of children. Use medicines only as directed on the label or by a physician.
- Use cleaners, pesticides, and other dangerous substances only in areas with proper ventilation. Store them out of the reach of children.
- Never operate a vehicle in an enclosed space. Have your furnace inspected yearly. Use caution with any substance that produces potentially toxic fumes, such as kerosene. If appropriate, install carbon monoxide detectors.
- Keep poisonous plants out of the reach of young children. These include azalea, oleander, rhododendron, wild mushrooms, daffodil and hyacinth bulbs, mistletoe berries, apple seeds, morning glory seeds, wisteria seeds, and the leaves and stems of potato, rhubarb, and tomato plants.

To be prepared in case of poisoning:

- Keep the number of the nearest Poison Control Center (or emergency room) in an accessible location.
- Keep a bottle of syrup of ipecac (this induces vomiting) on hand. Use it only on the advice of the Poison Control Center or your doctor.

Emergency first aid for poisonings:

1. Remove the poison from contact with eyes, skin, or mouth, or remove the victim from contact with poisonous fumes or gases.
2. Call the Poison Control Center immediately for instructions. Have the container with you.
3. Do not follow emergency instructions on labels. Some may be out of date and carry incorrect treatment information.
4. If you are instructed to go to an emergency room, take the poisonous substance or its container with you.
5. If advised by the Poison Control Center or a physician, administer syrup of ipecac to induce vomiting.

Guidelines for specific types of poisons:

- *Swallowed poisons.* If the person is awake and able to swallow, give water only; then call the Poison Control Center or a physician for advice.
- *Poisons on the skin.* Remove any affected clothing. Flood affected parts of the skin with warm water, wash with soap and water, and rinse. Then call for advice.
- *Poisons in the eye.* For children, flood the eye with lukewarm water poured from a pitcher held 3–4 inches above the eye for 15 minutes; alternatively, irrigate the eye under a faucet. For adults, get in the shower and flood the eye with a gentle stream of lukewarm water for 15 minutes. Then call for advice.
- *Inhaled poisons.* Immediately carry or drag the person to fresh air and, if necessary, give mouth-to-mouth resuscitation. If the victim is not breathing easily, call 911 for help. Ventilate the area. Then call for advice.

Fires

Each year about 80% of fire deaths and 65% of fire injuries occur in the home. Careless smoking is the leading cause of fire deaths.

To prevent fires:

- Dispose of all cigarettes in ashtrays. Never smoke in bed.
- Do not overload electrical outlets. Do not place extension cords under rugs or where people walk. Replace worn or frayed extension cords.
- Place a wire screen in front of fireplaces and wood stoves. Remove ashes carefully and store them in airtight metal containers, not paper bags.
- Properly maintain electrical appliances, kerosene heaters, and furnaces. Clean flues and chimneys annually.
- Keep portable heaters at least 3 feet away from curtains, bedding, towels, or anything that might catch fire. Never leave heaters on when you're out of the room or sleeping.

To be prepared for a fire:

- Plan at least two escape routes out of each room. Designate a location outside the home as a meeting place.
- Install a smoke-detection device on every level of your home. Clean the detectors and test batteries once a month and replace the batteries at least once a year.
- Keep a fire extinguisher in your home and know how to use it.

To prevent injuries from fire:

- Get out as quickly as possible and go to the designated meeting place. Don't stop for a keepsake or a pet. Never hide in a closet or under a bed. Once outside, count heads to see if everyone is out. If you think someone is still inside the burning building, tell the firefighters. Never go back inside a burning building.
- If you're trapped in a room, feel the door. If it is hot or if smoke is coming in through the cracks, don't open it; use

the alternative escape route. If you can't get out of a room, go to the window and shout or wave for help.

- Smoke inhalation is the largest cause of death and injury in fires. To avoid inhaling smoke, crawl along the floor away from the heat and smoke. Cover your mouth and nose, ideally with a wet cloth, and take short, shallow breaths.
- If your clothes catch fire, don't run. Drop to the ground, cover your face, and roll back and forth to smother the flames. Remember: stop-drop-roll.

Suffocation and Choking

Suffocation accounts for nearly 4000 deaths annually in the United States. Young children account for nearly half of these deaths. Children can suffocate if they put small items in their mouths, get tangled in their crib bedding, or get trapped in airtight appliances like old refrigerators. Keep small objects out of reach of children under age 3, and don't give them raw carrots, hot dogs, popcorn, or hard candy. Examine toys carefully for small parts that could come loose; don't give plastic bags or balloons to small children.

Adults can also become choking victims, especially if they fail to chew food properly, eat hurriedly, or try to talk and eat at the same time. Many choking victims can be saved with the Heimlich maneuver (Figure A.1, p. A-8). Infants who are choking can be saved with blows to the upper back, followed by chest thrusts if necessary.

Incidents Involving Firearms

Firearms pose a significant threat of unintentional injury, especially to people between ages 15 and 24.

To prevent firearm injuries:

- Never point a loaded gun at something you do not intend to shoot.
- Store unloaded firearms under lock and key in a place separate from ammunition.
- Inspect firearms carefully before handling them.
- Follow the safety procedures advocated in firearm safety courses.

LEISURE INJURIES

Leisure injuries take place in public places (but do not involve motor vehicles) and include recreational, sports, and transportation injuries. Many injuries in this category involve such recreational activities as boating and swimming, play-ground activities, in-line skating, and sports.

Drowning and Boating Injuries

Although most drownings are reported in lakes, ponds, rivers, and oceans, more than half the drownings of young children take place in residential pools. Among adolescents and adults, alcohol plays a significant role in many boating injuries and drownings.

To prevent drowning and boating injuries:

- Develop adequate swimming skill and make sure children learn to swim.
- Make sure residential pools are fenced and that children are never allowed to swim without supervision.
- Don't swim alone or in unsupervised places.
- Use caution when swimming in unfamiliar surroundings or for an unusual length of time. Avoid being chilled by water colder than 70°F.
- Don't swim or boat under the influence of alcohol or other drugs. Don't chew gum or eat while in the water.
- Check the depth of water before diving.
- When on a boat, use a life jacket (personal flotation device).

In-Line Skating and Scooter Injuries

Most in-line skating injuries occur because users are not familiar with the equipment and do not wear appropriate safety gear. Injuries to the wrist and head are the most common. To reduce your risk of being injured while skating, wear a helmet, elbow and knee pads, wrist guards, a long-sleeved shirt, and long pants.

Wearing a helmet and knee and elbow pads is also important for preventing scooter injuries. The rise in popularity of lightweight scooters has seen a corresponding increase in associated injuries. Scooters should not be viewed as toys, and young children should be closely supervised. Be sure that handlebars, steering column, and all nuts and bolts are securely fastened. Ride on smooth, paved surfaces away from motor vehicle traffic. Avoid streets and surfaces with water, sand, gravel, or dirt.

Sports Injuries

Since more people have begun exercising to improve their health, there has been an increase in sports-related injuries.

To prevent sports injuries:

- Develop the skills required for the activity. Recognize and guard against the hazards associated with it.
- Always warm up and cool down.
- Make sure facilities are safe.
- Follow the rules and practice good sportsmanship.
- Use proper safety equipment, including, where appropriate, helmets, eye protection, knee and elbow pads and wrist guards. Wear correct footwear.
- When it is excessively hot and humid, avoid heat stress by following the guidelines given in the box "Exercising in Hot Weather" in Chapter 3.

WORK INJURIES

Many aspects of workplace safety are monitored by the Occupational Safety and Health Administration (OSHA), a federal agency. The highest rate of work-related injuries occurs among laborers, whose jobs usually involve extensive manual labor and lifting—two areas not addressed by OSHA safety standards. Back injuries are the most common work injury.

To protect your back when lifting:

- Don't try to lift beyond your strength. If you need it, get help.
- Get a firm footing, with your feet shoulder-width apart. Get a firm grip on the object.

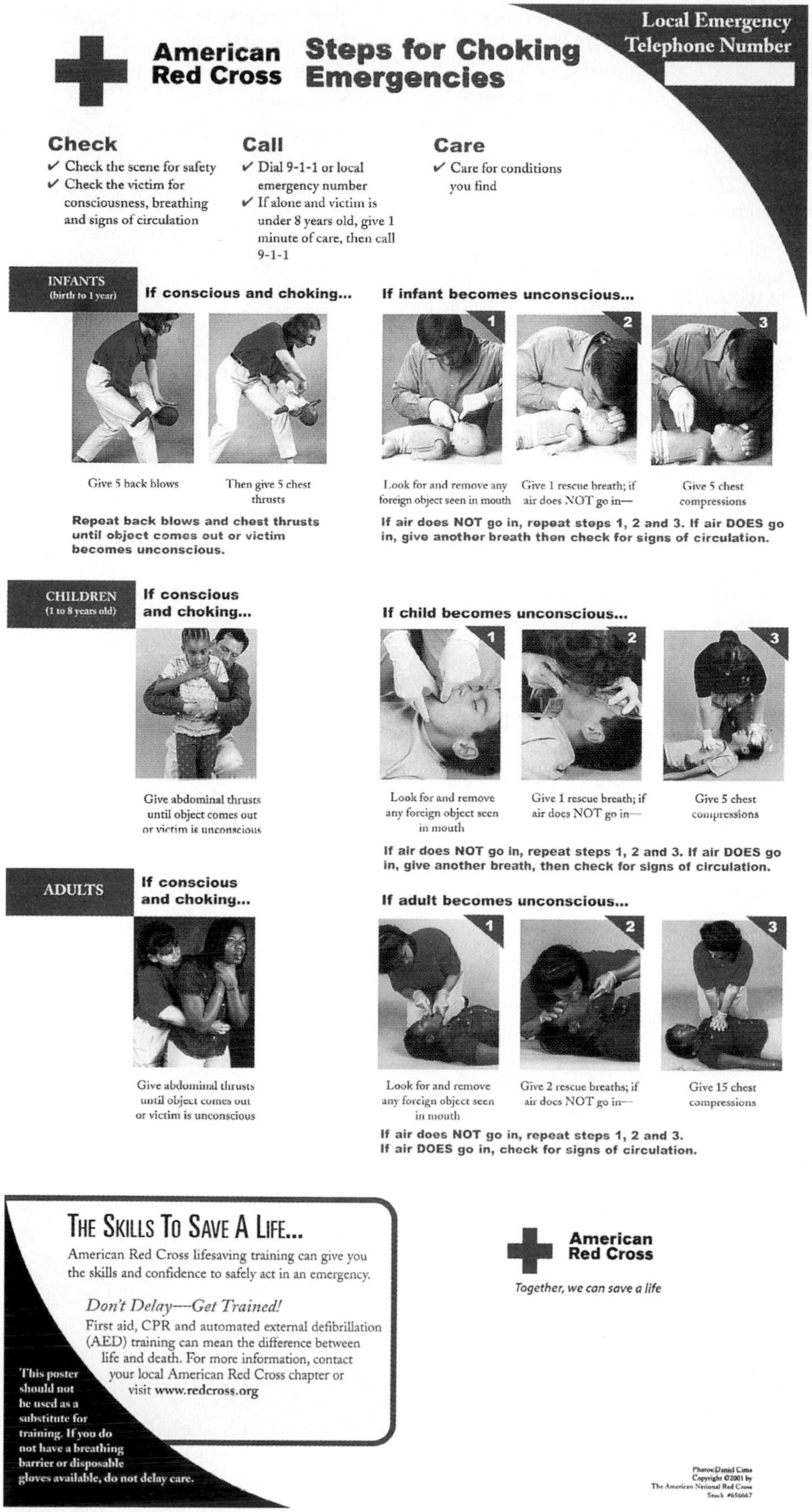
American Red Cross
Steps for Choking Emergencies
Local Emergency Telephone Number
Check
✔ Check the scene for safety
✔ Check the victim for consciousness, breathing and signs of circulation
Call
✔ Dial 9-1-1 or local emergency number
✔ If alone and victim is under 8 years old, give 1 minute of care, then call 9-1-1
Care
✔ Care for conditions you find
INFANTS (birth to 1 year)
If conscious and choking...
Give 5 back blows
Then give 5 chest thrusts
Repeat back blows and chest thrusts until object comes out or victim becomes unconscious.
If infant becomes unconscious...
1
2
3
Look for and remove any foreign object seen in mouth
Give 1 rescue breath; if air does NOT go in—
Give 5 chest compressions
If air does NOT go in, repeat steps 1, 2 and 3. If air DOES go in, give another breath then check for signs of circulation.
CHILDREN (1 to 8 years old)
If conscious and choking...
Give abdominal thrusts until object comes out or victim is unconscious
If child becomes unconscious...
1
2
3
Look for and remove any foreign object seen in mouth
Give 1 rescue breath; if air does NOT go in—
Give 5 chest compressions
If air does NOT go in, repeat steps 1, 2 and 3. If air DOES go in, give another breath, then check for signs of circulation.
ADULTS
If conscious and choking...
Give abdominal thrusts until object comes out or victim is unconscious
If adult becomes unconscious...
1
2
3
Look for and remove any foreign object seen in mouth
Give 2 rescue breaths; if air does NOT go in—
Give 15 chest compressions
If air does NOT go in, repeat steps 1, 2 and 3.
If air DOES go in, check for signs of circulation.
THE SKILLS TO SAVE A LIFE...
American Red Cross lifesaving training can give you the skills and confidence to safely act in an emergency.
Don't Delay—Get Trained!
First aid, CPR and automated external defibrillation (AED) training can mean the difference between life and death. For more information, contact your local American Red Cross chapter or visit www.redcross.org
This poster should not be used as a substitute for training. If you do not have a breathing barrier or disposable gloves available, do not delay care.
American Red Cross
Together, we can save a life

Figure A.1 Rescue breathing, first aid for choking, and ways to control bleeding: procedures recommended by the American Red Cross.

A

- Keep your torso in a relatively upright position and crouch down, bending at the knees and hips. Avoid bending at the waist. To lift, stand up or push up with your leg muscles. Lift gradually, keeping your arms straight. Keep the object close to your body.
- Don't twist. If you have to turn with an object, change the position of your feet.
- Put the object down gently, reversing the rules for lifting.

Another type of work-related injury is damage to the musculoskeletal system from repeated strain on the hand, arm, wrist, or other part of the body. Such repetitive-strain injuries are proliferating due to increased use of computers. One type, carpal tunnel syndrome, is characterized by pain and swelling in the tendons of the wrists and sometimes numbness and weakness.

To prevent carpal tunnel syndrome:

- Maintain good posture at the computer. Use a chair that provides back support and place the feet flat on the floor or on a foot rest.
- Position the screen at eye level and the keyboard so the hands and wrists are straight.
- Take breaks periodically to lessen the cumulative effects of stress.

VIOLENCE AND INTENTIONAL INJURIES

With more than 2 million Americans victims of violent injury each year, violence is a major public health concern. It includes assault, sexual assault, homicide, domestic violence, suicide, and child abuse. Compared with rates of violence in other industrialized countries, U.S. rates are abnormally high in two areas: homicide and firearm-related deaths.

Assault

Assault is the use of physical force to inflict injury or death on another person. Most assaults occur during arguments or in connection with another crime, such as robbery. Poverty, urban settings, and the use of alcohol and drugs are associated with higher rates of assault. Homicide is the fifteenth leading cause of death in the United States. Homicide victims are most likely to be male, between ages 19 and 24, and members of minority groups. Most homicides are committed with a firearm; the murderer and the victim usually know each other.

To protect yourself at home:

- Secure your home with good lighting and effective locks, preferably deadbolts. Make sure that all doors and windows are securely locked.
- Get a dog or post "Beware of Dog" signs.
- Don't hide keys in obvious places and don't give anyone the chance to duplicate your keys.
- Install a peephole in your front door. Don't open your door to people you don't know.
- If you or a family member owns a weapon, store it securely. Store guns and ammunition separately.
- If you are a woman living alone, use your initials rather than your full name in the phone directory. Don't use a greeting on your answering machine that implies you live alone or are not home.
- Teach everyone in the household how to obtain emergency assistance.
- Know your neighbors. Work out a system for alerting each other in case of an emergency.
- Establish a neighborhood watch program.

To protect yourself on the street:

- Avoid walking alone, especially at night. Stay where people can see and hear you.
- Walk on the outside of the sidewalk, facing traffic. Walk purposefully. Act alert and confident. If possible, keep at least two arm lengths between yourself and a stranger.
- Know where you are going. Appearing to be lost increases your vulnerability.
- Carry valuables in a fanny pack, pants pocket, or shoulder bag strapped diagonally across the chest.
- Always have your keys ready as you approach your vehicle or home.
- Carry a whistle to blow if you are attacked or harassed. If you feel threatened, run and/or yell. Go into a store or knock on the door of a home. If someone grabs you, yell "Help!" or "Fire!"

To protect yourself in your car:

- Keep your car in good working condition, carry emergency supplies, and keep the gas tank at least half full.
- When driving, keep doors locked and windows rolled up at least three-quarters of the way.
- Park your car in well-lighted areas or parking garages, preferably those with an attendant or a security guard.
- Lock your car when you leave it and check the interior before opening the door when you return.
- Don't pick up strangers. Don't stop for vehicles in distress; drive on and call for help.
- Note the location of emergency call boxes along highways and in public facilities. If you travel alone frequently, consider investing in a cellular phone.
- If your car breaks, down, raise the hood and tie a white cloth to the antenna or door handle. Wait in the car with the doors locked and windows rolled up. If someone approaches to offer help, open a window only a crack and ask the person to call the police or a towing service.
- When you stop at a light or stop sign, leave enough room to maneuver if you need an escape route.
- If you are involved in a minor automobile crash and you think you have been bumped intentionally, don't leave your car. Motion to the other driver to follow you to the nearest police station. If confronted by a person with a weapon, give up your car.

To protect yourself on public transportation:

- While waiting, stand in a populated, well-lighted area.
- Make sure that the bus, subway, or train is bound for your destination before you board it. Sit near the driver or conductor in a single seat or an outside seat.

- If you flag down a taxi, ensure that it's from a legitimate service. When you reach your destination, ask the driver to wait until you are safely inside the building.

To protect yourself on campus:

- Ensure that door and window locks are secure and that halls and stairwells have adequate lighting.
- Don't give dorm or residence keys to anybody.
- Don't leave your door unlocked or allow strangers into your room.
- Avoid solitary late-night trips to the library or laundry room. Take advantage of on-campus escort services.
- Don't exercise outside alone at night. Don't take shortcuts across campus that are unfamiliar or seem unsafe.
- If security guards patrol the campus, know the areas they cover and stay where they can see or hear you.

Sexual Assault—Rape and Date Rape

The use of force and coercion in sexual relationships is one of the most serious problems in human interactions. The most extreme manifestation of sexual coercion—forcing a person to submit to another's sexual desires—is rape. Taking advantage of circumstances that render a person incapable of giving consent (such as when drunk) is also considered sexual assault or rape. Coerced sexual activity in which the victim knows or is dating the rapist is often referred to as date rape.

At least 3.5 million females are raped annually in the United States, and some males—perhaps 10,000 annually—are raped each year by other males. Rape victims suffer both physical and psychological injury. The psychological pain can be substantial and long-lasting.

To protect yourself against rape:

- Following the guidelines listed earlier for protecting yourself against assault.
- Trust your gut feeling. If you feel you are in danger, don't hesitate to run and scream.
- Think out in advance what you would do if you were threatened with rape. However, no one knows what he or she will do when scared to death. Trust that you will make the best decision at the time—whether to scream, run, fight, or give in to avoid being injured or killed.

To protect yourself against date rape:

- Believe in your right to control what you do. Set limits and communicate them clearly, firmly, and early. Be assertive; men often interpret passivity as permission.
- If you are unsure of a new acquaintance, go on a group date or double date. If possible, provide your own transportation.
- Remember that some men think flirtatious behavior or sexy clothing indicates an interest in having sex.
- Remember that alcohol and drugs interfere with judgment, perception, and communication about sex.
- Use the statement that has proven most effective in stopping date rape: "This is rape and I'm calling the cops!"

If you are raped:

- Tell what happened to the first friendly person you meet.
- Call the police. Tell them you were raped and give your location.
- Try to remember everything you can about your attacker and write it down.
- Don't wash or douche before the medical exam. Don't change your clothes, but bring a new set with you if you can.
- At the hospital you will have a complete exam. Show the physician any bruises or scratches.
- Tell the police exactly what happened. Be honest and stick to your story.
- If you do not want to report the rape to the police, see a physician as soon as possible. Be sure you are checked for pregnancy and STDs.
- Contact an organization with skilled counselors so you can talk about the experience. Look in the telephone directory under "Rape" or "Rape Crisis Center" for a hotline number.

Guidelines for men:

- Be aware of social pressure. It's OK not to "score."
- Understand that "No" means "No." Stop making advances when your date says to stop. Remember that she has the right to refuse sex.
- Don't assume that flirtatious behavior or sexy clothing means a woman is interested in having sex, that previous permission for sex applies to the current situation, or that your date's relationships with other men constitute sexual permission for you.
- Remember that alcohol and drugs interfere with judgment, perception, and communication about sex.

Stalking and Cyberstalking

Stalking is characterized by harassing behaviors such as following or spying on a person and making verbal, written, or implied threats. It is estimated that 1 million U.S. women and 400,000 men are stalked each year; most stalkers are men. Cyberstalking, the use of electronic communications devices to stalk another person, is becoming more common. Cyberstalkers may send harassing or threatening e-mails or chat room messages to the victim, or they may encourage others to harass the victim by posting inflammatory messages and personal information on bulletin boards or chat rooms.

To protect yourself online:

- Never use your real name as an e-mail user name or chat room nickname. Select an age-and gender-neutral identity.
- Avoid filling out profiles for accounts related to e-mail use or chat room activities with information that could be used to identify you.
- Do not share personal information in public spaces anywhere online or give it to strangers.
- Learn how to filter unwanted e-mail messages.
- If you do experience harassment online, do not respond to the harasser. Log off or surf elsewhere. Save all communications for evidence. If harassment continues, report it to the harasser's Internet service provider, your Internet service provider, and the local police.
- Don't agree to meet someone you've met online face to face unless you feel completely comfortable about it. Schedule a

A

series of phone conversations first. Meet initially in a very public place and bring along a friend to increase your safety.

Coping after Terrorism or Mass Violence

For many Americans, the September 11, 2001, terrorist attacks were the first major national catastrophe they have experienced. Some people suffered the loss of relatives or friends; many others were robbed of their sense of security. Each person reacts differently to this type of traumatic disaster, and it is normal to experience a variety of responses. Reactions may include disbelief and shock, fear, anger and resentment, anxiety about the future, difficulty concentrating or making decisions, mood swings, irritability, sadness and depression, panic, guilt, apathy, feelings of isolation or powerlessness, and many of the behaviorial signs such as headaches or insomnia that are associated with excess stress (see Chapter 10). Reactions may occur immediately or may be delayed until weeks or months after the event.

Taking positive steps can help you cope with powerful emotions. Consider the following strategies:

- Share your experiences and emotions with friends and family members. Be a supportive listener. Reassure children and encourage them to talk about what they are feeling.
- Take care of your mind and body. Choose a healthy diet, exercise regularly, get plenty of sleep, and practice relaxation techniques. Don't turn to unhealthy coping techniques such as using alcohol or other drugs.
- Take a break from media reports and images, and try not to develop nightmare scenarios for possible future events.
- Reestablish your routines at home, school, and work.
- Find ways to help others. Donating money, blood, food, clothes, or time can ease difficult emotions and give you a greater sense of control.

Everyone copes with tragedy in a different way and recovers at a different pace. If you feel overwhelmed by your emotions, seek professional help. Additional information about coping with terrorism and violence is available from the Federal Emergency Management Agency (www.fema.gov), the U.S. Department of Justice (www.usdoj.gov), and the National Mental Health Association (www.nmha.org).

PROVIDING EMERGENCY CARE

You can improve someone else's chances of surviving if you are prepared to provide emergency help. A course in first aid offered by the American Red Cross and on many college campuses can teach you to respond appropriately when someone needs help. Emergency rescue techniques can save the lives of people who have stopped breathing, who are choking, or whose hearts have stopped beating. Pulmonary resuscitation (also known as rescue breathing, artificial respiration, or mouth-to-mouth resuscitation) is used when a person is not breathing (see Figure A.1). Cardiopulmonary resuscitation (CPR) is used when a pulse can't be found. Training is required before a person can perform CPR. Courses are offered by the American Red Cross and the American Heart Association.

When you have to provide emergency care:

- Remain calm and act sensibly. The basic pattern for providing emergency care is check-call-care.
- *Check the situation.* Make sure the scene is safe for both you and the injured person. Don't put yourself in danger; if you get hurt too, you will be of little help to the injured person.
- *Check the victim.* Conduct a quick head-to-toe examination. Assess the victim's signs and symptoms, such as level of responsiveness, pulse, and breathing rate. Look for bleeding and any indications of broken bones or paralysis.
- *Call for help.* Call 911 or a local emergency number. Identify yourself and give as much information as you can about the condition of the victim and what happened.
- *Care for the victim.* If the situation requires immediate action (no pulse, shock, etc.), provide first aid if you are trained to do so (see Figure A.1).

SELECTED BIBLIOGRAPHY

AAA Foundation for Traffic Safety. 1997. *Road Rage: How to Avoid Aggressive Driving.* Washington, D.C.: AAA Foundation for Traffic Safety.

American Academy of Pediatrics. 2002. Skateboard and scooter injuries. *Pediatrics* 103(3): 542–543.

Burt, C. W., and M. D. Overpeck. 2001. Emergency visits for sports-related injuries. *Annals of Emergency Medicine* 37(3): 301–308.

Centers for Disease Control and Prevention. 2001. Surveillance for fatal and nonfatal firearm-related injuries. *CDC Surveillance Summaries* 50(SS2).

Centers for Disease Control and Prevention. 2000. Prevalence and health consequences of stalking. *Morbidity and Mortality Weekly Report* 49(29): 653–655.

Federal Bureau of Investigation. 2001. *Crime in the United States: Uniform Crime Reports, 2000.* Washington, D.C.: U.S. Department of Justice.

Li, G., et al. 2001. Use of alcohol as a risk factor for bicycling injury. *Journal of the American Medical Association* 285(7): 893–896.

National Institutes of Health. 2001. Coping with terrorism. *Word on Health,* December.

National Mental Health Association. 2001. *Coping with Disaster: Tips for College Students* (http://www.nmha.org/reassurance/collegetips.cfm; retrieved April 30, 2002).

National Safety Council. 2001. *Injury Facts.* Itasca, Ill.: National Safety Council.

New York State Department of Motor Vehicles. 2000. *Aggressive Driving* (http://www.nysgtsc.state.ny.us/aggr-ndx.htm; retrieved December 27, 2000).

Philip, P., et al. 2001. Fatigue, alcohol, and serious road crashes in France. *British Medical Journal* 322(7290): 829–830.

U.S. Department of Justice. 1999. *1999 Report on Cyberstalking: A New Challenge for Law Enforcement and Industry* (http://www.usdoj.gov:80/criminal/cybercrime/cyberstalking.htm; retrieved December 17, 2000).

Williamson, A. M., and A. M. Feyer. 2000. Moderate sleep deprivation produces impairments in cognitive and motor performance equivalent to legally prescribed levels of alcohol intoxication. *Occupational and Environmental Medicine* 57(10): 649–655.

Nutritional Content of Common Foods

APPENDIX

B

For this food composition table, foods are listed within the following groups, corresponding to the Food Guide Pyramid: (1) breads, cereals, rice, and pasta; (2) vegetables; (3) fruit; (4) milk, yogurt, and cheese; (5) meat, poultry, fish, dry beans, eggs, and nuts; and (6) fats, oils, sweets, and alcoholic beverages.

Data are provided for a variety of nutrients. For planning and easy reference, complete the following chart with your approximate daily goals or limits; refer to Table 8.2 and the Nutrition Resources section that follows Chapter 8. Fill in the daily totals that apply to your approximate daily calorie intake, sex, and age.

TOTAL DAILY GOAL OR LIMIT			
Total energy	______ calories	**Cholesterol**	300 mg
Protein	______ grams	**Sodium**	2400 mg
Carbohydrate	______ grams	**Vitamin A**	______ RE
Dietary fiber	20–35 grams	**Vitamin C**	______ mg
Total fat	______ grams	**Calcium**	______ mg
Saturated fat	______ grams	**Iron**	______ mg

This appendix contains information on the same nutrients found on most food labels, so you can make easy comparisons. On food labels, percent Daily Values without corresponding units are usually provided for vitamins and minerals. For reference, the Daily Values are as follows: 5000 IU of vitamin A, 60 mg of vitamin C, 1000 mg of calcium, and 18 mg of iron.

BREADS, CEREALS, RICE, AND PASTA

The Food Guide Pyramid recommends 6–11 servings per day. One serving is equivalent to 1 slice of bread, about 1 cup of ready-to-eat cereal, or ½ cup of cooked cereal, rice, or pasta.

Name	Amount	Weight (g)	Energy (calories)	Protein (g)	Carbohydrate (g)	Fiber (g)	Total fat (g)	Saturated fat (g)	Cholesterol (mg)	Sodium (mg)	Vitamin A (RE)	Vitamin C (mg)	Calcium (mg)	Iron (mg)
Bagel, plain	1 bagel, 4″ dia.	89	245	9.3	47.5	2.0	1.4	0.2	0	475	0	0	216	3.2
Barley, pearled, cooked	½ cup	79	97	1.8	22.2	3.0	0.3	0.1	0	2	1	0	9	1.0
Bulgur, cooked	½ cup	83	110	3.0	23.5	4.5	0.1	0	0	4	0	0	11	0.5
Biscuit	1 biscuit, 2½″ dia.	27	93	1.8	12.8	0.4	4.0	1.0	0	325	0	0	5	0.7
Bread, corn	1 piece	60	188	4.3	28.9	1.4	6.0	1.6	37	467	26	0	44	1.1
Bread, French	1 slice	64	175	5.6	33.2	1.9	1.9	0.4	0	390	0	0	48	1.6
Bread, oatmeal	1 slice	27	73	2.3	13.1	1.1	1.2	0.2	0	162	1	0	18	0.67
Bread, pita, white	1 pita, 6½″ dia.	60	165	5.5	33.4	1.3	0.7	0.1	0	322	0	0	52	1.6
Bread, pita, whole wheat	1 pita, 6½″ dia.	64	170	6.3	35.2	4.7	1.7	0.3	0	340	0	0	10	2.0
Bread, pumpernickel	1 slice	26	65	2.3	12.3	1.7	0.8	0.1	0	174	0	0	18	0.7
Bread, raisin	1 slice	32	88	2.5	16.7	1.4	1.4	0.3	0	125	0	0	21	0.9
Bread, rye	1 slice	32	83	2.7	15.5	1.9	1.1	0.2	0	211	0	0.1	23	0.9
Bread sticks	2 sticks, 7⅝″ x ⅝″	20	82	2.4	13.6	0.6	1.9	0.3	0	131	0	0	4	0.8
Bread stuffing	½ cup	100	178	3.2	21.7	2.9	8.6	1.7	0	543	81	0	32	1.1
Bread, white	1 slice	30	80	2.5	14.9	0.7	1.1	0.2	0	161	0	0	32	0.9

B

Name	Amount	Weight (g)	Energy (calories)	Protein (g)	Carbohydrate (g)	Fiber (g)	Total fat (g)	Saturated fat (g)	Cholesterol (mg)	Sodium (mg)	Vitamin A (RE)	Vitamin C (mg)	Calcium (mg)	Iron (mg)
Bread, whole grain	1 slice	32	80	3.2	14.8	2.0	1.2	0.3	0	156	0	0.1	29	1.1
Bread, whole wheat	1 slice	28	69	2.7	12.9	1.9	1.2	0.3	0	148	0	0	20	0.9
Buckwheat groats, cooked	½ cup	84	77	2.8	16.8	2.3	0.5	0.1	0	3	0	0	6	0.7
Bun, hamburger/hot dog	1 roll	43	123	3.7	21.6	1.2	2.2	0.5	0	241	0	0	60	1.4
Cake, angelfood	1/12 of 10″ cake	50	129	3.1	29.4	0.1	0.2	0	0	255	0	0	42	0.1
Cake, chocolate w/frosting	⅛ of 18 oz cake	64	235	2.6	34.9	1.8	10.5	3.1	27	214	16	0.1	28	1.4
Cake, yellow w/icing	⅛ of 18 oz cake	64	243	2.4	35.5	1.2	11.1	3.0	35	216	21	0	23	1.3
Cereal, All-Bran	½ cup	30	53	3.7	22.7	15.3	0.9	0.2	0	127	260	17.3	116	5.2
Cereal, Bran Chex	⅗ cup	28	90	2.9	22.6	4.6	0.8	0.1	0	200	6	15.0	17	8.1
Cereal, Cheerios	1 cup	30	110	3.1	22.9	2.6	1.8	0.4	0	284	375	15.0	55	8.1
Cereal, corn flakes	1 cup	28	102	1.8	24.2	0.8	0.2	0.1	0	298	210	14.0	1	8.7
Cereal, Cream of Wheat	½ cup	126	67	1.9	13.8	0.9	0.3	0	0	168	0	0	25	5.1
Cereal, Frosted Flakes	¾ cup	31	119	1.2	28.3	0.6	0.2	0.1	0	200	225	15.0	1	4.5
Cereal, granola	½ cup	31	135	3.0	22.4	1.9	4.2	0.6	0	8	0	0.1	24	1.3
Cereal, raisin bran	1 cup	61	186	5.6	47.1	8.2	1.5	0	0	354	250	0	35	5.0
Cereal, Total	¾ cup	30	105	3.0	23.9	2.6	0.7	0.2	0	199	375	60.0	258	18.0
Cereal, Wheaties	1 cup	30	110	3.2	0.9	2.1	0.9	0.2	0	222	225	15.0	55	8.1
Coffee cake w/topping	1 piece	63	263	4.3	29.4	1.3	14.7	3.7	20	221	21	0.2	34	1.2
Cookie, chocolate chip	1 medium cookie	16	78	0.9	9.3	0.4	4.5	1.3	5	58	26	0	6	0.4
Cookie, fig bar	1 cookie	16	56	0.6	11.3	0.7	1.2	0.2	0	56	1	0	10	0.5
Cookie, fortune	1 cookie	8	30	0.3	6.7	0.1	0.2	0.1	0	22	0	0	1	0.1
Cookie, oatmeal	1 large cookie	18	81	1.1	12.4	0.5	3.3	0.8	0	69	0	0.1	7	0.5
Cookie, sandwich	1 cookie	10	47	0.5	7.0	0.3	0.3	0.4	0	60	0	0	3	0.4
Corn meal, dry	¼ cup	35	126	2.9	26.8	2.6	0.6	0.1	0	1	14	0	2	1.4
Corn grits, cooked	½ cup	121	73	1.7	15.7	0.2	0.2	0	0	0	7	0	0	0.8
Couscous, cooked	½ cup	79	88	3.0	18.2	1.1	0.1	0	0	4	0	0	6	0.3
Cracker, crispbread, rye	3 crispbreads	30	110	2.4	24.7	5.0	0.4	0	0	79	0	0	9	0.7
Cracker, Goldfish	24 goldfish	12	70	1.0	8.0	1.0	4.0	0	0	100	0	0	8	0.4
Cracker, graham	3 squares	28	119	2.0	21.3	1.0	2.8	0.4	0	185	0	0	22	1.2
Cracker, matzo	1 matzo	28	112	2.8	23.7	0.9	0.4	0.1	0	1	0	0	4	0.9
Cracker, melba toast	6 pieces	30	117	3.6	23.0	1.9	1.0	0.1	0	249	0	0	28	1.1
Cracker, Ritz	5 crackers	16	79	1.2	10.3	0.3	3.7	0.6	0	124	0	0	24	0.6
Cracker, saltine	10 squares	30	130	2.8	21.5	0.9	3.5	0.9	0	390	0	0	36	1.6
Cracker, whole wheat	6 crackers	24	106	2.1	16.5	2.5	4.1	0.8	0	158	0	0	24	0.7
Croissant, butter	1 medium	57	231	4.7	26.1	1.5	12.0	6.6	38	424	106	0.1	21	1.2
Danish pastry, cheese	1 pastry	71	266	5.7	26.4	0.7	15.5	4.8	11	320	32	0	25	1.1
Doughnut, glazed	1 medium	45	192	2.3	22.9	0.7	10.3	2.7	14	181	1	0	27	0.5
English muffin, plain	½ muffin	29	67	2.2	13.1	0.8	0.5	0.1	0	132	0	0	50	0.7
French toast	1 slice	65	149	5.0	16.3	0	7.0	1.8	75	311	86	0.2	65	1.1
Macaroni, cooked	½ cup	70	99	3.3	19.8	0.9	0.5	0.1	0	1	0	0	5	1.0
Muffin, blueberry	2″ by 2¾″	57	158	3.1	27.4	1.5	3.7	0.8	17	255	5	0.6	32	0.9
Muffin, oatbran	2¼″ by 2½″	57	154	4.0	27.5	2.6	4.2	0.6	0	224	0	0	36	2.4
Noodles, chow mein	½ cup	23	119	1.9	12.9	0.9	6.9	1.0	0	99	2	0	5	1.1
Noodles, egg, cooked	½ cup	80	106	3.8	19.9	0.9	1.2	0.2	53	6	5	0	10	1.3
Noodles, Japanese soba	½ cup	57	56	2.9	12.2	0	0.1	0	0	34	0	0	2	0.3
Oats, uncooked	¼ cup	20	78	3.2	27.1	2.1	1.3	0.2	0	1	2	0	11	0.9
Oatmeal, instant	1 packet	155	153	4.1	31.4	2.6	1.8	0.4	0	234	302	0	105	3.9
Pancake	4″ pancake	38	74	2.0	13.9	0.5	1.0	0.2	5	239	12	0.1	48	0.6
Pasta, cooked	½ cup	57	75	2.9	14.2	0	0.6	0.1	19	3	3	0	3	0.7
Popcorn, air-popped	2 cups	16	61	1.9	12.5	2.4	0.7	0.1	0	1	3	0	2	0.4
Popcorn, oil-popped	2 cups	22	110	1.9	12.6	2.2	6.2	1.0	0	194	3	0	2	0.6
Pretzels	10 twists	60	229	5.5	47.5	1.9	2.1	0.5	0	1029	0	0	22	2.6
Quinoa, uncooked	¼ cup	43	159	5.6	29.3	2.5	2.5	0.3	0	9	0	0	26	3.9
Roll, dinner	1 roll, 2″ square	28	84	2.4	14.1	0.8	2.0	0.5	0	146	0	0	33	0.9
Rice, brown, cooked	½ cup	71	109	2.3	22.9	1.8	0.8	0.3	0	1	0	0	10	0.5
Rice cake	1 cake	9	35	0.7	7.3	0.4	0.3	0	0	29	0	0	1	0.1
Rice, white, cooked	½ cup	93	121	2.2	26.6	0.3	0.2	0.1	0	0	0	0	3	1.4
Rice, wild, cooked	½ cup	82	83	3.3	17.5	1.5	0.3	0	0	3	0	0	2	0.5
Spaghetti, cooked	½ cup	70	99	3.3	19.8	1.2	0.5	0.1	0	70	0	0	5	1.0

Name	Amount	Weight (g)	Energy (calories)	Protein (g)	Carbohydrate (g)	Fiber (g)	Total fat (g)	Saturated fat (g)	Cholesterol (mg)	Sodium (mg)	Vitamin A (RE)	Vitamin C (mg)	Calcium (mg)	Iron (mg)
Taco shell	1 medium	13	62	1.0	8.3	1.0	3.0	0.4	0	49	0	0	21	0.3
Tortilla chips	1 oz.	28	142	2.0	17.8	1.8	7.4	1.4	0	150	6	0	44	0.4
Tortilla, corn	1 medium	26	58	1.5	12.1	1.4	0.7	0.1	0	42	0	0	46	0.4
Tortilla, flour	1 medium	49	159	4.3	27.2	1.6	3.5	0.9	0	234	0	0	61	1.6
Wheat germ, toasted	¼ cup	28	108	8.3	14.1	3.7	3.0	0.5	0	1	0	1.7	13	2.6

VEGETABLES The Food Guide Pyramid recommends 3–5 servings per day. One serving is equivalent to 1 cup of raw leafy vegetables, ½ cup of other raw or cooked vegetables, or ¾ cup of vegetable juice.

Name	Amount	Weight (g)	Energy (calories)	Protein (g)	Carbohydrate (g)	Fiber (g)	Total fat (g)	Saturated fat (g)	Cholesterol (mg)	Sodium (mg)	Vitamin A (RE)	Vitamin C (mg)	Calcium (mg)	Iron (mg)
Artichoke, cooked	1 medium	120	60	4.2	13.4	6.5	0.2	0	0	114	22	12.0	54	1.5
Arugula, raw	1 cup	20	5	0.5	0.7	0.3	0.1	0	0	3	24	3.0	16	0.1
Asparagus, cooked	6 spears	90	22	2.3	3.8	1.4	0.3	0	0	10	49	9.7	18	0.7
Bamboo shoots, canned	½ cup	66	13	1.1	2.1	0.9	0.3	0.1	0	5	1	0.7	5	0.2
Bean sprouts, raw	½ cup	35	43	4.6	3.3	0.4	2.3	0.3	0	5	0	5.4	23	0.7
*Beans, baked (plain)	½ cup	127	118	6.1	26.0	6.4	0.6	0.1	0	504	22	3.9	64	0.4
*Beans, black, cooked	½ cup	86	114	7.6	20.4	7.5	0.5	0.1	0	1	1	0	23	1.8
*Beans, fava, cooked	½ cup	85	94	6.5	16.7	4.6	0.3	0.1	0	4	2	0.3	31	1.3
Beans, green snap, cooked	½ cup	63	22	1.2	4.9	2.0	0.2	0	0	2	42	6.1	29	0.8
*Beans, kidney, cooked	½ cup	89	112	7.7	20.2	6.5	0.4	0.1	0	2	0	1.1	25	2.6
*Beans, lentils, cooked	½ cup	99	115	8.9	19.9	7.8	0.4	0.1	0	2	1	1.5	19	3.3
* Beans, lima, cooked	½ cup	94	108	7.3	19.6	6.6	0.4	0.1	0	2	0	0	16	2.2
*Beans, navy, cooked	½ cup	91	129	7.9	23.9	5.8	0.5	0.1	0	1	0	0.8	64	2.3
*Beans, pinto, cooked	½ cup	86	117	7.0	21.9	7.4	0.4	0.1	0	2	0	1.8	41	2.2
*Beans, refried	½ cup	126	118	6.9	19.6	6.7	1.6	0.6	10	377	0	7.6	44	2.1
Beans, yellow snap, cooked	½ cup	63	22	1.2	4.9	2.1	0.2	0	0	2	5	6.1	29	0.8
Beet greens, cooked	½ cup	144	39	3.7	7.9	4.2	0.3	0	0	347	734	35.9	164	2.7
Beets, cooked	½ cup	74	37	1.4	8.5	1.7	0.2	0	0	65	3	3.1	14	0.7
Broccoli spears, cooked	2 spears	78	22	2.3	3.9	2.3	0.3	0	0	20	108	58.2	36	0.7
Brussels sprouts, cooked	4 sprouts	84	33	2.1	7.3	2.2	0.4	0.1	0	18	60	52.1	30	1.0
Cabbage, cooked	½ cup	75	17	0.8	3.3	1.7	0.3	0	0	6	10	15.1	23	0.1
Cabbage, raw	½ cup	45	11	0.6	2.4	1.0	0.1	0	0	8	6	14.3	21	0.3
Carrot, juice	¾ cup	177	71	1.7	16.4	1.4	0.3	0	0	51	1938	15.0	42	0.8
Carrots, cooked	½ cup	78	35	0.9	8.2	2.6	0.1	0	0	51	1915	1.8	24	0.5
Carrots, raw	1 medium	61	26	0.6	6.2	1.8	0.1	0	0	21	1716	5.6	16	0.3
Cauliflower, cooked	½ cup	62	14	1.1	2.5	1.7	0.3	0	0	9	1	27.4	10	0.2
Celery, raw	8 sticks	32	5	0.2	1.2	0.5	0	0	0	28	4	2.2	13	0.1
Chard, cooked	½ cup	88	18	1.6	3.6	1.8	0.1	0	0	156	275	15.8	51	2.0
Coleslaw, homemade	½ cup	60	41	0.8	7.4	0.9	1.6	0.2	5	14	49	19.6	27	0.4
Collards, cooked	½ cup	95	25	2.0	4.7	2.7	0.3	0	0	9	297	17.3	113	0.4
Corn, yellow, cooked	½ cup	82	89	2.7	20.6	2.3	1.1	0.2	0	14	18	5.1	2	0.5
Cucumber, raw	½ cup	52	7	0.4	1.4	0.4	0.1	0	0	1	11	2.8	7	0.1
Eggplant, cooked	½ cup	50	14	0.4	3.3	1.2	0.1	0	0	1	3	0.6	3	0.2
Endive, raw	½ cup	25	4	0.3	0.8	0.8	0.1	0	0	6	51	1.6	13	0.2
Hominy, canned	½ cup	83	94	1.2	11.8	2.1	0.7	0.1	0	173	0	0	8	0.5
Kale, cooked	½ cup	65	18	1.2	3.6	1.3	0.3	0	0	15	481	26.7	47	0.6
Lettuce, iceberg	1 cup	55	7	0.6	1.1	0.8	0.1	0	0	5	18	2.1	10	0.3
Lettuce, looseleaf	1 cup	56	10	0.7	2.0	1.1	0.2	0	0	5	106	10.1	38	0.8
Lettuce, romaine	1 cup	56	8	0.9	1.3	1.0	0.1	0	0	4	152	13.4	20	0.6
Mushrooms, raw	½ cup	35	9	1.0	1.4	0.4	0.1	0	0	1	0	0.8	2	0.4
Mushrooms, cooked	½ cup	78	21	1.7	4.0	1.7	0.3	0	0	2	0	3.1	5	1.4
Mustard greens, cooked	½ cup	70	11	1.6	1.5	1.4	0.2	0	0	11	212	17.7	52	0.5
Okra, cooked	½ cup	92	26	1.9	5.3	2.6	0.3	0.1	0	3	47	11.2	88	0.6
Onion, raw	½ cup	80	30	0.9	6.9	1.4	0.1	0	0	2	0	5.1	16	0.2
Parsnip, raw	½ cup	67	50	0.8	12.0	3.2	0.2	0	0	7	0	11.3	24	0.4
*Peas, blackeye, cooked	½ cup	86	100	6.6	17.9	5.6	0.5	0.1	0	3	1	0.3	21	2.2
*Peas, chickpeas (garbanzos)	½ cup	82	134	7.3	22.5	6.2	2.1	0.2	0	6	2	1.1	40	2.4
Peas, edible, podded	10 pea pods	34	14	1.0	2.6	0.9	0.1	0	0	1	5	20.4	15	0.7

Name	Amount	Weight (g)	Energy (calories)	Protein (g)	Carbohydrate (g)	Fiber (g)	Total fat (g)	Saturated fat (g)	Cholesterol (mg)	Sodium (mg)	Vitamin A (RE)	Vitamin C (mg)	Calcium (mg)	Iron (mg)
Peas, green	½ cup	80	62	4.1	11.4	4.4	0.2	0	0	70	54	7.9	19	1.2
*Peas, split, cooked	½ cup	98	116	8.2	20.6	8.1	0.4	0.1	0	2	1	0.4	14	1.3
Pepper, green chili, canned	½ cup	70	15	0.5	3.2	1.2	0.2	0	0	276	9	23.8	25	0.9
Pepper, sweet green, raw	1 small	74	20	0.7	4.8	1.3	0.1	0	0	1	47	66.1	7	0.3
Pepper, sweet red, raw	1 small	74	20	0.7	4.8	1.5	0.1	0	0	1	422	140.6	7	0.3
Pickle, dill	1 medium	65	12	0.4	2.7	0.8	0.1	0	0	21	833	1.2	6	0.3
Potato, mashed w/milk	½ cup	105	81	2.0	18.4	2.1	0.6	0.3	2	318	6	7.0	27	0.3
Potato salad	½ cup	125	179	3.4	14.0	1.6	10.3	1.8	85	661	41	12.5	24	0.8
Potato, baked w/skin	1 medium	173	188	4.0	43.5	4.1	0.2	0	0	14	0	22.3	17	2.3
Potato, boiled	1 potato, 2½″ dia.	136	118	2.5	27.4	2.4	0.1	0	0	5	0	17.7	7	0.4
Potato, french fries	10 fries	50	109	1.7	17.0	1.6	4.1	1.9	0	141	0	4.8	5	0.7
Pumpkin, canned	½ cup	123	42	1.3	9.9	3.6	0.3	0.2	0	6	2702	5.1	32	1.7
Radish	13 medium	58	12	0.3	2.1	0.9	0.3	0	0	13.9	1	13.2	12	0.2
Rutabaga, mashed	½ cup	120	47	1.5	10.5	2.2	0.3	0	0	24	67	22.6	58	0.6
Sauerkraut, drained	½ cup	121	13	0.6	3.0	1.8	0.1	0	0	469	1	10.5	21	1.0
Soybeans, green, boiled	½ cup	90	127	11.1	9.9	3.8	5.8	0.7	0	13	14	15.3	131	2.3
Spinach, raw	1 cup	30	7	0.9	1.1	0.8	0.1	0	0	24	202	8.4	30	0.8
Spinach, cooked	½ cup	95	27	3.0	5.1	2.9	0.2	0	0	82	739	11.7	139	1.4
Squash, summer, raw	½ small squash	59	12	0.7	2.6	1.1	0.1	0	0	1	12	8.7	12	0.3
Squash, summer, cooked	½ cup	90	18	0.8	3.9	1.3	0.3	0	0	1	26	5.0	24	0.3
Squash, winter	½ cup	100	39	0.9	8.8	2.8	0.6	0.1	0	1	356	9.6	14	0.3
Sweet potato, baked	½ cup	100	103	1.7	24.3	3.0	0.1	0	0	10	2182	24.6	28	0.5
Sweet potato, canned w/syrup	½ cup	100	108	1.3	25.4	3.0	0.3	0.1	0	39	716	10.8	17	1.0
Tomato, raw	1 medium	123	26	1.0	5.7	1.4	0.4	0.1	0	11	76	23.5	6	0.6
Tomato sauce	½ cup	123	37	1.6	1.7	1.7	0.2	0	0	741	120	16.0	17	0.9
Tomato juice	¾ cup	182	31	1.4	7.7	1.5	1.4	0	0	18	102	33.3	16	1.1
Turnip, cooked, mashed	½ cup	115	24	0.8	5.6	2.3	0.1	0	0	108	0	13.3	25	0.3
Vegetable juice	¾ cup	182	35	1.1	8.3	1.5	0.2	0	0	491	213	50.4	20	0.8
Vegetables, mixed	½ cup	91	54	2.6	11.9	4.0	0.1	0	0	32	389	2.9	23	0.7
Vegetable soup	1 cup	241	72	2.1	12.0	0.5	1.9	0.3	0	822	301	1.4	22	1.1
Water chestnuts	½ cup	70	35	0.6	8.7	1.8	0	0	0	6	0	0.9	3	0.6

*Dry beans and peas (legumes) can be counted as servings of vegetables or as servings from the meat, poultry, fish, dry beans, eggs, and nuts group. They are listed here and marked with an asterisk.

FRUIT

The Food Guide Pyramid recommends 2–4 servings per day. One serving is equivalent to 1 medium apple, banana, orange, or pear; ½ cup of chopped, cooked, or canned fruit; or ¾ cup of fruit juice.

Name	Amount	Weight (g)	Energy (calories)	Protein (g)	Carbohydrate (g)	Fiber (g)	Total fat (g)	Saturated fat (g)	Cholesterol (mg)	Sodium (mg)	Vitamin A (RE)	Vitamin C (mg)	Calcium (mg)	Iron (mg)
Apple	1 medium	138	81	0.3	21.0	3.7	0.5	0.1	0	0	7	7.9	10	0.2
Apple juice	¾ cup	179	84	0.3	20.7	0.2	0.2	0	0	13	0	44.8	11	0.5
Apple sauce, unsweetened	½ cup	122	52	0.2	13.8	1.5	0.1	0	0	2	4	25.9	4	0.1
Apricots	2 medium	70	34	1.0	7.8	1.7	0.3	0	0	1	183	7.0	10	0.4
Apricots, dried	9 halves	32	75	1.2	19.4	2.8	0.1	0	0	3	228	0.8	14	1.5
Avocado	1 medium	173	306	3.7	12.0	8.5	30.0	4.5	0	21	105	13.7	19	2.0
Banana	1 medium	118	109	1.2	27.6	2.8	0.6	0.2	0	1	9	10.7	7	0.4
Blackberries	½ cup	72	37	0.5	9.2	3.8	0.3	0	0	0	12	15.1	23	0.4
Blueberries	½ cup	73	41	0.5	10.2	2.0	0.3	0	0	4	7	9.4	4	0.1
Cantaloupe	¼ melon, 5″ dia.	138	48	1.2	11.5	1.1	0.4	0.1	0	12	444	58.2	15	0.3
Carambola (starfruit)	1 small	70	23	0.4	5.5	1.9	0.2	0	0	1	34	14.8	3	0.2
Cherries, sweet, raw	11 cherries	75	54	0.9	2.3	1.7	0.7	0.2	0	0	16	5.2	11	0.3
Cherries, canned in syrup	½ cup	128	116	0.9	29.8	1.4	0.1	0	0	9	91	2.6	13	1.7
Cranberries, raw	½ cup	48	23	0.2	6.0	2.0	0.1	0	0	1	2	6.4	3	0.1
Cranberry juice cocktail	¾ cup	190	108	0	27.3	0.2	0.2	0	0	4	0	67.1	6	0.3
Cranberry sauce	¼ cup	139	105	0.1	26.9	0.7	0.1	0	0	20	1	1.4	3	0.2
Currants, dried	¼ cup	36	109	1.5	26.7	2.4	0.1	0	0	3	3	1.7	31	1.2
Dates, dried	¼ cup	45	122	0.9	32.7	3.3	0.2	0.1	0	1	2	0	14	0.5
Figs, raw	2 medium	100	74	0.8	19.2	3.3	0.3	0.1	0	1	14	2.0	35	0.4
Fruit cocktail, heavy syrup	½ cup	124	91	0.5	23.4	1.2	0.1	0	0	7	25	2.4	7	0.4

Name	Amount	Weight (g)	Energy (calories)	Protein (g)	Carbohydrate (g)	Fiber (g)	Total fat (g)	Saturated fat (g)	Cholesterol (mg)	Sodium (mg)	Vitamin A (RE)	Vitamin C (mg)	Calcium (mg)	Iron (mg)
Fruit cocktail, light syrup	½ cup	121	69	0.5	18.1	1.2	0.1	0	0	7	25	2.3	7	0.4
Fruit cocktail, juice	½ cup	119	55	0.5	14.1	1.2	0	0	0	5	37	3.2	9	0.3
Grapefruit	½ medium	128	41	0.8	10.3	1.4	0.1	0	0	0	15	44.0	15	0.1
Grapfruit juice	¾ cup	185	70	1.0	16.6	0.2	0.2	0	0	2	2	54.1	13	0.4
Grapes	12 grapes	60	43	0.4	10.7	0.6	0.3	0	0	1	4	6.5	7	0.2
Guava	1 fruit	90	46	0.7	10.7	4.9	0.5	0.2	0	3	71	165.2	18	0.3
Honeydew	⅛ melon, 5¼″ dia.	125	44	0.6	11.5	0.8	0.1	0	0	13	5	31.0	8	0.1
Kiwifruit	1 large	91	56	0.9	13.5	3.1	0.4	0	0	5	16	68.3	24	0.4
Kumquats	5 fruits	100	63	0.9	16.4	6.6	0.1	0	0	6	30	37.4	44	0.4
Lemon, with peel	1 fruit	108	22	1.3	11.6	5.1	0.3	0	0	3	3	83.2	66	0.8
Lemon juice	2 tablespoons	31	6	0.1	2.0	0.1	0.1	0	0	6	1	7.6	3	0
Mango	½ medium	103	65	0.5	17.0	1.8	0.3	0.1	0	2	389	27.7	10	0.1
Nectarine	1 fruit	136	67	1.3	16.0	2.2	0.6	0.1	0	0	101	7.3	7	0.2
Olives, ripe	10 large	44	51	0.3	2.8	1.4	4.7	0.6	0	383	18	0.4	39	1.5
Orange	1 medium	131	62	1.2	15.4	3.1	0.2	0	0	0	28	69.7	52	0.1
Orange juice	¾ cup	187	82	1.5	18.8	0.4	0.5	0.1	0	2	15	61.6	19	0.3
Papaya	½ medium	152	59	0.9	14.9	2.7	0.2	0.1	0	5	43	93.9	36	0.2
Passion fruit	½ cup	118	114	2.6	27.6	12.3	0.8	0.1	0	33	83	35.4	14	1.9
Peach, raw	1 medium	98	42	0.7	10.9	2.0	0.1	0	0	0	53	6.5	5	0.1
Peach, canned in juice	½ cup	124	55	0.8	14.3	1.6	0	0	0	5	47	4.4	7	0.3
Pear, raw	1 medium	166	98	0.6	25.1	4.0	0.7	0	0	0	3	6.6	18	0.4
Pear, canned	½ cup	124	62	0.4	16.0	2.0	0.1	0	0	5	1	2.0	11	0.4
Pineapple, canned in juice	½ cup	125	75	0.5	19.5	1.0	0.1	0	0	1	5	11.8	17	0.3
Pineapple, raw	1 slice, 3½″ x 3¼″	84	41	0.3	10.4	1.0	0.4	0	0	1	2	12.9	6	0.3
Plantain, raw	1 medium	179	218	2.3	57.1	4.1	0.7	0.3	0	7	6	2.3	5	1.1
Plums	1½ medium	99	55	0.8	13.0	1.5	0.6	0	0	0	32	9.5	4	0.1
Prune juice	¾ cup	192	136	1.2	33.5	1.9	0.1	0	0	8	0	7.9	23	2.3
Prunes, dried	5 prunes	42	80	1.1	26.3	3.0	0.2	0	0	2	84	1.4	21	1.0
Raisins	¼ cup	43	129	1.4	34.0	1.7	0.2	0.1	0	5	0	1.4	21	0.9
Raspberries	½ cup	62	30	0.6	7.1	4.2	0.3	0	0	0	8	15.4	14	0.4
Rhubarb, raw	1 stalk	51	11	0.5	2.3	0.9	0.1	0	0	2	5	4.1	44	0.1
Strawberries	5 large	90	27	0.6	6.3	2.1	0.3	0	0	1	3	51.0	13	0.3
Tangerine	1 medium	84	40	0.5	9.4	1.9	0.2	0	0	1	77	25.9	12	0.1
Watermelon	1⁄16 melon	286	92	1.8	20.5	1.4	1.2	0.1	0	6	106	27.5	23	0.5

MILK, YOGURT, AND CHEESE

The Food Guide Pyramid recommends 2–3 servings per day. One serving is equivalent to 1 cup milk or yogurt, 1½ ounces of natural cheese, or 2 ounces of processed cheese.

Name	Amount	Weight (g)	Energy (calories)	Protein (g)	Carbohydrate (g)	Fiber (g)	Total fat (g)	Saturated fat (g)	Cholesterol (mg)	Sodium (mg)	Vitamin A (RE)	Vitamin C (mg)	Calcium (mg)	Iron (mg)
Buttermilk, lowfat	1 cup	245	98	8.1	11.7	0	2.2	1.3	10	257	20	2.5	284	0.1
Cheese, American	2 oz.	57	186	11.1	4.1	0	13.9	8.8	36	905	124	0	325	0.5
Cheese, blue	1½ oz.	43	150	9.1	1.0	0	12.2	7.9	32	593	97	0	225	0.1
Cheese, cheddar	1½ oz.	43	171	10.6	0.5	0	14.1	9.0	45	264	118	0	307	0.3
Cheese, cottage, creamed	1 cup	210	216	26.2	5.6	0	9.5	6.0	32	850	101	0	126	0.3
Cheee, cottage, lowfat (1%)	1 cup	226	163	28.0	6.1	0	2.3	1.5	9	918	25	0	138	0.3
Cheese, cottage, fat free	1 cup	145	123	25.0	2.7	0	0.6	0.4	10	19	12	0	46	0.3
Cheese, cream	2 oz.	57	198	4.3	1.5	0	19.8	12.5	62	168	216	0	45	0.7
Cheese, cream, fat free	2 oz.	57	55	8.2	3.3	0	0.8	0.5	5	311	159	0	105	0.1
Cheese, feta	1½ oz.	43	112	6.0	1.7	0	9.0	6.4	38	475	54	0	210	0.3
Cheese, Mexican	1½ oz.	43	151	9.6	1.2	0	12.0	7.6	45	279	27	0	281	0.2
Cheese, Monterey	1½ oz.	43	159	10.4	0.3	0	12.9	8.1	38	228	108	0	317	0.3
Cheese, mozzarella, part skim	1½ oz.	43	108	10.3	1.2	0	6.8	4.3	25	198	75	0	275	0.1
Cheese, Parmesan, grated	2 tablespoons	10	46	4.2	0.4	0	3.0	1.9	8	186	17	0	138	0.1
Cheese, process spread	2 oz.	56	170	9.1	5.5	0	12.3	8.1	45	839	100	0.1	261	0.1
Cheese, provolone	1½ oz.	43	149	10.9	0.9	0	11.3	7.3	29	373	112	0	321	0.2
Cheese, ricotta, part skim	½ cup	124	171	14.1	6.4	0	9.8	6.1	38	155	140	0	337	0.5
Cheese, Swiss	1½ oz.	43	160	12.1	1.4	0	11.7	7.6	39	111	19	0	409	0.1
Ice cream, chocolate	1 cup	132	285	5.0	37.2	1.6	14.2	9.0	45	100	157	0.9	144	1.2

Name	Amount	Weight (g)	Energy (calories)	Protein (g)	Carbohydrate (g)	Fiber (g)	Total fat (g)	Saturated fat (g)	Cholesterol (mg)	Sodium (mg)	Vitamin A (RE)	Vitamin C (mg)	Calcium (mg)	Iron (mg)
Ice cream, vanilla, rich	1 cup	148	357	5.2	33.2	0	24.0	14.8	90	83	272	1.0	173	0.1
Ice cream, vanilla, light	1 cup	132	183	5.0	30.0	0	5.7	3.5	18	112	62	1.1	183	0.1
Ice cream, vanilla, soft serve	1 cup	172	370	7.1	38.2	0	22.4	12.9	157	105	265	1.4	225	0.4
Milk, chocolate	1 cup	250	208	7.9	25.9	2.0	8.5	5.3	30	150	73	2.3	280	0.6
Milk, fat free (nonfat)	1 cup	245	86	8.4	11.9	0	0.4	0.3	5	127	149	2.5	301	0.1
Milk, lowfat (1%)	1 cup	244	102	8.0	11.7	0	2.6	1.6	10	124	144	2.4	300	0.1
Milk, reduced fat (2%)	1 cup	244	122	8.1	11.7	0	4.7	2.9	20	122	139	2.4	298	0.1
Milk, whole	1 cup	244	149	8.0	11.4	0	8.2	5.1	34	120	76	2.2	290	0.1
Pudding, made with milk	½ cup	142	158	4.5	25.6	1.4	4.8	3.0	17	146	37	1.0	158	0.5
Yogurt, frozen, vanilla	1 cup	144	229	5.8	34.8	0	8.1	4.9	3	125	82	1.2	206	0.4
Yogurt, lowfat, plain	8 oz. container	227	143	11.9	16.0	0	3.5	2.3	14	159	36	1.8	415	0.2
Yogurt, lowfat, with fruit	8 oz. container	227	238	11.0	42.2	0	3.2	2.1	14	148	136	1.6	384	0.2
Yogurt, nonfat, plain	8 oz. container	227	127	13.0	17.4	0	0.4	0.3	5	175	5	2.0	452	0.2

MEAT, POULTRY, FISH, DRY BEANS, EGGS, AND NUTS The Food Guide Pyramid recommends 2–3 servings per day for a total of 5–7 ounces. One serving is equivalent to 2–3 ounces of cooked lean meat, poultry, or fish. The following count as equivalents of 1 ounce of meat: ½ cup of cooked dry beans or tofu, 2½ ounces of soyburger, 1 egg, 2 tablespoons of peanut butter, ⅓ cup of nuts, or ¼ cup of seeds.

Name	Amount	Weight (g)	Energy (calories)	Protein (g)	Carbohydrate (g)	Fiber (g)	Total fat (g)	Saturated fat (g)	Cholesterol (mg)	Sodium (mg)	Vitamin A (RE)	Vitamin C (mg)	Calcium (mg)	Iron (mg)
Bacon, Canadian	2 slices	47	86	11.3	0.6	0	3.9	1.3	27	719	0	0	5	0.4
Beef, ½″ fat	3 oz.	85	344	19.9	0	0	28.7	11.9	78	48	0	0	9	2.1
Beef, lean, fat trimmed	3 oz.	85	179	25.4	0	0	7.9	3.0	73	56	0	0	7	2.5
Beef, corned	3 oz.	85	213	23.0	0	0	12.7	5.3	73	856	0	0	10	1.8
Beef, ground, extra lean, broiled	3 oz.	85	218	21.6	0	0	13.9	5.5	71	60	0	0	6	2.0
Beef, ground, lean, broiled	3 oz.	85	231	21.0	0	0	15.7	6.2	74	65	0	0	9	1.8
Beef, ground, regular, broiled	3 oz.	85	246	20.5	0	0	17.6	6.9	77	71	0	0	9	2.1
Beef liver, braised	3 oz.	85	137	20.7	2.9	0	4.2	1.6	331	60	9011	19.6	6	5.8
Beef ribs, broiled	3 oz.	85	306	18.7	0	0	25.1	10.2	70	53	0	0	10	1.8
Chicken breast, w/skin, rst	½ breast	98	193	29.2	0	0	7.6	2.1	82	70	26	0	14	1.0
Chicken, dk mt, w/skin, rst	3 oz.	85	215	22.1	0	0	13.4	3.7	77	74	49	0	13	1.2
Chicken, dk mt, w/o skin, rst	3 oz.	85	168	22.2	0	0	7.9	2.2	76	76	18	0	12	1.1
Chicken, dk mt, w/skin, fried	3 oz.	85	253	18.6	8.0	0	15.8	4.2	76	251	26	0	18	1.2
Chicken, drumstick, w/skin, rst	1 drumstick	52	112	14.1	0	0	5.8	1.6	47	47	16	0	6	0.7
Chicken, lt mt, w/skin, rst	3 oz.	85	189	24.7	0	0	9.2	2.6	71	64	27	0	13	1.0
Chicken, lt mt, w/o skin, rst	3 oz.	85	147	26.3	0	0	3.8	1.1	72	65	8	0	13	0.9
Chicken, lt mt, w/skin, fried	3 oz.	85	235	20.0	8.1	0	13.1	3.5	71	243	20	0	17	1.1
Chicken, thigh, w/skin, rst	1 thigh	62	153	15.5	0	0	9.6	2.7	58	52	30	0	7	0.8
Chicken, wing, w/skin, rst	1 wing	34	99	9.1	0	0	6.6	1.9	29	28	16	0	5	0.4
Chicken liver, chopped	½ cup	70	110	17.1	0.8	0	3.8	1.3	442	36	3439	11.1	10	5.9
Egg white, large	1 egg white	33	17	3.5	0.3	0	0	0	0	55	0	0	2	0
Egg, whole, large	1 egg	50	75	6.2	0.6	0	5.1	1.6	213	63	97	0	25	0.7
Egg yolk, large	1 yolk	17	59	2.8	0.3	0	5.1	1.6	213	7	97	0	23	0.6
Fish, catfish, baked/broiled	3 oz.	85	129	15.9	0	0	6.8	1.5	54	68	13	0.7	8	0.7
Fish, cod, baked/broiled	3 oz.	85	89	19.5	0	0	0.7	0.1	40	77	9	2.6	7	0.3
Fish, halibut, baked/broiled	3 oz.	85	119	22.7	0	0	2.5	0.4	35	59	46	0	51	0.9
Fish, salmon, baked/broiled	3 oz.	85	175	18.8	0	0	10.5	2.1	54	52	13	3.1	13	0.3
Fish, salmon, canned	3 oz.	85	130	17.4	0	0	6.2	1.4	37	457	45	0	203	0.9
Fish, salmon, smoked	3 oz.	85	99	15.5	0	0	3.7	0.8	20	1700	22	0	9	0.7
Fish, sardine, canned in oil	1 can (3.75 oz.)	92	191	22.7	0	0	10.5	1.4	131	465	62	0	351	2.7
Fish, snapper, baked/broiled	3 oz.	85	109	22.3	0	0	1.5	0.3	40	48	30	1.4	34	0.2
Fish sticks	3 sticks	84	228	13.1	19.9	0	10.3	2.6	94	489	26	0	17	0.6
Fish, swordfish, baked/broiled	3 oz.	85	132	21.6	0	0	4.4	1.2	43	98	35	0.9	5	0.9
Fish, trout, baked/broiled	3 oz.	85	162	22.6	0	0	7.2	1.3	63	57	16	0.4	47	1.6
Fish, tuna, canned in oil	3 oz.	85	158	22.6	0	0	6.9	1.4	26	337	20	0	3	0.6
Fish, tuna, canned in water	3 oz.	85	109	20.1	0	0	2.5	0.7	36	320	5	0	12	0.8
Ham, extra lean	3 oz.	85	116	18.0	0.4	0	4.1	1.4	26	965	0	0	5	0.8

Name	Amount	Weight (g)	Energy (calories)	Protein (g)	Carbohydrate (g)	Fiber (g)	Total fat (g)	Saturated fat (g)	Cholesterol (mg)	Sodium (mg)	Vitamin A (RE)	Vitamin C (mg)	Calcium (mg)	Iron (mg)
Ham, regular	3 oz.	85	192	17.5	0.4	0	12.9	4.3	53	800	0	11.9	7	1.2
Lamb, trimmed	3 oz.	85	218	20.8	0	0	14.3	6.7	74	65	0	0	14	1.6
Lunch meat, beef pastrami	3 oz.	85	297	14.7	2.6	0	24.8	8.9	79	1043	0	0	8	1.6
Lunch meat, beef, sliced	3 oz.	85	151	23.9	4.9	0	3.3	1.4	35	1224	0	0	9	0.8
Lunch meat, bologna (beef)	3 slices	85	265	10.4	0.7	0	24.2	10.3	49	834	0	0	10	1.4
Lunch meat, bologna (turkey)	3 slices	85	169	11.7	0.8	0	12.9	4.3	84	747	0	0	71	1.3
Lunch meat, chicken breast	3 oz.	85	108	14.3	1.9	0	4.7	1.2	50	1005	0	0	14	1.3
Lunch meat, franks (beef)	1 frank	57	180	6.8	1.0	0	16.2	6.9	35	585	0	0	11	0.8
Lunch meat, franks (chicken)	1 frank	45	116	5.8	3.1	0	8.8	2.5	45	617	17	0	43	0.9
Lunch meat, ham, lean, sliced	3 slices	85	111	16.5	0.8	0	4.2	1.4	40	1215	0	0	6	0.6
Lunch meat, liverwurst	3 oz.	85	277	12.0	1.9	0	24.2	9.0	134	731	7059	0	22	5.4
Lunch meat, salami, dry	8 slices	80	334	18.3	2.1	0	27.5	9.8	63	1488	0	0	6	1.2
Lunch meat, turkey breast	3 oz.	85	94	19.1	0	0	1.3	0.4	35	1216	0	0	6	0.3
Nuts, almonds	⅓ cup	47	274	10.1	9.3	5.6	24.0	1.8	0	0	0	0	117	2.0
Nuts, cashews, dry roasted	⅓ cup	46	262	7.0	14.9	1.4	21.2	4.2	0	7	0	0	21	2.7
Nuts, chestnuts, roasted	⅓ cup	48	117	1.5	25.2	2.4	1.0	0.2	0	1	1	12.4	14	0.4
Nuts, macadamia, dry roasted	⅓ cup	45	321	3.5	6.0	3.6	34.0	5.3	0	2	0	0.3	31	0.3
Nuts, pecans	⅓ cup	36	249	3.3	5.0	3.5	25.9	2.2	0	0	3	0.4	25	0.9
Nuts, pine	⅓ cup	45	257	10.9	6.4	2.0	23.0	3.5	0	2	1	0.8	12	4.2
Nuts, pistachios, dry roasted	⅓ cup	43	244	9.1	11.8	4.4	19.6	2.4	0	4	23	1.0	47	1.8
Nuts, walnuts	⅓ cup	40	262	6.1	5.5	2.7	26.1	2.5	0	1	2	0.5	39	1.2
Peanut butter, chunky	2 tablespoons	32	188	7.7	6.9	2.1	16.0	3.1	0	156	0	0	13	0.7
Peanut butter, smooth	2 tablespoons	32	190	8.1	6.2	1.9	16.3	3.3	0	149	0	0	12	0.6
Peanuts, dry roasted	⅓ cup	49	285	11.5	10.5	3.9	24.2	3.4	0	3	0	0	26	1.1
Pork chop, pan fried	3 oz.	85	190	23.5	0	0	10.0	3.7	60	44	2	0.3	4	0.7
Pork ribs, braised	3 oz.	85	337	24.7	0	0	25.8	9.5	103	79	3	0	40	1.6
Pork roast	3 oz.	85	214	22.9	0	0	12.9	4.5	69	41	3	0	5	0.8
Pumpkin seeds, roasted	¼ cup	57	296	18.7	7.6	2.2	23.9	4.5	0	10	22	1.0	24	8.5
Sausage, beef	1 sausage	43	134	6.1	1.0	0	11.6	4.9	29	486	0	0	3	0.8
Sausage, pork	1 sausage	67	216	13.4	1.0	0	17.2	6.1	52	618	0	1.3	16	1.0
Sausage, smoked links	3 2″ links	48	161	6.4	0.7	0	14.6	5.1	34	454	0	0	5	0.7
Shellfish, clams, canned	3 oz.	85	126	21.7	4.4	0	1.7	0.2	57	95	145	18.8	78	23.8
Shellfish, clams, steamed	10 clams	95	140	24.3	4.9	0	1.9	0.2	64	106	542	21.0	87	26.6
Shellfish, crab, steamed	3 oz.	85	82	16.4	0	0	1.3	0.1	45	911	8	6.5	50	0.6
Shellfish, oysters, fried	6 medium	88	173	7.7	10.2	0	11.1	2.8	71	367	79	3.3	55	6.1
Shellfish, shrimp, canned	3 oz.	85	102	19.6	0.9	0	1.7	0.3	147	144	15	2.0	50	2.3
Shellfish, shrimp, fried	4 large	30	73	6.4	3.4	0.1	3.7	0.6	53	103	17	0.5	20	0.4
Sunflower seeds, dry roasted	¼ cup	32	186	6.2	7.7	3.6	15.9	1.7	0	1	0	0.4	22	1.2
Tempeh	½ cup	83	160	15.4	7.8	0	9.0	1.8	0	7	0	0	92	2.2
Tofu, firm	½ cup	126	183	19.9	5.4	2.9	11.0	1.6	0	18	21	0.3	861	13.2
Turkey, dk mt, w/o skin, rst	3 oz.	85	138	24.5	0	0	3.7	1.2	95	67	0	0	22	2.0
Turkey, dk mt, w/skin, rst	3 oz.	85	155	23.5	0	0	6.0	1.8	99	65	0	0	23	2.0
Turkey, lt mt, w/o skin, rst	3 oz.	85	119	25.7	0	0	1.0	0.3	73	48	0	0	13	1.3
Turkey, lt mt, w/skin, rst	3 oz.	85	139	24.5	0	0	3.9	1.1	81	48	0	0	15	1.4
Veal, sirloin, roasted	3 oz.	85	172	21.4	0	0	8.9	3.8	87	71	0	0	11	0.8
Vegetarian bacon, cooked	1 oz.	16	50	1.7	1.0	0.4	4.7	0.7	0	234	1	0	4	0.4
Vegetarian franks	1 frank	51	118	12.1	1.5	1.5	7.1	0.8	0	224	0	0	10	1.0
Vegetarian patties	1 patty	67	119	11.2	10.2	4.0	3.8	0.5	0	382	76	0	48	1.2
Vegetarian sausage	1 patty	38	97	7.0	3.7	1.1	6.9	1.1	0	337	24	0	24	1.4

FATS, OILS, SWEETS, AND ALCOHOLIC BEVERAGES

The total amount of fats, oils, and sweets you consume should be determined by your overall energy needs. Foods from this group should not replace foods from the other groups because they tend to provide calories but few nutrients.

Alcoholic beverage, beer	1 can or bottle	356	146	1.1	13.2	0.7	0	0	0	18	0	0	18	0.1
Alcoholic beverage, liquor	1.5 oz.	42	97	0	0	0	0	0	0	0	0	0	0	0
Alcoholic beverage, wine	5 oz.	148	103	0	2.1	0	0	0	0	12	0	0	12	0.5

Name	Amount	Weight (g)	Energy (calories)	Protein (g)	Carbohydrate (g)	Fiber (g)	Total fat (g)	Saturated fat (g)	Cholesterol (mg)	Sodium (mg)	Vitamin A (RE)	Vitamin C (mg)	Calcium (mg)	Iron (mg)
Bacon	3 slices	19	109	5.7	0.1	0	9.4	3.3	19	303	0	0	2	0.3
Beverage, fruit punch	1 cup	247	114	0	28.9	0.2	0	0	0	10	2	108.4	10	0.2
Beverage, kiwi-strawberry drink	1 cup	236	113	0.2	27.8	0	0	0	0	10	0	0	0	0
Beverage, cola	1 can	370	152	0	38.5	0	0	0	0	15	0	0	11	0.1
Beverage, lemon-lime soda	1 can	368	147	0	38.3	0	0	0	0	40	0	0	7	0.3
Beverage, tea, bottled, sweetened	1 bottle	480	178	0	40.8	0	0	0	0	0	0	0	0	0
Butter	1 tablespoon	14	102	0.1	0	0	11.5	7.1	31	117	107	0	3	0
Candy, caramels	1 piece	10	39	0.5	7.8	0.1	0.8	0.7	1	25	1	0.1	14	0
Candy, fudge	1 piece	17	65	0.3	13.5	0.1	1.4	0.9	2	11	8	0	7	0.1
Candy, jelly beans	10 large	28	104	0	26.4	0	0.1	0	0	7	0	0	1	0.3
Candy, milk chocolate	1 bar	44	226	3.0	26.0	1.5	13.5	8.1	10	36	24	0.2	84	0.6
Chocolate syrup	2 tablespoons	38	105	0.8	24.4	0.7	0.4	0.2	0	27	1	0.1	5	0.8
Cream, half and half	2 tablespoons	30	39	0.9	1.3	0	3.5	2.2	11	12	32	0.3	32	0
Cream, heavy, whipped	½ cup	60	206	1.2	1.7	0	22.1	13.8	82	23	252	0.4	39	0
Cream, sour	1 tablespoon	12	26	0.4	0.5	0	2.5	1.6	5	6	23	0.1	14	0
Frosting, chocolate	1/12 package	38	151	0.4	24.0	0.2	6.7	2.1	0	70	75	0	3	0.5
Honey	1 tablespoon	21	64	0.1	17.3	0	0	0	0	1	0	0.1	1	0.1
Jam/preserves	1 tablespoon	20	56	0.1	13.8	0.2	0	0	0	6	0	1.8	4	0.1
Lard	1 tablespoon	13	115	0	0	0	12.8	5.0	12	0	0	0	0	0
Marmalade	1 tablespoon	20	49	0.1	13.3	0	0	0	0	11	1	1.0	8	0
Margarine, hard	1 tablespoon	14	101	0.1	0.1	0	11.4	2.1	0	133	113	0	4	0
Margarine, liquid	1 tablespoon	14	102	0.3	0	0	11.4	1.9	0	111	113	0	9	0
Margarine, soft	1 tablespoon	14	101	0.1	0	0	11.3	2.0	0	152	113	0	4	0
Margarine-like spread	1 tablespoon	14	50	0.1	0.1	0	5.6	1.1	0	138	115	0	3	0
Mayonnaise, regular	1 tablespoon	15	57	0.1	3.5	0	4.9	0.7	4	105	12	0	2	0
Mayonnaise, fat free	1 tablespoon	16	11	0	2.0	0.3	0.4	6.1	2	120	1	0	1	0
Oil, canola	1 tablespoon	14	124	0	0	0	14.0	1.0	0	0	0	0	0	0
Oil, corn	1 tablespoon	14	120	0	0	0	13.6	1.7	0	0	0	0	0	0
Oil, olive	1 tablespoon	14	119	0	0	0	13.5	1.8	0	0	0	0	0	0.1
Popsicle	1 single stick	88	63	0	16.6	0	0	0	0	11	0	9.4	0	0
Salad dressing, blue cheese	2 tablespoons	31	154	1.5	2.3	0	16.0	3.0	5	335	20	0.6	25	0.1
Salad dressing, French	2 tablespoons	31	134	0.2	5.5	0	12.8	3.0	0	427	40	0	3	0.1
Salad dressing, Italian	2 tablespoons	29	137	0.2	3.0	0	14.2	2.1	0	231	7	0	3	0
Salad dressing, Italian, light	2 tablespoons	30	32	0	1.5	0	2.9	0.4	2	236	0	0	1	0.1
Sherbet	½ cup	74	102	0.8	22.5	0	1.5	0.9	0	34	10	2.3	40	0.1
Shortening, vegetable	1 tablespoon	13	113	0	0	0	12.8	3.2	0	0	0	0	0	0
Sugar, brown	1 tablespoon	14	52	0	13.4	0	0	0	0	5	0	0	12	0.3
Sugar, white	1 tablespoon	13	49	0	12.6	0	0	0	0	0	0	0	0	0
Syrup, corn	1 tablespoon	20	56	0	15.3	0	0	0	0	24	0	0	1	0
Syrup, maple	¼ cup	79	206	0	52.9	0	0.2	0	0	7	0	0	53	0.9

DATA SOURCE: U.S. Department of Agriculture, Agricultural Research Service. 2001. *USDA Nutrient Database for Standard Reference, Release 14* (http://www.nal.usda.gov/fnic/foodcomp).

APPENDIX C

Nutritional Content of Popular Items from Fast-Food Restaurants

Arby's

	Serving size	Calories	Protein	Total fat	Saturated fat	Total carbohydrate	Sugars	Fiber	Cholesterol	Sodium	Vitamin A	Vitamin C	Calcium	Iron	% calories from fat
	g		g	g	g	g	g	g	mg	mg	% Daily Value				
Regular roast beef	154	388	23	19	7	33	N/A	3	43	1009	N/A	N/A	N/A	N/A	44
Super roast beef	247	523	25	27	9	50	N/A	5	43	1189	N/A	N/A	N/A	N/A	46
French dip	195	475	30	22	8	40	N/A	3	55	1411	N/A	N/A	N/A	N/A	41
Junior roast beef	126	324	17	14	5	35	N/A	2	30	779	N/A	N/A	N/A	N/A	39
Roast chicken Caesar sandwich	300	660	41	24	5	70	N/A	N/A	80	1900	N/A	N/A	N/A	N/A	33
Roast turkey & swiss	327	630	42	30	8	52	N/A	N/A	80	1670	N/A	N/A	N/A	N/A	43
Breaded chicken fillet	205	536	28	28	5	46	N/A	5	45	1016	N/A	N/A	N/A	N/A	47
Ham 'n cheese	169	359	24	14	5	34	N/A	2	53	1283	N/A	N/A	N/A	N/A	35
Jalapeño bites	110	330	7	21	9	29	N/A	2	40	670	N/A	N/A	N/A	N/A	57
Cheddar curly fries	120	333	5	18	4	40	N/A	0	3	1016	N/A	N/A	N/A	N/A	49
Potato cakes	85	204	2	12	2	20	N/A	0	0	397	N/A	N/A	N/A	N/A	53
Red ranch dressing	14	75	0	6	1	5	N/A	0	0	115	N/A	N/A	N/A	N/A	72
French-toastix	124	430	10	21	5	52	N/A	3	0	550	N/A	N/A	N/A	N/A	44

N/A: not available.

SOURCE: Arby's © 2001, Arby's, Inc. Used with permission of Arby's, Inc. Nutritional information contained in this Arby's, Inc. brochure was obtained from independent lab analysis; Genesis Nutrition and Diet Software; supplier information, and the USDA Handbook #8. Information on Arby's products contained herein is based on laboratory and calculated analysis of Arby's ingredients as of July 25, 2001. Actual nutritional information may differ based on regional variability in product availability and in individual unit compliance with Arby's Standard Operating Procedures. Information is not to be used by individuals with special dietary needs in lieu of professional medical advice.

Burger King

	Serving size	Calories	Protein	Total fat	Saturated fat	Total carbohydrate	Sugars	Fiber	Cholesterol	Sodium	Vitamin A	Vitamin C	Calcium	Iron	% calories from fat
	g		g	g	g	g	g	g	mg	mg	% Daily Value				
Original Whopper®	304	760	35	46	14	52	11	4	100	1000	20	15	15	40	54
Original Double Whopper® w/cheese	426	1150	64	76	30	53	11	4	210	1530	25	15	30	50	59
Original Whopper Jr.®	158	390	17	22	7	32	6	2	45	570	10	6	8	20	51
BK Homestyle™ Griller	242	480	26	27	11	35	5	2	75	760	10	10	6	25	51
BK Big Fish® sandwich	262	710	24	39	15	66	7	4	50	1160	2	0	8	20	49
Chicken Whopper®	272	580	26	37	5	50	7	3	85	1600	15	15	8	160	57
Chicken Tenders® (8 pieces)	123	340	22	19	5	20	0	<1	50	840	2	0	2	4	50
BK Veggie™ Burger	173	330	14	10	1.5	45	6	4	0	770	8	10	6	35	27
French fries (large, salted)	160	500	6	25	7	63	1	5	0	880	0	20	2	6	45
Onion rings (medium)	91	320	4	16	4	40	5	3	0	460	0	0	10	0	45
Chicken caesar salad w/o dressing	288	300	24	19	5	10	5	3	55	1220	15	15	15	100	57
Dutch apple pie	113	340	2	14	3	52	23	1	1	470	2	2	0	8	37
Croissan'wich® w/sausage, egg & cheese	157	520	19	39	14	24	4	1	210	1090	10	0	30	25	68
French toast sticks (5)	112	390	6	20	4.5	46	11	2	0	440	0	0	6	10	46
Chocolate shake (medium)	425	790	15	42	27	89	75	2	125	380	30	0	45	6	48

SOURCE: Burger King Brands, Inc. 2002. Burger King® trademarks, trade name, and Nutritional Guide are reproduced with permission from Burger King Brands, Inc.

Domino's Pizza

(1 serving = 2 of 8 slices or ¼ of 14-inch pizza; 2 of 8 slices or ¼ of 12-inch pizza; 1 6-inch pizza)

	Serving size	Calories	Protein	Total fat	Saturated fat	Total carbohydrate	Sugars	Fiber	Cholesterol	Sodium	Vitamin A	Vitamin C	Calcium	Iron	% calories from fat
	g		g	g	g	g	g	g	mg	mg	% Daily Value				
14-inch lg. hand-tossed cheese	219	516	21	15	7	75	6	4	32	1080	18	0	26	23	26
14-inch lg. thin crust cheese	148	382	17	17	7	43	6	2	32	1172	18	0	32	8	40
14-inch lg. deep dish cheese	257	677	26	30	11	80	9	5	41	1575	21	<1	33	31	40
12-inch med. hand-tossed cheese	159	375	15	11	5	55	5	3	23	776	13	0	19	17	26
12-inch med. thin crust cheese	106	273	12	12	5	31	4	2	23	835	13	0	23	5	40
12-inch med. deep dish cheese	181	482	19	22	8	56	6	3	30	1123	15	<1	24	22	41
6-inch deep dish cheese	216	598	23	28	10	68	7	4	36	1341	17	<1	30	30	42
Toppings: pepperoni	*	98	5	9	3	<1	<1	<1	20	364	†	†	†	†	83
ham	*	31	5	2	<1	<1	<1	<1	12	292	†	†	†	†	58
Italian sausage	*	110	5	9	3	3	<1	<1	22	342	†	†	†	†	74
bacon	*	153	8	13	4	<1	<1	<1	22	424	†	†	†	†	77
beef	*	111	6	10	4	<1	<1	<1	21	309	†	†	†	†	81
anchovies	*	45	9	2	<1	<1	<1	<1	18	791	†	†	5	6	40
extra cheese	*	68	6	6	3	<1	<1	<1	15	228	11	†	12	†	79
cheddar cheese	*	71	5	6	3	<1	<1	<1	18	110	4	†	13	†	76
Barbeque buffalo wings	25	50	6	2	<1	2	1	<1	26	175	†	†	†	†	36
Breadsticks (1 stick)	37	116	3	4	<1	17	1	1	0	152	†	†	†	†	31
Double cheesy bread	43	142	4	6	2	18	<1	<1	6	183	†	†	†	†	38

* Topping information is based on minimal portioning requirements for one serving of a 14-inch large pizza; add the values for toppings to the values for a cheese pizza. The following toppings supply fewer than 15 calories per serving: green and yellow peppers, onion, olives, mushrooms, pineapple.
† Contains less than 2% of the Daily Value of these nutrients.

SOURCE: Domino's Pizza, 2002, http://www.dominos.com. Reproduced with permission from Domino's Pizza LLC.

Jack in the Box

	Serving size	Calories	Protein	Total fat	Saturated fat	Total carbohydrate	Sugars	Fiber	Cholesterol	Sodium	Vitamin A	Vitamin C	Calcium	Iron	% calories from fat
	g		g	g	g	g	g	g	mg	mg	% Daily Value				
Breakfast Jack®	133	310	14	14	5	34	5	1	210	770	N/A	N/A	N/A	N/A	41
Supreme croissant	172	540	18	35	9	41	5	1	240	860	N/A	N/A	N/A	N/A	58
Hamburger	104	250	12	9	3.5	30	5	2	30	610	N/A	N/A	N/A	N/A	32
Jumbo Jack® w/cheese	270	650	25	40	16	47	10	2	75	1180	N/A	N/A	N/A	N/A	55
Sourdough Jack®	228	660	27	47	16	33	4	3	75	950	N/A	N/A	N/A	N/A	64
Chicken fajita pita	230	330	24	11	4.5	35	4	3	55	910	N/A	N/A	N/A	N/A	30
Grilled chicken fillet	216	430	23	22	6	34	6	2	60	910	N/A	N/A	N/A	N/A	46
Chicken supreme	300	710	30	39	11	62	5	4	70	1440	N/A	N/A	N/A	N/A	49
Jack's Spicy Chicken®	253	580	24	31	6	53	7	3	60	950	N/A	N/A	N/A	N/A	48
Chicken teriyaki bowl	461	550	26	3	0.5	103	27	3	35	1710	N/A	N/A	N/A	N/A	5
Monster taco	125	280	10	17	6	22	2	3	20	310	N/A	N/A	N/A	N/A	55
Egg rolls (3)	170	400	14	19	6	44	4	6	15	920	N/A	N/A	N/A	N/A	43
Chicken breast pieces (5)	150	360	27	17	3	24	0	1	80	970	N/A	N/A	N/A	N/A	43
Stuffed jalapeños (7)	168	530	15	30	13	51	5	4	45	1600	N/A	N/A	N/A	N/A	51
Barbeque dipping sauce	28	45	1	0	0	11	4	0	0	330	N/A	N/A	N/A	N/A	0
Seasoned curly fries	125	400	6	23	5	45	1	5	0	890	N/A	N/A	N/A	N/A	52
Onion rings	119	500	6	30	5	51	3	3	0	420	N/A	N/A	N/A	N/A	54
Side salad	131	50	3	3	1.5	5	3	2	10	65	N/A	N/A	N/A	N/A	54
Thousand Island dressing	57	160	1	12	2	12	10	0	15	490	N/A	N/A	N/A	N/A	68

N/A: not available.

SOURCE: Jack in the Box, Inc. 2001 (http://www.jackinthebox.com). The following trademarks are owned by Jack in the Box, Inc.: Breakfast Jack,® Jumbo Jack,® Sourdough Jack,® Jack in the Box.® Reproduced with permission from Jack in the Box, Inc.

KFC

	Serving size (g)	Calories	Protein (g)	Total fat (g)	Saturated fat (g)	Total carbohydrate (g)	Sugars (g)	Fiber (g)	Cholesterol (mg)	Sodium (mg)	Vitamin A (% Daily Value)	Vitamin C (% Daily Value)	Calcium (% Daily Value)	Iron (% Daily Value)	% calories from fat
Original Recipe® breast	153	400	29	24	6	16	0	1	135	1116	*	*	4	6	54
Original Recipe® thigh	91	250	16	18	4.5	6	0	1	95	747	*	*	2	4	65
Extra crispy chicken breast	168	470	39	28	8	17	0	<1	160	874	*	*	2	6	54
Extra crispy chicken thigh	118	380	21	27	7	14	0	<1	118	625	*	*	2	6	64
Hot & spicy breast	180	505	38	29	8	23	9	1	162	1170	*	*	6	6	52
Hot & spicy thigh	107	355	19	26	7	13	0	1	126	630	*	*	2	4	66
Tender Roast sandwich w/sauce	211	350	32	15	3	26	1	1	75	880	4	*	4	10	39
Tender Roast sandwich w/o sauce	177	270	31	5	1.5	23	<1	1	65	690	*	*	4	10	17
Hot wings (6 pieces)	135	471	27	33	8	18	0	2	150	1230	*	*	4	8	63
Colonel's Crispy Strips™ (3)	115	300	26	16	4	18	1	1	56	1165	2	*	*	6	48
Chunky chicken pot pie	368	770	29	42	13	69	8	5	70	2160	80	2	10	10	49
Corn on the cob	162	150	5	1.5	0	35	8	2	0	20	2	6	*	*	9
Mashed potatoes w/gravy	136	120	1	6	1	17	0	2	,1	440	*	*	*	2	45
BBQ baked beans	156	190	6	3	1	33	13	6	5	760	8	*	8	10	14
Cole slaw	142	232	2	13.5	2	26	20	3	8	284	9	57	3	*	52
Biscuit (1)	56	180	4	10	2.5	20	2	<1	0	560	*	*	2	6	50
Potato salad	160	230	4	14	2	23	9	3	15	540	10	*	2	15	55

*Contains less than 2% of the Daily Value of these nutrients.

SOURCE: KFC Corporation, 2001, http://www.kfc.com. Reproduced with permission from Kentucky Fried Chicken Corporation.

Taco Bell

	Serving size (g)	Calories	Protein (g)	Total fat (g)	Saturated fat (g)	Total carbohydrate (g)	Sugars (g)	Fiber (g)	Cholesterol (mg)	Sodium (mg)	Vitamin A (% Daily Value)	Vitamin C (% Daily Value)	Calcium (% Daily Value)	Iron (% Daily Value)	% calories from fat
Taco	78	170	9	10	4	13	1	3	25	320	6	2	8	6	53
Taco Supreme®	113	220	9	14	6	15	2	3	35	330	8	6	10	6	57
Soft taco, beef	99	220	10	10	4	21	2	3	25	560	6	0	8	6	41
Soft taco Supreme,® chicken	134	240	14	11	5	21	3	2	45	490	6	6	10	4	41
Gordita Supreme,® steak	152	300	15	14	5	28	4	3	35	570	4	6	15	10	42
Gordita Baja,® chicken	153	340	16	18	4	28	4	3	40	720	4	10	15	10	48
Chalupa Supreme, beef	152	370	13	25	8	26	4	4	35	570	6	6	15	10	61
Chalupa Supreme, chicken	152	350	16	21	7	24	3	2	45	490	4	6	15	8	54
Bean burrito	198	370	13	11	3.5	56	3	10	5	1100	45	0	15	10	27
Burrito Supreme,® chicken	247	420	20	15	6	50	4	7	45	1140	45	8	15	10	32
Grilled stuffed burrito, beef	325	730	28	35	10	78	5	11	55	2010	30	15	20	20	43
Tostada	169	250	10	10	4	29	2	9	15	670	50	2	15	10	36
Taco salad with salsa	531	830	29	51	14	66	10	13	60	1760	150	40	30	35	55
Steak quesadilla	183	550	26	31	12	39	3	2	75	1370	10	0	50	15	51
Nachos Supreme	194	470	13	28	9	40	3	7	30	890	8	8	10	10	54
Nachos BellGrande®	307	810	20	48	14	76	4	12	30	1500	10	8	15	20	53
Pintos 'n cheese	127	180	9	7	3.5	20	1	7	15	660	45	0	15	10	35
Mexican rice	130	190	5	10	4	21	<1	1	15	760	90	6	15	6	47
Breakfast quesadilla	155	420	15	21	8	38	2	1	210	1100	40	2	30	15	45

SOURCE: Taco Bell Corporation, 2002, http://www.tacobell.com. Reproduced with permission from the Taco Bell Corporation.

Wendy's

	Serving size	Calories	Protein	Total fat	Saturated fat	Total carbohydrate	Sugars	Dietary Fiber	Cholesterol	Sodium	Vitamin A	Vitamin C	Calcium	Iron	% calories from fat
	g		g	g	g	g	g	g	mg	mg	% Daily Value				
Classic Single® w/everything	218	410	24	19	7	37	8	2	70	890	6	15	10	30	42
Big Bacon Classic®	282	570	34	29	12	46	11	3	100	1460	15	25	20	30	46
Jr. hamburger	117	270	14	9	3	34	6	2	30	600	2	6	10	20	30
Jr. bacon cheeseburger	165	380	20	18	7	34	6	2	55	890	8	15	15	20	43
Grilled chicken sandwich	188	300	24	7	1.5	36	8	2	55	740	4	15	8	15	21
Spicy chicken sandwich	217	430	27	15	3	47	6	3	60	1240	4	15	10	15	31
Chicken breast fillet sandwich	207	430	27	16	3	46	6	2	55	750	4	20	10	15	33
Caesar side salad (no dressing)	99	70	7	4	2	2	1	1	15	250	45	35	15	6	51
Chicken BLT salad (no toppings)	376	310	33	16	8	10	4	4	60	1100	50	50	30	10	46
Taco salad (no toppings)	495	360	27	17	9	29	8	8	65	1090	50	45	35	20	43
Creamy ranch dressing	71	250	1	25	4.5	5	3	0	15	640	0	0	6	0	90
Reduced fat creamy ranch dressing	71	110	1	9	1.5	7	3	1	15	610	0	0	6	0	74
Biggie® fries	159	440	5	19	3.5	63	0	7	0	380	0	6	2	10	39
Baked potato w/broccoli & cheese	411	480	9	14	3	81	6	9	5	510	35	120	20	25	26
Baked potato w/bacon & cheese	380	580	18	22	6	79	6	7	40	950	10	70	20	20	34
Chili, small, plain	227	200	17	6	2.5	21	5	5	35	870	15	4	8	10	27
Chili, large w/cheese	357	370	29	14	7	31	7	7	65	1410	25	6	25	20	34
Crispy Chicken Nuggets™ (5)	75	220	11	14	3	13	0	0	35	480	0	2	2	4	57
Barbecue sauce (1 packet)	28	40	1	0	0	10	7	0	0	160	0	0	0	4	0
Frosty,™ medium	298	440	11	11	7	73	56	0	50	260	20	0	41	8	23

SOURCE: Wendy's International, Inc., 2002, http://www.wendys.com. Reproduced with permission from Wendy's International, Inc.

Information on additional foods and restaurants is available online:

Arby's: http://www.arbysrestaurant.com
Burger King: http://www.burgerking.com
Domino's Pizza: http://www.dominos.com
Hardees: http://www.hardees.com
Jack in the Box: http://www.jackinthebox.com
KFC: http://www.kfc.com
McDonald's: http://www.mcdonalds.com
Subway: http://www.subway.com
Taco Bell: http://www.tacobell.com
Wendy's: http://www.wendys.com
White Castle: http://www.whitecastle.com

Monitoring Your Progress

APPENDIX

D

NAME ______________________ SECTION ______________ DATE ______________

As you completed the 11 labs listed below, you enterd the results in the Preprogram Assessment column of this lab. Now that you have been involved in a fitness and wellness program for some time, do the labs again and enter your new results in the Postprogram Assessment column. You will probably notice improvement in several areas. Congratulations! If you are not satisfied with your progress thus far, refer to the tips for successful behavior change in Chapter 1 and throughout this book. Remember—fitness and wellness are forever. The time you invest now in developing a comprehensive, individualized program will pay off in a richer, more vital life in the years to come.

	Preprogram Assessment	Postprogram Assessment
LAB 2.1 Activity Profile	Sleep: _____ hours Light activity: _____ hours Moderate activity: _____ hours Vigorous activity: _____ hours Stairs climbed: _____ flights	Sleep: _____ hours Light activity: _____ hours Moderate activity: _____ hours Vigorous activity: _____ hours Stairs climbed: _____ flights
LAB 3.1 Cardiorespiratory Endurance		
1-mile walk test	$\dot{V}O_{2max}$: _____ Rating: _______	$\dot{V}O_{2max}$: _____ Rating: _______
3-minute step test	$\dot{V}O_{2max}$: _____ Rating: _______	$\dot{V}O_{2max}$: _____ Rating: _______
1.5-mile run-walk test	$\dot{V}O_{2max}$: _____ Rating: _______	$\dot{V}O_{2max}$: _____ Rating: _______
Åstrand-Rhyming test	$\dot{V}O_{2max}$: _____ Rating: _______	$\dot{V}O_{2max}$: _____ Rating: _______
LAB 4.1 Muscular Strength		
Maximum bench press test	Weight: _____ lb Rating: _____	Weight: _____ lb Rating: _____
Maximum leg press test	Weight: _____ lb Rating: _____	Weight: _____ lb Rating: _____
Hand grip strength test	Weight: _____ kg Rating: _____	Weight: _____ kg Rating: _____
LAB 4.2 Muscular Endurance		
Curl-up test	Number: _____ Rating: _______	Number: _____ Rating: _______
Push-up test	Number: _____ Rating: _______	Number: _____ Rating: _______
YMCA bench press test	Number: _____ Rating: _______	Number: _____ Rating: _______
LAB 5.1 Flexibility		
Sit-and-reach test	Score: _____ in. Rating: _______	Score: _____ in. Rating: _______

	Preprogram Assessment	Postprogram Assessment
LAB 5.3 Low-Back Muscular Endurance Side bridge endurance test	Right: ______ sec Rating: ________ Left: ______ sec Rating: ________	Right: ______ sec Rating: ________ Left: ______ sec Rating: ________
LAB 6.1 Body Composition Body mass index Skinfold measurements (or other method for determining percent body fat) Waist circumference Waist-to-hip-circumference ratio	BMI: ______ kg/m^2 Rating: ______ Sum of 3 skinfolds: ______ mm % body fat: ______ % Rating: ______ Circumference: ________ Rating (√ high risk): ________ Ratio: ________ Rating (√ high risk): ________	BMI: ______ kg/m^2 Rating: ______ Sum of 3 skinfolds: ______ mm % body fat: ______ % Rating: ______ Circumference: ________ Rating (√ high risk): ________ Ratio: ________ Rating (√ high risk): ________
LAB 8.1 Daily Diet Number of servings Number of servings Number of servings Number of servings Number of servings	Milk, cheese, etc.: ________ Meat, poultry, fish, etc.: ________ Fruits: ________ Vegetables: ________ Breads, cereals, rice, etc.: ________	Milk, cheese, etc.: ________ Meat, poultry, fish, etc.: ________ Fruits: ________ Vegetables: ________ Breads, cereals, rice, etc.: ________
LAB 8.2 Dietary Analysis Percentage of calories Percentage of calories Percentage of calories Percentage of calories	From protein: ________% From fat: ________% From saturated fat: ________% From carbohydrate: ________%	From protein: ________% From fat: ________% From saturated fat: ________% From carbohydrate: ________%
LAB 9.1 Daily Energy Balance	Approximate daily energy expenditure: ________ cal/day	Approximate daily energy expenditure: ________ cal/day
LAB 10.1 Identifying Stressors	Average weekly stress score: ________	Average weekly stress score: ________
LAB 11.1 Cardiovascular Health CVD risk assessment Hostility assessment	Score: ______ Estimated risk: ______ Score: ________ Rating: ________	Score: ______ Estimated risk: ______ Score: ________ Rating: ________
LAB 12.1 Cancer Prevention Diet: Number of servings Skin cancer	Fruits/vegetables: ________ Score: ________ Risk: ________	Fruits/vegetables: ________ Score: ________ Risk: ________

Behavior Change Workbook

This workbook is designed to take you step by step through the process of behavior change. The first eight activities in the workbook will help you develop a successful plan—beginning with choosing a target behavior and moving through the program planning steps described in Chapter 1, including the completion and signing of a behavior change contract. The final seven activities will help you work through common obstacles to behavior change and maximize your program's chances of success.

Part 1 Developing a Plan for Behavior Change and Completing a Contract

1. Choosing a Target Behavior
2. Gathering Information About Your Target Behavior
3. Monitoring Your Current Patterns of Behavior
4. Setting Goals
5. Examining Your Attitudes About Your Target Behavior
6. Choosing Rewards
7. Breaking Behavior Chains
8. Completing a Contract for Behavior Change

Part 2 Overcoming Obstacles to Behavior Change

9. Building Motivation and Commitment
10. Managing Your Time Successfully
11. Developing Realistic Self-Talk
12. Involving the People Around You
13. Dealing with Feelings
14. Overcoming Peer Pressure: Communicating Assertively
15. Maintaining Your Program over Time

ACTIVITY 1 CHOOSING A TARGET BEHAVIOR

Use your knowledge of yourself and the results of Lab 1-2 (Lifestyle Evaluation) to identify five behaviors that you could change to improve your level of wellness. Examples of target behaviors include smoking cigarettes, not exercising regularly, eating candy bars every night, not getting enough sleep, getting drunk frequently on weekends, and not wearing a safety belt when driving or riding in a car. List your five behaviors below.

1. ______________________________
2. ______________________________
3. ______________________________
4. ______________________________
5. ______________________________

For successful behavior change, it's best to focus on one behavior at a time. Review your list of behaviors and select one to start with. Choose a behavior that is important to you and that you are strongly motivated to change. If this will be your first attempt at behavior change, start with a simple change, such as wearing your bicycle helmet regularly, before tackling a more difficult change, such as quitting smoking. Circle the behavior on your list that you've chosen to start with; this will be your target behavior throughout this workbook.

ACTIVITY 2 GATHERING INFORMATION ABOUT YOUR TARGET BEHAVIOR

Take a close look at what your target behavior means to your health, now and in the future. How is it affecting your level of wellness? What diseases or conditions does this behavior place you at risk for? What will changing this behavior mean to you? To evaluate your behavior, use information from this text, from the resources listed in the For Further Exploration section at the end of each chapter, and from other reliable sources.

Health behaviors have short-term and long-term benefits and costs associated with them. For example, in the short term, an inactive lifestyle allows for more time to watch TV and hang out with friends but leaves a person less able to participate in recreational activities. In the long term, it increases risk for cardiovascular disease, cancer, and premature death. Fill in the blanks below with the benefits and costs of continuing your current behavior and of changing to a new, healthier behavior. Pay close attention to the short-term benefits of the new behavior—these are an important motivating force behind successful behavior change programs.

Target (current) behavior ______________________________

Benefits *Short-Term* ______________________ *Long-Term* ______________________

______________________ ______________________

Costs *Short-Term* ______________________ *Long-Term* ______________________

______________________ ______________________

New behavior ______________________________

Benefits *Short-Term* ______________________ *Long-Term* ______________________

______________________ ______________________

Costs *Short-Term* ______________________ *Long-Term* ______________________

______________________ ______________________

ACTIVITY 3 MONITORING YOUR CURRENT PATTERNS OF BEHAVIOR

To develop a successful behavior change program, you need detailed information about your own behavior patterns. You can obtain this information by developing a system of record keeping geared toward your target behavior. Depending on your target behavior, you may want to monitor a single behavior, such as your diet, or you may want to keep daily activity records to determine how you could make time for exercise or another new behavior. Consider tracking factors such as the following:

- The behavior
- When and for how long it occurs
- Where it occurs
- What else you were doing at the time
- What other people you were with and how they influenced you
- Your thoughts and feelings
- How strong your urge for the behavior was (for example, how hungry you were or how much you wanted to watch TV)

Figure 1.5 (p. 13) shows a sample log for tracking daily diet. Below, create a format for a sample daily log for monitoring the behavior patterns relating to your target behavior. Then use this sample log to monitor your behavior for a day. Evaluate the log you've created as you use it. Ask yourself if you are tracking all the key factors that influence your behavior; make any necessary adjustments to the format of your log. Once you've developed an appropriate format for your log, use a separate notebook (your health journal) to keep records of your behavior for a week or two. These records will provide solid information about your behavior that will help you develop a successful behavior change program. Later activities in this workbook will ask you to analyze your records.

ACTIVITY 4 SETTING GOALS

For your behavior change program to succeed, you must set meaningful, realistic goals. In addition to an ultimate goal, set some intermediate goals—milestones that you can strive for on the way to your final objective. For example, if your overall goal is to run a 5K road race, an intermediate goal might be to successfully complete 2 weeks of your fitness program. If you set a final goal of eating 5 servings of fruits and vegetables every day, an intermediate goal would be to increase your daily intake from 2 to 3 servings. List your intermediate and final goals below. Don't strive for immediate perfection. Allow an adequate amount of time to reach each of your goals.

Intermediate Goals	Target Date
______________________________	____________________
______________________________	____________________
______________________________	____________________
______________________________	____________________
______________________________	____________________

Final Goal

______________________________	____________________

ACTIVITY 5 EXAMINING YOUR ATTITUDES ABOUT YOUR TARGET BEHAVIOR

Your attitudes toward your target behavior can determine whether your behavior change program will be successful. Consider your attitudes carefully by completing the following statements about how you think and feel about your current behavior and your goal.

1. I like ______________________ because ______________________
   (current behavior)
   ____

2. I don't like ______________________ because ______________________
   (current behavior)
   ____

3. I like ______________________ because ______________________
   (behavior goal)
   ____

4. I don't like ______________________ because ______________________
   (behavior goal)
   ____

5. I don't ______________________ now because ______________________
   (behavior goal)
   ____

6. I would be more likely to ______________________ if ______________________
   (behavior goal)
   ____

If your statements indicate that you have major reservations about changing your behavior, work to build your motivation and commitment before you begin your program. Look carefully at your objections to changing your behavior. How valid and important are they? What can you do to overcome them? Can you adopt any of the strategies you listed under statement 6? Review the facts about your current behavior and your goals.

ACTIVITY 6 CHOOSING REWARDS

Make a list of objects, activities, and events you can use as rewards for achieving the goals of your behavior change program. Rewards should be special, relatively inexpensive, and preferably unrelated to food or alcohol: for example, tickets to a ball game, a CD, or a long-distance phone call to a family member or friend—whatever is meaningful for you. Write down a variety of rewards you can use when you reach milestones in your program and your final goal.

Many people also find it helpful to give themselves small rewards daily or weekly for sticking with their behavior change program. These could be things like a study break, a movie, or a Saturday morning bike ride. Make a list of rewards for maintaining your program in the short term.

And don't forget to congratulate yourself regularly during your behavior change program. Notice how much better you feel. Savor how far you've come and how you've gained control of your behavior.

ACTIVITY 7 BREAKING BEHAVIOR CHAINS

Use the records you collected about your target behavior in Activity 3 and in your health journal to identify what leads up to your target behavior and what follows it. By tracing these chains of events, you'll be able to identify points in the chain where you can make a change that will lead to your new behavior. The sample behavior chain on the next page shows a sequence of events for a person who wants to add exercise to her daily routine—but who winds up snacking and watching TV instead. By examining the chain carefully, one can identify ways to break it at every step. After you review the sample, go through the same process for a typical chain of events involving your target behavior. Use the blank behavior chain on the following page.

Some general strategies for breaking behavior chains include the following:

- *Control or eliminate environmental cues that provoke the behavior.* Stay out of the room where your television is located. Go out for an ice cream cone instead of keeping a half gallon of ice cream in your freezer.
- *Change behaviors or habits that are linked to your target behavior.* If you always smoke in your car when you drive to school, try taking public transportation instead.
- *Add new cues to your environment to trigger your new behavior.* Prepare easy-to-grab healthy snacks and carry them with you to class or work. Keep your exercise clothes and equipment in a visible location.

See also the suggestions in Chapter 1.

continued

Chain of Events	Strategies for Breaking the Chain
Come home from class	You had planned an afternoon walk as part of your exercise program.
Feel tired, not like exercising	Tell yourself you'll feel better and more alert after working out.
Look for walking shoes; can'tfind them	Put shoes and clothes for exercise in an obvious place the night before.
Feel annoyed	Remind yourself of your program goals, and tell yourself that you can stick with your program.
Go to kitchen, see food	Stay out of kitchen unless you will be fixing or eating a planned meal or snack.
Feel hungry	Look at the picture of a healthy exerciser that you've put on the refrigerator to remind you of your goals.
Grab a soda and bag of chips	Have a glass of water or a pre-prepared healthy snack.
Turn on TV and sit down	Turn on the radio instead; listen to news or music while you get ready to exercise.
Eat chips, watch TV	If you really like to watch TV in the afternoon, plan to work out in the morning or exercise on a stationary bike or treadmill in front of the TV.
Feel guilty	Even if you do have occasional lapses, don't beat yourself up. Think positively about how you'll resume your program the next day.

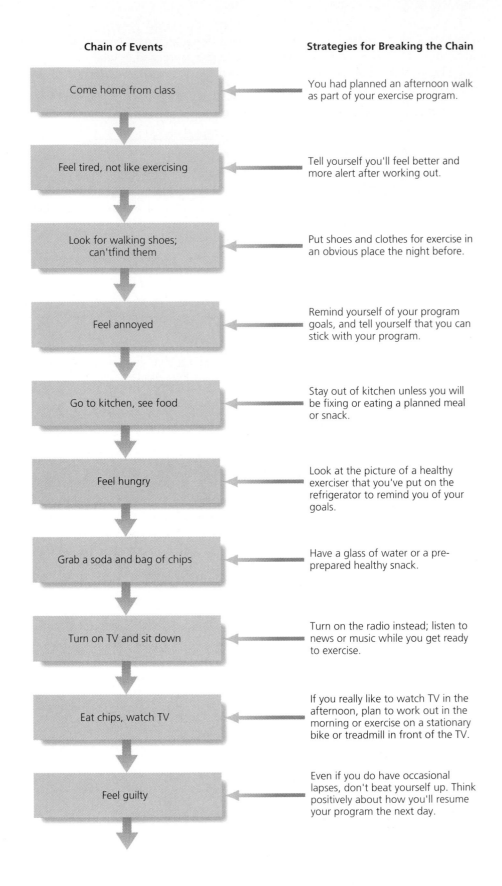

Chain of Events | **Strategies for Breaking the Chain**

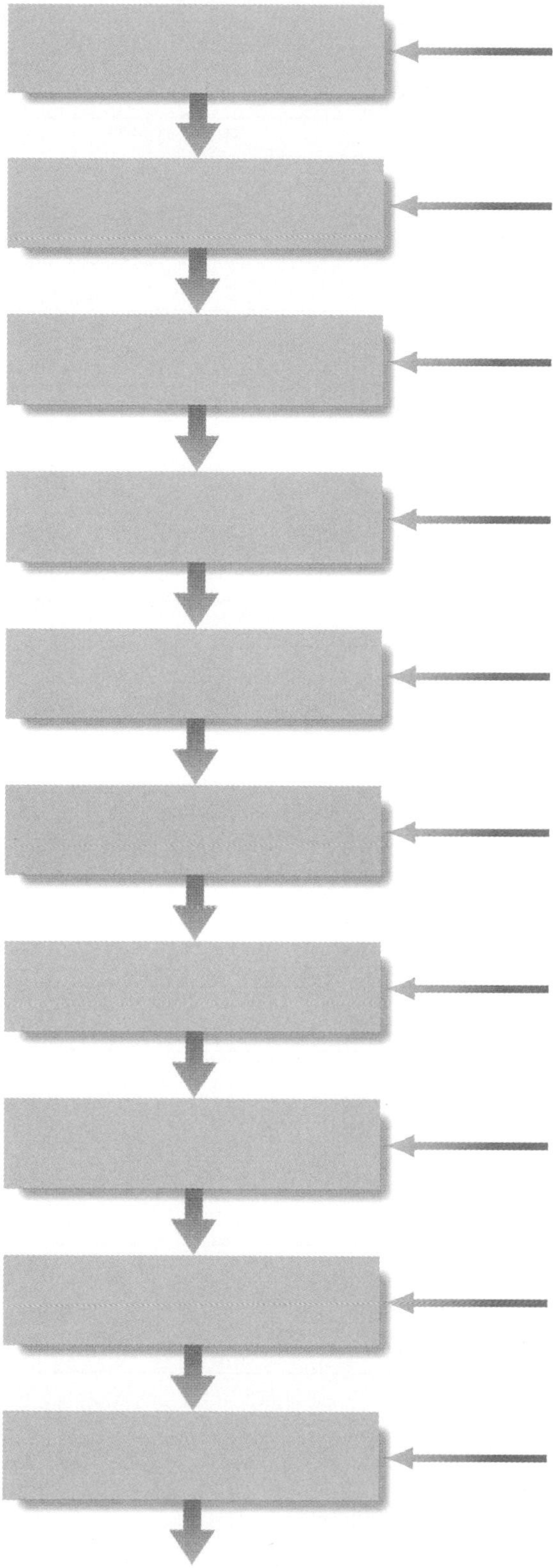

ACTIVITY 8 COMPLETING A CONTRACT FOR BEHAVIOR CHANGE

Your next step in creating a successful behavior change program is to complete and sign a behavior change contract. Your contract should include details of your program and indicate your commitment to changing your behavior. Use the information from previous activities in this workbook to complete the following contract. (If your target behavior relates to exercise, you may want to use the program plan and contract for a fitness program in Lab 7-1.)

1. I, ______________________ (name), agree to ______________________ (specify behavior you want to change)

____

2. I will begin on ____________ (start date) and plan to reach my goal of ______________________ (specify final goal)

______________________ by ____________

3. To reach my final goal, I have devised the following schedule of mini-goals. For each step in my program, I will give myself the reward listed.

______________________ (mini-goal 1) ____________ (target date) ____________ (reward)

______________________ (mini-goal 2) ____________ (target date) ____________ (reward)

______________________ (mini-goal 3) ____________ (target date) ____________ (reward)

______________________ (mini-goal 4) ____________ (target date) ____________ (reward)

______________________ (mini-goal 5) ____________ (target date) ____________ (reward)

My overall reward for reaching my final goal will be ______________________

4. I have gathered and analyzed data on my target behavior and have identified the following strategies for changing my behavior: ______________________

____

____

5. I will use the following tools to monitor my progress toward reaching my final goal:

______________________ (list any charts, graphs, or journals you plan to use)

____

I sign this contract as an indication of my personal commitment to reach my goal.

______________________ (your signature) ____________ (date)

I have recruited a helper who will witness my contract and ______________________

______________________ (list any way in which your helper will participate in your program)

______________________ (your signature) ____________ (date)

Describe in detail any special strategies you will use to help change your behavior (refer to Activity 7).

Create a plan below for any charts, graphs, or journals you will use to monitor your progress. The log format you developed in Activity 3 may be appropriate, or you may need to develop a more detailed or specific record-keeping system. Examples of journal formats are included in Labs 3-2, 4-3, 5-2, 8-1, and 10-1. You might also want to develop a graph to show your progress; posting such a graph in a prominent location can help keep your motivation strong and your program on track. Depending on your target behavior, you could graph the number of push-ups you can do, the number of servings of vegetables you eat each day, or your average daily stress level.

ACTIVITY 9 BUILDING MOTIVATION AND COMMITMENT

Complete the following checklist to determine whether you are motivated and committed to changing your behavior. Check the statements that are true for you.

_______ I feel responsible for my own behavior and capable of managing it.

_______ I am not easily discouraged.

_______ I enjoy setting goals and then working to achieve them.

_______ I am good at keeping promises to myself.

_______ I like having a structure and schedule for my activities.

_______ I view my new behavior as a necessity, not an optional activity.

_______ Compared with previous attempts to change my behavior, I am more motivated now.

_______ My goals are realistic.

_______ I have a positive mental picture of the new behavior.

_______ Considering the stresses in my life, I feel confident that I can stick to my program.

_______ I feel prepared for lapses and ups-and-downs in my behavior change program.

_______ I feel that my plan for behavior change is enjoyable.

_______ I feel comfortable telling other people about the change I am making in my behavior.

Did you check most of these statements? If not, you need to boost your motivation and commitment. Consider these strategies:

- Review the potential benefits of changing your behavior and the costs of not changing it (see Activity 2). Pay special attention to the short-term benefits of changing your behavior, including feelings of accomplishment and self-confidence. Post a list of these benefits in a prominent location.
- Visualize yourself achieving your goal and enjoying its benefits. For example, if you want to manage time more effectively, picture yourself as a confident, organized person who systematically tackles important tasks and sets aside time each day for relaxation, exercise, and friends. Practice this type of visualization regularly.
- Put aside obstacles and objections to change. Counter thoughts such as "I'll never have time to exercise" with thoughts like "Lots of other people do it and so can I."
- Bombard yourself with propaganda. Take a class dealing with the change you want to make. Read books and watch television shows on the subject. Post motivational phrases or pictures on your refrigerator or over your desk. Talk to people who have already made the change.
- Build up your confidence. Remind yourself of other goals you've achieved. At the end of each day, mentally review your good decisions and actions. See yourself as a capable person, one who is in charge of her or his behavior.

List two strategies for boosting your motivation and commitment; choose from the list above or develop your own. Try each strategy, and then describe how well it worked for you.

Strategy 1: ____

How well it worked: ____

____

Strategy 2: ____

How well it worked: ____

____

ACTIVITY 10 MANAGING YOUR TIME SUCCESSFULLY

"Too little time" is a common excuse for not exercising or engaging in other healthy behaviors. Learning to manage your time successfully is crucial if you are to maintain a wellness lifestyle. The first step is to examine how you are currently spending your time; use the following grid broken into blocks to track your activities.

Time	Activity	Time	Activity
6:00 A.M.		6:00 P.M.	
6:30 A.M.		6:30 P.M.	
7:00 A.M.		7:00 P.M.	
8:00 A.M.		8:00 P.M.	
9:00 A.M.		9:00 P.M.	
10:00 A.M.		10:00 P.M.	
11:00 A.M.		11:00 P.M.	
12:00 P.M.		12:00 A.M.	
1:00 P.M.		1:00 A.M.	
2:00 P.M.		2:00 A.M.	
3:00 P.M.		3:00 A.M.	
4:00 P.M.		4:00 A.M.	
5:00 P.M.		5:00 A.M.	

continued

Next, list each type of activity and the total time you engaged in it on a given day in the chart below (for example, sleeping, 7 hours; eating, 1.5 hours; studying, 3 hours; working, 3 hours; and so on). Take a close look at your list of activities. Successful time management is based on prioritization. Assign a priority to each of your activities according to how important it is to you: essential (A), somewhat important (B), or not important (C). Based on these priority rankings, make changes in your schedule by adding and subtracting hours from different categories of activities; enter a duration goal for each activity. Add your new activities to the list and assign a priority and duration goal to each.

Activity	Current Total Duration	Priority (A, B, or C)	Goal Total Duration

Prioritizing in this manner will involve tradeoffs. For example, you may choose to reduce the amount of time you spend watching television, listening to music, and chatting on the telephone while you increase the amount of time spent sleeping, studying, and exercising. Don't feel that you have to miss out on anything you enjoy. You can get more from less time by focusing on what you are doing. Strategies for managing time more productively and creatively are described in Chapter 10.

ACTIVITY 11 DEVELOPING REALISTIC SELF-TALK

Self-talk is the ongoing internal dialogue we have with ourselves throughout much of the day. Our thoughts can be accurate, positive, and supportive, or they can be exaggerated and negative. Self-talk is closely related to self-esteem and self-concept. Realistic self-talk can help maintain positive self-esteem, the belief that one is a good and competent person, worthy of friendship and love. A negative internal dialogue can reinforce negative self-esteem and can make behavior change very difficult. Substituting realistic self-talk for negative self-talk can help you build and maintain self-esteem and cope better with the challenges in your life.

First, take a closer look at your current pattern of self-talk. Use your health journal to track self-talk, especially as it relates to your target behavior. Does any of your self-talk fall into the common patterns of distorted negative self-talk shown in Chapter 10 (p. 296)? If so, use the examples of realistic self-talk from Chapter 10 to develop more accurate and rational responses. Write your current negative thoughts in the left-hand column, and then record more realistic responses in the right-hand column.

Current Self-Talk About Target Behavior	More Realistic Self-Talk

ACTIVITY 12 INVOLVING THE PEOPLE AROUND YOU

Your behavior change program will be more successful if the people around you are supportive and involved—or at least are not sabotaging your efforts. Use your health journal to track how other people influence your target behavior and your efforts to change it. For example, do you always skip exercising when you're with certain people? Do you always drink or eat too much when you socialize with certain friends? Are friends and family members offering you enthusiastic support for your efforts to change your behavior, or do they make jokes about your program? Have they even noticed your efforts? Summarize the reactions of those around you in the chart below.

Target behavior ____________________

Person	Typical Effect on Target Behavior	Involvment in/Reaction to Program

It may be difficult to change the actions and reactions of the people who are close to you. For them to be involved in your program, you may need to develop new ways of interacting with them (for example, taking a walk rather than going out to dinner as a means of socializing). Most of your friends and family members will want to help you—if they know how. Ask for exactly the type of help or involvement you want. Do you want feedback, praise, or just cooperation? Would you like someone to witness your contract or to be involved more directly in your program? Do you want someone to stop sabotaging your efforts by inviting you to watch TV, eat rich desserts, and so on? Look for ways that the people who are close to you can share in your behavior change program. They can help to motivate you and to maintain your commitment to your program. Develop a way that each individual you listed above can become involved in your program in a positive way.

Person	Target Involvement in Behavior Change Program

Choose one person on your list to tackle first. Talk to that person about her or his current behavior and how you would like her or him to be involved in your behavior change program. Below, describe this person's reaction to your talk and her or his subsequent behavior. Did this individual become a positive participant in your behavior change program?

____

____

____

____

ACTIVITY 13 DEALING WITH FEELINGS

Longstanding habits are difficult to change in part because many represent ways people have developed to cope with certain feelings. For example, people may overeat when bored, skip their exercise sessions when frustrated, or drink alcoholic beverages when anxious. Developing new ways to deal with feelings can help improve the chance that a behavior change program will succeed.

Review the records on your target behavior that you kept in your health journal. Identify the feelings that are interfering with the success of your program and develop new strategies for coping with them. Some common problematic feelings are listed below, along with one possible coping strategy for each. Put a check mark next to those that are influencing your target behavior and fill in additional strategies. Add the other feelings that are significant road-blocks in your program to the bottom of the chart, along with coping strategies for each.

✔	Feeling	Coping Strategies
	Stressed out	Go for a 10-minute walk.
	Anxious	Do one of the relaxation exercises described in Chapter 10.
	Bored	Call a friend for a chat.
	Tired	Take a 20-minute nap.
	Frustrated	Identify the source of the feeling and deal with it constructively.

- Julia is trying to give up smoking; her friend Marie continues to offer her cigarettes whenever they are together.
- Emilio is planning to exercise in the morning; his roommates tell him he's being antisocial by not having brunch with them.
- Tracy's boyfriend told her that in high school he once experimented with drugs and shared needles; she wants him to have an HIV test, but he says he's sure the people he shared needles with were not infected.

Peer pressure is the common ingredient in these situations. To successfully maintain your behavior change program, you must develop effective strategies for resisting peer pressure. Assertive communication is one such strategy. By communicating assertively—firmly, but not aggressively—you can stick with your program even in the face of pressure from others. Review your health journal to determine how other people affect your target behavior. If you find that you often do give in to peer pressure, try the following strategies for communicating more assertively:

- Collect your thoughts, and plan in advance what you will say. You might try out your response on a friend to get some feedback.
- State your case—how you feel and what you want—as clearly as you can.
- Use "I" messages—statements about how you feel—rather than statements beginning with "You."
- Focus on the behavior rather than the person. Suggest a solution, such as asking the other person to change his or her behavior toward you. Avoid generalizations. Be specific about what you want.
- Make clear, constructive requests. Focus on your needs ("I would like . . .") rather than the mistakes of others ("You always . . .").
- Avoid blaming, accusing, and belittling. Treat others with the same respect you'd like to receive yourself.
- Ask for action ahead of time. Tell others what you would like to happen; don't wait for them to do the wrong thing and then get angry at them.
- Ask for a response to what you have proposed. Wait for an answer and listen carefully to it. Try to understand other people's points of view, just as you would hope that others would understand yours.

With these strategies in mind, review your health journal and identify three instances in which peer pressure interfered with your behavior change program. For each of these instances, write out what you might have said to deal with the situation more assertively. (If you can't find three situations from your own experiences, choose one or more of the three scenarios described at the beginning of this activity.)

1. ______________________________

2. ______________________________

3. ______________________________

Assertive communication can help you achieve your behavior change goals in a direct way by helping you keep your program on track. It can also provide a boost for your self-image and increase your confidence in your ability to successfully manage your own behavior.

ACTIVITY 15 MAINTAINING YOUR PROGRAM OVER TIME

If you maintain your new behavior for at least 6 months, you've reached the maintenance stage and your chances of lifetime success are greatly increased. However, you may find yourself sliding back into old habits at some point. If this happens, there are some things you can do to help maintain your new behavior.

- Remind yourself of the goals of your program (list them here).

____

____

____

____

____

- Pay attention to how your new pattern of behavior has improved your wellness status. List the major benefits of changing your behavior, both now and in the future.

____

____

____

____

____

- Consider the things you enjoy most about your new pattern of behavior. List your favorite aspects.

____

____

____

____

____

- Think of yourself as a problem solver. If something begins to interfere with your program, devise strategies for dealing with it. Take time out now to list things that have the potential to derail your program and develop possible coping mechanisms.

Problem	**Solution**
____________	____________
	____________
____________	____________
	____________
____________	____________
	____________
____________	____________
	____________

- Remember the basics of behavior change. If your program runs into trouble, go back to keeping records of your behavior to pinpoint problem areas. Make adjustments in your program to deal with new disruptions. And don't feel defeated if you lapse. The best thing you can do is renew your commitment and continue with your program.

INDEX